Human Placental Trophoblasts

Impact of Maternal Nutrition

Human Placental Trophoblasts

Impact of Maternal Nutrition

Edited by
Asim K. Duttaroy
University of Oslo
Norway

Sanjay Basak
National Institute of Nutrition (ICMR)
Hyderabad, India

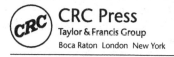

CRC Press
Taylor & Francis Group
Boca Raton London New York

CRC Press is an imprint of the
Taylor & Francis Group, an **informa** business

CRC Press
Taylor & Francis Group
6000 Broken Sound Parkway NW, Suite 300
Boca Raton, FL 33487-2742

First issued in paperback 2021

© 2016 by Taylor & Francis Group, LLC
CRC Press is an imprint of Taylor & Francis Group, an Informa business

No claim to original U.S. Government works

ISBN-13: 978-1-4822-5428-0 (hbk)
ISBN-13: 978-1-03-217962-9 (pbk)
DOI: 10.1201/b19151

Publisher's Note

The publisher has gone to great lengths to ensure the quality of this reprint but points out that some imperfections in the original copies may be apparent.

Visit the Taylor & Francis Web site at
http://www.taylorandfrancis.com

and the CRC Press Web site at
http://www.crcpress.com

Contents

SECTION I Early Placentation: Regulation of Trophoblast Growth and Development

SECTION II Maternal Nutrition and Fetal Growth and Development

SECTION III   Vitamins, Minerals, and Placentation

SECTION IV   Regulation of Trophoblast Angiogenesis and Invasion

SECTION V *Environmental and Lifestyle Factors in Pregnancy*

SECTION VI *Epigenetics, microRNA, and Placental Gene Expression*

Preface

During fetal life, maternal nutrition plays a critical role in the programming of susceptibility to adult disease. The placental supply of maternal nutrients to the fetus is critically important for fetal growth and development. The placenta is the highly specialized organ of pregnancy that supports the normal growth and development of the fetus. Apart from maternal nutrition status, the fetal supply is influenced by placental surface area and availability of specific nutrient transporters on the membranes. Therefore, the growth and function of the placenta are precisely regulated and coordinated to ensure the optimum exchange of nutrients and waste products between the maternal and fetal circulatory systems. In fact, more and more evidence suggests that placental growth and function contribute to fetus growth and health outcome in adult life.

In this book, we sought to cover a broad range of evidence in the areas of placental growth and function and its impact on fetoplacental outcome. We were fortunate to recruit subject-specialized authors who play leading roles within their discipline. These individuals gladly shared their insights into various aspects of placenta research. In Sections I and II, the book chapters include placenta size, structure, and organization; molecular regulation of early placentation; epigenetic regulation and placentation; trophoblast invasion, angiogenesis, maternal nutrition, epidemiology, and fetal outcome; amino acid transport; fatty acid uptake, metabolism, and transport; maternal fatty acid metabolism and fetoplacental growth; maternal long-chain fatty acids and size and function of the placenta; cholesterol transport and trophoblast growth and development; fatty acid and placentation; maternal micronutrients, placental growth, and fetal outcome. Section III lists topics involved with; folic acid uptake and its regulation in the placenta; effects of vitamin D on pregnancy and the placenta; maternal choline and placental trophoblast; and calcium and early development of placenta. Sections IV and V focus on regulation of trophoblast invasion and angiogenesis by lifestyle and environmental factors such as maternal obesity and placental vascular function; placental dysfunction and future maternal cardiovascular disease; trophoblast–natural killer cell interactions; hyperglycemia factors and its effects on angiogenesis; the role of cytokines in healthy and pathological pregnancies; the impact of aryl hydrocarbon on human trophoblasts; and synthetic chemicals and placentation. Section VI includes gene expression of the placenta in normal and pathological human pregnancy and regulation of microRNA expression and function of human placentas.

A book like this one, however, cannot be comprehensive, exhaustive, and specific by all means; the editors had to select from a large number of nutrients and an even larger number of effects of nutrients at the cellular and molecular level to understand their importance in fetoplacental outcome. For each topic that it is included in this book, another equally important topic may have been left out. We believe that this book will be helpful to all those who are working in these areas of maternal–fetal health and reproductive research.

Our thanks go to all the scientists who contributed chapters for this book. These individuals created time in their busy schedule to produce chapters of outstanding quality. Also, we thank Jill J. Jurgensen, senior project coordinator of the CRC Press, Taylor & Francis Group, for her continued support during the preparation of the manuscript.

Asim K. Duttaroy
Sanjay Basak

Editors

Dr. Asim K. Duttaroy was educated in India and the United States. Currently, he is the professor and group leader of chronic disease at the Department of Nutrition, Faculty of Medicine, at the University of Oslo, Norway. After his fellowship at the Thrombosis Research Centre, Temple University Medical School, Philadelphia, Pennsylvania, he joined as an assistant professor of medicine and biochemistry at the Wright State University and senior health scientist at the VA Medical Centre, Dayton, Ohio. He then moved to the Rowett Research Institute of Aberdeen University, Scotland, UK, as a professor and principal scientist. In 2001, he was appointed as professor and group leader at the University of Oslo, Norway. His research program focuses on the roles of dietary components on growth and development, as well as in the prevention of cardiovascular disease. He is investigating the mechanisms responsible for cellular growth, function, and metabolism of dietary lipids in the fetoplacental unit. He holds several international patents. His discovery, Fruitflow, is scientifically proven to inhibit platelet aggregation, a known cause of heart attack, stroke, and venous thrombosis. It became the first product in Europe to obtain an approved positive health claim under the European Food Safety Authority regulations.

Professor Duttaroy is a member of several international societies and editorial boards of several international journals. Recently, he was appointed as the editor-in-chief of *Food and Nutrition Research* journal.

His scientific work has been published in over 175 original contributions, reviews, books, book chapters, and editorials. He has supervised 25 PhD/MD students so far. He has a personal website, http://www.asimduttaroy.com, where his activities are regularly updated.

Dr. Sanjay Basak is a researcher. At present, he is working as a scientist at the Division of Molecular Biology, National Institute of Nutrition (ICMR), India. After receiving his PhD in biochemistry, he joined this institute as a research officer. Recently, he completed his research training fellowship in nutrition, physiology, and molecular biology from the Institute of Basic Medical Sciences, University of Oslo, Norway.

His research is actively involved in the molecular aspects of nutrition, trophoblast growth, development, and placentation. He secured a competitive overseas research fellowship grant (BOYSCAST) from the government of India. He was a recipient of the Henrik Homans Memorial Scholarship, Norway. Currently, he is associated as an editorial member of the peer-reviewed international journal *Food and Nutrition Research*, Co-action Publisher, Sweden.

To date, he has published 16 research articles, two review papers, and one book chapter. Most of his work is available at https://scholar.google.com/citations?user=Sxz3LsMAAAAJ&hl=en.

Contributors

Ganesh Acharya
Women's Health and Perinatology Research
    Group
UiT—The Arctic University of Norway
and
Department of Obstetrics and Gynecology
University Hospital of North Norway
Tromsł, Norway

Christiane Albrecht
Institute of Biochemistry and Molecular
    Medicine
and
Swiss National Center of Competence
    in Research
NCCR TransCure
University of Bern
Bern, Switzerland

João R. Araújo
Institut Pasteur
INSERM U786
Unité de Pathogénie Microbienne Moléculaire
Paris, France

Sanjay Basak
Molecular Biology Division
National Institute Nutrition
Indian Council of Medical Research
Hyderabad, India

Louiza Belkacemi
Department of Biology and Biochemistry
University of Houston
Houston, Texas

Judith N. Bulmer
Reproductive and Vascular Biology Group
Institute of Cellular Medicine
Newcastle University
Newcastle upon Tyne, UK

Manuela Cardellicchio
Unit of Obstetrics and Gynecology
Department of Biomedical and Clinical
    Sciences
Hospital L. Sacco
University of Milan
Milan, Italy

Marie A. Caudill
Division of Nutritional Sciences
Cornell University
Ithaca, New York

Irene Cetin
Unit of Obstetrics and Gynecology
Department of Biomedical and Clinical
    Sciences
Hospital L. Sacco
University of Milan
Milan, Italy

Saumitra Chakravarty
Department of Pathology
Bangabandhu Sheikh Mujib Medical University
Dhaka, Bangladesh

Bryanne Colvin
Department of Pediatrics
Division of Newborn Medicine
and
Department of Obstetrics and Gynecology
Washington University School of Medicine
    in St. Louis
St. Louis, Missouri

Mrinal K. Das
Male Reproductive Health
Department of Natural Health
Faculty of Health Sciences
Oslo and Akershus University College
    of Applied Sciences
Oslo, Norway

Mina Desai
Department of Obstetrics and Gynecology
David Geffen School of Medicine
University of California
and
Perinatal Research Laboratories
Los Angeles Biomedical Research Institute
    at Harbor-UCLA Medical Center
Los Angeles, California

Nur Duale
Norwegian Institute of Public Health
Division of Environmental Medicine
Department of Chemicals and Radiation
Oslo, Norway

Evemie Dubé
Département des Sciences Biologiques
and
Centre de Recherche BioMed
Universitø du Quøbec ⊠ Montrøl (UQ⊠ M)
Montrøl, Canada

Asim K. Duttaroy
Department of Nutrition
Institute for Basic Medical Sciences
University of Oslo
Oslo, Norway

Kristine Bjerve Gutzkow
Norwegian Institute of Public Health
Division of Environmental Medicine
Department of Chemicals and Radiation
Oslo, Norway

Christine Henriksen
Department of Nutrition
IMB
Faculty of Medicine
University of Oslo
Oslo, Norway

Tore Henriksen
Women and Children⊠ Division
Section of Obstetrics
Oslo University Hospital
Oslo, Norway

Emilio Herrera
Department of Biochemistry
Molecular Biology and Cell Biology
Faculties of Pharmacy and Medicine
Universidad San Pablo-CEU
Madrid, Spain

Tim Hofer
Norwegian Institute of Public Health
Division of Environmental Medicine
Department of Chemicals and Radiation
Oslo, Norway

M.B. Holm
Women and Children⊠ Division
Section of Obstetrics
Oslo University Hospital
Oslo, Norway

A.M. Holme
Women and Children⊠ Division
Section of Obstetrics
Oslo University Hospital
Oslo, Norway

H. Horne
Women and Children⊠ Division
Section of Obstetrics
Oslo University Hospital
Oslo, Norway

Arjun Jain
Institute of Biochemistry and Molecular
    Medicine
and
Swiss National Center of Competence
    in Research
NCCR TransCure
University of Bern
Bern, Switzerland

Sadhana Joshi
Interactive Research School for Health Affairs
Bharati Vidyapeeth University
Pune, India

Elisa Keating
Department of Biochemistry (I3S)
Faculty of Medicine
University of Porto
and
Centre of Biotechnology and Fine Chemistry
School of Biotechnology
Portuguese Catholic University
Porto, Portugal

Julia H. King
Division of Nutritional Sciences
Cornell University
Ithaca, New York

Martin Knöfler
Department of Obstetrics and Fetal⊠Maternal
    Medicine
Reproductive Biology Unit
Medical University of Vienna
Vienna, Austria

Sze Ting (Cecilia) Kwan
Division of Nutritional Sciences
Cornell University
Ithaca, New York

Julie Lafond
Dǿpartement des Sciences Biologiques
and
Centre de Recherche BioMed
Universitǿdu Quǿbec ⊠ Montrǿal (UQ⊠M)
Montrǿal, Canada

Gendie E. Lash
Reproductive and Vascular Biology Group
Institute of Cellular Medicine
Newcastle University
Newcastle upon Tyne, UK

Birgitte Lindeman
Norwegian Institute of Public Health
Division of Environmental Medicine
Department of Chemicals and Radiation
Oslo, Norway

Mark S. Longtine
Department of Pediatrics
Division of Newborn Medicine
and
Department of Obstetrics and Gynecology
Washington University School of Medicine
    in St. Louis
St. Louis, Missouri

Chiara Mandò
Unit of Obstetrics and Gynecology
Department of Biomedical and Clinical
    Sciences
Hospital L. Sacco
University of Milan
Milan, Italy

Fátima Martel
Department of Biochemistry (I3S)
Faculty of Medicine
University of Porto
Porto, Portugal

Akshaya Meher
Interactive Research School for Health Affairs
Bharati Vidyapeeth University
Pune, India

T.M. Michelsen
Women and Children⊠ Division
Section of Obstetrics
Oslo University Hospital
Oslo, Norway

Kohzoh Mitsuya
Center for Pregnancy and Newborn Research
University of Texas Health Science Center
    San Antonio
Department of Obstetrics and Gynecology
San Antonio, Texas

Leslie Myatt
Center for Pregnancy and Newborn Research
University of Texas Health Science Center
    San Antonio
Department of Obstetrics and Gynecology
San Antonio, Texas

D. Michael Nelson
Department of Pediatrics
Division of Newborn Medicine
and
Department of Obstetrics and Gynecology
Washington University School of Medicine
    in St. Louis
St. Louis, Missouri

Henar Ortega-Senovilla
Department of Biochemistry
Molecular Biology and Cell Biology
Faculties of Pharmacy and Medicine
Universidad San Pablo-CEU
Madrid, Spain

Abhilash D. Pandya
Nutrition and Chronic Diseases Group
Department of Nutrition
Institute of Basic Medical Sciences
Faculty of Medicine
University of Oslo
Oslo, Norway

Petr Pavek
Department of Pharmacology and Toxicology
Faculty of Pharmacy in Hradec Krá̄ovØ
Charles University in Prague
Hradec Krá̄ovØ Czech Republic

Jürgen Pollheimer
Department of Obstetrics and Fetal⊠Maternal
    Medicine
Reproductive Biology Unit
Medical University of Vienna
Vienna, Austria

Theresa L. Powell
Department of Pediatrics
Neonatology Division
School of Medicine
University of Colorado
Aurora, Colorado

Alka Rani
Interactive Research School for Health Affairs
Bharati Vidyapeeth University
Pune, India

Christopher W.G. Redman
University of Oxford
Oxford, UK

Johannes Rolin
Tynset Community Hospital
Tynset, Norway

Michael G. Ross
Department of Obstetrics and Gynecology
David Geffen School of Medicine
University of California
and
Perinatal Research Laboratories
Los Angeles Biomedical Research Institute
    at Harbor-UCLA Medical Center
Los Angeles, California

Allison L.B. Shapiro
Department of Epidemiology
Colorado School of Public Health
University of Colorado
Aurora, Colorado

Vasilis Sitras
Department of Obstetrics and Gynecology
Oslo University Hospital
Oslo, Norway

Tomas Smutny
Department of Pharmacology and Toxicology
Faculty of Pharmacy in Hradec Krá̄ovØ
Charles University in Prague
Hradec Krá̄ovØ Czech Republic

Anne Cathrine Staff
Department of Obstetrics and Gynaecology
Oslo University Hospital, Ullev⊠l
and
Faculty of Medicine
University of Oslo
Oslo, Norway

Daniel Vaiman
Institut Cochin
INSERM U 1016
CNRS UMR8104
UniversitØParis Descartes
Paris, France

Nisha Wadhwani
Interactive Research School for Health Affairs
Bharati Vidyapeeth University
Pune, India

Yuping Wang
Department of Obstetrics and Gynecology
Louisiana State University Health and Sciences
   Center
Shreveport, Louisiana

Section I

Early Placentation: Regulation
of Trophoblast Growth and Development

1 Human Placenta Development, Structure, and Organization in Relation to Function and Fetal Development

Tore Henriksen, A.M. Holme, H. Horne,
M.B. Holm, and T.M. Michelsen

CONTENTS

ABSTRACT

The placenta is a temporary but advanced organ with respiratory, nutritional, and endocrine functions. It controls the developmental conditions of the fetus by securing the supply of oxygen and nutrients and by partially shielding the fetus from exposure to compounds with potentially adverse effects. An important part of the placental endocrine properties is to modify maternal physiology in a way that supports fetal nutritional needs. However, the placenta itself is also under metabolic and endocrine influence both from the mother and the fetus. The increasing interest in the placenta is largely a result of the current understanding of the influence of fetal development conditions on the future health of the newborn.

The placenta develops from the blastocyst; thus, placental cells are genetically fetal and foreign to the maternal immune system. The development of the placenta has features of a growing tumor both in terms of angiogenesis and cellular invasion of adjacent tissue. However, development of the placenta differs from a tumor by a strict control of both invasion and angiogenesis. This control involves immunological mechanisms that are specific to placental development.

Invasion of placental cells (trophoblasts) into the uterine tissue effectuates an expanding remodeling of uterine end arteries, which secures sufficient maternal blood supply to the placenta. On the fetal side of the placenta, an extensive angiogenesis ensures sufficient fetal blood flow to the placenta. Closely linked to this angiogenic activity is the development of the villous apparatus that results in 10–12 m^2 membranous interphase (the interhemal layer) between the maternal and fetal blood circulation. This huge interphase area, together with numerous transport proteins situated in the interhemal layer, plays a fundamental role in the transfer of nutrients to the fetus.

Adverse placental development, especially disturbance of its vasculature, may result in impaired fetal growth and maturation and also (fetal) demise. There is also evidence that variation in placental function within a normal range may affect the future health of the newborn.

KEY WORDS

Mature intermediate villi (MIV), syncytium, placental maturation, hemodynamics and placenta, placental insufficiency.

1.1 INTRODUCTION

The nutritional and environmental conditions under which an individual develops from conception to birth have significant impact on the future health of the newborn child. In particular, inadequate nutrition in the fetal period of life may increase the risk of cardiovascular diseases, diabetes, overweight, and certain cancers (Godfrey, Gluckman, and Hanson 2010; Hanson and Gluckman 2011). Other environmental factors, including toxic compounds, may have long-term consequences for the developing individual, also in absence of structural malformations. The placenta is the organ that ultimately governs the environmental conditions of the developing fetus. First, virtually all substances reaching the fetal circulation have passed through or have their origin in the placental parenchymal cells. Second, the placenta secretes a variety of hormones and growth factors that modify maternal and fetal metabolism. The placenta is sensitive to maternal and fetal signals and may, within certain limits, adapt its properties to support fetal development. The ability of the placenta to adapt is reflected in size, structure, and functional properties (Fowden, Forhead, Sferruzzi-Perri, Burton, and Vaughan 2015; Sandovici, Hoelle, Angiolini, and Constancia 2012). The placenta is considered, in general, to have a significant reserve capacity. It has been claimed that a third of the placenta parenchyma may be nonfunctional before clinically evident effects on the fetus may be observed. However, there is now ample evidence that differences in the conditions under which the fetus grows, also within the normal range, may affect the future health of the newborn.

A variety of maternal factors may influence placental properties and fetal developmental conditions. First, the maternal immune system plays a fundamental role in the formation of the placenta by its interaction with the invading trophoblast cells during the first half of pregnancy and, thereby, in establishing the uteroplacental circulation (Moffett and Colucci 2014). Second, a number of maternal factors, including obesity and other malnutritional states, disturbances in glucose and lipid metabolism, diseases affecting the vasculature, like hypertension and certain autoimmune diseases, endocrine functions, infections, and exposure to toxic compounds, may all affect placental properties (Higgins, Greenwood, Wareing, Sibley, and Mills 2011; Jansson et al. 2008; Jeve, Konje, and Doshani 2015). The large majority of studies of the association between maternal factors and newborn properties have not included placental parameters. However, more recent studies of this kind, where placental physical characteristics have been included in the statistical models, indicate that the effect of maternal factors on newborn properties is markedly modified (Ouyang et al. 2013; Roland et al. 2014; Salafia et al. 2007). One study showed that the effect of maternal body mass index and plasma glucose on newborn body fat stores disappeared after adjusting for placental weight (Friis et al. 2013).

The ways by which placental properties may affect maternal influence on fetal development may broadly be divided into two. The first way is by the structural properties of placenta (Fowden, Sferruzzi-Perri, Coan, Constancia, and Burton 2009). The vascular structures both on the maternal and fetal sides are major determinants of blood flow and, therefore, of placental functional capacity. Closely linked to the microvasculature on the fetal side of the placenta are the structural features of the layers dividing maternal and fetal blood flow (the interhemal layer). The second main way by which placenta may affect maternal influence on fetal developmental conditions is by its specific functional properties, including activity of its transporters of nutrients, placenta's own metabolism, and its endocrine activity (Fowden, Sferruzzi-Perri, Coan, Constancia, and Burton 2009).

The fetus itself may also affect placental properties and, thereby, its own developmental conditions. Among the placental properties influenced by the fetus is the activity of nutrient transporters in the two cell layers (syncytium and endothelial cells) that separate the maternal and fetal circulations (Sandovici, Hoelle, Angiolini, and Constancia 2012).

In sum, placental development and functional properties are affected by both maternal and fetal factors and the placenta itself acts back on both the maternal and fetal organism. A pregnancy may be considered a 38-week interplay among three "individuals": mother, placenta, and fetus.

1.2 EARLY DEVELOPMENT OF THE PLACENTAL VASCULATURE

Establishment of the two placental circulations, the uteroplacental and the fetoplacental, is a sine qua non for a successful pregnancy.

The structural establishment of both the fetoplacental and uteroplacental circulations starts within 2 weeks after implantation in the human. The fetoplacental circulation continues a structural and functional development until term, whereas the structural adaption (remodeling) of the uteroplacental vascular structures are considered to be completed shortly after 20–22 weeks of human pregnancy (Benirschke, Burton, and Baergen 2012c).

At the time of implantation (6–7 days postcoitum [pc]), the fertilized egg has reached the blastocyst stage and consists of an outer cell mass of trophoblastic cells destined to develop into placenta and an inner cell lineage that becomes the embryo. Implantation is the process by which the blastocyst is embedded in the uterine endometrium (decidua). During the first 2–4 weeks after implantation, the trophoblastic (placental) cells dominate in terms of tissue mass and development. The trophoblast at this stage consists of two layers, the outer syncytial layer, to which the maternal decidual tissue is exposed, and the inner cytotrophoblastic layer surrounding the embryo. The syncytium may be considered a gigantic multinucleated cell that covers a huge area. The cytotrophoblastic layer consists of separate cells in contrast to the surrounding syncytium. Both layers are involved in establishing the uteroplacental circulation, but in different ways at different stages.

One very initial step in establishing the uteroplacental circulation (and the fetoplacental circulation as well, see below) is formation of lacunae in the syncytiotrophoblast (Huppertz 2008). The lacunae are primarily enclosed lakes within the syncytial layer, starting as small vacuole-like structures that coalesce. Eventually, the lacunae open into each other, only partially separated by trabecular-like connections formed by the remaining syncytium (the trabecular stage of placenta). This confluent lacunar system is reached at 8–12 days pc and later becomes the intervillous space.

Within the following week, two predominating processes start. First, the lacunae establish open connections with the luminae of the highly active endometrial glandulae. Glandular secretes can be seen entering the syncytial lacunae. This phenomenon is considered of major importance in the nutrition of the fetoplacental unit during the first two thirds of first trimester (histiotrophic nutrition, see below).

Second, the cytotrophoblasts start to proliferate and migrate into the trabecular syncytium separating the lacunae (Kingdom, Huppertz, Seaward, and Kaufmann 2000). Initially, the proliferating cytotrophoblasts form protrusions into the lacunar space covered by syncytium. These protrusions are designated primary villi and are observed from 12 to 14 days pc. Within a week (16–20 days pc), secondary villi are formed, characterized by ingrowth of mesenchymal tissue derived from the loose mesenchyme separating the embryonic unit from the placenta. Thus, the secondary villi consist of a central core of mesenchymal tissue, an adjacent cytotrophoblast layer covered by lacunar syncytium.

At this stage, quite a few of proliferating and migrating cytotrophoblasts form columns that penetrate the syncytial layer completely and reach the decidual tissue. They then spread laterally at the border between the syncytium and decidua (Huppertz and Peeters 2005). The cytotrophoblast replaces the syncytium at the decidual border and form the so-called trophoblastic shell. Now, the lacunar syncytium with the growing villi is separated from both the decidual and embryonic tissues by cytotrophoblastic cells. The cytotrophoblastic columns penetrating the syncytium later become the anchoring villi of placenta (see below).

1.3   ESTABLISHMENT OF FETOPLACENTAL CIRCULATION

A few days later, i.e., 19–21 days pc (clinically 5 weeks of pregnancy), extensive capillary formations (vasculogenesis) can be seen in the mesenchymal core of the secondary villi (Benirschke, Burton, and Baergen 2012a). The endothelial cells forming the capillary walls are derived from hemangioblastic stem cells in the mesenchyme. Some of the same stem cells are "trapped" within the lumen of the capillaries and become hematopoietic stem cells.

By the formation of the capillary structures, the secondary villi become, by definition, tertiary villi. The tertiary villus is the complete type of villus as it contains all its elements, i.e., syncytium, cytotrophoblast, vessels, and mesenchyme. Any villus in the later (growth of) placenta may be considered a type of tertiary villus (mesenchymal villi, immature intermediate villi [IIV], stem villi, mature intermediate villi [MIV], or terminal villi). The various types of villi are described below.

The capillary network of the tertiary villi establishes contact with the vessels formed around allantois in the connecting stalk of the fetus (the future umbilical cord) and eventually with the vessel of the developing fetus. A connecting fetoplacental vascular system is established between 25 and 30 days pc (around 6 weeks of pregnancy). However, the fetoplacental circulation first starts gradually 2–3 weeks later, i.e., 8–9 weeks of pregnancy. Initially, the villous capillaries are filled with nucleated erythrocytes that make the blood viscous and resistance to flow high. Toward the end of first trimester (12 weeks of pregnancy), nonnucleated read cells become predominant and the fetoplacental circulation is fully established.

The fundamental structure of the tertiary villus, where the fetal capillaries are separated from the intervillous (previously lacunar) space by a complete syncytium and partially by a subsyncytial trophoblast cells, as well as mesenchymal tissue, remains until term. However, extensive formation of new villi is a predominant feature of the growing placenta throughout pregnancy, and angiogenic mechanisms are essential. This expansion of the villous tree increases the area between the maternal and fetal circulations and secures, together with maturation of the terminal villi, a sufficient capacity to meet the requirements of the growing fetus.

1.4   ESTABLISHMENT OF UTEROPLACENTAL CIRCULATION

1.4.1   Structural Aspects

The increasing metabolic needs of the growing fetus require both a large exchange area between the maternal and fetal circulations and a sufficient maternal blood flow through the uterus. Around 2% of the cardiac output passes through the uterus in a nonpregnant state, whereas in the last half of pregnancy the percentage is increased to around 15% percent (Battaglia and Meschia 2013). The major cause of this large redistribution of maternal aortic blood flow is an extensive remodeling of the uterine end arteries (the spiral arteries), combined with a shunt-like low-resistance flow through the placental intervillous space (Pijnenborg, Vercruysse, and Hanssens 2006). In addition, there is a 40%–50% increase in maternal plasma volume and cardiac output. Around 50% of the gestational increase in cardiac output takes place in the first half of pregnancy (20–24 weeks), i.e., very much over the same period that remodeling of the spiral arteries take place (Desai, Moodley, and Naidoo 2004).

The remodeling process transforming the spiral arteries is unique to the uteroplacental unit and is not observed in any other human tissues. The number of end (spiral) arteries in the uterine vasculature has been estimated to be 50–80 (Burton, Woods, Jauniaux, and Kingdom 2009).

During pregnancy, most of these arteries undergo remodeling of various degrees, which results in an increase the average luminal area (Benirschke, Burton, and Baergen 2012a; Pijnenborg, Vercruysse, and Hanssens 2006). This enhances the exchange surface area of the placenta. The process of remodeling involves destruction and/or impairment of the smooth muscle layer of spiral arteries, making them less sensitive to vasoconstricting agents.

The cytothrophoblasts play a fundamental role in remodeling of the spiral arteries. At the sites where the cytotrophoblastic columns have penetrated the syncytium, the attachment sites of the anchoring villi, a subgroup of cytotrophoblastic cells (extravillous trophoblasts), start to move into the decidual interstitial tissue and become interstitial trophoblasts. The invasion of the extravillous trophoblast has been compared with the process seen in invading malignant tumors. However, in contrast to many malignant cells, the invading trophoblasts stop proliferating at the time they leave the proliferative zone of the anchoring villi. The process of trophoblast invasion is initiated within 2–3 weeks pc.

Parallel to this process, changes in the walls of the spiral arteries can be observed, including vacuolation of the endothelial cells and swelling of the smooth muscle cells. This is a phenomenon that may be independent of the invading trophoblasts (Craven, Morgan, and Ward 1998).

In the following weeks, the interstitial trophoblasts approach and eventually invade the muscular wall of the spiral arteries. This process is accompanied by disorganization of the vascular smooth muscle layers. Trophoblast cells are also observed within the lumen of the spiral arteries. These endovascular trophoblasts expand and move in the direction of the myometrium, a phenomenon named endovascular trophoblast invasion. At the ends of the spiral arteries, close to the trophoblastic shell, the endovascular trophoblasts usually fill the whole vascular lumen and obliterate the vessel. This plugging of the spiral arteries prevails until the end of the first trimester (Pijnenborg, Vercruysse, and Hanssens 2006).

The origin of the endovascular trophoblasts is not settled. Most probably, the endovascular trophoblasts invade the arteries from distal openings close to the trophoblastic shell or anchoring villi. The endovascular trophoblasts may also be derived from the interstitial trophoblasts that have crossed the vascular wall through the disorganized smooth muscle layers. By the end of the first trimester and in the following weeks, both the endovascular and the interstitial trophoblasts continue to move toward the inner third of the myometrium. The density of the cells decreases with the distance from the trophoblastic shell.

The endothelial lining of the spiral arteries is disrupted and apparently replaced in many areas by the endovascular trophoblastic cells. There is evidence that endovascular trophoblasts may acquire endothelial properties in terms of adhesion molecules (Zhou et al. 1997). It remains unresolved to which extent the trophoblasts may become fully endothelial cells and whether they contribute as cellular elements in the reendothelialization that occurs after transformation of the spiral arteries (Lyall et al. 2001). Current evidence indicates, however, that maternal endothelial cells are the main cellular source during reendothelialization (Pijnenborg, Vercruysse, and Hanssens 2006).

The remodeling of the spiral arteries is accompanied by depositions of fibrinoid material in the intimal and medial layers of the vessel wall. The fibrinoid material more or less replaces the smooth muscular cells. During the second trimester, this results in reendothelialization of the intima along with areas of subintimal thickening due to the appearance of cells with myofibroblastic features.

This remodeling process is grossly completed just after 20 weeks of gestation in the human, and the overall result is a marked broadening of the lumen of the majority of the spiral arteries. The luminal expansion may extend right to the inner third of the myometrium, although there are regional and individual variations. Importantly, in hypertensive disorders of pregnancy with placental insufficiency, especially preeclampsia combined with fetal growth restriction, the remodeling of the spiral arteries are, on average, reduced particularly in the deeper decidual and myometrial parts of the spiral arteries (Benirschke, Burton, and Baergen 2012a; Brosens and Khong 2010). This incomplete remodeling is assumed to explain the increased resistance in the uteroplacental blood flow often observed in preeclamptic patients as higher resistance indexes in sonographic Doppler measurements.

It is important to notice that even in normal pregnancies, the degree of remodeling of the spiral arteries varies between individuals and along each single spiral artery. Accordingly, there is an overlap in terms of the degree of spiral artery remodeling between normal pregnancy, preeclampsia and/or intrauterine growth restriction (IUGR) (Pijnenborg, Vercruysse, and Hanssens 2006). Within the group of preeclamptic disorders, early-onset preeclampsia exhibits a higher proportion of poorly remodeled spiral arteries than late-onset variants do.

In addition to the remodeling of the spiral arteries, there is evidence for changes in the functional properties of the uterine arteries proximal to the spiral arteries (radial and arcuate arteries). They become markedly dilated, as illustrated by the observation that the diameter of the arcuate arteries may exceed that of the uterine artery (Burchell 1967). In addition, there also seem to be a certain degree of arteriovenous shunting within the myometrium.

1.4.2 Functional Aspects

There is no flow of maternal blood into the intervillous space until the end of the first trimester, which is weeks after the remodeling of the spiral arteries started (Benirschke, Burton, and Baergen 2012c). This raises two questions. First, why is there a "delay" in the commencement of the uteroplacental (intervillous) circulation? Second, how is the fetoplacental unit nourished in the first trimester?

The first trimester absence of intervillous blood flow is believed to be effectuated by the cytotrophoblastic plugging of the terminal ends of the spiral arteries in the vicinity of the anchoring villi (Huppertz and Peeters 2005). As a consequence of the initial obliteration of the intervillous blood flow, the embryo and the placenta are developing in an environment of low oxygen tension. This may protect the early fetoplacental unit against free radicals generated by high oxygen concentration in immature tissues with poor antioxidant capacity. In addition, low oxygen concentration may promote capillary proliferation and, thereby, growth of villous tissue, which is essential in the early development of the fetoplacental unit (Burton, Charnock-Jones, and Jauniaux 2009).

It is believed that the plugging of the spiral arteries is less extensive in the areas closer to the endometrial surface (Huppertz 2008). This assumption is based on observations indicating that the start of the intervillous flow occurs in these peripheral areas. Introduction of maternal blood into the intervillous space increases the oxygen concentration markedly. The oxidative stress that follows leads to villous damage and degeneration in the peripheral parts of the placenta, which regresses to form chorion leave. Eventually, also the remaining deeper central part of villous mass becomes perfused with maternal blood. It is not well understood how this part of villous tissue resists the oxidative stress and therefore can develop to the definitive placenta. It may be speculated that cellular antioxidants are induced as the intervillous perfusion progresses from the periphery. The oxygen concentration may also be lower in this area because of a more efficient transfer of oxygen to the fetoplacental circulation, which is established a little ahead of the uteroplacental (intervillous) circulation.

As a consequence of the "delayed" onset of the uteroplacental circulation, the fetoplacental unit must be nourished by other mechanisms than direct transfer of nutrients from maternal blood. The intervillous space is filled with a clear fluid before the maternal circulation is established. This fluid may be derived from two sources. First, endometrial glands have been shown to open into the lacunar and, eventually, intervillous space. At this stage, the endometrial glands are highly secretory. Second, it is also suggested that maternal plasma enters the intervillous space as a filtrate of maternal blood passing through the intercellular space of plugs of the spiral arteries. Proteins and other contents of the glandular secretions and plasma filtrates are phagocytized by the syncytium and degraded in lysosomes to nutritional elements that may be transferred to the cells of the early fetoplacental unit. Thus, during a major part of the first trimester, the fetoplacental tissue is hypoxic and nourished by a system designated histiotrophic nutrition (Burton, Watson, Hempstock, Skepper, and Jauniaux 2002).

1.5 IMMUNOLOGICAL AND CELLULAR ASPECTS OF EARLY PLACENTAL DEVELOPMENT

During placentation, a complex interaction takes place among the trophoblast, the decidual tissue, the spiral arteries, and the maternal immune system (Moffett and Colucci 2014). This interaction is exceptional in the sense that it comprises both a tolerance to and regulation of invading semi-allogenic cells. Parallels have been drawn to immune responses to invasive cancers and organ transplants, but the biological mechanisms during placentation seem even more complex. A detailed discussion of these issues is beyond the scope of this chapter, but a few comments are given to the two fundamental biological processes involved, cellular invasion and the immune responses.

Cellular invasion requires cellular migration. As described above, cytotrophoblasts invade the decidual maternal tissue, first into the interstitium, then the vascular lumen of the spiral arteries, and continue an endovascular invasive process. Invasive migration of cells requires stimuli to invade and release of enzymes that degrade extracellular matrix to an extent that allow the cytotrophoblast to migrate. Many of the factors that stimulate cytotrophoblast migration into maternal tissue must come from the decidua itself. There are a large variety of factors that may mediate and control trophoblast migration, including transforming growth factor-β, fibroblast growth factor, insulin-like growth factor, vascular endothelial growth factor (VEGF), placental growth factor (PlGF), interferons, interleukins, hyperglycosylated human chorionic gonadotropin (HCG), leptin, nitric oxide (NO), and carbon monoxide (CO) (Benirschke, Burton, and Baergen 2012c). Many of these factors are present in the decidual tissue at the time of implantation, securing stimuli for invasion. As the trophoblast invasion progresses, gradients in decidual oxygen concentration may also promote trophoblast invasion.

In the degradation of matrix components, matrix metalloproteinases (MMPs) play a fundamental role. Both the cytotrophoblasts and other cells in the decidua secrete MMPs.

The cellular ability to invade also involves altered secretion of matrix proteins, like fibronectin, collagen IV, and laminin. The expression of matching cellular adhesion molecules will effectuate the binding to the matrix proteins and to other cells present at a given place at a given time. In the remodeling of the spiral arteries trophoblast migration, MMP-mediated extracellular matrix degradation, secretion of alternative extracellular matrix proteins, and a continuous shift in the expression of adhesion molecules are fundamental mechanisms.

The response of the maternal endometrial immune system in the first weeks of the placentation process operates conceivably along several paths serving different functions.

In the first trimester, a uterine population of natural killer cell (uNK) increases several-fold in the decidua (Zhang, Chen, Smith, and Croy 2011). Other important maternal immune cells are various types of macrophages. Accumulation of uNK cells is seen close to the adventitia of spiral arteries before any structural changes are obvious and seem to depart at the time trophoblast invasion appears. The macrophages, however, remain in the area of the vascular walls. It has therefore been hypothesized that uNK cells play a fundamental role (among other roles) in "destabilizing" the vascular wall and thereby mediate an obligatory preparation for the trophoblast-dependent remodeling of the spiral arteries. The very early vacuolization and swelling of the arterial endothelial and smooth muscle cells mentioned above may reflect an early destabilizing process.

A second path by which the maternal immune system operates is the response to foreign antigens on the trophoblast. The invading cytotrophoblast, in contrast to the syncytium, express unique human leukocyte antigen (HLA)-molecules, particularly HLA-G (Lynge, Djurisic, and Hviid 2014).

There is ample evidence that HLA-G plays a central role in the immunological tolerance against the partially allogeneic trophoblast as both trophoblast-bound and free HLA-G can bind to receptors on uNK, macrophages, and T-cells and thereby modify their responses. The interactions between maternal immune cells and the trophoblast may serve two main functions. First, it may prevent (too extensive) cytolytic destruction of the invading trophoblasts. Second, it may regulate the degree (deepness) of invasion of the trophoblasts.

1.6   PLACENTAL GROWTH IN THE SECOND AND THIRD TRIMESTER

Although the placentation process is finalized shortly after 20 weeks of gestation, the parenchymal part of the placenta continues to increase in size until term (Molteni, Stys, and Battaglia 1978). This increase is mainly a result of growth and maturation of the villous apparatus (Mayhew 2006).

As mentioned above, villous circulation starts at around 8–9 weeks of pregnancy (6–7 weeks pc). Doppler studies show the presence of end-diastolic flow at the beginning of the second trimester (12–14 weeks of pregnancy). Thereafter, end-diastolic flow increases throughout pregnancy, indicating reduced impedance in placental villous vasculature.

The first 12–14 weeks of the second trimester, i.e., until 24–26 weeks of pregnancy, a tertiary villus type now designated mesenchymal villi arises from existing villi by sequences similar to the ones seen during the initial development of placenta above (Benirschke, Burton, and Baergen 2012a). The mesenchymal villi appear to undergo a progressive transformation into IIV. These are characterized by a dense network of capillaries in a loose stroma and by the presence of canalicular structures containing macrophages (Hofbauer cells). The surface of IIV is covered by syncytium, underneath which there are layers of cytotrophoblasts (Langhans cells). Overall, IIV give a "swollen" and "edematous" appearance. At the surface of IIV, new mesenchymal villi are formed by proliferation of the cytotrophoblasts beneath the syncytium followed by a core of mesenchymal tissue and extensive capillary formation (angiogenesis). The older basal parts of the IIV generally transform into stem villi. During this transformation, the capillary and canalicular networks largely regress, and small arteries and veins with medial layers develop in the central part of the villus. Furthermore, along this transformation into stem villi, the mesenchymal tissue becomes more fibrotic, there are less cytotrophoblasts (Langhans cells), and the syncytium is replaced by fibrinoid material in many areas.

As the second half of pregnancy progresses, the number of IIV decreases and the mesenchymal villi now increasingly give rise to another type of villi, the MIV. MIV are different from IIV in several respects. They are slender villi, just slightly broader than the terminal villi to which they give rise. They are covered by syncytium, which overlay a richness of capillaries located mainly just beneath and has a loose connective tissue core mainly devoid of vessels. Cytotrophoblasts (Langhans cells) are regularly seen subsyncytially.

The terminal (distal) villi are the uttermost ends of the villous tree. They develop from the surface of the MIV in a grape-like fashion. The diameter of the terminal villi is in the range of 30–100 μm. They are covered by syncytium of variable thickness. The most conspicuous feature of the terminal villus is the abundance of capillaries. They occupy, on average, 50% of the volume of the villous stroma. The diameter of the capillaries varies because, frequently, they have a dilated sinusoid or bulbous appearance. At these sites, they are in tight contact with the overlying syncytium (see below). A few cytotrophoblastic (Langhans) cells are seen at distinct sites and in close contact with the overlying syncytium. The stroma is scant and macrophages (Hofbauer cells) are few.

Placental growth in the last trimester is dominated by expansion of the mature intermediate and terminal villi (Feneley and Burton 1991). Toward the end of pregnancy, the terminal villi constitute around 40% of the villous volume and more than 50% of total villous surface. At this stage of pregnancy, placental growth is driven by mechanisms that progressively increase the exchange surface between maternal and fetal blood as well as allowing more fetal blood to pass through the villous tree. It is therefore not surprising that growth and maturation of the terminal capillaries are main elements in the final development of the placenta.

During this period, longitudinal growth is a prominent feature of the capillary expansion, resulting in parallel capillary loops in the distal villi. However, various degrees of interconnections between the loops are also formed by budding or branching endothelial growth from the walls of the loops (Jirkovska et al. 2002; Mayhew 2009). This capillary growth is disproportionate to that of the villus as a whole, resulting in an intrusion of capillary loops toward the covering trophoblast, which becomes stretched, forming bulges in the intervillous space. This process results in a progressive reduction in the distance between maternal and fetal blood and enhances the efficacy of the transplacental transport of oxygen and nutrients.

1.7   PLACENTAL MATURATION

The term *maturation of placenta* refers, in general, to the process by which the villous tree attains a sufficient number and normal distribution of the final types of villi and to which extent the structural composition of each villus type is considered normal.

Thus, in the normal-term placenta, the villous picture is dominated by MIV from which numerous terminal villi branch (Benirschke, Burton, and Baergen 2012a). Maturation of the terminal villi refers to the final organization of the capillary network and is characterized by close approximation of the large proportion of capillary loops to the overlying syncytium. The mature terminal villus exhibits certain structural features of particular functional interest. The width of the capillary loops in the terminal villi varies, rendering a sinusoid picture. Flow of blood in these dilated segments is, as expected, decelerated, which increases the time for gas and nutrient exchanges. Many of the dilated capillary segments appear to stretch the overlying syncytium, which becomes very thin and free of nuclei and with few organelles. These areas are designated the vasculo-syncytial membrane, where maternal blood and fetal blood are separated only by thinned syncytium and endothelium between which fused basal membranes may be discerned. The layer between the maternal and fetal circulation (interhemal layer) varies in thickness. The thickness of the vasculo-syncytial membrane is only 2–3 µm, compared with an average of around 5 µm of the interhemal layer in the terminal villi. It has been estimated that the vasculo-syncytial membrane constitutes around one third of the surface of the terminal villi.

The vasculo-syncytial membrane is considered an area where exchange of gases and selected nutrients is particularly effective, both because of its thinness and presumed low metabolic activity (few organelles).

1.8   SYNCYTIUM AND SYNCYTIAL RENEWAL

Toward the very last weeks of pregnancy, the placenta normally reaches its full development, including maturation of the terminal villi. The weight of the placenta increases almost linearly up to term, reflecting continuous growth of the villous mass. Close to term, the area of the villous surfaces facing maternal blood (the apical syncytial surface) is considered to be 12–14 m². In addition, the apical syncytial membrane is microvillous, which makes the actual membranous surface several folds larger. The microvilli are structurally similar to microvilli in general; i.e., they are fingerlike protrusions of the cell membrane with a length at term of around 0.5–0.7 µm (Teasdale and Jean-Jacques 1985). They are present only on the apical surface of the syncytium. They cover the whole surface of the syncytium and are often so densely situated that the clefts between them are no larger than the diameter of the microvillus itself (0.10–0.2 µm). The microvilli are covered by a layer of glycocalyx consisting of proteoglycans and glycoproteins (Jones and Fox 1991). The glycocalyx layer is believed to play a role in preventing thrombus formation, in the immunological response of maternal immune cells to placental proteins, and in selection of components in maternal blood that reach the syncytial uptake machinery.

Most of the transport proteins are situated in the cell membrane of the microvilli.

It is believed that after having bound the ligand (e.g., a fatty acid), the transport protein/ligand complex is transported to the base of the microvillus, where coated pits mediate cytoplasmic uptake and further processing. It is not the scope of this chapter to discuss the large number and variety of the syncytial transport proteins beyond mentioning that glucose transporter (GLUT)-1 is the main glucose transporter after the first trimester and that amino acids and fatty acids are subject to active transport by a number of more or less specialized transport proteins. Transport proteins are also situated on the basal cell membrane of the syncytium. The density and relative abundance of the transport proteins differ from those of the microvillous membrane (Lager and Powell 2012).

In this context, the capillary endothelium beneath the syncytium needs to be mentioned because it is part of the path between maternal and fetal blood. The villous endothelium is of a nonfenestrated kind, where the endothelial cells are bridged by both adherent and tight types of junctions (Lievano, Alarcon, Chavez-Munguia, and Gonzalez-Mariscal 2006). Much less is known about the role of the endothelial layer, but emerging evidence indicates that the endothelial cells here, as elsewhere, are much more than a passive barrier. For example, during the last half of pregnancy, the villous endothelium expresses insulin receptors, exhibits specific interactions with fetal high-density lipoprotein (HDL) and acquires receptors for FcγRII (Elad, Levkovitz, Jaffa, Desoye, and Hod 2014; Simister, Jacobowitz, Ahouse, and Story 1997).

An intact syncytial layer is essential for effective exchange of gases and nutrients between maternal and fetal blood. The placental syncytium seems to have limited ability to renew and repair its cellular components. The syncytial nuclei do not exhibit proliferative activity and appears have overall low or selected transcriptional activity, and a large proportion of them have nuclei with condensed chromatin.

It is conceivable that the syncytium is exposed to mechanical trauma exerted by maternal blood, as well as metabolic stress due to the energy requiring nutrient transport, hormonal production, and the need for renewal of cellular components. In addition, syncytial damage due to oxidative stress seems to be present in normal pregnancies, but particularly in preeclamptic pregnancies. There is good evidence that the cytotrophoblasts (Langhans cells) are fundamental in the keeping of the overlying syncytium (Hempstock, Jauniaux, Greenwold, and Burton 2003; Siman, Sibley, Jones, Turner, and Greenwood 2001). The cell membrane of the apical part of cytotrophoblasts, i.e., the one facing the syncytium, is in direct contact with the basal cell membrane of the syncytium without any separating extracellular matrix. A variety of cellular adhesion proteins link the two cell membranes together in these areas. Syncytial expansion and renewal take place by a continuous process involving dissolution of the syncytial and cytotrophoblastic cell membranes at the sites of close contact, resulting in cell fusion and release of the cytotrophoblastic cytoplasm into the syncytium. A variety of membrane proteins are involved in the fusion process, including syncytins. At the time of cell fusion, the cytotrophoblast has differentiated from a proliferative cell to a cellular state characterized by a high content of organelles, proteins, and mRNA. This richness of cytoplasmic components ensures renewal of syncytial metabolic capacity after fusion. Conceivably, signals from the syncytium initiate the cytotrophoblastic differentiation, but this remains to be proven.

The nucleus of the cytotrophoblastic cells is also transferred into the syncytium. From that time on, the proliferative and transcriptional activities of the nucleus decline, the chromatin eventually becomes dense, and apoptotic features appear. It is, however, not clear to which extent apoptotic mechanisms are involved. Having reached the syncytium, the condensed nuclei gather under the apical syncytial cell membrane, where it forms protrusions into the intervillous space (designated "true syncytial knots") (Benirschke, Burton, and Baergen 2012b). It is believed that syncytial knots may eventually be released into the maternal circulation.

Besides renewing the syncytium, the cytotrophoblast may also repair disrupted syncytium. In these cases, fibrin will usually be deposited at the injured area. Cytotrophoblastic cells may proliferate and migrate over the fibrin layers and eventually fuse to form a new syncytium.

Taken together, the villous cytotrophoblasts are fundamental in ensuring the physical intactness and function of the syncytium.

In addition to the renewing function of the cytotrophoblast–syncytium interaction, another mechanism also seems to operate in securing the physical intactness of the maternal–fetal interphase. In normal placentas, fibrinoid material can be seen regularly at the villous surface at sites of damaged syncytium (Kaufmann, Huppertz, and Frank 1996). This material consists mainly of fibrin and is most probably derived from maternal fibrinogen, which is activated at sites of syncytial injury. It is believed that formation of villous fibrin-type fibrinoid is a rescue mechanism at sites where normal cytotrophoblastic sustainment of the syncytium fails. Although water, solutes, and certain nutrients may pass through the fibrinoid meshwork into the fetal circulation, it is conceivable that the fibrinoid represents areas of markedly reduced function in terms of placental transport and metabolism. It is unclear whether the sites of physiological villous surface fibrin may expand into larger thrombi and eventually cause local infarctions. Another type of villous fibrinoid is seen within the villus. This has another chemical composition and is probably part of villous degeneration.

1.9 HEMODYNAMIC AND RHEOLOGICAL ASPECTS OF PLACENTAL DEVELOPMENT

The development of both the uteroplacental and fetoplacental vasculature is a predominant feature of the placentation process. The structural characteristics that the vasculatures attain have rheological and hemodynamic consequences that are fundamental in optimizing placental function. Some of these have already been briefly discussed above.

The remodeling of the spiral arteries leads not only to a greater diameter but also to a change in shape (Burton, Woods, Jauniaux, and Kingdom 2009). The increase in diameter is largest distally, i.e., where the artery opens into the intervillous space. Accordingly, the three-dimensional shape of the spiral artery is that of a funnel. The maternal blood runs from the narrow part of the funnel through the wider and into the intervillous space. The consequence is a precipitous deceleration in speed of the blood flow, with a corresponding reduction in the momentum at which it enters the intervillous space. The effect of a slower blood flow is a more even distribution of the blood within the intervillous space, less risk of mechanical damage to the villi, and more time for gaseous and nutritional exchange with the fetoplacental blood.

Efficient placental transport of gases and nutrients is dependent on maintenance of the thinness of the vasculo-syncytial layer of the terminal villi. The thinness is preserved by dilated villous capillaries stretching the overlying syncytium. However, the dilated state of the capillaries can be maintained only if the blood pressure within the villous capillaries is higher than that of the intervillous space. How this fine-tuned pressure difference is maintained is not well understood. A main factor must be a low and stable intervillous pressure. Reasonably, the remodeling of the spiral arteries and the functional changes in the more proximal myometrial arteries must play a significant role. However, also the pressure of the uterine venous system affects the intervillous pressure. The regulation of the pressure within the villous capillaries has also been the subject of considerations but remains an elusive topic. It is conceivable that pressure disturbances in the pressure gradient across the vasculo-syncytial layer may underlie certain kinds of disturbed villous development, including avascular villi, with or without fibrinoid deposition and cases of impaired maturation. Another hemodynamic variable that may affect the development of the villous capillaries is the speed of the fetoplacental blood flow through changes in the sheer stress against the endothelial surface. Our insight into this topic is also highly limited, but in cases of fetal anemia, with increased maximum velocity of flow, disturbed villous development is prevalent.

1.10 OXYGEN AND PLACENTA

It is beyond the scope of this chapter to discuss in any detail, even a selection of the numerous bioactive compounds involved in placental development and maintenance. However, oxygen warrants a few remarks because it plays a fundamental role in development of placenta, beyond its role in mitochondrial energy production. In addition, oxygen has, under given conditions, the potential to induce tissue injury and therefore disturbed placental structure and function (Tuuli, Longtine, and Nelson 2011).

There is ample evidence that development of the villous tree occurs under low oxygen concentration until the intervillous blood flow is established by 10–12 weeks of pregnancy (Jauniaux et al. 2000).

Low oxygen tension stimulates angiogenesis, which is extensive during this period. Angiogenic and growth factors that respond to low oxygen include VEGF, PlGF and angiopoietins, all of which are considered essential in development and growth of the villous tree (Charnock-Jones, Kaufmann, and Mayhew 2004). During pregnancy, angiogenesis continues along with the growth of placenta, probably in response to local villous hypoxic and other stimuli. The role of low oxygen tension in stimulating villous capillary growth is illustrated in the placenta of pregnancies at high altitudes (Reshetnikova, Burton, and Milovanov 1994). The villous capillaries of these placentas exhibit larger surface areas and volumes than found in placentas from sea-level pregnancies. Furthermore, villi in the relative hypoxic periphery of placental lobules show more angiogenesis than do those situated centrally. Experimental animal studies support the role of low oxygen tension in villous capillary growth (Bacon et al. 1984).

Low oxygen tension also stimulates proliferation of cytotrophoblasts, both in the villi and in the cell columns of extravillous trophoblast (anchoring villi) (Red-Horse et al. 2004).

Oxygen, may, however, also mediate tissue damage trough generation of free radicals and induction oxidative stress. Placentae of preeclamptic pregnancies with poor remodeling of the spiral arteries show signs of oxidative stress. It has been proposed that in these cases, the incompletely remodeled spiral arteries have retained certain ability to contract (Burton, Woods, Jauniaux, and Kingdom 2009; Francis et al. 1998). This may lead to intermittent contraction and relaxation, resulting in repetitive placental ischemia (hypoxia) and reperfusion (reoxygenation), which is well known to induce oxidative stress (Cindrova-Davies, Spasic-Boskovic, Jauniaux, Charnock-Jones, and Burton 2007; Myatt 2010). Oxidative stress may injure the syncytium, causing reduced placenta capacity both by impaired syncytial function and by formation of thrombi resulting in villous infarction.

1.11 LOBULAR ORGANIZATION OF THE VILLOUS TREE

The placenta is organized in 30–50 lobules. Each lobuli usually has one spiral artery ending into its intervillous space (Schuhmann, Stoz, and Maier 1986). The villous types and mass are not evenly distributed within each lobule. The central part of the lobule has low density of villi, and these are predominantly of mature intermediate type. Toward the periphery, the density of the villi increases with a dominance of the terminal type. With this anatomical arrangement, the incoming geyser of maternal blood has space to slow down. Thereby, there is less risk of mechanical damage to the villous tree and the blood will be more evenly distributed between the villous branches of the lobule and at a low speed (transfer time 15–30 seconds). Thus, the lobular organization of the villous tree contributes to effective exchange between the maternal and fetal circulations.

1.12 THE TERMS PLACENTAL FUNCTION AND PLACENTAL INSUFFICIENCY

These are terms used extensively in the literature and in clinical work but lack good definitions.

The term *placental function* usually refers to the ability of placenta to provide the fetus with sufficient oxygen and nutrients. However, production of hormones and growth factors is also an essential placental function. So, placental function may as well be defined by the ability to produce sufficient amount and kinds of hormones and growth factors.

However, whichever of these two main functions of placenta is used in the/as definition, they are not operative. In fact, a general operative definition of placental function is inconceivable.

Meaningful operative definitions may be achieved only when they are context related, but they are then limited to certain aspects of the function of placenta. In experimental in vivo animal work, placental function may, for example, be defined as mass of selected nutrients transferred from mother to fetus per unit time.

Both in epidemiological and experimental work, the ratio between birth weight and placenta weight has been used as an indicator of placenta function (Fowden, Sferruzzi-Perri, Coan, Constancia, and Burton 2009; Molteni, Stys, and Battaglia 1978). This definition has birth weight as denominator. Birth weight is a crude indicator of the newborn nutritional and metabolic state and accordingly also a rough parameter of placental function. Evaluation of placental function is an integrate part of a more specialized antenatal care. Estimating placental size or form in utero has so far proven to be of little use in clinical work. Clinically, the term *placental insufficiency* is used rather than *normal placenta function* because in this setting, diagnostic and explaining definitions are more useful. Reduced fetal growth (i.e., growth less than expected) is generally a core criterion in the diagnosis of placental insufficiency, after exclusion of causes of reduced fetal growth that do not primarily involve decreased placental function (like fetal malformation, chromosomal aberrations, genetic diseases, maternal malnutrition, certain maternal diseases, etc.). Additional indicators of placental insufficiency may be obtained by monitoring other vital signs, like fetal blood flow patterns, heart rate variations, movements, and amount of amniotic fluid. Practically, parameters that can be obtained by sonography (ultrasound) are used to diagnose placenta insufficiency. Use of biochemical parameters has so far not proven clinically useful. Three kinds of sonographic parameters are used. The first is size parameters, including abdominal circumference versus head circumference and long bones, like the femur. Second, measurements of blood velocity parameters in the fetal circulation are widely used. The vessels mostly assessed are umbilical artery, middle cerebral artery, and ductus venosus. Third, heart rate variations are registered by cardiotocography.

Indications of placental insufficiency may also be obtained by measuring blood velocity patterns in the uterine artery. In cases of impaired transformation of the spiral arteries, which is associated with reduced placental function, increased resistance to flow in the uterine artery is often found.

It should be noted that the term *placental insufficiency* is rarely used until the second half of pregnancy. This does not mean that insufficient placental function is not an important cause of abortions in the first half of pregnancy, but clinical diagnosis of placental insufficiency in early pregnancy is a challenging task.

There is no general agreement on how many or which combinations of sonographic parameters should be abnormal before the term *placental insufficiency* may be used.

In fact, even reduced fetal growth may not necessarily be present to attribute a poor fetal outcome to insufficient placenta. For example, intrauterine fetal death of fetuses large for gestational age has been explained by a relative insufficiency of a usually large placenta. Hypoxic damage to the normally grown fetus during delivery (asphyxia) may be caused by a kind of placental insufficiency that is unmanifested until challenged by the extra demands after uterine contractions. After delivery, histopathological, microbiological, and genetic investigations may add important information to a final judgment of the role of the placenta in explaining the fetal outcome.

In experimental work, one specific aspect of placental function, for example, capacity to transport amino acids, may be studied under defined conditions. In a clinical setting, placental insufficiency is usually the result of a long-term process (weeks to months) that affects more or less simultaneously all the main determinants of placental function. The main determinants of placental function are the following:

1. Blood flow on both side of placenta, i.e., in the intervillous space and in the villous capillaries
2. The surface area of the villous syncytio-endothelial layer (interhemal layer)
3. The functional capacity of the interhemal layer per unit surface

    Given that the structural and metabolic integrity of the interhemal layer is intact, its functional capacity in terms of transport of oxygen and nutrients is determined by the following:

    a. The thickness of the interhemal layer, especially in the areas made up by vasculo-syncytial membrane
    b. The density and function of transport proteins

Placental function in terms of ability to produce hormones, growth factors, and other signal molecules is similarly dependent on the structural and metabolic integrity of the cellular elements, especially in the villous tissue but also in the placenta bed with its mixture of decidual cells and interstitial trophoblast.

Studies of placental functions have two aspects. The first is to understand how the main determinants mentioned above contribute to the "overall" placental function under physiological (normal) conditions. Central research issues are studies of transport proteins and placenta's own energy metabolism, including their genetic and epigenetic regulation and the effects of maternal and fetal factors on placental functions (Fowden, Sferruzzi-Perri, Coan, Constancia, and Burton 2009). This kind of insight is essential in the understanding of fetal developmental conditions, also within a range that may be considered normal. There is increasing evidence that variations in the fetal developmental conditions within a normal range may affect the future health of the newborn. Accordingly, understanding variations in normal placental functions is of interest beyond that of pure physiology.

The second aspect of placental studies is clinical and concerns which aspects of placental function or properties are the main contributors to poor fetal outcome, including fetal growth deviations (growth restriction, newborn overweight), malformations, cerebral dysfunctions, and death. As discussed above, this kind of insight is obtained by sonographic studies, combined with histopathological, genetic, and microbiological investigations of placenta and the fetus. Based on numerous publications of clinical material, the main explanation of placental insufficiency is disturbances in the uteroplacental circulation, which may also be named maternal malperfusion of the placenta. The structural features that reflect malperfusion include increased deposition of fibrin in the intervillous space and within the villi, combined with intervillous hemorrhage, presence of thrombi, and necrosis of villous tissue (infarction). Depending on the time interval and degree of malperfusion, fibrinoid depositions are present in the intervillous area or within the villi. Changes that are considered compensatory to malperfusion are often present, like syncytial knots, increased branching (density) in the capillaries in the terminal (distal) villi, and a hypoplastic appearance of many distal villi.

A major cause of the maternal malperfusion is insufficient remodeling of the spiral arteries often associated with atherotic changes. The latter may further compromise blood flow and accentuate ischemia (hypoxia). Disturbances in the uteroplacental circulation may also be caused by retained sensitivity to vasoconstricting agents, leading to hypoxia and reoxygenation in the intervillous space (see above).

Another cause of disturbed perfusion of the intervillous space is increased coagulability of the maternal blood, like that found in women with antiphospholipid antibodies and other procoagulant disorders. In these cases, thrombus formation may lead to an extent of placental infarctions that cause the clinical manifestations of placental insufficiency. Whether hypertension per se, independent of poor remodeling of the spiral arteries, may injure the villous apparatus is unknown, but not inconceivable. On the fetal side, circulatory disturbances caused by placenta may include abnormal insertion of the umbilical (allantoic) vessels and thrombotic processes in the vessels of the chorionic plate or umbilicus. In these cases, regions with avascular and fibrotic villi are regularly present. In general, the causes of disturbed fetoplacental circulation are less understood than those on the maternal side.

Another placental histological finding that may underlie placental insufficiency is delayed maturation of the villous apparatus (see above for the term *maturation*) (Higgins, McAuliffe, and Mooney 2011). This will lead to reduced areas with vasculo-syncytial membranes, more central placement of the capillaries in the villi, and an overall increase in the thickness of the interhemal layers.

Delayed maturation of the villi is usually found near term, often in cases with normal or even large fetuses, and is associated with fetal death. Placenta from women with diabetes in pregnancy may exhibit the combination of delayed maturation and large fetus. The increased risk of fetal death in diabetic pregnancies has been attributed to "relative placental insufficiency," i.e., that maturation of placenta has not kept up with the metabolic requirements of the often large fetus.

1.13 CONCLUDING REMARKS

Variation in placental function has two aspects. First, there may be a degree of disturbance that is of immediate clinical significance because it leads to fetal growth restriction, fetal hypoxia, prematurity, cerebral injuries, and death. Disturbances in the uteroplacental and/or fetoplacental circulations, as well as impaired maturation of the distal villous apparatus, are the main causes of placental insufficiency in a clinical setting. The common denominator of these causes is reduced capacity of vasculo-syncytial (interhemal) layers to transport oxygen and nutrients. The circulatory disturbances cause reduced interhemal area because of fibrin deposition, thrombus formation, and infarction, whereas delayed maturation lead to increased thickness of the interhemal layers.

Second, variation in placental function within what is considered a normal range may affect the development of the fetus. This may not be of immediate clinical significance but may have long-term effects on the future health of the newborn (Godfrey, Gluckman, and Hanson 2010; Hanson and Gluckman 2011). Accordingly, research aiming at understanding the normal range of placental function, as well as studies leading to better understanding and treatment of the causes of the placental circulatory changes and factors governing villous maturation, is of clinical interest.

REFERENCES

Bacon BJ, Gilbert RD, Kaufmann P, Smith AD, Trevino FT, and Longo LD. 1984. Placental anatomy and diffusing capacity in guinea pigs following long-term maternal hypoxia. *Placenta* 5 (6): 475–487.

Battaglia FC and Meschia G. 2013. Review of studies in human pregnancy and umbilical blood flows. *Developmental Period Medicine* 17 (4): 287–292.

Benirschke K, Burton GJ, and Baergen RN. 2012a. Architecture of normal villous trees. In *Pathology of the Human Placenta*, eds. K Benirschke, GJ Burton, and RN Baergen, 101–144. Berlin Heidelberg: Springer.

Benirschke K, Burton GJ, and Baergen RN. 2012b. Villous maldevelopment. In *Pathology of the Human Placenta*, eds. K Bernischke, GJ Burton, and RN Baergen, 411–427. Springer Berlin Heidelberg.

Benirschke K, Burton GJ, and Baergen RN. 2012c. Nonvillous parts and trophoblast invasion. In *Pathology of the Human Placenta*, eds. K Bernischke, Burton GJ, and RN Baergen, 157–240. Springer Berlin Heidelberg.

Brosens I and Khong TY. 2010. Defective sprial artery remodeling. In *Placental Bed Disorders: Basic Science and its Translation to Obstetrics*, eds. R Pijnenborg, I Brosens, and R Romero, 97–107. Cambridge: Cambridge University Press.

Burchell RC. 1967. Arterial blood flow into the human intervillous space. *American Journal of Obstetrics and Gynecology* 98 (3): 303–311.

Burton GJ, Watson AL, Hempstock J, Skepper JN, and Jauniaux E. 2002. Uterine glands provide histiotrophic nutrition for the human fetus during the first trimester of pregnancy. *The Journal of Clinical Endocrinology and Metabolism* 87 (6): 2954–2959.

Burton GJ, Charnock-Jones DS, and Jauniaux E. 2009. Regulation of vascular growth and function in the human placenta. *Reproduction* 138 (6): 895–902.

Burton GJ, Woods AW, Jauniaux E, and Kingdom JC. 2009. Rheological and physiological consequences of conversion of the maternal spiral arteries for uteroplacental blood flow during human pregnancy. *Placenta* 30 (6): 473–482.

Charnock-Jones DS, Kaufmann P, and Mayhew TM. 2004. Aspects of human fetoplacental vasculogenesis and angiogenesis. I. Molecular regulation. *Placenta* 25 (2–3): 103–113.

Cindrova-Davies T, Spasic-Boskovic O, Jauniaux E, Charnock-Jones DS, and Burton GJ. 2007. Nuclear factor-kappa B, p38, and stress-activated protein kinase mitogen-activated protein kinase signaling pathways regulate proinflammatory cytokines and apoptosis in human placental explants in response to oxidative stress: Effects of antioxidant vitamins. *American Journal of Pathology* 170 (5): 1511–1520.

Craven CM, Morgan T, and Ward K. 1998. Decidual spiral artery remodelling begins before cellular interaction with cytotrophoblasts. *Placenta* 19 (4): 241–252.

Desai DK, Moodley J, and Naidoo DP. 2004. Echocardiographic assessment of cardiovascular hemodynamics in normal pregnancy. *Obstetrics and Gynecology* 104 (1): 20–29.

Elad D, Levkovitz R, Jaffa AJ, Desoye G, and Hod M. 2014. Have we neglected the role of fetal endothelium in transplacental transport? *Traffic* 15 (1): 122–126.

Feneley MR and Burton GJ. 1991. Villous composition and membrane thickness in the human placenta at term: A stereological study using unbiased estimators and optimal fixation techniques. *Placenta* 12 (2): 131–142.

Fowden AL, Sferruzzi-Perri AN, Coan PM, Constancia M, and Burton GJ. 2009. Placental efficiency and adaptation: Endocrine regulation. *The Journal of Physiology* 587 (Pt 14): 3459–3472.

Fowden AL, Forhead AJ, Sferruzzi-Perri AN, Burton GJ, and Vaughan OR. 2015. Endocrine regulation of placental phenotype. *Placenta* 36 (Suppl. 1): S50–S59. doi: 10.1016/j.placenta.

Francis ST, Duncan KR, Moore RJ, Baker PN, Johnson IR, and Gowland PA. 1998. Non-invasive mapping of placental perfusion. *Lancet* 351 (9113): 1397–1399.

Friis CM, Qvigstad E, Paasche Roland MC, Godang K, Voldner N, Bollerslev J, and Henriksen T. 2013. Newborn body fat: Associations with maternal metabolic state and placental size. *PLoS One* 8 (2): e57467.

Godfrey KM, Gluckman PD, and Hanson MA. 2010. Developmental origins of metabolic disease: Life course and intergenerational perspectives. *Trends in Endocrinology & Metabolism* 21 (4): 199–205.

Hanson M and Gluckman P. 2011. Developmental origins of noncommunicable disease: Population and public health implications. *American Journal of Clinical Nutrition* 94 (6 Suppl): 1754S–1758S.

Hempstock J, Jauniaux E, Greenwold N, and Burton GJ. 2003. The contribution of placental oxidative stress to early pregnancy failure. *Human Pathology* 34 (12): 1265–1275.

Higgins L, Greenwood SL, Wareing M, Sibley CP, and Mills TA. 2011. Obesity and the placenta: A consideration of nutrient exchange mechanisms in relation to aberrant fetal growth. *Placenta* 32 (1): 1–7.

Higgins M, McAuliffe FM, and Mooney EE. 2011. Clinical associations with a placental diagnosis of delayed villous maturation: A retrospective study. *Pediatric and Developmental Pathology* 14 (4): 273–279.

Huppertz B. 2008. The anatomy of the normal placenta. *Journal of Clinical Pathology* 61 (12): 1296–1302.

Huppertz B and Peeters LL. 2005. Vascular biology in implantation and placentation. *Angiogenesis* 8 (2): 157–167.

Jansson N, Nilsfelt A, Gellerstedt M, Wennergren M, Rossander-Hulthen L, Powell TL, and Jansson T. 2008. Maternal hormones linking maternal body mass index and dietary intake to birth weight. *American Journal of Clinical Nutrition* 87 (6): 1743–1749.

Jauniaux E, Watson AL, Hempstock J, Bao YP, Skepper JN, and Burton GJ. 2000. Onset of maternal arterial blood flow and placental oxidative stress. A possible factor in human early pregnancy failure. *American Journal of Pathology* 157 (6): 2111–2122.

Jeve YB, Konje JC, and Doshani A. 2015. Placental dysfunction in obese women and antenatal surveillance strategies. *Best Practice & Research. Clinical Obstetrics & Gynaecology* 29 (3): 350–364.

Jirkovska M, Kubinova L, Janacek J, Moravcova M, Krejci V, and Karen P. 2002. Topological properties and spatial organization of villous capillaries in normal and diabetic placentas. *Journal of Vascular Research* 39 (3): 268–278.

Jones CJ and Fox H. 1991. Ultrastructure of the normal human placenta. *Electron Microscopy Reviews* 4 (1): 129–178.

Kaufmann P, Huppertz B, and Frank HG. 1996. The fibrinoids of the human placenta: Origin, composition and functional relevance. *Annals of Anatomy* 178 (6): 485–501.

Kingdom J, Huppertz B, Seaward G, and Kaufmann P. 2000. Development of the placental villous tree and its consequences for fetal growth. *European Journal of Obstetrics, Gynecology, and Reproductive Biology* 92 (1): 35–43.

Lager S and Powell TL. 2012. Regulation of nutrient transport across the placenta. *Journal of Pregnancy* 2012: 179827.

Lievano S, Alarcon L, Chavez-Munguia B, and Gonzalez-Mariscal L. 2006. Endothelia of term human placentae display diminished expression of tight junction proteins during preeclampsia. *Cell and Tissue Research* 324 (3): 433–448.

Lyall F, Bulmer JN, Duffie E, Cousins F, Theriault A, and Robson SC. 2001. Human trophoblast invasion and spiral artery transformation: The role of PECAM-1 in normal pregnancy, preeclampsia, and fetal growth restriction. *American Journal of Pathology* 158 (5): 1713–1721.

Lynge NL, Djurisic S, and Hviid TV. 2014. Controlling the immunological crosstalk during conception and pregnancy: HLA-G in reproduction. *Frontiers in immunology* 5: 198.

Mayhew TM. 2006. Allometric studies on growth and development of the human placenta: Growth of tissue compartments and diffusive conductances in relation to placental volume and fetal mass. *Journal of Anatomy* 208 (6): 785–794.

Mayhew TM. 2009. A stereological perspective on placental morphology in normal and complicated pregnancies. *Journal of Anatomy* 215 (1): 77–90.

Moffett A and Colucci F. 2014. Uterine NK cells: Active regulators at the maternal–fetal interface. *Journal of Clinical Investigation* 124 (5): 1872–1879.

Molteni RA, Stys SJ, and Battaglia FC. 1978. Relationship of fetal and placental weight in human beings: Fetal/placental weight ratios at various gestational ages and birth weight distributions. *Journal of Reproductive Medicine* 21 (5): 327–334.

Myatt L. 2010. Review: Reactive oxygen and nitrogen species and functional adaptation of the placenta. *Placenta* 31 Suppl: S66–S69.

Ouyang F, Parker M, Cerda S, Pearson C, Fu L, Gillman MW, Zuckerman B, and Wang X. 2013. Placental weight mediates the effects of prenatal factors on fetal growth: The extent differs by preterm status. *Obesity (Silver Spring)* 21 (3): 609–620.

Pijnenborg R, Vercruysse L, and Hanssens M. 2006. The uterine spiral arteries in human pregnancy: Facts and controversies. *Placenta* 27 (9–10): 939–958.

Red-Horse K, Zhou Y, Genbacev O, Prakobphol A, Foulk R, McMaster M, and Fisher SJ. 2004. Trophoblast differentiation during embryo implantation and formation of the maternal–fetal interface. *Journal of Clinical Investigation* 114 (6): 744–754.

Reshetnikova OS, Burton GJ, and Milovanov AP. 1994. Effects of hypobaric hypoxia on the fetoplacental unit: The morphometric diffusing capacity of the villous membrane at high altitude. *American Journal of Obstetrics and Gynecology* 171 (6): 1560–1565.

Roland MC, Friis CM, Godang K, Bollerslev J, Haugen G, and Henriksen T. 2014. Maternal factors associated with fetal growth and birthweight are independent determinants of placental weight and exhibit differential effects by fetal sex. *PLoS One* 9 (2): e87303.

Salafia CM, Zhang J, Miller RK, Charles AK, Shrout P, and Sun W. 2007. Placental growth patterns affect birth weight for given placental weight. *Birth Defects Research. Part A, Clinical and Molecular Teratology* 79 (4): 281–288.

Sandovici I, Hoelle K, Angiolini E, and Constancia M. 2012. Placental adaptations to the maternal–fetal environment: Implications for fetal growth and developmental programming. *Reproductive Biomedicine Online* 25 (1): 68–89.

Schuhmann R, Stoz F, and Maier M. 1986. [Histometric studies of placentones of the human placenta]. *Zeitschrift fur Geburtshilfe und Perinatologie* 190 (5): 196–203.

Siman CM, Sibley CP, Jones CJ, Turner MA, and Greenwood SL. 2001. The functional regeneration of syncytiotrophoblast in cultured explants of term placenta. *American Journal of Physiology. Regulatory, Integrative and Comparative Physiology* 280 (4): R1116–R1122.

Simister NE, Jacobowitz IE, Ahouse JC, and Story CM. 1997. New functions of the MHC class I-related Fc receptor, FcRn. *Biochemical Society Transactions* 25 (2): 481–486.

Teasdale F and Jean-Jacques G. 1985. Morphometric evaluation of the microvillous surface enlargement factor in the human placenta from mid-gestation to term. *Placenta* 6 (5): 375–381.

Tuuli MG, Longtine MS, and Nelson DM. 2011. Review: Oxygen and trophoblast biology—A source of controversy. *Placenta* 32 Suppl 2: S109–S118.

Zhang J, Chen Z, Smith GN, and Croy BA. 2011. Natural killer cell-triggered vascular transformation: Maternal care before birth? *Cellular & Molecular Immunology* 8 (1): 1–11.

Zhou Y, Fisher SJ, Janatpour M, Genbacev O, Dejana E, Wheelock M, and Damsky CH. 1997. Human cytotrophoblasts adopt a vascular phenotype as they differentiate. A strategy for successful endovascular invasion? *Journal of Clinical Investigation* 99 (9): 2139–2151.

2 Molecular Regulation of Human Extravillous Trophoblast Development

Jürgen Pollheimer and Martin Knöfler

CONTENTS

ABSTRACT

Development of the human placenta and its different trophoblasts subtypes plays an essential role in determining successful pregnancy outcome. These particular epithelial cells fulfill diverse functions such as adaption of the implanted blastocyst to the uterine environment, remodeling of maternal spiral arteries, and nutrition of the developing fetus. Failures in placentation and function of trophoblasts during early stages of gestation are associated with numerous pregnancy diseases such as miscarriage, preeclampsia, and intrauterine growth restriction, eventually affecting health in later life through fetal programming. However, sequential events and regulatory mechanisms controlling human trophoblast development are poorly understood. Because of ethical considerations, our knowledge is based largely on the histological analyses of early placental specimens obtained from pregnant women who underwent hysterectomy. Moreover, analyses of placental tissues from legal pregnancy terminations between the 6th and 12th weeks of gestation provided first insights into the putative role of regulatory signaling pathways controlling early trophoblast differentiation. In this chapter, we review our present knowledge about localization and the structure of different trophoblast subtypes arising during the first weeks of gestation. In particular, development of the extravillous trophoblast (EVT) lineage and its invasive subtypes, interacting with different maternal uterine cells, will be discussed. Furthermore, we describe genes and key regulatory mechanisms that could regulate the intrinsic differentiation program of EVT in the placental anchoring villus.

KEY WORDS

Human placenta, trophoblast development, extravillous trophoblast, trophoblast invasion, differentiation, key regulatory transcription factors, trophoblast signaling.

2.1 INTRODUCTION

2.1.1 SPECIFICATION OF HUMAN TROPHOBLAST LINEAGES

Anatomic description of placental material at early embryonic stages led to the identification of different trophoblast cell types arising during the first weeks of gestation (Hamilton and Boyd 1960). Shortly after implantation, stem cells of the trophectoderm, forming the outermost layer of the blastocyst, generate miscellaneous trophoblast subtypes, which give rise to the early placental structures. Around day 7 postimplantation, cell fusion of trophoectodermal stem cells creates the so-called primitive syncytium likely representing the earliest invasive cell type of human placentation (Figure 2.1). Around day 8, vacuoles appear in the expanding syncytial mass to form a system of lacunae. At later stages of pregnancy, the lacunae system develops into the intervillous space, which is (first) flooded with maternal blood around the 10th to 12th week of pregnancy, at a time when embryonic growth has a high demand for nutrients and oxygen. Apart from syncytial structures, the trophectodermal progenitors generate proliferative cell columns (CCs) consisting of mononuclear cytotrophoblasts (CTBs), which break through the primitive syncytium around days 12 to 15 after conception. These primary villi contact the underlying maternal decidua and, like the early multinuclear structures, eventually erode uterine blood vessels and glands. At this stage, proliferating CTBs at distal sites also expand laterally and thereby form the trophoblastic shell, which represents the outermost site of placenta encircling the embryo. The shell lacks maternal cell types and is thought to be critical for anchorage of the placenta to the maternal uterus and protection of the embryo from oxidative stressors. Moreover, it forms the basal plate of the placenta in conjunction with the decidua basalis, the uterine cell layer underneath the implantation site.

Thereafter, primary villi are transformed into secondary villi and tertiary villi upon formation of a mesenchymal villous core and subsequent vascularization, respectively. Briefly, placental branching morphogenesis, starting around day 14, involves migration of extraembryonic mesenchymal cells into the primary villi as well as expansion of the epithelial surface by continuous proliferation and cell fusion of villous cytotrophoblasts (vCTBs). The latter process generates the multinuclear syncytium, the interface between mother and fetus controlling nutrient transport and gas exchange. After day 20 postimplantation, vascularization of these secondary villi begins, at a time when the fetal allantois fuses with the chorionic plate. Subsequent formation of the placental vascular network involves growth of capillaries in length and diameter as well as angiogenesis. These events finally connect placental vessels with the vasculature of the fetus after the fourth week of pregnancy (Burton, Charnock-Jones, and Jauniaux 2009). Tertiary villi undergo dramatic developmental changes during gestation, resulting in various types of villi differing in structure and function. In terminal villi, the syncytial layer gets in close contact with the placental capillaries and decreases in thickness thereby facilitating oxygen and nutrient transport to the fetus (Jones and Fox 1991).

In early placental development, lateral cell fusion of mononuclear CTBs likely contributes to the formation of early placental structures such as the primitive syncytium or the cytotrophoblastic shell. However, during later gestation, multinuclear syncytiotrophoblasts (STBs) of floating villi are generated by asymmetrical cell division, differentiation, and fusion of vCTBs with the preexisting syncytium (Aplin 2010). STBs secrete different pregnancy-specific hormones such as chorionic gonadotropin, pregnancy-specific glycoprotein, and placental lactogen thereby adapting the maternal environment to pregnancy (Evain-Brion and Malassine 2003). Adhesion molecules, proteases, cell fusion proteins, and numerous growth factors are thought to control syncytialization (Huppertz and Borges 2008; Morrish, Dakour, and Li 1998).

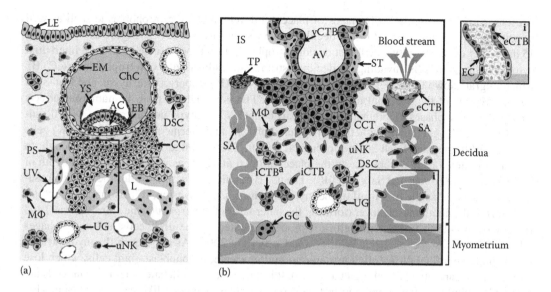

FIGURE 2.1 Early stages of human placental development. (a) Formation of the primitive syncytium and primary villi. Shortly after implantation, trophectodermal stem cells give rise to the primitive syncytium, in which the lacunae system is formed. Primary villi consisting of proliferating cytotrophoblast CCs break through the multinucleated structure and contact the underlying maternal decidua. Uterine glands and vessels are eroded by these early trophoblast subtypes. (b) Formation of differentiated trophoblasts. Tertiary villi are generated upon migration of extraembryonic mesodermal cells into the primary villi and subsequent vascularization. The two-layered epithelium of placental floating villi consists of underlying vCTB progenitors generating the syncytiotrophoblast by cell fusion. At the tips of anchoring villi, cytotrophoblasts detach from the columns and invade spiral arteries and the decidual stroma. During the first weeks of pregnancy, plugging of the spiral arteries by trophoblasts creates a hypoxic environment promoting placental and fetal development. Later on, iCTBs approach the spiral arteries from outside and eventually integrate into the vessel wall. Various uterine cell types such as macrophages, uterine NK cells, and decidual stromal cells interact with the iCTBs, thereby controlling time and depth of trophoblast invasion as well as artery remodeling. Eventually, iCTBs aggregate and form giant cells as the end stage of the invasive differentiation pathway. After the 10th week of pregnancy, dissolving of the plugs initiates blood flow into the intervillous space. Deep endovascular invasion of spiral arteries in the decidual layer and first third of the myometrium, replacement of maternal endothelial cells by trophoblasts, and disruption of the vessel wall represent typical features of the remodeling process. (i) Cross-section of a maternal vessel undergoing remodeling. eCTBs replace maternal endothelial cells. Intramural cytotrophoblasts reside in the vessel wall. iCTBs and maternal cell types such as uNK cells provoke degradation of the muscular wall. AC, amniotic cavity; AV, anchoring villus; CC, cell column; CCT, cell column trophoblast; ChC, chorionic cavity; CT, chorionic trophoblast; DSC, decidual stromal cell; EB, embryoblast; EC, endothelial cells; eCTB, endovascular cytotrophoblast; EM, extraembryonic mesoderm; GC, giant cell; iCTB, interstitial cytotrophoblast; iCTBa, interstitial cytotrophoblast aggregate; IS, intervillous space; L, lacunae; LUE, luminal uterine epithelium; MΦ, macrophage; PS, primitive syncytium; SA, spiral artery; ST, syncytiotrophoblast; TP, trophoblast plug; UG, uterine gland; uNK, uterine NK cell; UV, uterine vessel; vCTB, villous cytotrophoblast; YS, yolk sac.

2.1.2 Development of Extravillous Trophoblast (EVT)

The focus of this article is to specifically discuss function and development of extravillous trophoblasts (EVTs), representing placental cells that detach from anchoring villi and invade the maternal uterus and its vessels (Red-Horse et al. 2004). Transformation of the maternal endometrium into the decidua, the endometrium of pregnancy, is a prerequisite for successful formation and differentiation of EVTs. Decidualization involves changes in morphology and the secretory activity of stromal cells and glands as well as structural changes of the spiral arteries (Gellersen, Brosens, and

Brosens 2007). During the early stages of placental development, the trophoblastic shell as well as primary villi, both attached to the decidua, give rise to invasive EVTs (Figure 2.1b). Already 15 days after conception, two different decidual trophoblast subtypes can be identified: interstitial cytotrophoblasts (iCTBs) invading the decidual stroma and endovascular cytotrophoblasts (eCTB), which migrate down the lumen of maternal spiral arteries (Pijnenborg, Vercruysse, and Hanssens 2006). Invasion of the maternal uterine tissue by iCTBs is thought to provoke numerous effects during the early phases of pregnancy. This particular EVT subtype communicates with decidual stromal cells, glandular epithelial cells, macrophages, and uterine natural killer (uNK) cells (Bulmer, Williams, and Lash 2010; Moser et al. 2010). These cellular interactions are thought to regulate immunological acceptance of the placental/fetal allograft as well as timing and depth of iCTB invasion (Redman and Sargent 2010). The iCTB population deeply invades the decidua basalis reaching as far as the first third of the myometrium. During invasion, iCTBs induce apoptosis of the arterial smooth muscle layer (forming the outer layer of maternal uterine spiral arteries) and thereby contribute to vessel remodeling, a process initiated by the uNK cells and macrophages (Harris 2011; Robson et al. 2012; Whitley and Cartwright 2009). As they reach the myometrium, iCTBs undergo a final differentiation step into multinucleated trophoblast giant cells, which lose their invasive capacity (Pijnenborg et al. 1980). It is still a matter of debate whether giant cells are formed by cellular fusion or endoreplication. However, their formation likely represents a mechanism that may prevent deeper penetration into the uterine wall (Moffett-King 2002). Invasion of the maternal spiral arteries by eCTBs is critical for physiological adaptations during pregnancy and thus essential for successful fetal–placental development. Within the decidua and the first third of the myometrium, these vessels are subject to extensive remodeling, allowing for a precise control of blood flow to the intervillous space (Pijnenborg et al. 1981). Briefly, during the first weeks of pregnancy, eCTBs occlude the decidual arteries to prevent precocious onset of the maternal–placental circulation (Burton, Jauniaux, and Watson 1999; Pijnenborg, Vercruysse, and Hanssens 2006). It is thought that a premature rise in oxygen levels results in oxidative damage of the fetal–placental unit owing to the generation of reactive oxygen radicals. Indeed, disorganized early onset of blood flow and incomplete plugging of the maternal vessels are features of miscarried pregnancies (Hustin, Jauniaux, and Schaaps 1990; Khong, Liddell, and Robertson 1987). At the periphery, however, degeneration of the trophoblast layer in a hyperoxic environment could represent a mechanism for physiological regression of villi, resulting in the formation of the mature, discoidal structure of the placenta (Burton, Jauniaux, and Charnock-Jones 2010). In normal pregnancies, the utero-placental circulation is not established before 10th to 12th weeks of gestation (Burton, Jauniaux, and Charnock-Jones 2010). During this period, trophoblastic plugs dissolve and eCTBs further migrate down the lumen of the maternal spiral arteries and replace the endothelial cell lining. Moreover, elastolysis and degradation of the muscular vessel wall by iCTBs, uNK cells, and macrophages are key events of uterine artery remodeling (Harris 2011). These processes finally lead to the transformation of narrow vessels with relatively high resistance into highly dilated, low-resistance conduits (Brosens, Pijnenborg, and Brosens 2002). The establishment of a vascular connection between mother and fetus by the end of the first trimester marks the transition from histiotrophic to hemotrophic nutrition (Burton, Jauniaux, and Charnock-Jones 2010). In humans, the placenta is therefore referred to as hemochorial since placental villi are in direct contact with maternal blood, which has filled the intervillous space (Moffett and Loke 2006). Constant rates of low-pressure blood flow into the intervillous space ensure adequate transport of oxygen and nutrients to the growing embryo. In contrast, elevated blood pressure and vessel contractility could provoke hypoxia reoxygenation injuries of placental villi (Burton, Jauniaux, and Charnock-Jones 2010). As a consequence, the oxidatively stressed placenta may release various antiangiogenic factors, such as soluble Fms-like tyrosine kinase-1, soluble endoglin, and STB microparticles, that could injure the maternal endothelium (Redman, Sargent, and Staff 2014; Redman et al. 2012). Indeed, abnormal placentation and failures in spiral artery remodeling are characteristic signs of pathological pregnancies such as severe forms of fetal growth restriction, stillbirth, and preeclampsia, a hypertensive disorder of the mother (Pijnenborg et al. 1991; Pijnenborg, Vercruysse, and Hanssens 2006). Moreover, typical features of the latter condition are abnormal serum levels of vasoactive factors, elevated shedding of trophoblast microvesicles, acute atherosis, and an excessive maternal systemic inflammatory response (Redman and Sargent 2004; Redman, Sargent, and Staff 2014). Multiple factors are thought to contribute to the pathogenesis and subsequent clinical characteristics of these pregnancy diseases. Failures in the development, differentiation, and function of EVTs could represent an underlying cause (Whitley et al. 2007; Zhou, Damsky, and Fisher 1997; Zhou et al. 2013).

2.2 AUTOCRINE AND PARACRINE CONTROL OF HUMAN EVT

2.2.1 THE ROLE OF ENDOMETRIAL GLANDS

Because of the absence of maternal blood into the intervillous space during the first trimester, development of placenta and fetus depends on alternative sources such as nutrients and growth factors secreted from decidual glands (Burton, Jauniaux, and Charnock-Jones 2007). The identification of connections between these glands and the lacunae system through channels formed in the cytotrophoblastic shell enforce this assumption (Hamilton and Boyd 1960). Moreover, the histological appearance of the glands as well as peak serum levels of glycodelin A, one of their major products, at the end of the first trimester, suggest a high glandular secretory activity during the early phase of gestation (Burton et al. 2002; Seppala et al. 1988). Glycodelin A rapidly drops thereafter, at a time when the uteroplacental circulation starts. The identification of different secretory products, expressed in endometrial glands during the second half of the menstrual cycle (Bell 1988), led to the assumption that these proteins could also promote histiotrophic nutrition of the developing fetus during the early phase of pregnancy. In addition, other glycoproteins, such as uteroglobin and whey acidic protein, have been detected, which could feed the embryo and have additional immune-modulatory effects (Burton, Jauniaux, and Charnock-Jones 2007). Moreover, growth factors secreted by the glands, for example, epidermal growth factor (EGF), endocrine gland-derived vascular endothelial growth factor (EG-vEGF), and leukemia inhibitory factor, could have pivotal functions in trophoblast development and differentiation (Hempstock et al. 2004). Although the influence of these factors on early human trophoblast subtypes cannot be functionally tested, different experiments with trophoblast cultures from later stages of gestation supported their beneficial roles. Indeed, stimulation of first trimester villous explant cultures with EGF or EG-vEGF was shown to increase vCTB/CC trophoblast (CCT) proliferation and/or survival (Brouillet et al. 2013; Maruo et al. 1992). Hence, it can be assumed that these and other glandular products are critical for high rates of trophoblast growth and differentiation during early pregnancy, thereby promoting expansion of the syncytial area of floating placental villi (Burton, Jauniaux, and Charnock-Jones 2007). Similarly, proliferation of CCTs could also be induced by these factors, which might constantly feed the CCs to maintain their size and integrity, at a time when EVT formation, detachment, and invasion into the maternal uterine tissue take place.

2.2.2 DECIDUA- AND TROPHOBLAST-DERIVED FACTORS

Interactions of anchoring CC and (newly formed) iCTBs with decidual macrophages and uNK cells play a critical role in successful implantation and immunological acceptance of the fetal allograft. Key proteins involved in the latter process, such as human leukocyte antigen G (HLA-G) and HLA-C expressed by iCTBs, the role of different leukocyte populations, as well as genetic aspects of normal and failed implantation and miscarriage are discussed elsewhere (Erlebacher 2013; Hunt et al. 2005; Moffett and Colucci 2014). In addition, decidual cell-derived soluble proteins may also, besides their immune-modulatory properties, regulate growth and differentiation of villi anchored at the basal plate of the placenta. Indeed, decidual stromal cells, uNK cells, macrophages, and the developing trophoblast express a vast range of molecules such as prosta-glandins, growth factors, cytokines, chemokines, and angiogenic factors, which were shown to control trophoblast proliferation and/or motility in vitro (Knöfler 2010; Knöfler and Pollheimer 2012; Lala and Graham 1990; Pollheimer and Knöfler 2005). Different signaling cascades have been identified which are thought to regulate trophoblast function in an autocrine or paracrine manner (Knöfler 2010; Pollheimer and Knöfler 2005). For example, EGF, interleukin-1 (IL-1), insulin-like growth factor (IGF), and hepatocyte growth factor increased trophoblast invasion, whereas tumor necrosis factor, endostatin, IL-10, and transforming growth factor β (TGF-β) had inhibitory effects (Knöfler and Pollheimer 2012). Moreover, trophoblast-derived hormones such as human chorionic gonadotrophin and placental lactogen were also shown to promote tropho-blast migration and invasion (Lacroix et al. 2005; Prast et al. 2008). However, most studies using soluble proteins have been conducted in trophoblast cell lines and primary CTBs isolated from first-trimester placenta, the latter representing a mixture of vCTBs, CCTs, and EVTs. Therefore, differential effects by these secreted proteins on individual trophoblast subtypes remain largely elusive. Along those lines, only a few factors have been analyzed with respect to their specific effects on CCT proliferation by using first-trimester villous explants (Fock et al. 2013; Velicky et al. 2014). Spontaneous trophoblast outgrowth has been observed in these cultures upon seeding onto extracellular matrix (ECM) (Genbacev, Schubach, and Miller 1992). In principle, utiliza-tion of villous explant cultures allows discriminating between vCTB and CCT proliferation, but stimulation of cell migration can be hardly discerned from proliferative effects. Using this system EGF, IGF, and activin were shown to increase trophoblast outgrowth, whereas TGF-β2 showed inhibitory effects. Moreover, IL-33 expressed by decidual macrophages has recently been shown to increase CCT proliferation, suggesting a beneficial role of the particular IL in CC growth and development (Fock et al. 2013). On the other hand, tumor necrosis factor, released by the uter-ine macrophages, blocked detachment of EVTs from anchoring villi and cell invasion (Bauer et al. 2004; Renaud et al. 2005), indicating that balanced activation of these cells is necessary for successful placentation. Moreover, subsequent to the colonization of the primary villi by the extraembryonic mesoderm, factors present in the villous core could modulate CC formation and EVT differentiation. IGF-I, for example, expressed in the placental mesenchyme could control trophoblast proliferation and migration (Forbes et al. 2008; Lacey et al. 2002). In summary, the present literature suggests that the decidua produces a variety of factors stimulating or inhibit-ing CCT proliferation, detachment of distal CCTs from the column, and trophoblast migration. In vitro, many of the above-mentioned factors induce the secretion of ECM-degrading proteases from CTBs, such as matrix metalloproteinases and urokinase plasminogen activator, thereby pro-moting invasion into the uterine tissue (Knöfler and Pollheimer 2012; Lala and Graham 1990). In contrast, the respective inhibitory factors expressed by decidual cells, tissue inhibitors of metal-loproteinases and plasminogen activator inhibitors, might limit depth of trophoblast invasion (Knöfler and Pollheimer 2012; Lala and Graham 1990).

EVT differentiation is characterized by a time- and distance-dependent induction of marker genes such as HLA-G and specific integrins, the latter controlling adhesive properties and cell migration of iCTBs (Damsky et al. 1994; McMaster et al. 1995). However, regulators of integrin switching and EVT marker expression are largely unknown. It is likely that the intrinsic molecular features of EVTs and the contact of the CC with the decidual matrix are the main triggers of the invasive differentiation program of trophoblasts (see Section 2.3). In contrast, soluble decidual fac-tors might play a minor role.

2.2.3 REGULATION BY OXYGEN LEVELS

Because of the lack of maternal blood flow, trophoblast development during early pregnancy occurs in a hypoxic environment (Burton, Jauniaux, and Watson 1999). At this period of gestation, main-tenance of a trophoblast stem cell niche and massive CC proliferation are necessary for successful placentation. This has led to the assumption that hypoxia could be the main trigger of early trophoblast growth. Indeed, villous explant cultures cultivated under low oxygen conditions showed increased numbers of outgrowing villi and elevated proliferation (Genbacev et al. 1997). The effects on trophoblast growth under low oxygen conditions may be driven by hypoxia-inducible factor 1α (HIF1α)-induced expression of TGF-β3. The latter inhibits trophoblast differentiation toward the invasive phenotype (Caniggia et al. 2000). These data supported the view that increased oxygen levels after the 10th to 11th week of pregnancy could inhibit EVT differentiation, once blood flow to the intervillous space commences. However, data describing the function of TGF-β molecules or interpreting the role of hypoxia are controversial (James, Stone, and Chamley 2006; Prossler et al. 2014). HIF1α expression has been detected throughout pregnancy, and proliferation of CTBs occurs until term, although at lower rates (Mayhew and Barker 2001; Rajakumar and Conrad 2000). Moreover, there is evidence that hypoxia could also stimulate invasiveness, suggesting different functions depending on the period of gestation and the trophoblast subtype (James, Stone, and Chamley 2006). In addition, how a high-oxygen environment after the 20th week of pregnancy may contribute to the decline in trophoblast invasion remains elusive. Hence, the view that low oxygen promotes proliferation at the expense of EVT formation and invasion is maybe too simplistic. It is likely that in early pregnancy, low oxygen effectively stimulates proliferation to guarantee integrity and maintenance of CCs. Continuous formation of CCTs, in turn, leads to increased rates of EVT differentiation and invasion, both of which are induced by matrix contact and intrinsic cellular programs. Once the placenta switches to hemotrophic nutrition, rising oxygen concentrations might slow down proliferation of CCTs and, as a consequence, the formation of invasive EVTs. The decreasing secretory activity of glands after the first trimester of pregnancy could also contribute to this phenomenon (Burton, Jauniaux, and Charnock-Jones 2007).

2.3 KEY REGULATORS OF EVT DIFFERENTIATION

2.3.1 MARKER PROTEINS AND TRANSCRIPTIONAL REGULATORS

EVT differentiation requires the presence of the decidual ECM, which provokes detachment of trophoblasts from the tips of anchoring villi; generation of EVT subtypes, such as iCTBs and eCTBs; and migration into tissues and vessel. Differentiated EVTs invading the decidua lose their epithelial polarity, characterized by the loss of E-cadherin and integrin α6β4, and start to express critical marker genes, including HLA-G, specific proteases, for example, a disintegrin and metalloproteinase 12 (ADAM12), and adhesion molecules such as integrin α1β1 and integrin α5β1 (Biadasiewicz et al. 2014; Damsky et al. 1994; McMaster et al. 1995). Whereas HLA-G has immune-modulatory properties, proteases and adhesion molecules are thought to control trophoblast invasion and migration upon interaction with diverse decidual matrix proteins. For example, integrin α1β1 and integrin α5β1 comprise cellular receptors for collagen IV and fibronectin, respectively. Both matrix proteins are expressed by decidual stromal cells as well as by invasive trophoblasts (Aplin, Charlton, and Ayad 1988; Earl, Estlin, and Bulmer 1990; Oefner et al. 2015). In addition, eCTBs, involved in vessel remodeling, acquire a vascular adhesion phenotype, which could be abnormal in preeclampsia (Zhou, Damsky, and Fisher 1997). Moreover, primary CTBs isolated from preeclamptic placentae failed to induce the characteristic marker proteins being expressed during in vitro differentiation on ECM (Lim et al. 1997; Zhou et al. 2013). These data suggest that pathological changes in EVT development could contribute to the pathogenesis of the particular pregnancy disease.

However, our knowledge about critical steps controlling CC formation and EVT differentiation remains only scarce. Contact of the anchoring villus with the decidual matrix is likely important, but whether it is sufficient to promote formation of the different EVT subtypes remains unknown. Growth factors originating from glands and other decidual cell types could be partly involved. On the other hand, there is convincing evidence that EVT differentiation is controlled by an efficient intrinsic program, since the induction of the above-mentioned marker proteins occurs independently of the surrounding environment. Trophoblast implantation at ectopic sites, such as tubal pregnancies, displays normal differentiation, although the size of CCs might be increased (Goffin et al. 2003). Moreover, similar to the in vivo situation, purified primary CTBs as well as differentiating villous explant cultures induce EVT markers in a time- and/or distance-dependent manner (Damsky et al. 1994; Vicovac, Jones, and Aplin 1995). Expression of HLA-G, integrin α (ITGA) 1, ITGA, or ADAM12 in adherent placental explants occurs in the absence of serum, under high oxygen levels, and independently of the matrix conditions (Bauer et al. 2004; Vicovac, Jones, and Aplin 1995).

On the other hand, proteins expressed in the mesenchymal core of the villous, such as IGF-1, might control the proliferative capacity of CCs and induce migration and differentiation once the signaling activity decreases at distal sites. This concept might be strengthened by the fact that floating villous explant cultures, eventually forming trophoblast outgrowth in the absence of matrix, show expression of EVT markers at the tips of their CCs.

Considering the fact that access to placental material of early human pregnancy is limited, little is known about key regulatory transcription factors involved in EVT differentiation. Although many different transcriptional activators and repressors have been shown to control invasion of trophoblast cell lines and primary CTBs (Knöfler, Vasicek, and Schreiber 2001; Loregger, Pollheimer, and Knöfler 2003), their putative functions in column proliferation and EVT formation have been poorly investigated. Indeed, only few factors were satisfactorily analyzed in support of their role as regulators of the invasive differentiation process. For example, storkhead box-1 (STOX-1) and HIF-1α may promote CTB proliferation but inhibit trophoblast invasion (Caniggia et al. 2000; van Dijk and Oudejans 2011). In contrast, expression of glial cells missing 1 (GCM1), a critical regulator of branching morphogenesis and syncytialization in mouse and human, could abolish trophoblast growth but foster invasion (Baczyk et al. 2009). Therefore, the regulatory roles of these transcription factors might suggest that CC proliferation and EVT differentiation are mutually exclusive processes, an assumption that, however reasonable, has not been proven.

Most of our understanding regarding trophoblast formation and differentiation has been obtained from studies in animal models, particularly in mice. Different key regulatory transcription factors involved in early trophectoderm development, spongiotrophoblast formation, and giant cell differentiation have been identified (Cross et al. 2003; Rossant and Tam 2009). Based on the roles of these critical genes and the expression pattern of their counterparts in CCs and EVTs, analogous functions in human placentation were proposed. For example, key factors of early murine trophoblast lineage specification such as ELF5 and Cdx2 (Donnison et al. 2005; Strumpf et al. 2005) are also expressed in CCs of first trimester pregnancies but have not been functionally tested yet (Hemberger et al. 2010). Along those lines, the basic helix-loop-helix proteins Mash-2 and Hand1 were shown to control murine spongiotrophoblast maintenance and giant cell formation, respectively (Cross et al. 2003). Expression of Hand1 was also detectable in outer cells of early human blastocysts but was absent from trophoblasts of first-trimester placentae (Knöfler et al. 1998, 2002). These data suggest that the expression of some of the putative key regulators of human EVT differentiation may rapidly cease during the early phase of placentation.

2.3.2 DEVELOPMENTAL PATHWAYS

Despite considerable efforts, human trophoblast stem cells have not been successfully isolated and maintained in culture. To gain insights into the early steps of human trophoblast differentiation, model systems involving treatment of embryonic stem cells (hESCs) with morphogenetic proteins (BMPs) or the formation of hESC embryoid bodies have been developed (Golos, Giakoumopoulos, and Gerami-Naini 2013; James, Carter, and Chamley 2012). However, unexpected effects of BMP on different hESC clones, such as the induction of mesodermal genes, have been observed

(Bernardo et al. 2011). Moreover, since comparative studies are hampered by the fact that early human trophoblast populations cannot be isolated, it remains uncertain whether the BMP-induced hESCs represent useful equivalents of in vivo trophoblasts. Along those lines, characterization of CTB progenitors of first-trimester placental tissue and their potential to develop into the differentiated trophoblast subtypes remains poorly understood. Bipotential trophoblast precursors, capable of differentiating both into sncytiotrophoblast and EVT, as well as separate progenitors of the two lineages have been proposed (Baczyk et al. 2006; James, Stone, and Chamley 2005). Based on the observation that the primitive syncytium, CCT and EVT are formed during early pregnancy, a common stem cell/precursor of STB and invasive trophoblast can be assumed. However, it is not known whether and, if so, at which time during gestation these cells might get lost. It is likely that the number of putative trophoblast stem cells decreases after the first trimester of pregnancy, a process that may eventually be accompanied by the rise in oxygen levels and downregulation of the proliferative capacity of the placenta. Indeed, recent evidence suggested that expression of Cdx2 as well as of the stem cell marker Notch1 in CCTs rapidly declines after the first trimester (Haider et al. 2014; Hemberger et al. 2010; Hunkapiller et al. 2011).

Key regulatory pathways, such as Notch, Wingless (Wnt), Hippo, and EGF/EGFR, are known to control embryogenesis, cell lineage determination, and differentiation. Therefore, it is not surprising that these critical signaling cascades are also involved in trophoblast development and placentation. For example, knockout mice harboring homozygous deletions of different Wnt signaling components show abnormalities in different trophoblast layers (Knöfler and Pollheimer 2013). On the other hand, Hippo and Notch play a crucial role in early murine trophectoderm specification (Rayon et al. 2014). Similar to Wnt signaling, Notch also regulates various steps of placentation, such as branching morphogenesis, labyrinth formation/function, and chorion-allantoic fusion in mice (Cross et al. 2006; Gasperowicz and Otto 2008). Putative functions of these key pathways in human placental developmental are based largely on the expression pattern of their critical components in different trophoblast subtypes. EGFR, Notch1, Notch3, and Notch4 are restricted to proliferative CCTs (Haider et al. 2014; Hunkapiller et al. 2011; Jokhi, King, and Loke 1994), suggesting a role in trophoblast proliferation and/or maintenance of precursors in the CC (Figure 2.2). In contrast, Notch2, a regulator of murine endovascular invasion, and the Wnt-dependent transcription factors T-cell factor (TCF)-3 and TCF-4 are predominantly expressed in differentiated CCTs and EVTs (Hunkapiller et al. 2011; Plessl et al. 2015; Pollheimer et al. 2006), indicating a role in invasive differentiation and/or trophoblast migration (Figure 2.2). Again, few functional studies with primary cultures have been conducted to support a role of these developmental genes in EVT differentiation. Silencing of TCF-4 inhibited trophoblast migration and expression of EVT-specific genes, suggesting that activation of the canonical Wnt pathway could be part of the EVT differentiation program (Meinhardt et al. 2014). The latter shares similarities with a process called epithelial–mesenchymal transition (EMT), occurring during development and cancerogenesis (Moustakas and Heldin 2007). Differentiating CCTs downregulates epithelial proteins of tight (zonula occludens 1, occludin) and adherens junctions (E-cadherin) and induces characteristic EMT markers such as mesenchymal genes (fibroblast specific protein 1, fibronectin) and activators of EMT (TCF-4 and Snail) (Knöfler and Pollheimer 2013). Interestingly, inhibition of canonical Notch activity and silencing of its critical transcriptional regulator, recombination signal binding protein for immunoglobulin kappa J region, elevated not only CCT proliferation but also EVT marker expression (Haider et al. 2014; Velicky et al. 2014). Likewise, EGF treatment increased trophoblast proliferation as well as EVT differentiation (Prast et al. 2008; Wright et al. 2010). These recent data support the idea that growth factor stimulation and manipulation of critical developmental genes might stimulate progenitors in the CC to enhance their mitotic rates, thereby increasing the efficiency of EVT formation and differentiation. This hypothesis would contradict the view that CTB proliferation occurs at the expense of trophoblast differentiation and invasion.

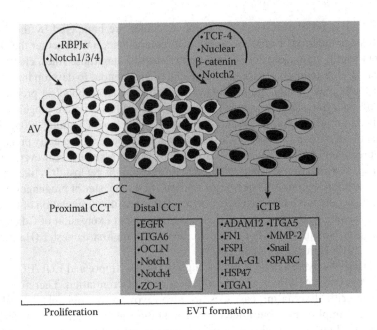

FIGURE 2.2 Schematic depiction of developmental signaling pathways involved in EVT differentiation. Proliferative CCT of the proximal cell column express RBPJκ and Notch1, 3, and 4 in vivo and in vitro. Whereas Notch1, 3, and 4 and the canonical Notch activity decrease during formation of distal CCTs/iCTBs, Notch2 increases. Along with the expression of HLA-G, ITGA1, and ITGA5, trophoblasts differentiating along the invasive pathway downregulate proteins involved in epithelial integrity (ZO-1, ITGA6, OCLN) and induce proteases (MMP-2, ADAM12) as well as regulators (Snail, TCF-4, nuclear β-catenin) and markers genes (SPARC, HSP47, FN1, FSP1) of EMT. Notch signaling in proximal CCTs could be required for balanced rates of proliferation and EVT differentiation. Activation of canonical Wnt signaling in EVTs promotes motility and controls expression of EVT markers and EMT-associated genes. ADAM12, a disintegrin and metalloproteinase 12; CCT, cell column trophoblast; EMT, epithelial-to-mesenchymal transition; FN1, fibronectin 1; FSP1, fibroblast-specific protein 1; HSP47, heat shock protein 47; iCTB, interstitial cytotrophoblast; integrin α, ITGA; MMP, matrix metalloproteinase; OCLN, occludin; SPARC, secreted protein acidic and rich in cysteine; TCF-4, T-cell factor 4; ZO-1, zonula occludens 1.

2.4 SUMMARY

In mice, different molecular mechanisms controlling development of trophectoderm and placenta have been identified. Hippo-dependent transcription enhancer domain protein 4 (TEAD4), the T-box transcription factor Eomes, and Cdx2 are expressed in outside cells at the morula stage, thereby determining trophoblast cell fate (Rossant and Tam 2009). Subsequently, numerous signaling molecules and key regulatory transcription factors control specification, maintenance, and differentiation of different trophoblast subtypes (Cross et al. 2003). In humans, limited availability of first-trimester placental material and the fact that very early stages of placentation cannot be functionally analyzed hamper our understanding of trophoblast lineage development and differentiation. Although different primary cells systems have been established, key regulatory transcription factors and signaling pathways remain poorly characterized. Despite considerable differences between mouse and human placentation, many of the critical regulators such as Cdx2, Elf5, or Hand1 are expressed at certain stages of EVT development, although their exact functions in trophoblast maintenance and differentiation have not been investigated. Similarly, the roles of developmental cascades such as Wnt and Notch and their critical transcriptional activators are only slowly emerging. Besides the need for a better understanding of the underlying network of transcriptional regulators, numerous other questions regarding EVT formation and differentiation have to be answered. For example, the influence of autocrine and paracrine factors on these processes and the precise role of oxygen and ECM proteins have to be unraveled. Establishment of human trophoblast stem cells and improvement of the current primary cell models should advance our knowledge about the formation and maintenance of CC progenitors and their differentiation into distinct EVT subtypes.

ACKNOWLEDGMENT

The present article is supported by funding of the Austrian Science Fund (grant P-22687-B13).

REFERENCES

Aplin, J. D. 2010. "Developmental cell biology of human villous trophoblast: Current research problems." *Int J Dev Biol* 54 (2–3):323–9. doi:10.1387/ijdb.082759ja.

Aplin, J. D., A. K. Charlton, and S. Ayad. 1988. "An immunohistochemical study of human endometrial extracellular matrix during the menstrual cycle and first trimester of pregnancy." *Cell Tissue Res* 253 (1):231–40.

Baczyk, D., C. Dunk, B. Huppertz, C. Maxwell, F. Reister, D. Giannoulias, and J. C. Kingdom. 2006. "Bi-potential behaviour of cytotrophoblasts in first trimester chorionic villi." *Placenta* 27 (4–5):367–74. doi:10.1016/j.placenta.2005.03.006.

Baczyk, D., S. Drewlo, L. Proctor, C. Dunk, S. Lye, and J. Kingdom. 2009. "Glial cell missing-1 transcription factor is required for the differentiation of the human trophoblast." *Cell Death Differ* 16 (5):719–27. doi:10.1038/cdd.2009.1.

Bauer, S., J. Pollheimer, J. Hartmann, P. Husslein, J. D. Aplin, and M. Knöfler. 2004. "Tumor necrosis factor-alpha inhibits trophoblast migration through elevation of plasminogen activator inhibitor-1 in first-trimester villous explant cultures." *J Clin Endocrinol Metab* 89 (2):812–22. doi:10.1210/jc.2003-031351.

Bell, S. C. 1988. "Secretory endometrial/decidual proteins and their function in early pregnancy." *J Reprod Fertil Suppl* 36:109–25.

Bernardo, A. S., T. Faial, L. Gardner, K. K. Niakan, D. Ortmann, C. E. Senner, E. M. Callery, M. W. Trotter, M. Hemberger, J. C. Smith, L. Bardwell, A. Moffett, and R. A. Pedersen. 2011. "BRACHYURY and CDX2 mediate BMP-induced differentiation of human and mouse pluripotent stem cells into embryonic and extraembryonic lineages." *Cell Stem Cell* 9 (2):144–55. doi:10.1016/j.stem.2011.06.015.

Biadasiewicz, K., V. Fock, S. Dekan, K. Proestling, P. Velicky, S. Haider, M. Knöfler, C. Frohlich, and J. Pollheimer. 2014. "Extravillous trophoblast-associated ADAM12 exerts pro-invasive properties, including induction of integrin beta 1-mediated cellular spreading." *Biol Reprod* 90 (5):101. doi:10.1095/biolreprod.113.115279.

Brosens, J. J., R. Pijnenborg, and I. A. Brosens. 2002. "The myometrial junctional zone spiral arteries in normal and abnormal pregnancies: A review of the literature." *Am J Obstet Gynecol* 187 (5):1416–23.

Brouillet, S., P. Murthi, P. Hoffmann, A. Salomon, F. Sergent, P. De Mazancourt, M. Dakouane-Giudicelli, M. N. Dieudonne, P. Rozenberg, D. Vaiman, S. Barbaux, M. Benharouga, J. J. Feige, and N. Alfaidy. 2013. "EG-VEGF controls placental growth and survival in normal and pathological pregnancies: Case of fetal growth restriction (FGR)." *Cell Mol Life Sci* 70 (3):511–25. doi:10.1007/s00018-012-1141-z.

Bulmer, J. N., P. J. Williams, and G. E. Lash. 2010. "Immune cells in the placental bed." *Int J Dev Biol* 54 (2–3):281–94. doi:10.1387/ijdb.082763jb.

Burton, G. J., E. Jauniaux, and A. L. Watson. 1999. "Maternal arterial connections to the placental intervillous space during the first trimester of human pregnancy: The Boyd collection revisited." *Am J Obstet Gynecol* 181 (3):718–24.

Burton, G. J., A. L. Watson, J. Hempstock, J. N. Skepper, and E. Jauniaux. 2002. "Uterine glands provide histiotrophic nutrition for the human fetus during the first trimester of pregnancy." *J Clin Endocrinol Metab* 87 (6):2954–9. doi:10.1210/jcem.87.6.8563.

Burton, G. J., E. Jauniaux, and D. S. Charnock-Jones. 2007. "Human early placental development: Potential roles of the endometrial glands." *Placenta* 28 Suppl A:S64–9.

Burton, G. J., D. S. Charnock-Jones, and E. Jauniaux. 2009. "Regulation of vascular growth and function in the human placenta." *Reproduction* 138 (6):895–902. doi:10.1530/REP-09-0092.

Burton, G. J., E. Jauniaux, and D. S. Charnock-Jones. 2010. "The influence of the intrauterine environment on human placental development." *Int J Dev Biol* 54 (2–3):303–12. doi:10.1387/ijdb.082764gb.

Caniggia, I., H. Mostachfi, J. Winter, M. Gassmann, S. J. Lye, M. Kuliszewski, and M. Post. 2000. "Hypoxia-inducible factor-1 mediates the biological effects of oxygen on human trophoblast differentiation through TGFbeta(3)." *J Clin Invest* 105 (5):577–87. doi:10.1172/JCI8316.

Cross, J. C., D. Baczyk, N. Dobric, M. Hemberger, M. Hughes, D. G. Simmons, H. Yamamoto, and J. C. Kingdom. 2003. "Genes, development and evolution of the placenta." *Placenta* 24 (2–3):123–30.

Cross, J. C., H. Nakano, D. R. Natale, D. G. Simmons, and E. D. Watson. 2006. "Branching morphogenesis during development of placental villi." *Differentiation* 74 (7):393–401. doi:10.1111/j.1432-0436.2006.00103.x.

Damsky, C. H., C. Librach, K. H. Lim, M. L. Fitzgerald, M. T. McMaster, M. Janatpour, Y. Zhou, S. K. Logan, and S. J. Fisher. 1994. "Integrin switching regulates normal trophoblast invasion." *Development* 120 (12):3657–66.

Donnison, M., A. Beaton, H. W. Davey, R. Broadhurst, P. L'Huillier, and P. L. Pfeffer. 2005. "Loss of the extraembryonic ectoderm in Elf5 mutants leads to defects in embryonic patterning." *Development* 132 (10):2299–308. doi:10.1242/dev.01819.

Earl, U., C. Estlin, and J. N. Bulmer. 1990. "Fibronectin and laminin in the early human placenta." *Placenta* 11 (3):223–31.

Erlebacher, A. 2013. "Immunology of the maternal-fetal interface." *Annu Rev Immunol* 31:387–411. doi:10.1146/annurev-immunol-032712-100003.

Evain-Brion, D. and A. Malassine. 2003. "Human placenta as an endocrine organ." *Growth Horm IGF Res* 13 Suppl A:S34–7.

Fock, V., M. Mairhofer, G. R. Otti, U. Hiden, A. Spittler, H. Zeisler, C. Fiala, M. Knöfler, and J. Pollheimer. 2013. "Macrophage-derived IL-33 is a critical factor for placental growth." *J Immunol* 191 (7):3734–43. doi:10.4049/jimmunol.1300490.

Forbes, K., M. Westwood, P. N. Baker, and J. D. Aplin. 2008. "Insulin-like growth factor I and II regulate the life cycle of trophoblast in the developing human placenta." *Am J Physiol Cell Physiol* 294 (6): C1313–22. doi:10.1152/ajpcell.00035.2008.

Gasperowicz, M., and F. Otto. 2008. "The notch signalling pathway in the development of the mouse placenta." *Placenta* 29 (8):651–9.

Gellersen, B., I. A. Brosens, and J. J. Brosens. 2007. "Decidualization of the human endometrium: Mechanisms, functions, and clinical perspectives." *Semin Reprod Med* 25 (6):445–53. doi:10.1055/s-2007-991042.

Genbacev, O., S. A. Schubach, and R. K. Miller. 1992. "Villous culture of first trimester human placenta—Model to study extravillous trophoblast (EVT) differentiation." *Placenta* 13 (5):439–61.

Genbacev, O., Y. Zhou, J. W. Ludlow, and S. J. Fisher. 1997. "Regulation of human placental development by oxygen tension." *Science* 277 (5332):1669–72.

Goffin, F., C. Munaut, A. Malassine, D. Evain-Brion, F. Frankenne, V. Fridman, M. Dubois, S. Uzan, P. Merviel, and J. M. Foidart. 2003. "Evidence of a limited contribution of feto–maternal interactions to trophoblast differentiation along the invasive pathway." *Tissue Antigens* 62 (2):104–16.

Golos, T. G., M. Giakoumopoulos, and B. Gerami-Naini. 2013. "Review: Trophoblast differentiation from human embryonic stem cells." *Placenta* 34 Suppl:S56–61. doi:10.1016/j.placenta.2012.11.019.

Haider, S., G. Meinhardt, P. Velicky, G. R. Otti, G. Whitley, C. Fiala, J. Pollheimer, and M. Knöfler. 2014. "Notch signaling plays a critical role in motility and differentiation of human first-trimester cytotropho-blasts." *Endocrinology* 155 (1):263–74. doi:10.1210/en.2013-1455.

Hamilton, W. J., and J. D. Boyd. 1960. "Development of the human placenta in the first three months of gestation." *J Anat* 94:297–328.

Harris, L. K. 2011. "IFPA Gabor Than Award lecture: Transformation of the spiral arteries in human pregnancy: Key events in the remodelling timeline." *Placenta* 32 Suppl 2:S154–8. doi:10.1016/j.placenta.2010.11.018.

Hemberger, M., R. Udayashankar, P. Tesar, H. Moore, and G. J. Burton. 2010. "ELF5-enforced transcriptional networks define an epigenetically regulated trophoblast stem cell compartment in the human placenta." *Hum Mol Genet* 19 (12):2456–67. doi:10.1093/hmg/ddq128.

Hempstock, J., T. Cindrova-Davies, E. Jauniaux, and G. J. Burton. 2004. "Endometrial glands as a source of nutrients, growth factors and cytokines during the first trimester of human pregnancy: A morphological and immunohistochemical study." *Reprod Biol Endocrinol* 2:58. doi:10.1186/1477-7827-2-58.

Hunkapiller, N. M., M. Gasperowicz, M. Kapidzic, V. Plaks, E. Maltepe, J. Kitajewski, J. C. Cross, and S. J. Fisher. 2011. "A role for Notch signaling in trophoblast endovascular invasion and in the pathogenesis of pre-eclampsia." *Development* 138 (14):2987–98. doi:10.1242/dev.066589.

Hunt, J. S., M. G. Petroff, R. H. McIntire, and C. Ober. 2005. "HLA-G and immune tolerance in pregnancy." *FASEB J* 19 (7):681–93. doi:10.1096/fj.04-2078rev.

Huppertz, B., and M. Borges. 2008. "Placenta trophoblast fusion." *Methods Mol Biol* 475:135–47. doi:10.1007/978-1-59745-250-2_8.

Hustin, J., E. Jauniaux, and J. P. Schaaps. 1990. "Histological study of the materno-embryonic interface in spontaneous abortion." *Placenta* 11 (6):477–86.

James, J. L., P. R. Stone, and L. W. Chamley. 2005. "Cytotrophoblast differentiation in the first trimester of pregnancy: Evidence for separate progenitors of extravillous trophoblasts and syncytiotrophoblast." *Reproduction* 130 (1):95–103. doi:10.1530/rep.1.00723.

James, J. L., P. R. Stone, and L. W. Chamley. 2006. "The regulation of trophoblast differentiation by oxygen in the first trimester of pregnancy." *Hum Reprod Update* 12 (2):137–44. doi:10.1093/humupd/dmi043.

James, J. L., A. M. Carter, and L. W. Chamley. 2012. "Human placentation from nidation to 5 weeks of gestation. Part II: Tools to model the crucial first days." *Placenta* 33 (5):335–42. doi:10.1016/j.placenta.2012.01.019.

Jokhi, P. P., A. King, and Y. W. Loke. 1994. "Reciprocal expression of epidermal growth factor receptor (EGF-R) and c-erbB2 by non-invasive and invasive human trophoblast populations." *Cytokine* 6 (4):433–42.

Jones, C. J., and H. Fox. 1991. "Ultrastructure of the normal human placenta." *Electron Microsc Rev* 4 (1):129–78.

Khong, T. Y., H. S. Liddell, and W. B. Robertson. 1987. "Defective haemochorial placentation as a cause of miscarriage: A preliminary study." *Br J Obstet Gynaecol* 94 (7):649–55.

Knöfler, M. 2010. "Critical growth factors and signalling pathways controlling human trophoblast invasion." *Int J Dev Biol* 54 (2–3):269–80. doi:10.1387/ijdb.082769mk.

Knöfler, M., and J. Pollheimer. 2012. "IFPA Award in Placentology lecture: Molecular regulation of human trophoblast invasion." *Placenta* 33 Suppl:S55–62. doi:10.1016/j.placenta.2011.09.019.

Knöfler, M., and J. Pollheimer. 2013. "Human placental trophoblast invasion and differentiation: A particular focus on Wnt signaling." *Front Genet* 4:190. doi:10.3389/fgene.2013.00190.

Knöfler, M., G. Meinhardt, R. Vasicek, P. Husslein, and C. Egarter. 1998. "Molecular cloning of the human Hand1 gene/cDNA and its tissue-restricted expression in cytotrophoblastic cells and heart." *Gene* 224 (1–2):77–86.

Knöfler, M., R. Vasicek, and M. Schreiber. 2001. "Key regulatory transcription factors involved in placental trophoblast development—A review." *Placenta* 22 Suppl A:S83–92. doi:10.1053/plac.2001.0648.

Knöfler, M., G. Meinhardt, S. Bauer, T. Loregger, R. Vasicek, D. J. Bloor, S. J. Kimber, and P. Husslein. 2002. "Human Hand1 basic helix-loop-helix (bHLH) protein: Extra-embryonic expression pattern, interaction partners and identification of its transcriptional repressor domains." *Biochem J* 361 (Pt 3):641–51.

Lacey, H., T. Haigh, M. Westwood, and J. D. Aplin. 2002. "Mesenchymally-derived insulin-like growth factor 1 provides a paracrine stimulus for trophoblast migration." *BMC Dev Biol* 2:5.

Lacroix, M. C., J. Guibourdenche, T. Fournier, I. Laurendeau, A. Igout, V. Goffin, J. Pantel, V. Tsatsaris, and D. Evain-Brion. 2005. "Stimulation of human trophoblast invasion by placental growth hormone." *Endocrinology* 146 (5):2434–44. doi:10.1210/en.2004-1550.

Lala, P. K., and C. H. Graham. 1990. "Mechanisms of trophoblast invasiveness and their control: The role of proteases and protease inhibitors." *Cancer Metastasis Rev* 9 (4):369–79.

Lim, K. H., Y. Zhou, M. Janatpour, M. McMaster, K. Bass, S. H. Chun, and S. J. Fisher. 1997. "Human cytotrophoblast differentiation/invasion is abnormal in pre-eclampsia." *Am J Pathol* 151 (6):1809–18.

Loregger, T., J. Pollheimer, and M. Knöfler. 2003. "Regulatory transcription factors controlling function and differentiation of human trophoblast—A review." *Placenta* 24 Suppl A:S104–10.

Maruo, T., H. Matsuo, K. Murata, and M. Mochizuki. 1992. "Gestational age-dependent dual action of epidermal growth factor on human placenta early in gestation." *J Clin Endocrinol Metab* 75 (5):1362–7. doi:10.1210/jcem.75.5.1430098.

Mayhew, T. M., and B. L. Barker. 2001. "Villous trophoblast: Morphometric perspectives on growth, differentiation, turnover and deposition of fibrin-type fibrinoid during gestation." *Placenta* 22 (7):628–38. doi:10.1053/plac.2001.0700.

McMaster, M. T., C. L. Librach, Y. Zhou, K. H. Lim, M. J. Janatpour, R. DeMars, S. Kovats, C. Damsky, and S. J. Fisher. 1995. "Human placental HLA-G expression is restricted to differentiated cytotrophoblasts." *J Immunol* 154 (8):3771–8.

Meinhardt, G., S. Haider, P. Haslinger, K. Proestling, C. Fiala, J. Pollheimer, and M. Knöfler. 2014. "Wnt-dependent T-cell factor-4 controls human etravillous trophoblast motility." *Endocrinology* 155 (5):1908–20. doi:10.1210/en.2013-2042.

Moffett, A., and C. Loke. 2006. "Immunology of placentation in eutherian mammals." *Nat Rev Immunol* 6 (8):584–94. doi:10.1038/nri1897.

Moffett, A., and F. Colucci. 2014. "Uterine NK cells: Active regulators at the maternal–fetal interface." *J Clin Invest* 124 (5):1872–9. doi:10.1172/JCI68107.

Moffett-King, A. 2002. "Natural killer cells and pregnancy." *Nat Rev Immunol* 2 (9):656–63. doi:10.1038/nri886.

Morrish, D. W., J. Dakour, and H. Li. 1998. "Functional regulation of human trophoblast differentiation." *J Reprod Immunol* 39 (1–2):179–95.

Moser, G., M. Gauster, K. Orendi, A. Glasner, R. Theuerkauf, and B. Huppertz. 2010. "Endoglandular trophoblast, an alternative route of trophoblast invasion? Analysis with novel confrontation co-culture models." *Hum Reprod* 25 (5):1127–36. doi:10.1093/humrep/deq035.

Moustakas, A., and C. H. Heldin. 2007. "Signaling networks guiding epithelial–mesenchymal transitions during embryogenesis and cancer progression." *Cancer Sci* 98 (10):1512–20. doi:10.1111/j.1349-7006 .2007.00550.x.

Oefner, C. M., A. Sharkey, L. Gardner, H. Critchley, M. Oyen, and A. Moffett. 2015. "Collagen type IV at the fetal–maternal interface." *Placenta* 36 (1):59–68. doi:10.1016/j.placenta.2014.10.012.

Pijnenborg, R., G. Dixon, W. B. Robertson, and I. Brosens. 1980. "Trophoblastic invasion of human decidua from 8 to 18 weeks of pregnancy." *Placenta* 1 (1):3–19.

Pijnenborg, R., J. M. Bland, W. B. Robertson, G. Dixon, and I. Brosens. 1981. "The pattern of interstitial trophoblastic invasion of the myometrium in early human pregnancy." *Placenta* 2 (4):303–16.

Pijnenborg, R., J. Anthony, D. A. Davey, A. Rees, A. Tiltman, L. Vercruysse, and A. van Assche. 1991. "Placental bed spiral arteries in the hypertensive disorders of pregnancy." *Br J Obstet Gynaecol* 98 (7):648–55.

Pijnenborg, R., L. Vercruysse, and M. Hanssens. 2006. "The uterine spiral arteries in human pregnancy: Facts and controversies." *Placenta* 27 (9–10):939–58. doi:10.1016/j.placenta.2005.12.006.

Pollheimer, J., and M. Knöfler. 2005. "Signalling pathways regulating the invasive differentiation of human trophoblasts: A review." *Placenta* 26 Suppl A:S21–30. doi:10.1016/j.placenta.2004.11.013.

Pollheimer, J., T. Loregger, S. Sonderegger, L. Saleh, S. Bauer, M. Bilban, K. Czerwenka, P. Husslein, and M. Knöfler. 2006. "Activation of the canonical wingless/T-cell factor signaling pathway promotes invasive differentiation of human trophoblast." *Am J Pathol* 168 (4):1134–47.

Prast, J., L. Saleh, H. Husslein, S. Sonderegger, H. Helmer, and M. Knöfler. 2008. "Human chorionic gonadotropin stimulates trophoblast invasion through extracellularly regulated kinase and AKT signaling." *Endocrinology* 149 (3):979–87. doi:10.1210/en.2007-1282.

Plessl, K., S. Haider, C. Fiala, J. Pollheimer, and M. Knöfler. 2015. Expression pattern and function of Notch2 in different subtypes of first trimester cytotrophoblast. *Placenta* 36 (4):365–371. doi:10.1016/j .placenta.2015.01.009.

Prossler, J., Q. Chen, L. Chamley, and J. L. James. 2014. "The relationship between TGFbeta, low oxygen and the outgrowth of extravillous trophoblasts from anchoring villi during the first trimester of pregnancy." *Cytokine* 68 (1):9–15. doi:10.1016/j.cyto.2014.03.001.

Rajakumar, A., and K. P. Conrad. 2000. "Expression, ontogeny, and regulation of hypoxia-inducible transcription factors in the human placenta." *Biol Reprod* 63 (2):559–69.

Rayon, T., S. Menchero, A. Nieto, P. Xenopoulos, M. Crespo, K. Cockburn, S. Canon, H. Sasaki, A. K. Hadjantonakis, J. L. de la Pompa, J. Rossant, and M. Manzanares. 2014. "Notch and hippo converge on Cdx2 to specify the trophectoderm lineage in the mouse blastocyst." *Dev Cell* 30 (4):410–22. doi:10.1016 /j.devcel.2014.06.019.

Red-Horse, K., Y. Zhou, O. Genbacev, A. Prakobphol, R. Foulk, M. McMaster, and S. J. Fisher. 2004. "Trophoblast differentiation during embryo implantation and formation of the maternal–fetal interface." *J Clin Invest* 114 (6):744–54. doi:10.1172/JCI22991.

Redman, C. W., and I. L. Sargent. 2004. "Preeclampsia and the systemic inflammatory response." *Semin Nephrol* 24 (6):565–70.

Redman, C. W., and I. L. Sargent. 2010. "Immunology of pre-eclampsia." *Am J Reprod Immunol* 63 (6):534–43. doi:10.1111/j.1600-0897.2010.00831.x.

Redman, C. W., D. S. Tannetta, R. A. Dragovic, C. Gardiner, J. H. Southcombe, G. P. Collett, and I. L. Sargent. 2012. "Review: Does size matter? Placental debris and the pathophysiology of pre-eclampsia." *Placenta* 33 Suppl:S48–54. doi:10.1016/j.placenta.2011.12.006.

Redman, C. W., I. L. Sargent, and A. C. Staff. 2014. "IFPA Senior Award Lecture: Making sense of pre-eclampsia—Two placental causes of preeclampsia?" *Placenta* 35 Suppl:S20–5. doi:10.1016/j .placenta.2013.12.008.

Renaud, S. J., L. M. Postovit, S. K. Macdonald-Goodfellow, G. T. McDonald, J. D. Caldwell, and C. H. Graham. 2005. "Activated macrophages inhibit human cytotrophoblast invasiveness in vitro." *Biol Reprod* 73 (2):237–43. doi:10.1095/biolreprod.104.038000.

Robson, A., L. K. Harris, B. A. Innes, G. E. Lash, M. M. Aljunaidy, J. D. Aplin, P. N. Baker, S. C. Robson, and J. N. Bulmer. 2012. "Uterine natural killer cells initiate spiral artery remodeling in human pregnancy." *FASEB J* 26 (12):4876–85. doi:10.1096/fj.12-210310.

Rossant, J., and P. P. Tam. 2009. "Blastocyst lineage formation, early embryonic asymmetries and axis patterning in the mouse." *Development* 136 (5):701–13. doi:10.1242/dev.017178.

Seppala, M., L. Riittinen, M. Julkunen, R. Koistinen, T. Wahlstrom, K. Iino, H. Alfthan, U. H. Stenman, and M. L. Huhtala. 1988. "Structural studies, localization in tissue and clinical aspects of human endometrial proteins." *J Reprod Fertil Suppl* 36:127–41.

Strumpf, D., C. A. Mao, Y. Yamanaka, A. Ralston, K. Chawengsaksophak, F. Beck, and J. Rossant. 2005. "Cdx2 is required for correct cell fate specification and differentiation of trophectoderm in the mouse blastocyst." *Development* 132 (9):2093–102. doi:10.1242/dev.01801.

van Dijk, M., and C. B. Oudejans. 2011. "STOX1: Key player in trophoblast dysfunction underlying early onset preeclampsia with growth retardation." *J Pregnancy* 2011:521826. doi:10.1155/2011/521826.

Velicky, P., S. Haider, G. R. Otti, C. Fiala, J. Pollheimer, and M. Knöfler. 2014. "Notch-dependent RBPJkappa inhibits proliferation of human cytotrophoblasts and their differentiation into extravillous trophoblasts." *Mol Hum Reprod* 20 (8):756–66. doi:10.1093/molehr/gau038.

Vicovac, L., C. J. Jones, and J. D. Aplin. 1995. "Trophoblast differentiation during formation of anchoring villi in a model of the early human placenta in vitro." *Placenta* 16 (1):41–56.

Whitley, G. S., and J. E. Cartwright. 2009. "Trophoblast-mediated spiral artery remodelling: A role for apoptosis." *J Anat* 215 (1):21–6. doi:10.1111/j.1469-7580.2008.01039.x.

Whitley, G. S., P. R. Dash, L. J. Ayling, F. Prefumo, B. Thilaganathan, and J. E. Cartwright. 2007. "Increased apoptosis in first trimester extravillous trophoblasts from pregnancies at higher risk of developing preeclampsia." *Am J Pathol* 170 (6):1903–9. doi:10.2353/ajpath.2007.070006.

Wright, J. K., C. E. Dunk, H. Amsalem, C. Maxwell, S. Keating, and S. J. Lye. 2010. "HER1 signaling mediates extravillous trophoblast differentiation in humans." *Biol Reprod* 83 (6):1036–45. doi:10.1095/biolreprod.109.083246.

Zhou, Y., C. H. Damsky, and S. J. Fisher. 1997. "Preeclampsia is associated with failure of human cytotrophoblasts to mimic a vascular adhesion phenotype. One cause of defective endovascular invasion in this syndrome?" *J Clin Invest* 99 (9):2152–64. doi:10.1172/JCI119388.

Zhou, Y., M. J. Gormley, N. M. Hunkapiller, M. Kapidzic, Y. Stolyarov, V. Feng, M. Nishida, P. M. Drake, K. Bianco, F. Wang, M. T. McMaster, and S. J. Fisher. 2013. "Reversal of gene dysregulation in cultured cytotrophoblasts reveals possible causes of preeclampsia." *J Clin Invest* 123 (7):2862–72. doi:10.1172/JCI66966.

3 Epigenetics and the Placenta
Impact of Maternal Nutrition

Leslie Myatt and Kohzoh Mitsuya

CONTENTS

ABSTRACT

The placenta has a central role not only in determining immediate pregnancy outcomes but also in mediating the process of fetal programming and subsequent development of disease later in life. Adverse maternal conditions, including level and type of nutrition, affect placental function and directly or indirectly program the fetus via epigenetic modifications in the placenta and fetus. Epigenetic modifications include histone methylation and acetylation, which, in turn, may facilitate differential DNA methylation and alter gene expression. The sexual dimorphism seen in epigenetic changes in placenta may underlie the different responses of male and female fetuses to the intrauterine environment. The zygote uniquely undergoes global demethylation early in gestation and is then remethylated, but the trophectoderm, which forms the placenta, is remethylated to a level below that of somatic tissues. The level and composition of nutrients and metabolic health (obesity, diabetes) can effect epigenetic changes in many organs. Currently, there is little direct evidence for nutrients affecting placental epigenetics; however, abundant data show altered epigenetics with adverse pregnancy outcomes, including diabetes, undernutrition and overnutrition, preeclampsia, and intrauterine growth restriction (IUGR). The mechanisms linking nutrition and epigenetic changes are slowly being revealed, including those between cellular metabolism and methylation–demethylation via the regulation of ten-eleven translocation enzymes by α-ketoglutarate, a product of the citric acid cycle. As the supply of methyl donors by the one-carbon cycle can regulate DNA methylation, manipulation of methyl donors may epigenetically alter fetal metabolic phenotype.

Other bioactive food compounds such as genistein, polyphenols, tea catechin, resveratrol, butyrate, and curcumin may also regulate enzymes involved in epigenesis.

KEY WORDS

Epigenetics, placenta, DNA methylation, histone methylation, histone acetylation, ten-eleven translocation, α-ketoglutarate.

3.1   INTRODUCTION: ROLE OF THE PLACENTA IN PREGNANCY OUTCOME AND FETAL PROGRAMMING

Pregnancy complications and adverse outcomes including stillbirth, preeclampsia, growth restriction, macrosomia, obesity, pregestational and gestational diabetes, and preterm and postterm birth affect a large proportion of the 211 million pregnancies worldwide each year. We have previously highlighted (Myatt 2006) that the placenta is recognized to be involved in most, if not all, of these complications and the associated adverse outcomes via its roles at the maternal–fetal interface, by regulating vascular supply and transport of nutrients, and as the "director" of pregnancy secreting peptide and steroid hormones that regulate maternal metabolism and fetal growth and development. In addition, adverse intrauterine environments lead to programming of the offspring for subsequent development of obesity, diabetes, cardiovascular disease, and neurodevelopmental and behavioral disorders (Chu et al. 2007; Frias et al. 2011; Rogers and Velten 2011; Yogev and Catalano 2009). At term, the placenta can be collected and serve as a diary of fetal exposure to adverse environments, including the level and type of nutrients and pollutants (Boekelheide et al. 2012), which may then be used to predict the development of disease in childhood and adult life in the offspring. While inappropriate placental developmental processes are involved in the etiology of pregnancy complications, placental function may also be affected as a consequence of a pregnancy condition, e.g., nutrition, pregestational and gestational diabetes, the oxidative stress of preeclampsia, or the abnormal metabolic milieu of obesity. Many investigators are seeking the mechanisms that link the adverse intrauterine environments of obesity, diabetes, preeclampsia, and other medical conditions to altered placental function and fetal programming (Myatt and Roberts 2006) to prevent the intergenerational transmission of disease.

3.2   INTERACTION OF GENES AND ENVIRONMENTAL FACTORS: EPIGENETICS

Epigenetics is the study of *heritable* changes in gene expression that are not mediated by DNA sequence alterations (Bird 2002) and are susceptible to environmental influences (Petronis 2001). Epigenetic information is conveyed in mammals via a synergistic interaction between mitotically heritable patterns of DNA methylation (Jones and Takai 2001) and chromatin structure (Rakyan et al. 2001). Local chromatin conformation regulates specific methylation patterns to control gene transcription (Cedar and Bergman 2009). An increasing number of diverse factors are known to epigenetically regulate genes, including age, lifestyle, inflammation, gender, genotype, stress, nutrition, metabolism, drugs, and infection, factors that are all involved in adverse pregnancy outcomes.

3.2.1   EPIGENETIC MECHANISMS

1. Histone modification

    Gene expression can be altered via posttranslational covalent modifications of chromatin by histone methylation or acetylation (Figure 3.1). This determines accessibility to transcription factors (Weinmann et al. 2001) leading to transcriptionally repressive or permissive chromatin structures (Kimura, Liebhaber, and Cooke 2004). Histone acetylation usually marks active genes as does dimethylation or trimethylation of lysine residue

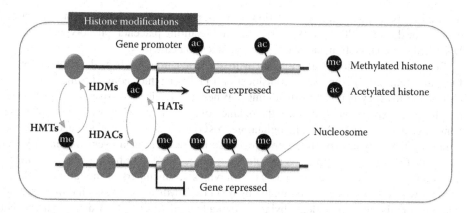

FIGURE 3.1 Chromatin-modifying enzymes involved in (a) histone and (b) DNA modifications. DNA demethylation process involves TET-mediated active or passive replication-dependent dilution mechanism. HMTs, histone methyltransferases; HDMs, histone demethylases; HATs, histone acetyltransferases; HDACs, histone deacetylases.

four of histone H3 (H3K4me2, K4me3), whereas H3K9me2/3 and H3K27me3 constitute repressive marks (Peterson and Laniel 2004; Sims and Reinberg 2006) implicated in guiding DNA methylation to specific chromatin regions (reviewed in Denis, Ndlovu, and Fuks 2011). Repressive histone modifications seem to confer short-term, flexible silencing important for developmental plasticity, whereas DNA methylation is believed to be a more stable, long-term silencing mechanism (Boyer et al. 2006; Reik 2007).

2. DNA methylation

DNA methylation is a well-studied modification (Figure 3.2), which involves the addition of methyl groups to the cytosine residues present in a Cytosine-phosphate-Guanine (CpG) dinucleotide (Jones and Takai 2001). CpG dinucleotides occur at low abundance throughout the eukaryotic genomes and tend to concentrate in CpG islands found in the promoter regions of genes. Hypermethylation of DNA in promoter regions typically is associated with transcriptional repression of genes, whereas hypomethylation leads to gene activity (Feinberg and Tycko 2004). Most tissue-specific differential methylation in normal tissue and cancer-specific single-copy differential methylation occurs at CpG island shores or shelves outside CpG islands (Heyn and Esteller 2012). Therefore, the entirety of DNA methylation across the genome needs to be considered. DNA methylation in the placenta

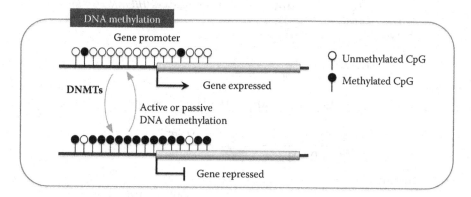

FIGURE 3.2 Chromatin-modifying enzymes involved in (a) histone and (b) DNA modifications. DNA demethylation process involves TET-mediated active or passive replication-dependent dilution mechanism. DNMTs, DNA methyltransferases.

has mainly been investigated in relation to transcription of imprinted and nonimprinted genes (Fowden et al. 2006; Reik et al. 2003) and resulting placental phenotype.

3. DNA hydroxymethylation and ten-eleven translocation enzymes

Recently, a novel modification, DNA hydroxymethylation, has been described (Branco, Ficz, and Reik 2012). Ten-eleven translocation (TET) enzymes convert 5-methylcytosine (5mC) to 5-hydroxymethylcytosine (5hmC). Whereas 5mC is repressive, 5hmC is permissive for gene expression. Therefore, the balance of 5mC to 5hmC at particular CpGs may control gene expression. Alpha ketoglutarate (αKG) (Iyer et al. 2009), produced from isocitrate by the enzyme isocitrate dehydrogenase in the citric acid cycle (Figure 3.3) and ascorbate (Minor et al. 2013), acts as cofactors, suggesting a link between cellular metabolism and epigenetic regulation. The TET enzymes are members of the family of dioxygenases whose activity can be regulated by αKG or 2-hydroxy glutarate and include JmjC domain containing histone demethylases (Tsukada et al. 2006), RNA demethylases (Niu et al. 2013), and prolyl hydroxylases (Epstein et al. 2001) that regulate hypoxia-inducible factor-1α degradation. Hence, αKG may mediate several aspects of epigenome.

4. DNA methyltransferase

In mammalian genomes, DNA methyltransferase (DNMT) enzymes mediate the transfer of methyl groups from S-adenosylmethionine to cytosine (Goll and Bestor 2005), establish and maintain DNA methylation patterns at specific regions of the genome, and contribute to gene regulation. Of the three active DNMTs, DNMT1 is primarily a maintenance methyltransferase preserving methylation patterns during cell division, while DNMT3 enzymes are responsible for de novo methylation. The catalytic activity of DNMT3A and DNMT3B is influenced by sequences next to target CG sites, suggesting sequence preference in human genomic methylation patterns (Handa and Jeltsch 2005). DNMTs apparently can read histone modifications, leading to their recruitment to nucleosomes carrying specific marks. There is a strong correlation between DNA methylation and histone H3K4 methylation in embryonic stem and somatic cells (Hodges et al. 2009). In neural stem cells, most DNMT3A is excluded from active chromatin marked by H3K4 trimethylation (H3K4me3)

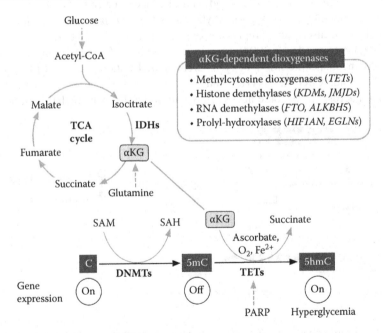

FIGURE 3.3 Relationship of cellular metabolism to the epigenome. αKG, alpha-ketoglutarate; DNMTs, DNA methyltransferases.

(Wu et al. 2010) and DNMT3A is located in gene bodies and intergenic regions, which is consistent with the observation that DNA methylation levels are high in gene bodies of actively transcribed genes (Laurent et al. 2010).

3.3 EPIGENETICS, IMPRINTED GENES, AND PLACENTAL DEVELOPMENT

3.3.1 Imprinted Genes and Placental Development

Genomic imprinting is a reiterative epigenetic process whereby a gene or genomic domain is biochemically marked differently depending on its parental origin. Whereas the vast majority of human genes in a diploid cell are expressed equally from both parental chromosomes, imprinted genes are expressed exclusively or preferentially on one of the two parental chromosomes but are repressed on the other (Reik and Walter 2001). To date, approximately 120 imprinted genes (less than 0.5% of the genome) have been described as being either paternally or maternally expressed and are found in humans and mice (for a complete list, see http://igc.otago.ac.nz/home.html or http://www.mousebook.org/mousebook-catalogs/imprinting-resource). It has long been established that genomic imprinting plays a critical role in fetoplacental development before birth and has biological and clinical implications. Most imprinted genes are expressed in both placenta and embryo, with a subset of imprinted genes being expressed predominantly in the placenta, and some genes more widely expressed but imprinted selectively in the placenta and not in the embryo (Coan, Burton, and Ferguson-Smith 2005; Monk et al. 2009). The gene ontology of imprinted genes indicates direct involvement in regulating the ability of placenta to support embryonic development and to transfer nutrients (Constancia, Kelsey, and Reik 2004). Among vertebrates, genomic imprinting is well described specifically in therian mammals (Cleaton, Edwards, and Ferguson-Smith 2014), where the allocation of maternal resources continues throughout embryonic development, indicating that imprinting arose at the time of evolution of lactation and placentation. In line with this, mouse models highlight that the most common functions of imprinted genes involve the regulation of placentation, embryonic growth, and energy homeostasis (Cleaton, Edwards, and Ferguson-Smith 2014). Indeed, the original historical perspectives on genomic imprinting revealed a unique link between imprinting and fetoplacental development (Barton, Surani, and Norris 1984). A series of pronuclear transplantation experiments performed in the 1980s were among the first to demonstrate that embryos with two paternal genomes (androgenotes) had poorly developed embryonic components but better developed extraembryonic tissues, whereas embryos with two maternal genomes (gynogenotes or parthogenotes) showed better embryonic development, although they were growth retarded with a failure of the extraembryonic lineages, which give rise to the placenta. In accordance with Haig's parental conflict theory (Moore and Haig 1991), paternally expressed genes generally increase resource transfer from the mother to the fetus, while maternally expressed genes limit this transfer in the womb to ensure the maternal well-being (Reik et al. 2003). There is evidence that the maternal and paternal metabolic environments, e.g., associated with famine (Tobi et al. 2009) or obesity (Soubry et al. 2013), can alter methylation of imprinted genes and also that methylation of imprinted genes such as insulin-like growth factor 2 at birth is associated with the development of metabolic disorders (Perkins et al. 2012), clearly showing a link between nutritional state and methylation of genes. This fits within the wider context of a potential role of imprinted genes for sensing environmental exposures, including nutritional status and toxic chemicals (Lambertini 2014). Recently, imprinted genes in mouse placenta have been shown to be susceptible to reduced methylation in association with caloric restriction (Chen et al. 2013).

3.3.2 DNA Demethylation in Early Development and Hypomethylation in Placenta

Epigenetic modifications contribute to the long-term maintenance of cellular phenotype or identity and are thereby generally stable in somatic cells, enabling fine control of gene expression. In early embryos, however, genome-wide reprogramming occurs with two opposing waves of DNA demethylation and subsequent de novo methylation. In mice, shortly after fertilization, global loss of DNA methylation takes place in the highly methylated genomes of mature sperm and oocyte. This genome-scale demethylation is then followed by de novo methylation occurring around the time of blastocyst implantation, but to a larger extent in the embryo than in the outer extraembryonic layer, which gives rise to the placenta (Rossant et al. 1986). This finding of DNA hypomethylation in the placenta has been confirmed by recent high-throughput sequencing studies, indicating that the placenta is globally demethylated with a methylation level of 40%–50% relative to that of somatic tissues (70%–85%) derived from the blastocyst in mice (Lee, Hore, and Reik 2014). There are also limited data available in humans suggesting a general DNA hypomethylation in the placenta (Fuke et al. 2004; Gama-Sosa et al. 1983). While the physiological significance of DNA hypomethylation in the placenta remains unknown, genome-scale epigenetic reprogramming in the early embryo is involved in acquisition of pluripotency or totipotency, transcriptional silencing of transposons (or mobile elements), and epigenetic inheritance across generations. Notably, many different genes that are transcribed at high levels specifically in the human placenta appear to originate from ancient transposable elements (Rawn and Cross 2008). For instance, the syncytin-1 gene, which encodes the endogenous retroviral envelope protein, is expressed primarily in placental villi and is involved in fusion of cytotrophoblast cells to form the syncytial surface of the placenta.

3.4   EVIDENCE FOR A ROLE FOR EPIGENETIC MODIFICATIONS IN THE PLACENTA AND WITH COMPLICATED PREGNANCIES

Histone modifying enzymes are involved in selective activation of placental-specific genes. The expression of the human transcription factor glial cell missing transcription factor a (GCMa), which regulates syncytin and trophoblast fusion, is regulated by histone deacetylase and histone acetlytransferases (HAT) (Chuang et al. 2006). The transcriptional activation of the placental-specific and pituitary-specific *hGH* genes is differentially regulated with roles for HAT and histone methyltransferase (HMT) coactivator complexes in each of these tissues (Kimura, Liebhaber, and Cooke 2004). There is evidence of differential histone modification occurring in a gender-specific manner (Strakovsky et al. 2014; Welstead et al. 2012), but overall, there are relatively little data (Nelissen et al. 2011) on histone modification in the human placenta per se and even less with pregnancy complications.

Global DNA methylation in the placenta increases with advancing gestational age (Chavan-Gautam et al. 2011; Novakovic et al. 2011), but with greater interindividual variation in the third trimester, suggesting that environmental influences may influence methylation, gene expression, and function of the placenta. Several recent publications (Koukoura, Sifakis, and Spandidos 2012) show variations in DNA methylation profiles in the term placenta in relation to pregnancy outcome. Methylation of specific gene loci was found to be predictive of IUGR and small-for-gestational-age (Banister et al. 2011), and an association between methylation of the glucocorticoid receptor and large-for-gestational-age infants has been described (Filiberto et al. 2011). Hypomethylation of CpGs at putative binding sites for hypoxia and inflammatory response elements and increased transcription of the *SERPINA3* gene has been found in placentas of IUGR and preeclamptic pregnancies (Chelbi et al. 2007). An association between *WNT2* promoter methylation and low-birth-weight percentile has been described, with a significant association being found between high promoter methylation and reduced gene expression (Ferreira et al. 2011). Epigenome-wide approaches have shown altered gene methylation in the placenta with preeclampsia (Yuen et al. 2009).

Administration of a single dose of 5′-aza-2′-deoxycytidine (a DNA methylation inhibitor) to pregnant rats at different stages of development disrupts trophoblast proliferation (Vlahovic et al. 1999), and in human choriocarcinoma-derived cell lines, 5′-aza-2′-deoxycytidine disrupts trophoblast migration (Rahnama et al. 2006). Furthermore, knockout mice studies of Dnmt1 and Dnmt3L have shown that the placentas of homozygous mice exhibit multiple morphological defects, like chorioallantoic fusion defects and lack of labyrinth formation (Bourc'his et al. 2001; Li, Bestor, and Jaenisch 1992).

3.5 EVIDENCE FOR THE INFLUENCE OF NUTRITION OR THE METABOLIC ENVIRONMENT ON EPIGENETIC MODIFICATIONS

There is now a large amount of evidence that not only can the diet alter DNA methylation and, hence, gene expression but also that individual nutrients or components of the diet can achieve this (reviewed in Choi and Friso 2010). During in utero development, the fetus and placenta respond and adapt continuously to changes in the maternal metabolic environment involving nutrients and metabolites, hormones, immune, or inflammatory mediators. Tight regulation of epigenetic changes is essential especially in the early phase of gestation, where global DNA demethylation in the zygote is seen but may subsequently be influenced by the maternal metabolic environment. Chromatin-modifying enzymes including DNMTs can sense and respond to alterations to the nutritional environment through their effects on intermediary metabolites (Gut and Verdin 2013). Differences in DNA methylation have been reported in individuals exposed to famine during the Dutch Hunger Winter (Heijmans et al. 2009; Tobi et al. 2009), showing that nutritional exposures in utero can induce epigenetic changes in offspring. In later life, the epigenome appears to be capable of responding to changes in nutrients, including deficiencies in methyl donors (Waterland et al. 2006), folic acid supplementation (Keyes et al. 2007), fat (Hoile et al. 2013), and caloric restriction (Hass et al. 1993). There are as yet little data on the effects of nutrients on DNA methylation in placenta; however, the dramatic changes in methylation seen in early gestation and the relative hypomethylation of the placenta suggest it to be susceptible to dietary influences. For example, ethanol-exposed mouse placentas and embryos are growth restricted with DNA methylation at the H19 imprinting control region (Haycock and Ramsay 2009), and long interspersed nuclear element 1 (LINE-1) methylation is related to maternal alcohol use in humans (Wilhelm-Benartzi et al. 2012). Recently, intrauterine caloric restriction in mice, which programs male offspring for glucose intolerance, increased fat mass, and hypercholesterolemia, has been shown to give a significant decrease in overall methylation throughout the placental genome (Chen et al. 2013). The level of demethylation was greater in placentas of male versus female mice and imprinted genes appeared to be more susceptible to methylation changes.

3.5.1 ONE-CARBON METABOLISM AND EPIGENETIC PROGRAMMING

DNA and histone methylation is coupled with a cellular cyclic pathway termed *one-carbon metabolism* in which folate, vitamin B12, methionine, choline, and betaine play essential roles (Scott and Weir 1998). In this cyclic pathway, *S*-adenosyl-methionine (SAM) is used as a methyl donor cofactor of DNA and HMTs (Figure 3.4). These methyltransferases transfer a methyl group from SAM to a substrate target such as DNA or histone macromolecules. Multiple experimental models in rodents have shown that methyl donor supplements can influence the degree of DNA methylation of specific genes during pregnancy (Waterland and Jirtle 2003) and can, to a certain extent, prevent a metabolic phenotype in the offspring induced by maternal dietary protein restriction (Lillycrop et al. 2005). Another product of one-carbon metabolism, *S*-adenosylhomocysteine, is a product inhibitor of methyltransferases. Whether these micronutrients confer relevant effects on the human epigenome remains unclear, but it is noted that the human genome encodes 208 methyltransferases, including 70 HMTs and four DNMTs (Petrossian and Clarke 2011). More recently, one-carbon metabolism has been reported to be essential for maintaining stem cell pluripotency and to modulate the levels of histone methylation (Shyh-Chang et al. 2013).

Biotin, niacin, and pantothenic acid, which are also water-soluble B vitamins, may have a role in epigenetic regulation as they are involved in histone modification (Kirkland 2009). Further, the activity of DNMTs and histone acetyltransferrases can be altered by bioactive food components

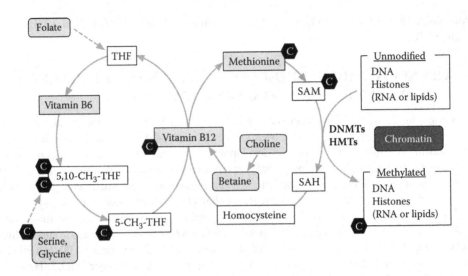

FIGURE 3.4 Effects of one-carbon metabolism on epigenetic modifications of the genome. DNMTs, DNA methyltransferases; HMTs, histone methyltransferases; SAM, S-adenosyl-L-methionine; SAH, S-adenosyl-L-homocysteine; THF, tetrahydrofolate; 5-CH₃-THF, 5-methyl-tetrahydrofolate; 5,10-CH₃-THF, 5,10-methylenetetrahydrofolate.

including genistein, polyphenols, tea catechin, resveratrol, butyrate, and curcumin (reviewed in Bacalini et al. 2014; Choi and Friso 2010). Thus, nutrients can influence epigenetics, including in the placenta, at several levels.

3.5.2 OBESITY AND DIABETES

In primates (Aagaard-Tillery et al. 2008) and rats (Strakovsky et al. 2011), consumption of a maternal high-fat diet gave altered histone modifications accompanied by altered expression of fetal hepatic genes. In primary aortic endothelial cells, 24-hour exposure to high glucose caused significant alterations in DNA methylation within 5kb of transcription start sites (Pirola et al. 2011). This was accompanied by broad changes in H3K9.K14 acetylation, which correlated well with DNA hypomethylation and gene induction. Indeed, variations in DNA methylation are correlated with many aspects of diabetes mellitus, including susceptibility (Ling et al. 2008), insulin resistance (Zhao et al. 2012), development of complications (Sapienza et al. 2011), and early detection (Akirav et al. 2011). Using a zebrafish model, Dhliwayo et al. (2014) showed that hyperglycemia induces poly(ADP-ribose) polymerase (Parp) enzymes, which in turn stimulate TET enzymes, leading to DNA demethylation and, in the zebrafish, persistent diabetes complications. This pathway could be blocked by Parp inhibition and suggests a central role for TET in hyperglycemia-induced demethylation and the transmission of diabetes.

In placentas of women exposed to gestational diabetes mellitus (GDM), Bouchard et al. found decreased DNA methylation of leptin and adiponectin genes with increasing blood glucose levels (Bouchard et al. 2012, 2010) and a correlation of leptin gene expression with its DNA methylation. A candidate gene approach studying metabolic programming found decreased methylation of the maternally imprinted gene *MEST*, which is essential for fetal and placental growth in placentas from GDM (El Hajj et al. 2013).

There is evidence that the metabolic/inflammatory milieu of obesity alters DNMT as expression of DNMT3a is increased in the adipose tissue of obese mice (Kamei et al. 2010) and correlates with gene suppression. In transgenic mice overexpressing DNMT3a, increased DNA methylation of the SFRP1 gene promoter was seen, accompanied by decreased gene expression (Kamei et al. 2010), suggesting that increased expression of DNMT3a in adipose tissue might be involved in obesity-related adipose tissue inflammation. A significant, positive correlation between serum tumor necrosis factor-α and pancreatic tissue levels of DNMTs was seen in rats with induced type 2 diabetes (El-Hadidy, Mohamed, and Mannaa 2014). However, there are little data available on DNMTs in human placenta.

3.6 SEXUAL DIMORPHISM, DEVELOPMENTAL PROGRAMMING, AND THE PLACENTA

Male and female fetuses respond differently to the adverse intrauterine environment, which may then relate to their risk of developing disease in adult life. Male fetuses show greater incidences of preterm birth, preterm premature rupture of membranes, placenta previa, lagging lung development, macrosomia with maternal glucose intolerance, and later stillbirths associated with pregestational diabetes (Eriksson et al. 2010), whereas the female neonate can more readily adapt to an adverse environment before delivery (Stark, Wright, and Clifton 2009). Sood et al. (2006) showed differential gene expression, especially of immune genes between male and female placentas, and a recent bioinformatics analysis from 11 microarray datasets showed that >140 genes were differentially expressed between male and female placentae (Buckberry et al. 2014). Of particular interest, higher female expression of genes involved in placental development, maintenance of pregnancy, and maternal immune tolerance of the conceptus were found. As previously mentioned, there is evidence of differential histone modification occurring in a gender-specific manner (Gagnidze et al. 2013; Strakovsky et al. 2014; Welstead et al. 2012), and maternal caloric restriction-induced decreased methylation in placenta was greater in the male than in the female fetus (Chen et al. 2013). Further, a sexual dimorphism in changes in gene expression in response to maternal inflammatory status (Clifton 2005; Osei-Kumah et al. 2011) or change in maternal diet (Mao et al. 2010) has been described. In an oligonucleotide microarray study, Radaelli et al. (2003) found significant alterations in the expression of genes related to inflammatory response, lipid metabolism, and extracellular matrix in the placenta with GDM. Overall, these data suggest that all epigenetic investigations of the placenta consider sexual dimorphism.

3.7 SUMMARY

In its position between mother and fetus, the placenta has a central role in both determining the immediate outcomes of pregnancy and in mediating the process of fetal programming and subsequent development of disease later in life in the offspring. Any adverse maternal condition, including level and quality of nutrition, will affect placental function and directly or indirectly program the fetus. Epigenetic modifications made in response to maternal condition will determine placental and fetal phenotype. These modifications can occur at several levels, including histone methylation and acetylation, which in turn can facilitate differential DNA methylation and alter gene expression (Figure 3.5). Importantly, sexual dimorphism has also been shown in epigenetic changes in placenta, which probably underlie the different responses of male and female placentas and fetuses to the intrauterine environment. Evidence is accruing that the level and composition of nutrients and metabolic health (obesity, diabetes) can effect epigenetic changes in many organs. Currently, there is little direct evidence for nutrients affecting epigenetics in the placenta; however, there are burgeoning data showing altered epigenetics with situations associated with adverse pregnancy outcomes, including diabetes, undernutrition and overnutrition, preeclampsia, and IUGR. The mechanisms underlying the link between nutrition and epigenetic changes are slowly being revealed, including that between cellular metabolism and methylation–demethylation via the regulation of TET enzymes by α-ketoglutarate, a product of the citric acid cycle (Figure 3.5). The one-carbon cycle is a major regulator of DNA methylation by supplying methyl donors, and manipulation of methyl donors is under investigation to epigenetically alter fetal metabolic phenotype. Given their intimate interaction as the fetoplacental unit, the regulation of the placental

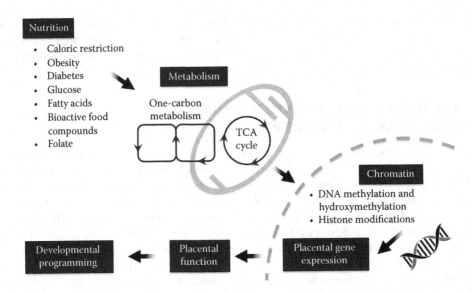

FIGURE 3.5 Maternal nutritional environment can influence the placental epigenome and thus affect placental function.

epigenome is crucial to determination of both placental and fetal phentotype and development of disease in later life.

REFERENCES

Aagaard-Tillery, K. M., K. Grove, J. Bishop, X. Ke, Q. Fu, R. McKnight, and R. H. Lane. 2008. "Developmental origins of disease and determinants of chromatin structure: Maternal diet modifies the primate fetal epigenome." *J Mol Endocrinol* 41 (2):91–102. doi:10.1677/JME-08-0025.

Akirav, E. M., J. Lebastchi, E. M. Galvan, O. Henegariu, M. Akirav, V. Ablamunits, P. M. Lizardi, and K. C. Herold. 2011. "Detection of beta cell death in diabetes using differentially methylated circulating DNA." *Proc Natl Acad Sci U S A* 108 (47):19018–23. doi:10.1073/pnas.1111008108.

Bacalini, M. G., S. Friso, F. Olivieri, C. Pirazzini, C. Giuliani, M. Capri, A. Santoro, C. Franceschi, and P. Garagnani. 2014. "Present and future of anti-ageing epigenetic diets." *Mech Ageing Dev* 136–137:101–15. doi:10.1016/j.mad.2013.12.006.

Banister, C. E., D. C. Koestler, M. A. Maccani, J. F. Padbury, E. A. Houseman, and C. J. Marsit. 2011. "Infant growth restriction is associated with distinct patterns of DNA methylation in human placentas." *Epigenetics* 6 (7):920–7. doi:10.4161/epi.6.7.16079.

Barton, S. C., M. A. Surani, and M. L. Norris. 1984. "Role of paternal and maternal genomes in mouse development." *Nature* 311 (5984):374–6.

Bird, A. 2002. "DNA methylation patterns and epigenetic memory." *Genes Dev* 16 (1):6–21. doi:10.1101/gad .947102.

Boekelheide, K., B. Blumberg, R. E. Chapin, I. Cote, J. H. Graziano, A. Janesick, R. Lane, K. Lillycrop, L. Myatt, J. C. States, K. A. Thayer, M. P. Waalkes, and J. M. Rogers. 2012. "Predicting later-life outcomes of early-life exposures." *Environ Health Perspect* 120 (10):1353–61. doi:10.1289/ehp.1204934.

Bouchard, L., M. F. Hivert, S. P. Guay, J. St-Pierre, P. Perron, and D. Brisson. 2012. "Placental adiponectin gene DNA methylation levels are associated with mothers' blood glucose concentration." *Diabetes* 61 (5):1272–80. doi:10.2337/db11-1160.

Bouchard, L., S. Thibault, S. P. Guay, M. Santure, A. Monpetit, J. St-Pierre, P. Perron, and D. Brisson. 2010. "Leptin gene epigenetic adaptation to impaired glucose metabolism during pregnancy." *Diabetes Care* 33 (11):2436–41. doi:10.2337/dc10-1024.

Bourc'his, D., G. L. Xu, C. S. Lin, B. Bollman, and T. H. Bestor. 2001. "Dnmt3L and the establishment of maternal genomic imprints." *Science* 294 (5551):2536–9. doi:10.1126/science.1065848.

Boyer, L. A., K. Plath, J. Zeitlinger, T. Brambrink, L. A. Medeiros, T. I. Lee, S. S. Levine, M. Wernig, A. Tajonar, M. K. Ray, G. W. Bell, A. P. Otte, M. Vidal, D. K. Gifford, R. A. Young, and R. Jaenisch. 2006. "Polycomb complexes repress developmental regulators in murine embryonic stem cells." *Nature* 441 (7091):349–53. doi:10.1038/nature04733.

Branco, M. R., G. Ficz, and W. Reik. 2012. "Uncovering the role of 5-hydroxymethylcytosine in the epigenome." *Nat Rev Genet* 13 (1):7–13. doi:10.1038/nrg3080.

Buckberry, S., T. Bianco-Miotto, S. J. Bent, G. A. Dekker, and C. T. Roberts. 2014. "Integrative transcriptome meta-analysis reveals widespread sex-biased gene expression at the human fetal–maternal interface." *Mol Hum Reprod* 20 (8):810–9. doi:10.1093/molehr/gau035.

Cedar, H. and Y. Bergman. 2009. "Linking DNA methylation and histone modification: Patterns and paradigms." *Nat Rev Genet* 10 (5):295–304. doi:10.1038/nrg2540.

Chavan-Gautam, P., D. Sundrani, H. Pisal, V. Nimbargi, S. Mehendale, and S. Joshi. 2011. "Gestation-dependent changes in human placental global DNA methylation levels." *Mol Reprod Dev* 78 (3):150. doi:10.1002/mrd.21296.

Chelbi, S. T., F. Mondon, H. Jammes, C. Buffat, T. M. Mignot, J. Tost, F. Busato, I. Gut, R. Rebourcet, P. Laissue, V. Tsatsaris, F. Goffinet, V. Rigourd, B. Carbonne, F. Ferre, and D. Vaiman. 2007. "Expressional and epigenetic alterations of placental serine protease inhibitors: SERPINA3 is a potential marker of preeclampsia." *Hypertension* 49 (1):76–83. doi:10.1161/01.HYP.0000250831.52876.cb.

Chen, P. Y., A. Ganguly, L. Rubbi, L. D. Orozco, M. Morselli, D. Ashraf, A. Jaroszewicz, S. Feng, S. E. Jacobsen, A. Nakano, S. U. Devaskar, and M. Pellegrini. 2013. "Intrauterine calorie restriction affects placental DNA methylation and gene expression." *Physiol Genomics* 45 (14):565–76. doi:10.1152/physiolgenomics.00034.2013.

Choi, S. W. and S. Friso. 2010. "Epigenetics: A new bridge between nutrition and health." *Adv Nutr* 1 (1):8–16. doi:10.3945/an.110.1004.

Chu, S. Y., S. Y. Kim, J. Lau, C. H. Schmid, P. M. Dietz, W. M. Callaghan, and K. M. Curtis. 2007. "Maternal obesity and risk of stillbirth: A metaanalysis." *Am J Obstet Gynecol* 197 (3):223–8. doi:10.1016/j.ajog.2007.03.027.

Chuang, H. C., C. W. Chang, G. D. Chang, T. P. Yao, and H. Chen. 2006. "Histone deacetylase 3 binds to and regulates the GCMa transcription factor." *Nucleic Acids Res* 34 (5):1459–69. doi:10.1093/nar/gkl048.

Cleaton, M. A., C. A. Edwards, and A. C. Ferguson-Smith. 2014. "Phenotypic outcomes of imprinted gene models in mice: Elucidation of pre- and postnatal functions of imprinted genes." *Annu Rev Genomics Hum Genet* 15:93–126. doi:10.1146/annurev-genom-091212-153441.

Clifton, V. L. 2005. "Sexually dimorphic effects of maternal asthma during pregnancy on placental glucocorticoid metabolism and fetal growth." *Cell Tissue Res* 322 (1):63–71. doi:10.1007/s00441-005-1117-5.

Coan, P. M., G. J. Burton, and A. C. Ferguson-Smith. 2005. "Imprinted genes in the placenta—A review." *Placenta* 26 Suppl A:S10–20. doi:10.1016/j.placenta.2004.12.009.

Constancia, M., G. Kelsey, and W. Reik. 2004. "Resourceful imprinting." *Nature* 432 (7013):53–7. doi:10.1038/432053a.

Denis, H., M. N. Ndlovu, and F. Fuks. 2011. "Regulation of mammalian DNA methyltransferases: A route to new mechanisms." *EMBO Rep* 12 (7):647–56. doi:10.1038/embor.2011.110.

Dhliwayo, N., M. P. Sarras Jr., E. Luczkowski, S. M. Mason, and R. V. Intine. 2014. "Parp inhibition prevents ten-eleven translocase enzyme activation and hyperglycemia-induced DNA demethylation." *Diabetes* 63 (9):3069–76. doi:10.2337/db13-1916.

El-Hadidy, W. F., A. R. Mohamed, and H. F. Mannaa. 2014. "Possible protective effect of procainamide as an epigenetic modifying agent in experimentally induced type 2 diabetes mellitus in rats." *Alexandria J Med*.

El Hajj, N., G. Pliushch, E. Schneider, M. Dittrich, T. Muller, M. Korenkov, M. Aretz, U. Zechner, H. Lehnen, and T. Haaf. 2013. "Metabolic programming of MEST DNA methylation by intrauterine exposure to gestational diabetes mellitus." *Diabetes* 62 (4):1320–8. doi:10.2337/db12-0289.

Epstein, A. C., J. M. Gleadle, L. A. McNeill, K. S. Hewitson, J. O'Rourke, D. R. Mole, M. Mukherji, E. Metzen, M. I. Wilson, A. Dhanda, Y. M. Tian, N. Masson, D. L. Hamilton, P. Jaakkola, R. Barstead, J. Hodgkin, P. H. Maxwell, C. W. Pugh, C. J. Schofield, and P. J. Ratcliffe. 2001. "C. elegans EGL-9 and mammalian homologs define a family of dioxygenases that regulate HIF by prolyl hydroxylation." *Cell* 107 (1):43–54.

Eriksson, J. G., E. Kajantie, C. Osmond, K. Thornburg, and D. J. Barker. 2010. "Boys live dangerously in the womb." *Am J Hum Biol* 22 (3):330–5. doi:10.1002/ajhb.20995.

Feinberg, A. P. and B. Tycko. 2004. "The history of cancer epigenetics." *Nat Rev Cancer* 4 (2):143–53. doi:10.1038/nrc1279.

Ferreira, J. C., S. Choufani, D. Grafodatskaya, D. T. Butcher, C. Zhao, D. Chitayat, C. Shuman, J. Kingdom, S. Keating, and R. Weksberg. 2011. "WNT2 promoter methylation in human placenta is associated with low birthweight percentile in the neonate." *Epigenetics* 6 (4):440–9.

Filiberto, A. C., M. A. Maccani, D. Koestler, C. Wilhelm-Benartzi, M. Avissar-Whiting, C. E. Banister, L. A. Gagne, and C. J. Marsit. 2011. "Birthweight is associated with DNA promoter methylation of the glucocorticoid receptor in human placenta." *Epigenetics* 6 (5):566–72.

Fowden, A. L., C. Sibley, W. Reik, and M. Constancia. 2006. "Imprinted genes, placental development and fetal growth." *Horm Res* 65 Suppl 3:50–8. doi:10.1159/000091506.

Frias, A. E., T. K. Morgan, A. E. Evans, J. Rasanen, K. Y. Oh, K. L. Thornburg, and K. L. Grove. 2011. "Maternal high-fat diet disturbs uteroplacental hemodynamics and increases the frequency of stillbirth in a nonhuman primate model of excess nutrition." *Endocrinology* 152 (6):2456–64. doi:10.1210/en.2010-1332.

Fuke, C., M. Shimabukuro, A. Petronis, J. Sugimoto, T. Oda, K. Miura, T. Miyazaki, C. Ogura, Y. Okazaki, and Y. Jinno. 2004. "Age related changes in 5-methylcytosine content in human peripheral leukocytes and placentas: An HPLC-based study." *Ann Hum Genet* 68 (Pt 3):196–204. doi:10.1046/j.1529-8817.2004.00081.x.

Gagnidze, K., Z. M. Weil, L. C. Faustino, S. M. Schaafsma, and D. W. Pfaff. 2013. "Early histone modifications in the ventromedial hypothalamus and preoptic area following oestradiol administration." *J Neuroendocrinol* 25 (10):939–55. doi:10.1111/jne.12085.

Gama-Sosa, M. A., R. M. Midgett, V. A. Slagel, S. Githens, K. C. Kuo, C. W. Gehrke, and M. Ehrlich. 1983. "Tissue-specific differences in DNA methylation in various mammals." *Biochim Biophys Acta* 740 (2):212–9.

Goll, M. G. and T. H. Bestor. 2005. "Eukaryotic cytosine methyltransferases." *Annu Rev Biochem* 74:481–514. doi:10.1146/annurev.biochem.74.010904.153721.

Gut, P. and E. Verdin. 2013. "The nexus of chromatin regulation and intermediary metabolism." *Nature* 502 (7472):489–98. doi:10.1038/nature12752.

Handa, V. and A. Jeltsch. 2005. "Profound flanking sequence preference of Dnmt3a and Dnmt3b mammalian DNA methyltransferases shape the human epigenome." *J Mol Biol* 348 (5):1103–12. doi:10.1016/j.jmb.2005.02.044.

Hass, B. S., R. W. Hart, M. H. Lu, and B. D. Lyn-Cook. 1993. "Effects of caloric restriction in animals on cellular function, oncogene expression, and DNA methylation in vitro." *Mutat Res* 295 (4–6):281–9.

Haycock, P. C. and M. Ramsay. 2009. "Exposure of mouse embryos to ethanol during preimplantation development: Effect on DNA methylation in the h19 imprinting control region." *Biol Reprod* 81 (4):618–27. doi:10.1095/biolreprod.108.074682.

Heijmans, B. T., E. W. Tobi, L. H. Lumey, and P. E. Slagboom. 2009. "The epigenome: Archive of the prenatal environment." *Epigenetics* 4 (8):526–31.

Heyn, H. and M. Esteller. 2012. "DNA methylation profiling in the clinic: Applications and challenges." *Nat Rev Genet* 13 (10):679–92. doi:10.1038/nrg3270.

Hodges, E., A. D. Smith, J. Kendall, Z. Xuan, K. Ravi, M. Rooks, M. Q. Zhang, K. Ye, A. Bhattacharjee, L. Brizuela, W. R. McCombie, M. Wigler, G. J. Hannon, and J. B. Hicks. 2009. "High definition profiling of mammalian DNA methylation by array capture and single molecule bisulfite sequencing." *Genome Res* 19 (9):1593–605. doi:10.1101/gr.095190.109.

Hoile, S. P., N. A. Irvine, C. J. Kelsall, C. Sibbons, A. Feunteun, A. Collister, C. Torrens, P. C. Calder, M. A. Hanson, K. A. Lillycrop, and G. C. Burdge. 2013. "Maternal fat intake in rats alters 20:4n-6 and 22:6n-3 status and the epigenetic regulation of Fads2 in offspring liver." *J Nutr Biochem* 24 (7):1213–20. doi:10.1016/j.jnutbio.2012.09.005.

Iyer, L. M., M. Tahiliani, A. Rao, and L. Aravind. 2009. "Prediction of novel families of enzymes involved in oxidative and other complex modifications of bases in nucleic acids." *Cell Cycle* 8 (11):1698–710.

Jones, P. A. and D. Takai. 2001. "The role of DNA methylation in mammalian epigenetics." *Science* 293 (5532):1068–70. doi:10.1126/science.1063852.

Kamei, Y., T. Suganami, T. Ehara, S. Kanai, K. Hayashi, Y. Yamamoto, S. Miura, O. Ezaki, M. Okano, and Y. Ogawa. 2010. "Increased expression of DNA methyltransferase 3a in obese adipose tissue: Studies with transgenic mice." *Obesity (Silver Spring)* 18 (2):314–21. doi:10.1038/oby.2009.246.

Keyes, M. K., H. Jang, J. B. Mason, Z. Liu, J. W. Crott, D. E. Smith, S. Friso, and S. W. Choi. 2007. "Older age and dietary folate are determinants of genomic and p16-specific DNA methylation in mouse colon." *J Nutr* 137 (7):1713–7.

Kimura, A. P., S. A. Liebhaber, and N. E. Cooke. 2004. "Epigenetic modifications at the human growth hormone locus predict distinct roles for histone acetylation and methylation in placental gene activation." *Mol Endocrinol* 18 (4):1018–32. doi:10.1210/me.2003-0468.

Kirkland, J. B. 2009. "Niacin status impacts chromatin structure." *J Nutr* 139 (12):2397–401. doi:10.3945/jn.109.111757.

Koukoura, O., S. Sifakis, and D. A. Spandidos. 2012. "DNA methylation in the human placenta and fetal growth (review)." *Mol Med Report* 5 (4):883–9. doi:10.3892/mmr.2012.763.

Lambertini, L. 2014. "Genomic imprinting: Sensing the environment and driving the fetal growth." *Curr Opin Pediatr* 26 (2):237–42. doi:10.1097/MOP.0000000000000072.

Laurent, L., E. Wong, G. Li, T. Huynh, A. Tsirigos, C. T. Ong, H. M. Low, K. W. Kin Sung, I. Rigoutsos, J. Loring, and C. L. Wei. 2010. "Dynamic changes in the human methylome during differentiation." *Genome Res* 20 (3):320–31. doi:10.1101/gr.101907.109.

Lee, H. J., T. A. Hore, and W. Reik. 2014. "Reprogramming the methylome: Erasing memory and creating diversity." *Cell Stem Cell* 14 (6):710–9. doi:10.1016/j.stem.2014.05.008.

Li, E., T. H. Bestor, and R. Jaenisch. 1992. "Targeted mutation of the DNA methyltransferase gene results in embryonic lethality." *Cell* 69 (6):915–26.

Lillycrop, K. A., E. S. Phillips, A. A. Jackson, M. A. Hanson, and G. C. Burdge. 2005. "Dietary protein restriction of pregnant rats induces and folic acid supplementation prevents epigenetic modification of hepatic gene expression in the offspring." *J Nutr* 135 (6):1382–6.

Ling, C., S. Del Guerra, R. Lupi, T. Ronn, C. Granhall, H. Luthman, P. Masiello, P. Marchetti, L. Groop, and S. Del Prato. 2008. "Epigenetic regulation of PPARGC1A in human type 2 diabetic islets and effect on insulin secretion." *Diabetologia* 51 (4):615–22. doi:10.1007/s00125-007-0916-5.

Mao, J., X. Zhang, P. T. Sieli, M. T. Falduto, K. E. Torres, and C. S. Rosenfeld. 2010. "Contrasting effects of different maternal diets on sexually dimorphic gene expression in the murine placenta." *Proc Natl Acad Sci U S A* 107 (12):5557–62. doi:10.1073/pnas.1000440107.

Minor, E. A., B. L. Court, J. I. Young, and G. Wang. 2013. "Ascorbate induces ten-eleven translocation (Tet) methylcytosine dioxygenase-mediated generation of 5-hydroxymethylcytosine." *J Biol Chem* 288 (19):13669–74. doi:10.1074/jbc.C113.464800.

Monk, D., P. Arnaud, J. Frost, F. A. Hills, P. Stanier, R. Feil, and G. E. Moore. 2009. "Reciprocal imprinting of human GRB10 in placental trophoblast and brain: Evolutionary conservation of reversed allelic expression." *Hum Mol Genet* 18 (16):3066–74. doi:10.1093/hmg/ddp248.

Moore, T. and D. Haig. 1991. "Genomic imprinting in mammalian development: A parental tug-of-war." *Trends Genet* 7 (2):45–9. doi:10.1016/0168-9525(91)90230-N.

Myatt, L. 2006. "Placental adaptive responses and fetal programming." *J Physiol* 572 (Pt 1):25–30. doi:10.1113/jphysiol.2006.104968.

Myatt, L. and V. H. Roberts. 2006. "Placental mechanisms and developmental origins of health and disease." In *Developmental Origins of Health and Disease*, edited by P. Gluckman and M. Hanson, 130–142. Cambridge: Cambridge University Press.

Nelissen, E. C., A. P. van Montfoort, J. C. Dumoulin, and J. L. Evers. 2011. "Epigenetics and the placenta." *Hum Reprod Update* 17 (3):397–417. doi:10.1093/humupd/dmq052.

Niu, Y., X. Zhao, Y. S. Wu, M. M. Li, X. J. Wang, and Y. G. Yang. 2013. "N6-methyl-adenosine (m6A) in RNA: An old modification with a novel epigenetic function." *Genomics Proteomics Bioinformatics* 11 (1):8–17. doi:10.1016/j.gpb.2012.12.002.

Novakovic, B., R. K. Yuen, L. Gordon, M. S. Penaherrera, A. Sharkey, A. Moffett, J. M. Craig, W. P. Robinson, and R. Saffery. 2011. "Evidence for widespread changes in promoter methylation profile in human placenta in response to increasing gestational age and environmental/stochastic factors." *BMC Genomics* 12:529. doi:10.1186/1471-2164-12-529.

Osei-Kumah, A., R. Smith, I. Jurisica, I. Caniggia, and V. L. Clifton. 2011. "Sex-specific differences in placental global gene expression in pregnancies complicated by asthma." *Placenta* 32 (8):570–8. doi:10.1016/j.placenta.2011.05.005.

Perkins, E., S. K. Murphy, A. P. Murtha, J. Schildkraut, R. L. Jirtle, W. Demark-Wahnefried, M. R. Forman, J. Kurtzberg, F. Overcash, Z. Huang, and C. Hoyo. 2012. "Insulin-like growth factor 2/H19 methylation at birth and risk of overweight and obesity in children." *J Pediatr* 161 (1):31–9. doi:10.1016/j.jpeds.2012.01.015.

Peterson, C. L. and M. A. Laniel. 2004. "Histones and histone modifications." *Curr Biol* 14 (14):R546–51. doi:10.1016/j.cub.2004.07.007.

Petronis, A. 2001. "Human morbid genetics revisited: Relevance of epigenetics." *Trends Genet* 17 (3):142–6.

Petrossian, T. C. and S. G. Clarke. 2011. "Uncovering the human methyltransferasome." *Mol Cell Proteomics* 10 (1):M110.000976. doi:10.1074/mcp.M110.000976.

Pirola, L., A. Balcerczyk, R. W. Tothill, I. Haviv, A. Kaspi, S. Lunke, M. Ziemann, T. Karagiannis, S. Tonna, A. Kowalczyk, B. Beresford-Smith, G. Macintyre, M. Kelong, Z. Hongyu, J. Zhu, and A. El-Osta. 2011. "Genome-wide analysis distinguishes hyperglycemia regulated epigenetic signatures of primary vascular cells." *Genome Res* 21 (10):1601–15. doi:10.1101/gr.116095.110.

Radaelli, T., A. Varastehpour, P. Catalano, and S. Hauguel-de Mouzon. 2003. "Gestational diabetes induces placental genes for chronic stress and inflammatory pathways." *Diabetes* 52 (12):2951–8.

Rahnama, F., F. Shafiei, P. D. Gluckman, M. D. Mitchell, and P. E. Lobie. 2006. "Epigenetic regulation of human trophoblastic cell migration and invasion." *Endocrinology* 147 (11):5275–83. doi:10.1210/en.2006-0288.

Rakyan, V. K., J. Preis, H. D. Morgan, and E. Whitelaw. 2001. "The marks, mechanisms and memory of epigenetic states in mammals." *Biochem J* 356 (Pt 1):1–10.

Rawn, S. M. and J. C. Cross. 2008. "The evolution, regulation, and function of placenta-specific genes." *Annu Rev Cell Dev Biol* 24:159–81. doi:10.1146/annurev.cellbio.24.110707.175418.

Reik, W. 2007. "Stability and flexibility of epigenetic gene regulation in mammalian development." *Nature* 447 (7143):425–32. doi:10.1038/nature05918.

Reik, W. and J. Walter. 2001. "Genomic imprinting: Parental influence on the genome." *Nat Rev Genet* 2 (1):21–32. doi:10.1038/35047554.

Reik, W., M. Constancia, A. Fowden, N. Anderson, W. Dean, A. Ferguson-Smith, B. Tycko, and C. Sibley. 2003. "Regulation of supply and demand for maternal nutrients in mammals by imprinted genes." *J Physiol* 547 (Pt 1):35–44. doi:10.1113/jphysiol.2002.033274.

Rogers, L. K. and M. Velten. 2011. "Maternal inflammation, growth retardation, and preterm birth: Insights into adult cardiovascular disease." *Life Sci* 89 (13–14):417–21. doi:10.1016/j.lfs.2011.07.017.

Rossant, J., J. P. Sanford, V. M. Chapman, and G. K. Andrews. 1986. "Undermethylation of structural gene sequences in extraembryonic lineages of the mouse." *Dev Biol* 117 (2):567–73.

Sapienza, C., J. Lee, J. Powell, O. Erinle, F. Yafai, J. Reichert, E. S. Siraj, and M. Madaio. 2011. "DNA methylation profiling identifies epigenetic differences between diabetes patients with ESRD and diabetes patients without nephropathy." *Epigenetics* 6 (1):20–8.

Scott, J. M. and D. G. Weir. 1998. "Folic acid, homocysteine and one-carbon metabolism: A review of the essential biochemistry." *J Cardiovasc Risk* 5 (4):223–7.

Shyh-Chang, N., J. W. Locasale, C. A. Lyssiotis, Y. Zheng, R. Y. Teo, S. Ratanasirintrawoot, J. Zhang, T. Onder, J. J. Unternaehrer, H. Zhu, J. M. Asara, G. Q. Daley, and L. C. Cantley. 2013. "Influence of threonine metabolism on S-adenosylmethionine and histone methylation." *Science* 339 (6116):222–6. doi:10.1126/science.1226603.

Sims, R. J. 3rd and D. Reinberg. 2006. "Histone H3 Lys 4 methylation: Caught in a bind?" *Genes Dev* 20 (20):2779–86. doi:10.1101/gad.1468206.

Sood, R., J. L. Zehnder, M. L. Druzin, and P. O. Brown. 2006. "Gene expression patterns in human placenta." *Proc Natl Acad Sci U S A* 103 (14):5478–83. doi:10.1073/pnas.0508035103.

Soubry, A., S. K. Murphy, F. Wang, Z. Huang, A. C. Vidal, B. F. Fuemmeler, J. Kurtzberg, A. Murtha, R. L. Jirtle, J. M. Schildkraut, and C. Hoyo. 2013. "Newborns of obese parents have altered DNA methylation patterns at imprinted genes." *Int J Obes (Lond)*. doi:10.1038/ijo.2013.193.

Stark, M. J., I. M. Wright, and V. L. Clifton. 2009. "Sex-specific alterations in placental 11beta-hydroxysteroid dehydrogenase 2 activity and early postnatal clinical course following antenatal betamethasone." *Am J Physiol Regul Integr Comp Physiol* 297 (2):R510–4. doi:10.1152/ajpregu.00175.2009.

Strakovsky, R. S., X. Zhang, D. Zhou, and Y. X. Pan. 2011. "Gestational high fat diet programs hepatic phosphoenolpyruvate carboxykinase gene expression and histone modification in neonatal offspring rats." *J Physiol* 589 (Pt 11):2707–17. doi:10.1113/jphysiol.2010.203950.

Strakovsky, R. S., X. Zhang, D. Zhou, and Y. X. Pan. 2014. "The regulation of hepatic Pon1 by a maternal high-fat diet is gender specific and may occur through promoter histone modifications in neonatal rats." *J Nutr Biochem* 25 (2):170–6. doi:10.1016/j.jnutbio.2013.09.016.

Tobi, E. W., L. H. Lumey, R. P. Talens, D. Kremer, H. Putter, A. D. Stein, P. E. Slagboom, and B. T. Heijmans. 2009. "DNA methylation differences after exposure to prenatal famine are common and timing- and sex-specific." *Hum Mol Genet* 18 (21):4046–53. doi:10.1093/hmg/ddp353.

Tsukada, Y., J. Fang, H. Erdjument-Bromage, M. E. Warren, C. H. Borchers, P. Tempst, and Y. Zhang. 2006. "Histone demethylation by a family of JmjC domain-containing proteins." *Nature* 439 (7078):811–6. doi:10.1038/nature04433.

Vlahovic, M., F. Bulic-Jakus, G. Juric-Lekic, A. Fucic, S. Maric, and D. Serman. 1999. "Changes in the placenta and in the rat embryo caused by the demethylating agent 5-azacytidine." *Int J Dev Biol* 43 (8):843–6.

Waterland, R. A. and R. L. Jirtle. 2003. "Transposable elements: Targets for early nutritional effects on epigenetic gene regulation." *Mol Cell Biol* 23 (15):5293–300.

Waterland, R. A., J. R. Lin, C. A. Smith, and R. L. Jirtle. 2006. "Post-weaning diet affects genomic imprinting at the insulin-like growth factor 2 (Igf2) locus." *Hum Mol Genet* 15 (5):705–16. doi:10.1093/hmg/ddi484.

Weinmann, A. S., S. M. Bartley, T. Zhang, M. Q. Zhang, and P. J. Farnham. 2001. "Use of chromatin immuno-precipitation to clone novel E2F target promoters." *Mol Cell Biol* 21 (20):6820–32. doi:10.1128/MCB .21.20.6820-6832.2001.

Welstead, G. G., M. P. Creyghton, S. Bilodeau, A. W. Cheng, S. Markoulaki, R. A. Young, and R. Jaenisch. 2012. "X-linked H3K27me3 demethylase Utx is required for embryonic development in a sex-specific manner." *Proc Natl Acad Sci U S A* 109 (32):13004–9. doi:10.1073/pnas.1210787109.

Wilhelm-Benartzi, C. S., E. A. Houseman, M. A. Maccani, G. M. Poage, D. C. Koestler, S. M. Langevin, L. A. Gagne, C. E. Banister, J. F. Padbury, and C. J. Marsit. 2012. "In utero exposures, infant growth, and DNA methylation of repetitive elements and developmentally related genes in human placenta." *Environ Health Perspect* 120 (2):296–302. doi:10.1289/ehp.1103927.

Wu, H., V. Coskun, J. Tao, W. Xie, W. Ge, K. Yoshikawa, E. Li, Y. Zhang, and Y. E. Sun. 2010. "Dnmt3a-dependent nonpromoter DNA methylation facilitates transcription of neurogenic genes." *Science* 329 (5990):444–8. doi:10.1126/science.1190485.

Yogev, Y. and P. M. Catalano. 2009. "Pregnancy and obesity." *Obstet Gynecol Clin North Am* 36 (2):285–300, viii. doi:10.1016/j.ogc.2009.03.003.

Yuen, R. K., L. Avila, M. S. Penaherrera, P. von Dadelszen, L. Lefebvre, M. S. Kobor, and W. P. Robinson. 2009. "Human placental-specific epipolymorphism and its association with adverse pregnancy outcomes." *PLoS One* 4 (10):e7389. doi:10.1371/journal.pone.0007389.

Zhao, J., J. Goldberg, J. D. Bremner, and V. Vaccarino. 2012. "Global DNA methylation is associated with insulin resistance: A monozygotic twin study." *Diabetes* 61 (2):542–6. doi:10.2337/db11-1048.

4 Maternal Diet, Trophoblast Biology, and Epigenetic Regulation

Daniel Vaiman

CONTENTS

ABSTRACT

The placenta is the pivotal interface regulating nutrient exchanges between the mother and the fetus in Therian mammals. The placenta contains specific cells called trophoblasts, originating from trophoblast stem cells and having several fates (in humans, they will evolve into villous trophoblasts, extravillous trophoblasts, and syncytiotrophoblasts) and indispensable functions. Maternal nutrition may impact on maternal blood composition in nutrients at the materno–fetal interface. The mammalian target of rapamycin pathway, together with the network of placental imprinted genes, is able to sense the content and composition in nutrients and regulate these materno–fetal exchanges. Revisiting microarray experiments by novel bioinformatics tools allowed identification of the key role played by epigenetic modulators in adjusting the fetal demand to the maternal offer. Two examples are analyzed; one is provided by placental gene expression in diet-restricted mothers during pregnancy, and the other one is based on the study of maternal supplementation by polyunsaturated fatty acid in the maternal diet, in humans. The identification of pivotal regulators of placental response may help to propose a rationale by which trophoblast biology is modified by the external environment to account for variation in nutrients. Finding these regulators will also help to understand the basis of a programmed metabolic response in permanent organs long after pregnancy in the offspring. This response may sometimes be abnormal when placental adjustment has been achieved at a non-null physiological cost.

KEY WORDS

Placenta, maternal diet, epigenetics, mTOR signaling cascade, imprinted genes, bioinformatics, gene networks.

4.1 INTRODUCTION

Fetal growth needs energy. In placental species, energy originates from the food intake of the mother, who transmits nutrients to the growing fetus. This process is allowed by a specific organ, varying in shape and structure throughout mammals, the placenta (for a recent review, see Furukawa, Kuroda, and Sugiyama 2014). The placenta is a fetal transitory organ, intimately interfaced with maternal tissue, featured in metatherian (marsupials) and eutherian mammalian species; besides its nutritional function, it has major immunological and endocrine roles during pregnancy (Garratt et al. 2013). Recurrent findings suggest that imprinted genes that are expressed from only one allele are often expressed at a high level in the placenta, stressing their role in the management of resources flowing from the mother to the fetus, in a potential context of genetic conflict stemming from partly contrasting Darwinian interests between the paternal and maternal genomes (Haig 1993). Interestingly, the sequencing of the platypus genome (*Ornithorhynchus anatinus*), an egg-laying mammal, revealed an apparent absence of imprinted genes correlated to limited acquisition of certain categories of repetitive elements (Renfree et al. 2009; Suzuki et al. 2011; Warren et al. 2008).

Environmental conditions will influence the genome to regulate its function through epigenetic mechanisms. Epigenetic mechanisms can be defined as a cell-based machinery able to induce reversible modifications of the chromatin (without changing the DNA sequence), leading to a heritable status of gene expression or gene repression at the transcriptional or posttranscriptional level. Briefly, three major epigenetic mechanisms are at work in mammalian cells; DNA methylation; histone posttranslational modification, often referred to as the histone code; and the presence of an important load of small regulatory RNAs, such as micro-RNA, able to inactivate genes before translation of the target mRNAs, defined as cognates owing to sequence identity or during their translation.

Imbalance or insufficiency in the food absorbed by the mother will bathe the placenta in an unwanted or suboptimal nutrient microenvironment. Consistent reports suggest that this environmental situation will trigger specific responses of the placenta, possibly to alleviate the detrimental effect of the environment. These responses are associated with epigenetic processes that can have extended effects toward the developing fetus, the young adult, or even toward the generations to come.

4.2 DIET-INDUCED EPIGENETIC ALTERATIONS AND PLACENTAL DEVELOPMENT

4.2.1 INTRODUCTORY EXAMPLE

In humans, a clear example of the epigenetic effect of female alimentation on the placenta is provided by the Dutch famine of 1944 (Lumey et al. 2007). This famine occurred during the winter of 1944–1945, and during this period, after a German blockade on alimentary products that triggered the death of ~20,000 persons, the mothers obtained often less than 1000 kilocalories per day. The authors studied DNA methylation in cells from whole blood, at the level of the differentially methylated region (DMR) of the imprinted gene *IGF2* (Heijmans et al. 2008), and showed that 60 years after exposure, there was a significant demethylation in individuals whose mothers were exposed during the early gestational period (but not at later gestation times). While in this example, the placenta could not be studied, it is probable that the epigenetic alterations of the blood cells reflect alterations "sensed" *in utero* and that the placenta played the role of a pivotal "sensory organ" that was firstly affected by epigenetic modifications. It is now well demonstrated that the placenta will respond to environmental/diet-induced stress through epigenetic alterations. The placenta will harbor marks of alterations that can be studied and could potentially be used to evaluate possible consequences on adult health (Myatt 2006).

4.2.2 STRUCTURE AND DEVELOPMENT OF THE PLACENTA

The mammalian placenta plays various roles as a transitory endocrine organ producing specific hormones (human chorionic gonadotrophin [hCG] and human placental lactogen [hPL]), promoting materno–fetal tolerance during gestation, and allowing for nutrient and gas exchanges during pregnancy. Trophoblasts are the placental-specific cell type, and in mice, it is known that trophoblast stem cells (TS cells) differentiate following various trajectories to constitute specific pools of cells located in specific zones and are important for placental function, namely, spongiotrophoblasts in the junctional zone, syncytiotrophoblast, and giant cells in the labyrinth region, closer to the embryo and where the exchanges occur (Maltepe, Bakardjiev, and Fisher 2010). In humans (Figure 4.1), the placenta exchange surface near term is composed of villi, branched up to the 16th rank, and is covered by a thin, multinucleated syncytium, the syncytiotrophoblast, on a surface estimated at ~10 m^2 (http://www.uvp5.univ-paris5.fr/campus-gyneco-obst/cycle3/poly/2600fra.asp). Located under the syncytiotrophoblast is a layer of villous cytotrophoblasts, which tend to decrease in number near the end of pregnancy (Rigourd et al. 2009).

Placental structure and function are directly determined by trophoblast biology. Trophoblasts derive from TS cells, characterized in particular by the expression of the transcription factor *Cdx2*, at the difference of the embryonic stem (ES) cells, where *Oct4* is a major transcriptional regulator and Cdx2/Oct4 acts as a molecular switch presiding to the fate of the cells toward either the embryo or

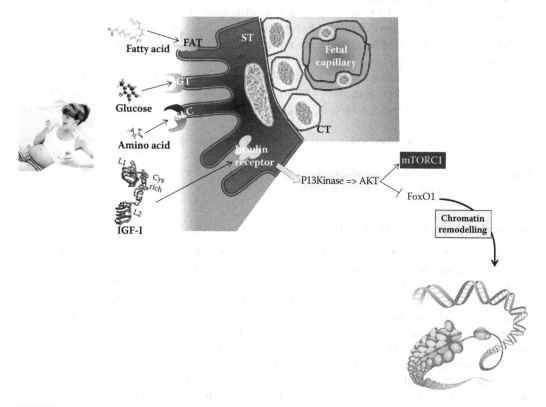

FIGURE 4.1 The placenta plays a pivotal role in sensing the nutritional environment provided by the mother's alimentation. Receptors to lipids (fatty acids), glucose, amino acids, and insulin growth-factor I are present on the syncytial villi. The nutrients provided in the blood by the mother can alter in quality and quantity the message received at the syncytiotrophoblast level. One major sensor of the nutritional environment in the placenta appears to be the mTOR kinase, itself dependent on phosphorylation through the PI3-kinase-AKT pathway. FoxO1 plays the role of an alternative target to mTOR phosphorylation and its deregulation may lead to abnormal chromatin remodeling and epigenetically driven alterations of gene expression.

the extraembryonic tissue, which will later generate the placenta and other embryo annexes (Niwa et al. 2005). A recent study showed that ES cells differ from TS cells by the methylation and expression of downstream genes (highly methylated and with a low expression specifically in ES cells, *Ezrin*, *Handl*, *Laspl*, *Map3k8*, *Plei1*, *Rin3*, *Sh2d3c*, *Tead4*, and *Tinagl1*). Apparently, they cannot completely be transdifferentiated toward the trophoblast lineage, thanks to the resistance of a TS-specific methylation of a set of genes, such as *Elf5* and *Ezr*, extremely refractory to reprogramming (Cambuli et al. 2014). Despite these fixed anchors, TS cells have to present a dose of plasticity since as mentioned before, several different lineages originate from them. Indeed, trophoblast biology is defined by two major functional axes: proliferation and invasion, together with differentiation in polynucleated structures in most mammalian species (syncytiotrophoblast). While the trajectories are less well identified in humans than in mice, trophoblast that originates from TS cells will differentiate in (1) syncytiotrophoblast, (2) villous cytotrophoblasts, and (3) extravillous cytotrophoblasts.

It is reasonable to think that in the human placenta, the syncytiotrophoblast is renewed from the underlying trophoblast layer throughout gestation, since fragments of this external layer of the placenta as well as small particles are known to be shed from the placenta into the maternal circulation throughout normal and pathological pregnancies (Chamley et al. 2014; Redman et al. 2012; Shetty, Patil, and Ghosh 2013). However, until now, it has not been possible to derive trophoblast progenitors from villous cytrophoblasts (Genbacev et al. 2013). Rather, it has recently been possible to develop trophoblast-like stem cells from the chorionic layer of the placenta. These cells constitute a promising model to study early defects of human placental development (Genbacev et al. 2011). Eventually, some cytotrophoblasts leave the villi to invade the maternal endometrium (invasive extravillous trophoblasts), and some replace the endothelial layer of the maternal uterine spiral arteries to a deepness reaching the first third of the myometrium. This invasion, specific to human pregnancy, has considerable importance for allowing a low-resistance vascular flow to reach the intervillous space (Kasiviswanathan, Collins, and Copeland 2012). All these trophoblast cells stem from the trophectoderm, the layer of cells surrounding the blastocyst at implantation (~7 days in humans).

Potentially, then, the complete gestation period, as well as periods beforehand, constitute critical time windows where maternal diet may have an influence on the outcome of pregnancy. Placental adaptation to harsh environmental conditions is reasonably thought to be due to epigenetic alterations/adaptation.

4.2.3 Impact of Food Availability on Placental Function

Food deprivation is known to have consequences on fetal growth. These consequences have been described long ago. In 1996, for instance, in a very thorough study, Malandro et al. (1996) exposed female rats to a low-protein isocaloric diet to evaluate the consequences on amino acid transport in the placenta. The authors showed decreased maternal, fetal, and placental weight. While maternal serum amino acids were not reduced, the fetuses were deprived of these nutrients. Isolating the apical and basal membranes of the placental trophoblasts, the authors showed a decreased activity of amino acid transport mechanisms for neutral and cationic amino acids. Specifically, EAAC1 and CAT1 systems had their mRNA levels decreased in the low-protein group. In 2001, the structure of the placenta was studied after diet restriction in a guinea pig model (Roberts et al. 2001). The authors showed a reduction in all the functional parameters of the placenta (fetal weight, density of the syncytiotrophoblast, volume of maternal blood space). Interestingly, they correlated these reductions with expression levels of proteins of the insulin-like growth factor (IGF) system (IGF1, IGF2, and IGFBP2). Among the major conclusions, the ratio IGF2/IGFBP2 was reduced by 75% near term, thus pointing to this growth axis as a relevant target, making a link between maternal diet and placental development. Another study using protein deprivation in the rat model revealed that in the placenta, genes involved in epigenetic modifications (DNA methyl transferase, histone deacetylases, chromodomain- and bromodomain-containing factors, histone acetyl transferases) were almost systematically up-regulated at the transcriptional level when the females were fed with a 9% protein chow (instead of 20%, in the normal chow) isocaloric diet (Buffat et al. 2007), this observation being paralleled with a ~10% decrease in the weight of the fetuses at 20 days post-fertilization. Interestingly, the transcriptome analysis of other tissues in the same animals (lung, liver, kidney, and heart) did not reveal a similar modification of imprinting-related genes that were either not affected or not systematically induced (Vaiman et al. 2011).

In line with this observation of gene expression modifications observed in the placenta and other tissues, several elements indicate that babies born from food-restricted mothers may suffer from long-term consequences in their adult health (with a higher propensity to metabolic diseases). This is the concept of fetal programming, brought forward and developed by the late David Barker.

4.3 REVISITING PLACENTAL GENE REGULATION PATHWAYS AFTER DIET-INDUCED GROWTH RESTRICTION IN THE RAT MODEL: AN EPIGENETIC OVERVIEW

For the present review, the placental microarray described above (Buffat et al. 2007) was reanalyzed using new bioinformatic approaches that were not readily available at the time of the publication, such as Gene Set Enrichment Analysis (GSEA; http://www.broadinstitute.org/gsea/index.jsp), developed by the Broad Institute (Johansson, Lindgren, and Berglund 2003; Subramanian et al. 2005), to discover putative epigenetic pathways that remained undetected in the 2007 analysis. Among the 23,456 initial transcripts of the Nimblegen rat array, 21,071 were collapsed to known transcripts and were further collapsed to 10,054 unique genes in the GSEA procedure. Consistent with the expected effect of diet restriction, only 3227 (32.1%) were induced in the placentas from protein-restricted females, while 6827 (67.9%) were repressed. A total of 4026 gene sets were screened with the GSEA procedure, fixing thresholds limiting the gene sets between 10 and 1000 genes. In the restriction protein up-regulated group, 184 gene sets were significant using a false discovery rate (FDR) of <0.25 (classically used in this type of analyses), while in the restriction protein down-regulated group, 1274 gene sets were significant with an FDR of <0.25. Therefore, there are 6.3-fold more significant clusters in the down-regulated genes while the genes themselves are only twice as many. This means that there is a more efficient possibility to clusterize these down-regulated genes than the up-regulated genes. In both GSEA groups, epigenetic modulator pathways appeared in the most significant clusters but belonged to different categories.

Among the up-regulated groups identified by GSEA, four groups of genes regulated through methylation at CpG island appear as strongly correlated with the intrauterine growth restriction (IUGR) data set (Figure 4.2). Also, groups of genes associated with histone methylation (H3K27Me3) are prominent in these GSEA clusters correlated with up-regulated placental genes (15 clusters identified) often linking DNA methylation at specific CpG islands (intermediate, high and low CpG density) and H3K27Me3. By contrast, no cluster of microRNA miR-regulated genes was evidenced.

On the other hand, when placental down-regulated gene clusters were analyzed, miR modulation appeared largely prominent. Indeed, one cluster of genes regulated by histone acetylation and four linked to DNA methylation appeared, while 19 clusters of genes modified by miRNA associated significantly with diet restriction induced down-regulation of gene expression in the placenta (regulated by miR-21, miR-30, miR-106b, miR-302a, miR-192, miR-215, miR-1, miR-16, miR-34a, miR-133, miR-34b, miR-34c, miR-15a, mir16.1, miR-31, Let7a), as exemplified for miR-21 and miR-30 in Figure 4.2. In addition, regulation by SMARCA2, part of the SWItch/Sucrose Non-Fermentable (SWI/SNF) epigenetic complex, was also significantly associated to down-regulation of placental genes (Figure 4.2). To summarize, the epigenetic mechanisms potentially involved in gene modulation in the placenta and the trophoblast are completely different for the up-regulated (prominence of chromatin modifications, based on alterations of the histone code and DNA methylation) and

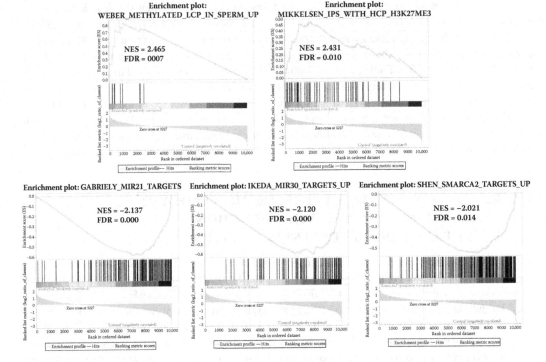

FIGURE 4.2 Diet restriction on the placenta targets genes that are also modified by players of the epigenetic regulation machinery. The figure represents a Gene Set Enrichment Analysis (GSEA) of the gene expression profile in rat placentas (20 days postfertilization) when the mothers were fed either a control diet (20% protein) or a protein-restricted diet (9% protein) during gestation, transcriptome data being extracted from Buffat and coworkers (2007). Briefly, the curve represents the enrichment of genes present in the cascade analyzed. NES is the normalized enrichment score, taking into account the number of genes present in the cluster. FDR is the false discovery rate, estimated through 1000 permutations of the data set. The two upper GSEA figures represent genes that are induced in the experimental data set (placental gene expression, restriction vs. normal), as well as in the data set scrutinized by the program. In this case, it means that genes that have a low density of CpG in the promoter that are methylated correlate with placental genes induced by diet restriction in the placenta (left, up). Similarly, genes with high CpG content (HCP) that are targets of H3K27Me3 in induced pluripotent stem (IPS) cells are also induced by protein restriction in the placenta (up, right). In the lower part of the figure are groups of genes correlating with genes that are down-regulated in the placenta after diet restriction. As examples, those correlate very strongly with MiR-21 and MiR-30 targets, as well as SMARCA2 targets, with SMARC being a component of the SWI/SNF complex, marks of active chromatin.

the down-regulated (very strong prominence of putative regulation by miR) genes. Since the same group of gene sets is used for both genes, this observation clearly reflects a genuine biological difference that was not perceived in the previous analysis carried out in the initial publication of the data. These observations point out that the miRNA system may be the first sentinel to detect a protein restriction in the maternal blood. It suggests that some specific miRNAs are induced at the transcriptional level and will tend to decrease several genes in a concerted fashion (Figure 4.3).

Studying the predicted targets of miR-21 and miR-30a using miRWalk2.0 (http://www.umm.uni-heidelberg.de/apps/zmf/mirwalk/) (Dweep et al. 2011) revealed enrichment of specific functions correlated with epigenetics regulation for miR-30a (DNMT3B, HDAC9, MLL).

Moving to gene function, network analysis of the genes through the use of STRING (Snel et al. 2000) and CYTOSCAPE (Shannon et al. 2003) revealed the existence of specific clusters of up-regulated and especially down-regulated genes (in accordance with the GSEA observations) involved

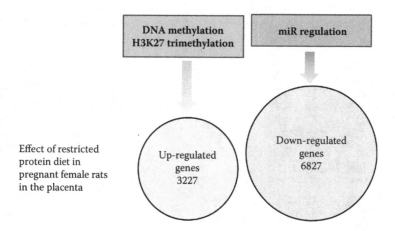

FIGURE 4.3 DNA methylation and H3K27 trimethylation targets are also genes associated with up-regulation in the placenta after diet restriction in the mother's regimen. miR-regulated targets are generally also genes that are down-regulated in the diet-restricted placenta.

in specific biological functions (Figure 4.4). Interestingly, the down-regulated gene cascade includes mitochondrial function, protein synthesis, and the cytokine network.

In addition to this epigenetic analysis of a 2007 diet-induced IUGR in the rat model, another recent study analyzed placental epigenetic alterations in the case of mild IUGR created by gestational protein deficiency, decreasing the ration from 21% to 9% for the protein content (Reamon-Buettner, Buschmann, and Lewin 2014). The restriction is quite similar to the one used by Buffat and coworkers (2007) and results in a mild decrease in placenta weight and fetal weight (~5%). In this paper, the authors studied the expression of a series of imprinted genes, *Cdkn1C*, *Gnas*, *Ilk*, *Nr3c1*, *Phlda2*, *Dhrc24*, *Plagl1*, *Dlk1*, *Gatm*, *Igf2*, *H19*, and *Wnt2*. The authors found a significant differential gene expression for *Wnt2* and *Dlk1*, with strong correlations between *Wnt2* expression and placental and fetal weight. Interestingly, *Wnt2* was also down-regulated in the work of Buffat and coworkers (expression restricted ~2.4-fold). Surprisingly, *Nr3c1*, increased more than ~4-fold in the Buffat study, was not obviously pinpointed in the second study. The methylation and hydroxymethylation analysis of the Wnt2 promoter was carried out by bisulphite sequencing and revealed a significant correlation between total methylation and fetal weight. The Wnt pathway is a conserved pathway known to be important in development and growth, and a very recent study associated abnormal Wnt2 expression with abnormal pregnancy, especially preeclampsia (Zhang et al. 2013).

Mechanistical aspects of the impact of caloric restriction in placental epigenetics have also been addressed recently in the mouse model (Chen et al. 2013; Ganguly et al. 2014). Chen et al. (2013) used a genome-wide approach to analyze the impact of calorie restriction on placental DNA methylation through the technique of reduced representation bisulfite sequencing (for an overview of methylation analysis techniques, see Calicchio et al. 2013). The analysis was coupled with a systematic study of gene expression that revealed quasi-systematic down-regulation of pregnancy-specific glycoprotein genes, as well as up-regulation of apolipoproteins in males, and deregulation of fatty acid binding proteins and cathepsin and granzyme genes. Differentially methylated genes (297) were found after calorie restriction, involved in embryonic and cardiovascular development, cell–cell signaling, and nervous system development. Overall, the placental genome was slightly demethylated in calorie restriction cases, consistent with a decreased expression of Dnmt1, but the demethylation was clusterized on the chromosomes, suggesting heterogeneous sensitivity to diet-induced methylation alterations. Imprinted genes were enriched in the list of deregulated genes, a recurrent feature of the effects of diet on epigenetic deregulation. In the same comprehensive study,

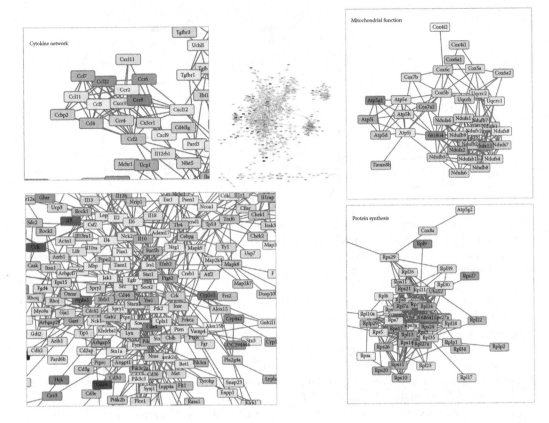

FIGURE 4.4 The diet-restricted placenta displays abnormal gene regulation in clusters. Among the clusters presenting a concerted modification of expression, cytokine signaling effectors (top, left) and mitochondrial function and oxydo-reduction regulation (top, right) are very clearly identified as discrete groups of genes. RNAs involved in the ribosome components, and thus involved in protein synthesis, are very consistently less abundant, suggesting a slowing down of protein synthesis after protein deprivation (bottom, right). A dense group of transcripts more abundant in protein-restricted placenta is presented at the bottom left. This cluster is centered on Cd44, Pik3, Ptgs2, and Stat5, suggesting activation of inflammatory cascade and apoptosis, response to wounding after diet restriction in the placenta. (From Buffat C., *J Pathol* 213 (3): 337–46, 2007.)

the methylation of miRNA-encoding genes was also affected, especially calorie restriction-induced methylation and overexpression of miR-149.

Ganguly and coworkers also studied the methylation of the 5′-flanking region of the glut3 gene (Slc2A3), an important component of materno–fetal regulation of nutrient exchanges (Constancia et al. 2005). They demonstrate a slightly increased methylation in the group exposed to caloric restriction, correlated with a decreased level of Glut3 mRNA in the placenta. The authors also addressed by chromatin immunoprecipitation-quantitative polymerase chain reaction (ChIP-qPCR) the interaction of the promoter with several DNA-interacting proteins and found an increased presence of MeCP2, DNMT3B, and HDAC2, while SP1 was reduced on the Glut3 promoter.

Except in exceptional situations, the epigenetic effects of diet-induced IUGR could not be scientifically analyzed in the human placenta. Nevertheless, there are abundant proofs showing associations between IUGR and human placental abnormal epigenetic regulation at specific genes. One of the first observations relates to the abnormal methylation of the chromosome 11 imprinted region encompassing IGF2 and H19 in cases of small for gestational age babies (SGA) (Wu, Starzinski-Powitz, and Guo 2008), correlated with a decreased expression of IGF2. These alterations of placental gene methylation are far from concerning only demonstrated imprinted genes: alterations of methylation in IUGR could be identified in Cullin genes, such as CUL4B and CUL7 (Gascoin-Lachambre et al. 2010). Cullins are proteins that are part of the ubiquitin–ligase complex, leading to the ubiquitinylation of target proteins. CUL4B and CUL7 mRNAs are increased in IUGR placentas, consistent with the idea that the shortage in nutrients induces an accelerated turnover of cellular proteins, allowing recycling of amino acids and using them to either generate energy or reconstruct novel proteins after coupling with matched tRNA by specific tRNA ligases. Genes involved in lipid metabolism, such as TBX15, are also found to be epigenetically deregulated (Chelbi et al. 2012), as well as proteins important for body and energy homeostasis, such as SERPINA3 (Chelbi et al. 2007, 2012).

4.4 SENSING DIET RESTRICTION/DIET ALTERATIONS

Identifying the effects of abnormal maternal diet on the placenta and trophoblast is relatively straightforward using high-throughput approaches available today. However, finding the key sensors of maternal nutritional exchanges remains a complex challenge. A recurrent pathway mentioned in diet-induced stress is the mammalian target of rapamycin (mTOR) pathway. The mTOR kinase is known to be sensitive to nutrients, energy availability, and growth factors, and this has been clearly and recurrently reported in the placenta, in various species (Kavitha et al. 2014; Kim et al. 2013; Knuth et al. 2015; Larque, Ruiz-Palacios, and Koletzko 2013; Rosario et al. 2011). This pathway has been shown to be central to trophoblast invasion and, thus, for placental success (Busch et al. 2009; Gonzalez et al. 2012; Ross et al. 2009). The last very elegant study by Gonzalez and coworkers shows unambiguously that arginin and leucin are indispensable for trophoblast outgrowth in culture, through the activation of mTOR but independently from its transcription, with these results making the link between "diet sensing" and trophoblast biology. This has recently been substantiated by a recent study by Knuth and coworkers that analyzes a cell model of first-trimester placenta (SW71), cultivated with rapamycin, with or without addition of the placental growth factor (PlGF). Phosphorylation of mTOR was decreased by rapamycin treatment, and this was associated with a decrease in trophoblast invasion, itself counterbalanced by PlGF treatment (Knuth et al. 2015). PlGF has an important impact on adipose tissue equilibrium (Lijnen et al. 2006) and the regulation of adipogenesis (Christiaens et al. 2007) and is thus an important regulator of nutrient exchanges and metabolism.

Besides this primary sensing of harsh conditions, it appears clearly that imprinted genes, functioning as a network (Varrault et al. 2006), constitute the major cellular machine able to "sense" perturbed dietary environment and able to react in modulating the nutrient flux (Keverne 2014). Interestingly, several imprinted genes are transporters of amino acids, such as Slc38a4 or slc22a2. Fowden and coworkers showed that maternal undernutrition modulates negatively IGF2P0, the placental-specific promoter of the IGF2 gene (Constancia et al. 2002) and Slc38a4, and up-regulates Slc38a2 (Fowden et al. 2011). Very recently, Iglesias-Platas et al. (2014) analyzed the imprinted transcription factor *PLAGL1* in human placentas from adequate of gestational age (AGA) and SGA pregnancies. The authors showed that there is a sex-specific difference in expression where *PLAGL1* is up-regulated in the placenta from girls. They also show an overall decrease in the expression of this gene associated with the use of assisted reproductive technologies, consistent with many earlier reports in mice showing that imprinted genes are affected by these technologies (Fauque et al. 2007; Fauque et al. 2010a,b). ChIP analysis revealed a direct interaction of PLAGL1 with the promoters and imprinting control region of H19 and with the promoter region of SLC2A4. Outside imprinted genes, PLAGL1 interacts with important metabolism-involved transcription factors, such as peroxisome proliferator-activated receptor gamma (PPARγ) and transcription factor 4 (TCF4). Analyzing the methylation of the PLAGL1 DMR in normal and SGA placentas did not reveal any alterations in the imprinted-characteristic hemimethylation profile of this DMR, suggesting that the expression differences are not linked to an imprinted defect.

4.5   ADDITIVE ALTERATIONS OF THE DIET (HIGH FAT, HIGH SUGAR FOOD, LONG POLYUNSATURATED FATTY ACIDS, AND EPIGENETIC MODULATORS)

It is now well demonstrated that placental structure and function are modified after food deprivation, with a specific modification of genes modulating epigenetic mechanisms. This suggests that these placenta modifications could follow adaption to inadequate environmental conditions triggered by food deprivation. Such modification can also be caused symmetrically by food excess or unbalanced food composition (low protein, high fat, high sugar–high fat, etc.). In two elegant papers, Gallou-Kabani and coworkers explored the putative epigenetic effects of high-fat diet consumed during pregnancy on the placentas of mice. After an evaluation of the global methylation pattern by the Luminometric Methylation Assay technique (Karimi et al. 2006), the study focused on the expression of 20 imprinted genes. Interestingly, the authors discovered expression and methylation differences that were sexually dimorphic (Gallou-Kabani et al. 2010). The placentas were larger and heavier in males and females from high-fat diet mothers, albeit the "male" placentas were larger in any case than the "female" placentas. The effect of diet was significant for *Rtl1* and three imprinted transporter genes, *Slc22a1*, *Slc22a2*, and *Slc22a3*. Sex-specific differences were also visible for *Peg10*, *Slc22a1*, and *Slc22a2*. Less stringent statistical analysis also revealed a female expression modification for *Dlk1* and *Dio3*. Also, independently from the diet, *Asb4*, *Peg3*, and *Ascl2* were found sexually dimorphic at the expression level. The global methylation analysis revealed that the placenta was overall demethylated, but exclusively in females. When focusing on a CpG island shared by Igf2R and Air on chromosome 17, the methylation was increased in female placenta when the mother was exposed to a high-fat diet, while no significant effect was detected in the male placentas. In the following paper of the same team (Gabory et al. 2012), the placentas were analyzed by a whole genome microarray approach. While numerous genes were deregulated in a sex-specific fashion (164 in the females and 171 in the males), only 11 were not influenced by the diet, 3 of them belonging to the X and 3 belonging to the Y chromosome. Only 16 genes were modified similarly in males and females. The study also reveals that the gene ontology pathways of modified genes are very different between the two sexes whose mothers were exposed to a high-fat diet during pregnancy. In a recent study (Kim et al. 2014), the mouse placenta of normal and obese mice was analyzed using various approaches (histology, flow cytometry, qPCR, and multiplex cytokine analysis), unfortunately not in terms of epigenetic questions. Nevertheless, another study using obesogenic diet in mice showed that together with very clear-cut phenotypical differences, alterations in the expression of imprinted genes were present in the placenta (Sferruzzi-Perri et al. 2013).

These results obtained in mice are comforted in several human studies. For instance, a recent series of papers by Lappas and coworkers analyzed the effects of maternal obesity on the placenta on genes involved in inflammation and apoptosis (SLIT2, NR4A receptors, and cIAP1 and cIAP2) (Lim and Lappas 2015; Lappas 2014a,b,c) and showed unambiguously that obesity triggers "negative" effects (increased inflammation and increased apoptosis mechanisms). The same cohort of patients was investigated for energy parameter anomalies such as placental mitochondrial activity (Hastie and Lappas 2014). This revealed a decrease in the number of mitochondria and activity of complex I, II, and III and an increase in H_2O_2, suggesting an altered placental function and increased oxidative stress. Another recent interventional study applied maternal omega-3 polyunsaturated acid diet, followed by transcriptome analysis of placental gene expression (Sedlmeier et al. 2014). The study incorporated 208 Western European women with body mass index of 18 and 30. One group received an n-3 supplementation (docosahéxaénoic acid [DHA], eicosapentaénoic acid [EPA]), in addition to an advised healthy diet. An interesting outcome, supporting the rodent results, showed a very clear and major effect of placental sex on gene expression, but this effect was more moderate in the omega-3 women (387 genes deregulated versus only 53, and only 12 in common). The intervention taking into account only the males resulted in 66 differential genes, 166 for the females and 133 when both sexes were considered as a whole. For the present review, a novel analysis of the dataset of the study (GSE53291) was performed (Figure 4.5). The gene network was produced using String and Cytoscape as described previously (Section 4.3, Figure 4.5a), and an essential network was calculated showing the topology of the network that revealed a central position for p53 (Figure 4.5b), also clearly visible when the network was restricted to the subset of the genes having a degree of connections above 10 (Figure 4.5c). Finally, analyzing the promoters of these minimal essential network genes revealed pivotal functions for transcription factors E2F6, DDX20, and FOXM1 (Figure 4.5d). Interestingly, FOXM1 is a major regulator of cell cycle and cell divisions (Kalin, Ustiyan, and Kalinichenko 2011). In terms of epigenetic regulators, a precise analysis revealed significant striking differences between the sexes. In the females, CHD4 (chromodomain-containing proteins generally associated to methylated histones and the RNA-induced transcriptional complex, and thus to chromatin silencing) was down-regulated and HDAC5 was upregulated. In males, BRD2 (bromodomain-containing proteins associated to acetylated

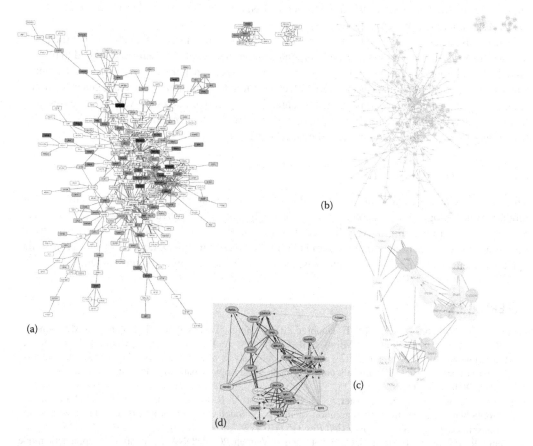

FIGURE 4.5 Reanalysis of the microarray data by Seldmeier and coworkers (effect of a polyunsaturated complemented diet on maternal placental expression, 2014) by Cytoscape. The network of interacting genes is shown in panel a, showing a cluster of heavily down-regulated genes (ANAPC4, CEP192, FGF2, SYCP2, RAD51AP, RFC3, and PCNA), centered around Tp53, itself mildly induced. Several of these genes are involved in mitosis regulation, suggesting a possible slowing of cell division processes and of proliferation. Topology analysis leading to identification of a minimal essential network (b and c) confirms this central position of TP53 as a major node of the network. (d) iREGULON promoter analysis pinpointed crucial transcription factors recognizing specific promoter motives in the modified genes, such as E2F6 and DDX20 and in particular FOXM1, putatively explaining the hierarchy of regulation leading to the down-regulation of cell-cycle-related genes.

lysine marks and therefore to open chromatin) was increased, while MBD2 (a methylated DNA binding protein, contributing to repressed expression) was down-regulated. In sum, this very recent study shows clearly that supplementation in the diet induces important effects on the placenta with a differential activation of the epigenetic machinery.

While protein alterations modify epigenetic modulators in the rat and other animal models, several teams attempted to adapt these modulations by the addition of specific molecules playing the role of donors in epigenetic cascades. Among those, nicotinamide (NAD; also called niacin or vitamin B3) is a major negative regulator in the production of *S*-adenosyl-methionine, since it enters in the cycle as a competitor for methyl groups; contrastingly, betaine is an important donor of methyl groups, not renewable, compared to other donors such as methionine or folate that come back in the cycle after reaction. Very recently, Tian et al. (2014) studied the effect of NAD supplementation on placental and liver development in the rat model. The expression of genes involved in epigenetic regulation, such as Dnmt1, and in proliferation and cell division (p53) was altered. The catalase expression was considerably augmented by NAD and even more by betaine. Expression of nicotinamide *N*-methyltransferase (*Nnmt*), a major actor of NAD transport, was significantly increased in the liver but not in the placenta.

While this review focuses on the maternal diet, there are now increasing evidence that the paternal diet plays also a very important role in pregnancy consequences, this being associated to placental defects and, thus, alterations of trophoblast biology. A recent paper showed that folate deficiency alters sperm methylation and is associated with expression deregulation of placental genes (Lambrot et al. 2013). Epigenetic alterations of the placenta, future putative marks of systemic diseases, may therefore come by both parents. In sum, both parents' ways of life and diet have impact on trophoblast biology, placental development, and health later in life.

4.6 CONCLUSIONS

This review attempts to sum up available data showing how trophoblast nutritional environment modulates its biology and, thus, on a larger scale, the biology/structure/function of the placenta. The available literature is still relatively limited, but it is clearly to be expected in the future that these questions will raise increasing interests and that the number of mechanistic studies dealing with the epigenetic sensors/modulators of trophoblast biology will become much better defined.

REFERENCES

Buffat, C., F. Mondon, V. Rigourd, F. Boubred, B. Bessieres, L. Fayol, J. M. Feuerstein, M. Gamerre, H. Jammes, R. Rebourcet, F. Miralles, B. Courbieres, A. Basire, F. Dignat-Georges, B. Carbonne, U. Simeoni, and D. Vaiman. 2007. "A hierarchical analysis of transcriptome alterations in intrauterine growth restriction (IUGR) reveals common pathophysiological pathways in mammals." *J Pathol* 213 (3):337–46. doi:10.1002/path.2233.

Busch, S., S. J. Renaud, E. Schleussner, C. H. Graham, and U. R. Markert. 2009. "mTOR mediates human trophoblast invasion through regulation of matrix-remodeling enzymes and is associated with serine phosphorylation of STAT3." *Exp Cell Res* 315 (10):1724–33. doi:10.1016/j.yexcr.2009.01.026.

Calicchio, R., L. Doridot, F. Miralles, C. Mehats, and D. Vaiman. 2013. "DNA methylation, an epigenetic mode of gene expression regulation in reproductive science." *Curr Pharm Des* 20 (11):1726–50.

Cambuli, F., A. Murray, W. Dean, D. Dudzinska, F. Krueger, S. Andrews, C. E. Senner, S. J. Cook, and M. Hemberger. 2014. "Epigenetic memory of the first cell fate decision prevents complete ES cell reprogramming into trophoblast." *Nat Commun* 5:5538. doi:10.1038/ncomms6538.

Chamley, L. W., O. J. Holland, Q. Chen, C. A. Viall, P. R. Stone, and M. Abumaree. 2014. "Review: Where is the maternofetal interface?" *Placenta* 35 Suppl:S74–80. doi:10.1016/j.placenta.2013.10.014.

Chelbi, S. T., F. Mondon, H. Jammes, C. Buffat, T. M. Mignot, J. Tost, F. Busato, I. Gut, R. Rebourcet, P. Laissue, V. Tsatsaris, F. Goffinet, B. Carbonne, F. Ferre, and D. Vaiman. 2007. "Expressional and epigenetic alterations of placental serine protease inhibitors: SERPINA3 is a potential marker of preeclampsia." *Hypertension* 49 (1):76–83. doi:10.1161/01.HYP.0000250831.52876.cb.

Chelbi, S. T., M. L. Wilson, A. C. Veillard, S. A. Ingles, J. Zhang, F. Mondon, G. Gascoin-Lachambre, L. Doridot, T. M. Mignot, R. Rebourcet, B. Carbonne, J. P. Concordet, S. Barbaux, and D. Vaiman. 2012. "Genetic and epigenetic mechanisms collaborate to control SERPINA3 expression and its association with placental diseases." *Hum Mol Genet* 21 (9):1968–78. doi:10.1093/hmg/dds006.

Chen, P. Y., A. Ganguly, L. Rubbi, L. D. Orozco, M. Morselli, D. Ashraf, A. Jaroszewicz, S. Feng, S. E. Jacobsen, A. Nakano, S. U. Devaskar, and M. Pellegrini. 2013. "Intrauterine calorie restriction affects placental DNA methylation and gene expression." *Physiol Genomics* 45 (14):565–76. doi:10.1152/physiolgenomics.00034.2013.

Christiaens, V., G. Voros, I. Scroyen, and H. R. Lijnen. 2007. "On the role of placental growth factor in murine adipogenesis." *Thromb Res* 120 (3):399–405. doi:10.1016/j.thromres.2006.10.007.

Constancia, M., M. Hemberger, J. Hughes, W. Dean, A. Ferguson-Smith, R. Fundele, F. Stewart, G. Kelsey, A. Fowden, C. Sibley, and W. Reik. 2002. "Placental-specific IGF-II is a major modulator of placental and fetal growth." *Nature* 417 (6892):945–8.

Constancia, M., E. Angiolini, I. Sandovici, P. Smith, R. Smith, G. Kelsey, W. Dean, A. Ferguson-Smith, C. P. Sibley, W. Reik, and A. Fowden. 2005. "Adaptation of nutrient supply to fetal demand in the mouse involves interaction between the Igf2 gene and placental transporter systems." *Proc Natl Acad Sci U S A* 102 (52):19219–24. doi:10.1073/pnas.0504468103.

Dweep, H., C. Sticht, P. Pandey, and N. Gretz. 2011. "miRWalk—Database: Prediction of possible miRNA binding sites by "walking" the genes of three genomes." *J Biomed Inform* 44 (5):839–47. doi:10.1016/j.jbi.2011.05.002.

Fauque, P., P. Jouannet, C. Lesaffre, M. A. Ripoche, L. Dandolo, D. Vaiman, and H. Jammes. 2007. "Assisted Reproductive Technology affects developmental kinetics, H19 Imprinting Control Region methylation and H19 gene expression in individual mouse embryos." *BMC Dev Biol* 7:116. doi:10.1186/1471-213X-7-116.

Fauque, P., F. Mondon, F. Letourneur, M. A. Ripoche, L. Journot, S. Barbaux, L. Dandolo, C. Patrat, J. P. Wolf, P. Jouannet, H. Jammes, and D. Vaiman. 2010a. "In vitro fertilization and embryo culture strongly impact the placental transcriptome in the mouse model." *PLoS One* 5 (2):e9218. doi:10.1371/journal.pone.0009218.

Fauque, P., M. A. Ripoche, J. Tost, L. Journot, A. Gabory, F. Busato, A. Le Digarcher, F. Mondon, I. Gut, P. Jouannet, D. Vaiman, L. Dandolo, and H. Jammes. 2010b. "Modulation of imprinted gene network in placenta results in normal development of in vitro manipulated mouse embryos." *Hum Mol Genet* 19 (9):1779–90. doi:10.1093/hmg/ddq059.

Fowden, A. L., P. M. Coan, E. Angiolini, G. J. Burton, and M. Constancia. 2011. "Imprinted genes and the epigenetic regulation of placental phenotype." *Prog Biophys Mol Biol* 106 (1):281–8. doi:10.1016/j.pbiomolbio.2010.11.005.

Furukawa, S., Y. Kuroda, and A. Sugiyama. 2014. "A comparison of the histological structure of the placenta in experimental animals." *J Toxicol Pathol* 27 (1):11–8. doi:10.1293/tox.2013-0060.

Gabory, A., L. Ferry, I. Fajardy, L. Jouneau, J. D. Gothie, A. Vige, C. Fleur, S. Mayeur, C. Gallou-Kabani, M. S. Gross, L. Attig, A. Vambergue, J. Lesage, B. Reusens, D. Vieau, C. Remacle, J. P. Jais, and C. Junien. 2012. "Maternal diets trigger sex-specific divergent trajectories of gene expression and epigenetic systems in mouse placenta." *PLoS One* 7 (11):e47986. doi:10.1371/journal.pone.0047986.

Gallou-Kabani, C., A. Gabory, J. Tost, M. Karimi, S. Mayeur, J. Lesage, E. Boudadi, M. S. Gross, J. Taurelle, A. Vige, C. Breton, B. Reusens, C. Remacle, D. Vieau, T. J. Ekstrom, J. P. Jais, and C. Junien. 2010. "Sex- and diet-specific changes of imprinted gene expression and DNA methylation in mouse placenta under a high-fat diet." *PLoS One* 5 (12):e14398. doi:10.1371/journal.pone.0014398.

Ganguly, A., Y. Chen, B. C. Shin, and S. U. Devaskar. 2014. "Prenatal caloric restriction enhances DNA methylation and MeCP2 recruitment with reduced murine placental glucose transporter isoform 3 expression." *J Nutr Biochem* 25 (2):259–66. doi:10.1016/j.jnutbio.2013.10.015.

Garratt, M., J. M. Gaillard, R. C. Brooks, and J. F. Lemaitre. 2013. "Diversification of the eutherian placenta is associated with changes in the pace of life." *Proc Natl Acad Sci U S A* 110 (19):7760–5. doi:10.1073/pnas.1305018110.

Gascoin-Lachambre, G., C. Buffat, R. Rebourcet, S. T. Chelbi, V. Rigourd, F. Mondon, T. M. Mignot, E. Legras, U. Simeoni, D. Vaiman, and S. Barbaux. 2010. "Cullins in human intra-uterine growth restriction: Expressional and epigenetic alterations." *Placenta* 31 (2):151–7. doi:10.1016/j.placenta.2009.11.008.

Genbacev, O., M. Donne, M. Kapidzic, M. Gormley, J. Lamb, J. Gilmore, N. Larocque, G. Goldfien, T. Zdravkovic, M. T. McMaster, and S. J. Fisher. 2011. "Establishment of human trophoblast progenitor cell lines from the chorion." *Stem Cells* 29 (9):1427–36. doi:10.1002/stem.686.

Genbacev, O., J. D. Lamb, A. Prakobphol, M. Donne, M. T. McMaster, and S. J. Fisher. 2013. "Human trophoblast progenitors: Where do they reside?" *Semin Reprod Med* 31 (1):56–61. doi:10.1055/s-0032-1331798.

Gonzalez, I. M., P. M. Martin, C. Burdsal, J. L. Sloan, S. Mager, T. Harris, and A. E. Sutherland. 2012. "Leucine and arginine regulate trophoblast motility through mTOR-dependent and independent pathways in the preimplantation mouse embryo." *Dev Biol* 361 (2):286–300. doi:10.1016/j.ydbio.2011.10.021.

Haig, D. 1993. "Genetic conflicts in human pregnancy." *Q Rev Biol* 68 (4):495–532.

Hastie, R., and M. Lappas. 2014. "The effect of pre-existing maternal obesity and diabetes on placental mitochondrial content and electron transport chain activity." *Placenta* 35 (9):673–83. doi:10.1016/j.placenta.2014.06.368.

Heijmans, B. T., E. W. Tobi, A. D. Stein, H. Putter, G. J. Blauw, E. S. Susser, P. E. Slagboom, and L. H. Lumey. 2008. "Persistent epigenetic differences associated with prenatal exposure to famine in humans." *Proc Natl Acad Sci U S A* 105 (44):17046–9. doi:10.1073/pnas.0806560105.

Iglesias-Platas, I., A. Martin-Trujillo, P. Petazzi, A. Guillaumet-Adkins, M. Esteller, and D. Monk. 2014. "Altered expression of the imprinted transcription factor PLAGL1 deregulates a network of genes in the human IUGR placenta." *Hum Mol Genet* 23 (23):6275–85. doi:10.1093/hmg/ddu347.

Johansson, D., P. Lindgren, and A. Berglund. 2003. "A multivariate approach applied to microarray data for identification of genes with cell cycle-coupled transcription." *Bioinformatics* 19 (4):467–73.

Kalin, T. V., V. Ustiyan, and V. V. Kalinichenko. 2011. "Multiple faces of FoxM1 transcription factor: Lessons from transgenic mouse models." *Cell Cycle* 10 (3):396–405.

Karimi, M., S. Johansson, D. Stach, M. Corcoran, D. Grander, M. Schalling, G. Bakalkin, F. Lyko, C. Larsson, and T. J. Ekstrom. 2006. "LUMA (LUminometric Methylation Assay)—A high throughput method to the analysis of genomic DNA methylation." *Exp Cell Res* 312 (11):1989–95. doi:10.1016/j.yexcr.2006.03.006.

Kasiviswanathan, R., T. R. Collins, and W. C. Copeland. 2012. "The interface of transcription and DNA replication in the mitochondria." *Biochim Biophys Acta* 1819 (9–10):970–8. doi:10.1016/j.bbagrm.2011.12.005.

Kavitha, J. V., F. J. Rosario, M. J. Nijland, T. J. McDonald, G. Wu, Y. Kanai, T. L. Powell, P. W. Nathanielsz, and T. Jansson. 2014. "Down-regulation of placental mTOR, insulin/IGF-I signaling, and nutrient transporters in response to maternal nutrient restriction in the baboon." *FASEB J* 28 (3):1294–305. doi:10.1096/fj.13-242271.

Keverne, E. B. 2014. "Genomic imprinting, action, and interaction of maternal and fetal genomes." *Proc Natl Acad Sci U S A*. doi:10.1073/pnas.1411253111.

Kim, J., G. Song, G. Wu, H. Gao, G. A. Johnson, and F. W. Bazer. 2013. "Arginine, leucine, and glutamine stimulate proliferation of porcine trophectoderm cells through the MTOR-RPS6K-RPS6-EIF4EBP1 signal transduction pathway." *Biol Reprod* 88 (5):113. doi:10.1095/biolreprod.112.105080.

Kim, D. W., S. L. Young, D. R. Grattan, and C. L. Jasoni. 2014. "Obesity during pregnancy disrupts placental morphology, cell proliferation, and inflammation in a sex-specific manner across gestation in the mouse." *Biol Reprod* 90 (6):130. doi:10.1095/biolreprod.113.117259.

Knuth, A., L. Liu, H. Nielsen, D. Merril, D. S. Torry, and J. A. Arroyo. 2015. "Placenta growth factor induces invasion and activates p70 during rapamycin treatment in trophoblast cells." *Am J Reprod Immunol.* 73 (4):330–40. doi:10.1111/aji.12327.

Lambrot, R., C. Xu, S. Saint-Phar, G. Chountalos, T. Cohen, M. Paquet, M. Suderman, M. Hallett, and S. Kimmins. 2013. "Low paternal dietary folate alters the mouse sperm epigenome and is associated with negative pregnancy outcomes." *Nat Commun* 4:2889. doi:10.1038/ncomms3889.

Lappas, M. 2014a. "Cellular inhibitors of apoptosis (cIAP) 1 and 2 are increased in placenta from obese pregnant women." *Placenta* 35 (10):831–8. doi:10.1016/j.placenta.2014.07.011.

Lappas, M. 2014b. "Markers of endothelial cell dysfunction are increased in human omental adipose tissue from women with pre-existing maternal obesity and gestational diabetes." *Metabolism* 63 (6):860–73. doi:10.1016/j.metabol.2014.03.007.

Lappas, M. 2014c. "The NR4A receptors Nurr1 and Nur77 are increased in human placenta from women with gestational diabetes." *Placenta* 35 (11):866–75. doi:10.1016/j.placenta.2014.08.089.

Larque, E., M. Ruiz-Palacios, and B. Koletzko. 2013. "Placental regulation of fetal nutrient supply." *Curr Opin Clin Nutr Metab Care* 16 (3):292–7. doi:10.1097/MCO.0b013e32835e3674.

Lijnen, H. R., V. Christiaens, I. Scroyen, G. Voros, M. Tjwa, P. Carmeliet, and D. Collen. 2006. "Impaired adipose tissue development in mice with inactivation of placental growth factor function." *Diabetes* 55 (10):2698–704. doi:10.2337/db06-0526.

Lim, R., and M. Lappas. 2015. "Slit2 exerts anti-inflammatory actions in human placenta and is decreased with maternal obesity." *Am J Reprod Immunol.* 73 (1): 66–78. doi:10.1111/aji.12334.

Lumey, L. H., A. D. Stein, H. S. Kahn, K. M. van der Pal-de Bruin, G. J. Blauw, P. A. Zybert, and E. S. Susser. 2007. "Cohort profile: The Dutch Hunger Winter families study." *Int J Epidemiol* 36 (6):1196–204. doi:10.1093/ije/dym126.

Malandro, M. S., M. J. Beveridge, M. S. Kilberg, and D. A. Novak. 1996. "Effect of low-protein diet-induced intrauterine growth retardation on rat placental amino acid transport." *Am J Physiol* 271 (1 Pt 1):C295–303.

Maltepe, E., A. I. Bakardjiev, and S. J. Fisher. 2010. "The placenta: Transcriptional, epigenetic, and physiological integration during development." *J Clin Invest* 120 (4):1016–25. doi:10.1172/JCI41211.

Myatt, L. 2006. "Placental adaptive responses and fetal programming." *J Physiol.* 572 (Pt 1):25–30.

Niwa, H., Y. Toyooka, D. Shimosato, D. Strumpf, K. Takahashi, R. Yagi, and J. Rossant. 2005. "Interaction between Oct3/4 and Cdx2 determines trophectoderm differentiation." *Cell* 123 (5):917–29. doi:10.1016/j.cell.2005.08.040.

Reamon-Buettner, S. M., J. Buschmann, and G. Lewin. 2014. "Identifying placental epigenetic alterations in an intrauterine growth restriction (IUGR) rat model induced by gestational protein deficiency." *Reprod Toxicol* 45:117–24. doi:10.1016/j.reprotox.2014.02.009.

Redman, C. W., D. S. Tannetta, R. A. Dragovic, C. Gardiner, J. H. Southcombe, G. P. Collett, and I. L. Sargent. 2012. "Review: Does size matter? Placental debris and the pathophysiology of pre-eclampsia." *Placenta* 33 Suppl:S48–54. doi:10.1016/j.placenta.2011.12.006.

Renfree, M. B., A. T. Papenfuss, G. Shaw, and A. J. Pask. 2009. "Eggs, embryos and the evolution of imprinting: Insights from the platypus genome." *Reprod Fertil Dev* 21 (8):935–42. doi:10.1071/RD09092.

Rigourd, V., S. Chelbi, C. Chauvet, R. Rebourcet, S. Barbaux, B. Bessieres, F. Mondon, T. M. Mignot, J. L. Danan, and D. Vaiman. 2009. "Re-evaluation of the role of STOX1 transcription factor in placental development and preeclampsia." *J Reprod Immunol* 82 (2):174–81. doi:10.1016/j.jri.2009.05.001.

Roberts, C. T., A. Sohlstrom, K. L. Kind, P. A. Grant, R. A. Earl, J. S. Robinson, T. Y. Khong, P. C. Owens, and J. A. Owens. 2001. "Altered placental structure induced by maternal food restriction in guinea pigs: A role for circulating IGF-II and IGFBP-2 in the mother?" *Placenta* 22 Suppl A:S77–82. doi:10.1053/plac.2001.0643.

Rosario, F. J., N. Jansson, Y. Kanai, P. D. Prasad, T. L. Powell, and T. Jansson. 2011. "Maternal protein restriction in the rat inhibits placental insulin, mTOR, and STAT3 signaling and down-regulates placental amino acid transporters." *Endocrinology* 152 (3):1119–29. doi:10.1210/en.2010-1153.

Ross, J. W., M. D. Ashworth, D. R. Stein, O. P. Couture, C. K. Tuggle, and R. D. Geisert. 2009. "Identification of differential gene expression during porcine conceptus rapid trophoblastic elongation and attachment to uterine luminal epithelium." *Physiol Genomics* 36 (3):140–8. doi:10.1152/physiolgenomics.00022.2008.

Sedlmeier, E. M., S. Brunner, D. Much, P. Pagel, S. E. Ulbrich, H. H. Meyer, U. Amann-Gassner, H. Hauner, and B. L. Bader. 2014. "Human placental transcriptome shows sexually dimorphic gene expression and responsiveness to maternal dietary n-3 long-chain polyunsaturated fatty acid intervention during pregnancy." *BMC Genomics* 15:941. doi:10.1186/1471-2164-15-941.

Sferruzzi-Perri, A. N., O. R. Vaughan, M. Haro, W. N. Cooper, B. Musial, M. Charalambous, D. Pestana, S. Ayyar, A. C. Ferguson-Smith, G. J. Burton, M. Constancia, and A. L. Fowden. 2013. "An obesogenic diet during mouse pregnancy modifies maternal nutrient partitioning and the fetal growth trajectory." *FASEB J* 27 (10):3928–37. doi:10.1096/fj.13-234823.

Shannon, P., A. Markiel, O. Ozier, N. S. Baliga, J. T. Wang, D. Ramage, N. Amin, B. Schwikowski, and T. Ideker. 2003. "Cytoscape: A software environment for integrated models of biomolecular interaction networks." *Genome Res* 13 (11):2498–504. doi:10.1101/gr.1239303.

Shetty, S., R. Patil, and K. Ghosh. 2013. "Role of microparticles in recurrent miscarriages and other adverse pregnancies: A review." *Eur J Obstet Gynecol Reprod Biol* 169 (2):123–9. doi:10.1016/j.ejogrb.2013.02.011.

Snel, B., G. Lehmann, P. Bork, and M. A. Huynen. 2000. "STRING: A web-server to retrieve and display the repeatedly occurring neighbourhood of a gene." *Nucleic Acids Res* 28 (18):3442–4.

Subramanian, A., P. Tamayo, V. K. Mootha, S. Mukherjee, B. L. Ebert, M. A. Gillette, A. Paulovich, S. L. Pomeroy, T. R. Golub, E. S. Lander, and J. P. Mesirov. 2005. "Gene set enrichment analysis: A knowledge-based approach for interpreting genome-wide expression profiles." *Proc Natl Acad Sci U S A* 102 (43):15545–50. doi:10.1073/pnas.0506580102.

Suzuki, S., G. Shaw, T. Kaneko-Ishino, F. Ishino, and M. B. Renfree. 2011. "The evolution of mammalian genomic imprinting was accompanied by the acquisition of novel CpG islands." *Genome Biol Evol* 3:1276–83. doi:10.1093/gbe/evr104.

Tian, Y. J., N. Luo, N. N. Chen, Y. Z. Lun, X. Y. Gu, Z. Li, Q. Ma, and S. S. Zhou. 2014. "Maternal nicotinamide supplementation causes global DNA hypomethylation, uracil hypo-incorporation and gene expression changes in fetal rats." *Br J Nutr* 111 (9):1594–601. doi:10.1017/S0007114513004054.

Vaiman, D., G. Gascoin-Lachambre, F. Boubred, F. Mondon, J. M. Feuerstein, I. Ligi, I. Grandvuillemin, S. Barbaux, E. Ghigo, V. Achard, U. Simeoni, and C. Buffat. 2011. "The intensity of IUGR-induced transcriptome deregulations is inversely correlated with the onset of organ function in a rat model." *PLoS One* 6 (6):e21222. doi:10.1371/journal.pone.0021222.

Varrault, A., C. Gueydan, A. Delalbre, A. Bellmann, S. Houssami, C. Aknin, D. Severac, L. Chotard, M. Kahli, A. Le Digarcher, P. Pavlidis, and L. Journot. 2006. "Zac1 regulates an imprinted gene network critically involved in the control of embryonic growth." *Dev Cell* 11 (5):711–22. doi:10.1016/j.devcel.2006.09.003.

Warren, W. C., L. W. Hillier, J. A. Marshall Graves, E. Birney, C. P. Ponting, F. Grutzner, K. Belov, W. Miller, L. Clarke, A. T. Chinwalla, S. P. Yang, A. Heger, D. P. Locke, P. Miethke, P. D. Waters, F. Veyrunes, L. Fulton, B. Fulton, T. Graves, J. Wallis, X. S. Puente, C. Lopez-Otin, G. R. Ordonez, E. E. Eichler, L. Chen, Z. Cheng, J. E. Deakin, A. Alsop, K. Thompson, P. Kirby, A. T. Papenfuss, M. J. Wakefield, T. Olender, D. Lancet, G. A. Huttley, A. F. Smit, A. Pask, P. Temple-Smith, M. A. Batzer, J. A. Walker, M. K. Konkel, R. S. Harris, C. M. Whittington, E. S. Wong, N. J. Gemmell, E. Buschiazzo, I. M. Vargas Jentzsch, A. Merkel, J. Schmitz, A. Zemann, G. Churakov, J. O. Kriegs, J. Brosius, E. P. Murchison, R. Sachidanandam, C. Smith, G. J. Hannon, E. Tsend-Ayush, D. McMillan, R. Attenborough, W. Rens, M. Ferguson-Smith, C. M. Lefevre, J. A. Sharp, K. R. Nicholas, D. A. Ray, M. Kube, R. Reinhardt, T. H. Pringle, J. Taylor, R. C. Jones, B. Nixon, J. L. Dacheux, H. Niwa, Y. Sekita, X. Huang, A. Stark, P. Kheradpour, M. Kellis, P. Flicek, Y. Chen, C. Webber, R. Hardison, J. Nelson, K. Hallsworth-Pepin, K. Delehaunty, C. Markovic, P. Minx, Y. Feng, C. Kremitzki, M. Mitreva, J. Glasscock, T. Wylie, P. Wohldmann, P. Thiru, M. N. Nhan, C. S. Pohl, S. M. Smith, S. Hou, M. Nefedov, P. J. de Jong, M. B. Renfree, E. R. Mardis, and R. K. Wilson. 2008. "Genome analysis of the platypus reveals unique signatures of evolution." *Nature* 453 (7192):175–83. doi:10.1038/nature06936.

Wu, Y., A. Starzinski-Powitz, and S. W. Guo. 2008. "Prolonged stimulation with tumor necrosis factor-alpha induced partial methylation at PR-B promoter in immortalized epithelial-like endometriotic cells." *Fertil Steril* 90 (1):234–7. doi:10.1016/j.fertnstert.2007.06.008.

Zhang, Z., L. Zhang, L. Jia, P. Wang, and Y. Gao. 2013. "Association of Wnt2 and sFRP4 expression in the third trimester placenta in women with severe preeclampsia." *Reprod Sci* 20 (8):981–9. doi:10.1177/1933719112472740.

Section II

Maternal Nutrition and Fetal Growth and Development

5 Placental Amino Acid Transport in Response to Maternal Nutrition during Pregnancy

Allison L.B. Shapiro and Theresa L. Powell

CONTENTS

ABSTRACT

The extent of fetal growth and infant size at birth result from underlying genetics as well as in utero exposures that include nutrient availability. The placenta is a unique organ that mediates the influence of maternal nutrient status on nutrient delivery to the fetus. Alterations in maternal nutrient availability such as nutrient deficit or excess impact placental transport of nutrients and, therefore, the growth of the fetus. In this chapter, we describe two well-studied placental amino acid (AA) transport systems, System A and System L, and how maternal nutritional status impacts the expression and activity of these transporters. Research to date has established a clear, mechanistic relationship between maternal nutrient deficiency such as overall calorie restriction or protein restriction during pregnancy and reductions in AA transport mediated by System A and System L. On the other side of the spectrum, research into maternal overnutrition, either through maternal obesity, gestational diabetes, or dietary fat excess, has produced more variable findings, therefore supporting a call for further research into the role of placental AA transport in pregnancies experiencing nutrient excess and fetal overgrowth.

KEY WORDS

Placenta, amino acid transport, nutrition, small for gestational age, intrauterine growth restriction, large for gestational age, System A, System L, obesity, gestational diabetes.

5.1   INTRODUCTION

The perinatal period is a sensitive period for fetal development, and perturbations in growth during this period have been associated with chronic disease risk in later life. Specifically, small for gestational age (SGA) and large for gestational age (LGA) neonates are at increased risk of obesity and metabolic-related diseases in adulthood (Arends et al., 2005; Boney et al., 2005; Mericq et al., 2009; Reinehr et al., 2009; Yu et al., 2013). Maternal nutritional experiences during pregnancy, such as food insecurity (undernourishment) or obesity (overnourishment), contribute to these abnormal patterns of fetal growth (Belkacemi et al., 2010; Campbell et al., 2012; Ehrenberg et al., 2004; Jariyapitaksakul and Tannirandorn, 2013; Shin and Song, 2014), making interventions that target maternal nutrition potentially important for the prevention of chronic diseases in future generations. Therefore, it is critical to understand the mechanisms mediating the effects of maternal undernutrition and overnutrition on fetal development and long-term health.

In recent decades, the placenta has emerged as a target for research focusing on the transmission of maternal exposures to the fetus. The placenta is a dynamic organ responsible for production of hormones and for nutrient transfer between the mother and her fetus. The key macronutrients transported to the fetus are glucose, lipids, and amino acids (AAs), which are derived from the maternal diet and metabolism. Glucose is a key source of energy, while lipids are essential for neurodevelopment and fat accretion and as structural components in, for example, plasma membranes. AAs constitute building blocks for proteins and are therefore required for muscle and lean tissue development, and a significant portion of fetal AA uptake is used for energy production.

AA transport across the placenta is dependent on several factors, including placental size and surface area, blood oxygen concentration (Regnault et al., 2013), and nutrient transporter distribution and activity. Importantly, each of these factors is likely to be impacted by maternal nutrient restriction or excess during pregnancy, therefore contributing to adverse fetal growth. In this review, we will focus primarily on AAs, their transport across the placental barrier, and consequences of dysregulation of their transport related to maternal nutritional status.

5.2 SYNCYTIOTROPHOBLAST AA TRANSPORTERS

Transplacental AA transfer from the mother to the fetus occurs across a unique epithelial cell layer called the syncytiotrophoblast. This is a polarized syncytial epithelium with the maternal-facing membrane lined with microvilli (microvillous membrane [MVM]), which are in direct contact with maternal blood in the intervillous space. The fetal-facing plasma membrane or basal membrane (BM) is juxtaposed with the fetal capillary. The syncytial nature of this epithelia means that there are no lateral walls or tight junctions; all nutrients and waste products must primarily pass through the syncytiotrophoblast. Nutrient transporters are localized in both the MVM and BM, and differential localization on these membrane surfaces allows for vectorial transport of nutrients toward the fetus while waste products are directed toward the maternal circulation.

While many of the known human AA transporters have been described in the placenta, two transport systems, System A and System L, have been most extensively studied. System A is responsible for transporting neutral AAs such as serine and alanine, and System L exchanges essential AAs such as leucine for nonessential AAs transported by System A. In this way, these two systems function in synergy, with System A's Na+-dependent active transport of neutral AAs across the MVM, supporting an intracellular concentration gradient that is needed by System L to exchange essential AAs in an Na+-independent mechanism (Verrey, 2003). These two systems create a concentration gradient with high cytoplasmic levels of both essential and nonessential AAs, which allows for diffusion across the BM to the fetal circulation (Cleal et al., 2007, 2011).

Placental AA uptake by System A involves activity of three protein isoforms, sodium-coupled neutral AA transporter (SNAT) 1, SNAT 2, and SNAT 4, with varying expressions throughout pregnancy. Recent studies have shown that SNAT 4 is significantly more active in early pregnancy compared with late pregnancy, whereas SNAT 1 and 2 are active from early pregnancy to term (Desforges et al., 2006, 2009). The consistency of SNAT 1 and 2 activity throughout pregnancy, along with differences in the binding affinities for AAs, suggests that these isoforms of System A are primarily responsible for maintaining the concentration gradient of neutral AAs within the syncytiotrophoblast, which is needed for continued exchange of essential AAs for use by the growing fetus. The role of SNAT 1 and 2 in maintaining the concentration gradient throughout pregnancy highlights the potential impact on essential AA delivery to the fetus through exchange by System L if either SNAT 1 or 2 expression and activity are altered.

System L is similarly composed of several protein isoforms. Unlike System A, System L transporters are heterodimers made up of a light chain protein, large neutral AA transporter (LAT) 1 or LAT 2, and a heavy chain protein 4f2hc/CD98 (Verrey, 2003). System L isoforms LAT 1 and LAT 2 are polarized in the syncytiotrophoblast, where LAT 1 is predominantly found on the maternal-facing MVM and LAT 2 is localized to the fetal-facing BM (Kudo and Boyd, 2001). This localization is believed to facilitate the exchange of essential AAs across the two membranes toward the fetus. Further, LAT 1 expression is significantly higher at term compared with midpregnancy (Okamoto et al., 2002), suggesting accelerated delivery of essential AAs as pregnancy progresses and fetal growth rates are maximal.

5.3 INFLUENCE OF MATERNAL NUTRIENT DEFICIENCY ON PLACENTAL AA TRANSPORTERS

Chronic food insecurity is experienced by 11.3% of the world's population, with the greatest burden shouldered by populations living in developing nations (Food and Agricultural Organization of the United Nations, 2014). However, in the United States, it was estimated that in 2013, 14.3% of households experienced food insecurity, and of those households, 5.6% were living with very low food security (Coleman-Jensen et al., 2014). These estimates highlight the continued global struggle in both developed and developing countries to provide adequate nutrition to individuals and families, including pregnant women.

Nutrient restriction during pregnancy is a well-established risk factor for the delivery of SGA and intrauterine growth restricted (IUGR) infants (Belkacemi et al., 2010; Campbell et al., 2012; Jariyapitaksakul and Tannirandorn, 2013). Many of the proposed mechanisms linking maternal nutrient restriction and restricted intrauterine fetal growth involve changes in placental function, with placental AA transport playing a major role (Lager and Powell, 2012; Sibley et al., 2005). In animal models, reduced expression and activity of the AA transport Systems A and L in response to global maternal nutrient deficit and isocaloric protein restriction have been consistently demonstrated (Coan et al., 2010; Jansson et al., 2006; Kavitha et al., 2014; Rosario et al., 2011). Further, animal models have provided evidence that disruption of fetal growth due to maternal undernourishment and placental AA transporter down-regulation is evident primarily in the later stages of pregnancy (Coan et al., 2010). These findings suggest that in maternal undernutrition, placental nutrient transport capacity becomes insufficient to meet the nutrient requirements to support normal growth during the period of rapid fetal growth in late gestation.

Reduced placental size in nutrient-restricted pregnancies may be a strong indicator of the placenta's failure to meet fetal growth demands. In a study by Coan and colleagues (2010), rat dams fed a globally restricted diet, which was 80% of the calories provided in the control diet, were found to have significantly smaller placentas by mass and volume (Coan et al., 2010). In human IUGR placentas, a parallel phenomenon is observed. Jansson et al. (2002a) found that placentas of human IUGR pregnancies weighed 40% less than placentas from uncomplicated pregnancies. This significant reduction in placental mass among IUGR pregnancies was also reported by Mahendran et al. (1993). The reduced size of the placenta limits the surface area across which AA transporters are expressed and distributed. Therefore, the fetus experiences a double-hit with AA transporter availability and activity per unit plasma membrane reduced in the IUGR placenta along with a reduced placental size. Both of these placental characteristics will contribute to reduce fetal nutrient availability and limit fetal growth.

Several studies have shown that the extent of AA transporter down-regulation, specifically System A in the MVM, is related to the severity of growth restriction (Glazier et al., 1997; Jansson et al., 2002a). Furthermore, specific isoforms of the System A transporter family are disproportionately affected. Mandò et al. (2013) found that the gene expression of System A isoform, SNAT 2, was significantly lower (–27%) in IUGR placentas compared with placentas from uncomplicated pregnancies, but the large difference was driven by the two most severe IUGR groups (IUGR with abnormal pulsatility index plus normal fetal heart rate or IUGR with abnormal pulsatility index plus abnormal fetal heart rate). While gestational age-dependent reductions in System A transporters and IUGR have not been consistently reported in human studies, several studies in the rat model have established that decreased placental System A transporter activity precedes growth restriction of the fetus in response to maternal protein restriction (Jansson et al., 2006; Rosario et al., 2011).

Placental System L transporters are also impacted by undernutrition, further disrupting the flux of AAs to the fetus, specifically essential AAs. Kavitha et al. (2014) demonstrated that protein expressions of System L isoforms LAT 1 and LAT 2 were significantly reduced in the placentas of diet-restricted baboons, and this paralleled the significantly lower fetal serum essential AA concentration. In human placentas, Jansson et al. (1998) measured the uptake of radiolabeled AA by System L in isolated membrane vesicles from IUGR pregnancies and found significant reductions in leucine uptake by both the MVM and BM. In contrast to the work of Jansson et al., Aiko et al. (2014) recently observed significant increases in the heavy chain protein, 4f2hc, and light chain protein, LAT 1, of System L in human IUGR placental explants. However, the increases in the System L proteins observed by Aiko and colleagues are difficult to relate to the activity of System L-mediated transport because the protein levels were measured in the cytosol and not in the cell membrane, suggesting that the proteins measured were not actively involved in the exchange of essential AAs. The increased protein expression in the cytosol, however, indicates that the mechanism of AA transporter protein translocation to the cell membrane may be an important process that is affected by restricted maternal nutrition. Further research is needed to corroborate the work of the Jansson group and to further explain the role of System L AA transporter proteins in the pathology of IUGR.

While global nutrient restriction has a demonstrated impact on fetal growth through reduction in AA transport, protein restriction alone can mimic these same consequences, suggesting that protein availability may be a significant nutritional signal to which the placenta responds. In the human BeWo cell line, exposure to media lacking nonessential AAs with physiological levels of essential AA significantly down-regulated expression of SNAT 1, but SNAT 2 expression and localization to the cell membrane were significantly increased (Jones et al., 2006), suggesting that SNAT 2 may be involved in compensatory AA transport when SNAT 1 is down-regulated. Jones and colleagues also found that the removal of nonessential AAs had no effect on System L transporters, possibly due to the up-regulation of SNAT 2, which may have maintained the intracellular nonessential AA levels needed for System L to continue essential AA exchange. These cell culture models suggest that placental AA transporters may adapt in response to AA deprivation. However, in vivo models afford a more holistic view of placental AA transporters and their response to whole-body (maternal) changes in the endocrine environment that result from nutrient deficit.

Observations in vivo using an isocaloric, protein-restricted pregnant rat model have shown similar results to the in vitro studies. Placental expressions of the System A isoform, SNAT 2, and System L isoforms, LAT 1 and LAT 2, were significantly lower in rat dams fed an isocaloric diet with 4% protein compared with dams fed a normal protein diet (18%). This reduction in expression was coupled with an overall reduction in System A and System L activity (Rosario et al., 2011). Malandro et al. (1996) also demonstrated that System A activity was significantly lower in both the MVM and BM of trophoblast from protein-restricted rat dams compared with dams on a protein-appropriate isocaloric diet. These data implicate dietary protein restriction as the key mechanism causing reduction in placental AA transport in maternal undernourishment, suggesting that from a nutritional standpoint, dietary protein supplementation may be an effective intervention for women experiencing food insecurity and who are at risk of suboptimal nutrition in pregnancy.

Undernutrition in pregnancy continues to present challenges to growth and development and results in a greater health risk throughout life for individuals who are born small. Understanding the mechanisms by which different dietary patterns or nutrition components contribute to the patho-physiology of placental AA transport that result in a small baby will help to drive the development of practical and effective interventions.

5.4 EFFECT OF MATERNAL NUTRIENT EXCESS ON PLACENTAL AA TRANSPORTERS

Overweight and obesity have been increasing over the past five decades and are now experienced by more than 60% of Americans (Flegal et al., 2010; Ogden et al., 2014) and a growing number of Europeans (Anonymous, 2010). Consequently over half of US women of reproductive age are overweight or obese (Flegal et al., 2010), making this the most prevalent pregnancy complication. The intrauterine environment of overweight and obese mothers imparts significant risk for the offspring (Boney et al., 2005; Yu et al., 2013), and these mothers are also at increased risk of preg-nancy complications (Avcı et al., 2014; Galtier-Dereure et al., 2000). While not every obese mother gives birth to an LGA neonate, the risk of fetal overgrowth among the pregnant obese population compared with lean pregnant women ranges between 1.4 and 18 (Galtier-Dereure et al., 2000). It has also been shown that overweight and obese mothers give birth to larger babies compared with weight-appropriate mothers (Catalano et al., 2009; Starling et al., 2015). Furthermore, the body composition of a neonate is dependent on the mother's body mass index (BMI), with higher pre-pregnancy BMI being significantly associated with higher fat mass but not lean mass (Catalano et al., 2009; Starling et al., 2015). The increased risk of LGA as well as the observed increased overall body mass and fat mass suggest that the nutrient-rich environment provided by overweight or obese mothers may enhance placental nutrient transport, providing a potential pathway to fetal overgrowth.

As in pregnancies where low placental weight contributes to the IUGR phenotype, higher placen-tal weight in overweight and obese pregnancies is also linked to fetal overgrowth. Placental hyper-trophy is more common in overweight and obese human pregnancies and is significantly related to higher birth weight (Wallace et al., 2012) and LGA (Jansson et al., 2002a). Larger placentas have also been linked to increases in AA transporter activity. In a study of human diabetic pregnancies, the placentas from the women with diabetes of any type weighed significantly more and were found to have significantly increased MVM System A activity compared with those from control preg-nancies (Jansson et al., 2002b). This suggested increased AA transporter activity, coupled with the observation that larger placentas are more likely to result from pregnancies experiencing obesity, provides a potential link between maternal obesity and increased nutrient transport of AAs and the resulting larger infant.

While the larger placenta and a corresponding increase in AA transport represent a possible double-hit to the fetus, reports on placental AA transport in maternal obesity are inconsistent. Farley and colleagues reported a significant reduction in activity of System A transporters in asso-ciation with maternal obesity in both human (Farley et al., 2010) and nonhuman primate (Farley et al., 2009) studies. Specifically, the expression of SNAT 4 in the MVM was significantly decreased in placentas of obese women compared with control pregnancies (Farley et al., 2010). Similarly, in the obese baboon, System A activity was suppressed and the fetal-to-maternal AA ratio was lower compared with controls (Farley et al., 2009), indicating that a global reduction in placental AA flux may be a consequence of obesity in pregnancy. However, despite the findings, the offspring in both studies by Farley and colleagues were of normal weight; therefore, the differences in System A transporter activity and expression are not directly reflective of the obese pregnancies that give rise to fetal overgrowth. This also suggests that there may be an additional factor that mediates the relationship between maternal obesity and fetal overgrowth, in addition to increased AA transport. Another study found that there was no difference in System A or L activity in the MVM of placen-tas from women in a high-BMI group compared with women in a normal-BMI group but that there was a significant, positive correlation between expression of SNAT 2 and maternal early pregnancy

BMI (Jansson et al., 2013). In the same study, the Jansson group also found that the MVM SNAT 2 expression and System A activity were significantly and positively correlated with birth weight, implicating AA transporter expression and activity as potential markers of increased fetal growth. Collectively, the available data on placental AA transport in maternal obesity are limited and inconsistent and do not allow firm conclusions. It is possible that placental AA transport is enhanced and contributes to fetal overgrowth in the subgroup of obese women that do deliver a large baby. However, further research is required to address this possibility.

Compared with overweight and obese women, women who have diabetes during pregnancy (type 1 [T1DM] or 2 diabetes mellitus or gestational diabetes [GDM]) are a group with a more severe spectrum of metabolic disease that can cause fetal overgrowth. Among women with GDM, the risk of having an LGA infant is twice that of women without diabetes in pregnancy and risk of macrosomia is 2.5 times greater (Bowers et al., 2013). One suggested mechanism to explain accelerated fetal growth involves increased fetal pancreatic insulin response (hyperinsulinemia) due to excess maternal glucose availability from the diabetic mother. However, AA transporters may also play a significant role. Among women who gave birth to LGA neonates and in all diabetes groups studied (GDM and T1DM), Jansson et al. (2002a) reported that System A activity in the MVM was increased 60%–80% above that in placentas from pregnancies that were not complicated by diabetes. Further, System L transport of leucine was also significantly increased in placentas from GDM pregnancies that gave rise to LGA offspring (Jansson et al., 2002a). From these data, the resulting LGA infant from a diabetic pregnancy may be due, in part, to an increase in AA transport through Systems A and L. However, it remains unclear whether the maternal diabetes is the cause of increased placental AA transporter expression and activity or if the LGA fetus is itself the driver of increased nutrient transport. Investigation of AA transporter activity and expression in pregnancies complicated by diabetes and that give rise to babies born on the higher end of the appropriate for gestational age spectrum is lacking in the literature and could provide further evidence for the mechanism of fetal overgrowth and the independent role of maternal diabetes as an overnutrition exposure during pregnancy.

Despite the work by Jansson and colleagues, conflicting results remain in both human and nonhuman pregnant models of diabetes. Kuruvilla et al. (1994) found a 49% reduction in MVM System A activity in the placentas of LGA infants born to diabetic mothers. In a study using pregnant rats exposed to acute hyperglycemic conditions in early and late pregnancy, Ericsson et al. (2007) observed no change in either System L or System A expression but a significant decrease in System A activity. Furthermore, in cell culture experiments with BeWo cells, exposure to diabetic conditions had no effect on System L transporter activity (Araújo et al., 2013). The inconsistency between human and animal models again highlights the need for further research on alterations in AA transport among human diabetic pregnancies.

Given the dramatic and ubiquitous shift to a high-fat diet (HFD) in developed countries such as the United States (Austin et al., 2011), it is pertinent to understand the relationship between dietary nutrient excess in the absence of overt obesity on placental transport. However, the contribution of an energy-rich diet and specific dietary components to placental transport of AAs independent of the maternal metabolic state is convoluted and difficult to establish. Unfortunately, few studies have attempted to identify the effect of diet on AA transport, but those that have done so find broadly consistent results. In the absence of maternal prepregnancy obesity, Lin et al. (2012) were able to demonstrate an up-regulation of System A expression in the placentas of pregnant rats fed an HFD throughout pregnancy with and without high fiber, suggesting that diet during pregnancy may have an important, additive role to maternal physiology on placental nutrient transport. Jones et al. (2009) have also found evidence of increased System A neutral AA transport in vivo as well as increased expression of the isoform SNAT 2 in a nonobese mouse model given an HFD before and during pregnancy.

Additionally, specific fatty acids have also been shown to impact AA transporter activity. Lager et al. (2013, 2014) found that treatment of cultured primary human trophoblast cells with oleic acid resulted in increased System A activity without affecting System L. Conversely, treatment of cultured trophoblast with docosahexaenoic acid (DHA) reduced System A activity (Lager et al., 2014). However, this is the only study investigating a specific nutrient's contribution to AA transport; therefore, the question remains whether it is the energy-rich diet or a specific component of the energy-rich diet that induces changes in placental transport of nutrients. Human studies of dietary excess and placental AA transport are also absent from the body of literature concerning placental response to overnutrition of specific dietary components.

Linking the evidence of increased AA transport as a result of dietary overnutrition to fetal overgrowth has proven to be more difficult. While Lin et al. (2012) and Jones et al. (2009) were able to demonstrate that the increase in AA transport paralleled increased fetal weight, models testing HFDs and overfeeding can produce variable results with regard to birth weight. Often, maternal HFD during pregnancy in animals can lead to a null change in offspring body weight above that of the control diet (Desai et al., 2014; Sun et al., 2012) and even IUGR (Tarrade et al., 2013). Furthermore, the lack of objective, unbiased, and accurate dietary recall tools makes the study of dietary overnutrition, and the impact on offspring growth, exceptionally difficult in humans.

5.5 REGULATION OF PLACENTAL SYSTEM A AND SYSTEM L ACTIVITY AND PROTEIN EXPRESSION

In addition to maternal nutritional fuels, maternal and placental metabolic factors that signal the availability of maternal nutrients such as insulin, leptin, and adiponectin also contribute to regulating AA transport across the placenta. In cultured trophoblast cells, both insulin and leptin have been shown to stimulate System A activity (Jansson et al., 2003; Von Versen-Höynck et al., 2009). Conversely, full-length adiponectin counters the stimulatory effect of insulin on System A activity (Jones et al., 2010) by reducing insulin sensitivity. In a study where full-length adiponectin was administered to pregnant mice during midgestation, both System A and L transport activity in the placenta was significantly repressed (−56% and −50%, respectively) with corresponding downregulation of SNAT 1, 2, and 4 and LAT 1 and 2 protein expression in the adiponectin-treated group versus the placebo group (Rosario et al., 2012). Fetal weights were also significantly lower in the adiponectin-treated group, corroborating the reductions in AA transporters.

Data supporting insulin's influence on System L expression and activity are less consistent. Roos et al. (2009b) found that insulin increased System L activity in cultured human trophoblast. However, in another study also using primary human trophoblast cell culture by Jones et al. (2010), insulin had a null effect on System L. Further, the impact of leptin and adiponectin on System L activity is currently unknown, highlighting a gap in knowledge that should be addressed by future research.

Novel cell signaling pathways involving protein kinases have also emerged as potentially important mechanisms influencing nutrient transport in the placenta. One in particular involves the mammalian target of rampamycin (mTOR). mTOR has been shown to function as a nutrient sensor in whole organ systems as well as individual cells (Wullschleger et al., 2006), and recently, the role of mTOR as a central regulator of placental nutrient transport has been suggested. Specifically, AA transporters are downstream targets of mTOR, and evidence suggests that mTOR may act to regulate their expression and membrane localization in the placenta in response to signals of nutrient availability (Roos et al., 2007, 2009). Roos et al. (2009) have shown that mTOR mediates the effect of insulin exposure in culture on System A and L activity in that when mTOR is blocked using rampamycin (a potent mTOR inhibitor), increasing insulin concentration ceases to increase the activity of System A and L. Furthermore, in cell culture, direct inhibition of mTOR significantly decreases the activity of both System A and L AA transport (Rosario et al., 2013), providing further in vivo evidence toward the regulatory mechanism of mTOR action in placental AA transport.

mTOR may also help to explain, in part, the link between IUGR and reduced placental AA transport. Recent studies of IUGR placentas have shown reduced mTOR protein levels and expression paralleling the reduced activity of System A and L (Roos et al., 2007). These studies remain associative, although research is ongoing to further understand the specific mechanisms of the mTOR signaling pathway and its role in placental dysfunction and perturbed fetal growth.

The response of placental AA transporters to factors that act as signals for nutrient availability provides a potential link between maternal nutrition and abnormal fetal growth, particularly in women who have diabetes or are obese during pregnancy (overnutrition) as these women generally have greater insulin resistance and higher insulin and leptin serum levels (Misra and Trudeau, 2011) as well as lower circulating adiponectin (Eriksson et al., 2010). In pregnancies that result in infants who are born small, placental mTOR appears to act as a strong nutrient sensor and it has been suggested that placental mTOR inhibition directly contributes to down-regulation of placental AA

TABLE 5.1
Expression and Activity of Placental Transporters in Response to Maternal Nutrient Deficit and Excess

	System A Activity and/or Expression	System L Activity and/or Expression	Supporting References
		Nutrient Deficit	
Calorie restriction with IUGR	↓a, b, c	↓d, e ↑f	a. Jansson et al., 2002a b. Glazier et al., 1997 c. Mandò et al., 2013 d. Kavitha et al., 2014 e. Jansson et al., 1998 f. Aiko et al., 2014
Protein restriction with IUGR	↓a, b, c	− c	a. Jansson et al., 2006 b. Rosario et al., 2011 c. Jones et al., 2006
		Nutrient Excess	
Obesity	↓a, b − c	− c	a. Farley et al., 2009 b. Farley et al., 2010 c. Jansson et al., 2013
Diabetes with LGA	↑a ↓b − c	↑a − c, d	a. Jansson et al., 2002a b. Kuruvilla et al., 1994 c. Ericsson et al., 2007 d. Araújo et al., 2013
High-fat diet	↑a, b	UK	a. Lin et al., 2012 b. Jones et al., 2009
Dietary oleic acid	↑a	UK	a. Lager et al., 2014
Dietary DHA	↓a	UK	a. Lager et al., 2014
		Regulatory Factors	
Insulin	↑a	↑b − c	a. Jansson et al., 2010 b. Roos et al., 2009 c. Jones et al., 2010
Leptin	↑a	UK	a. Von Versen-Höynck et al., 2009
Adiponectin[a]	↓a, b	↓b	a. Jones et al., 2010 b. Rosario et al., 2012
mTOR inhibition	↓a	↓a	a. Rosario et al., 2013

Note: ↑, Increased expression and/or activity; ↓, decreased expression and/or activity; −, no change observed; UK, unknown.

[a] Full-length adiponectin only.

transport in IUGR. The role of mTOR in obese and diabetic pregnancies has not yet been adequately addressed, although there is some evidence of increased mTOR signaling in placentas from obese pregnancies (Jansson et al., 2013). However, further research should investigate whether and how the mTOR signaling pathway mediates the relationship between obese and diabetic metabolism and placental AA transporter activity.

5.6 CONCLUDING REMARKS

Table 5.1 provides a summary of what is currently known about maternal nutritional status and placental AA transport systems. In summary, over the past decade, researchers have established a clear and consistent relationship between maternal undernutrition, both by overall calorie restriction and isocaloric protein restriction and reductions in placental AA transport with the resulting IUGR or SGA infant phenotype. The reduced AA transport, coupled with a smaller placenta, represents a double-hit to fetal growth in these pregnancies. The relationship between placental AA transport and nutrient excess is not as clear. While the risk of fetal overgrowth is higher in mothers who are obese and/or have diabetes during pregnancy, these are complex, multifaceted metabolic conditions with varying phenotypic profiles. Obesity, classified as having a BMI greater than 30 kg/m², may not accurately capture the maternal exposure that drives nutrient transport and the subsequent increased fetal growth. Maternal factors that are significantly related to obesity but that are not necessarily present at pathological levels in all obese women, such as higher insulin levels and lower adiponectin, may be the drivers of increased AA transport. Research that investigates maternal obesity with additional classification using maternal metabolic markers is needed to further understand the maternal phenotype that leads to placental AA transport-mediated accelerated fetal growth.

REFERENCES

Aiko, Y., D. J. Askew, S. Aramaki, M. Myoga, C. Tomonaga, T. Hachisuga, R. Suga, T. Kawamoto, M. Tsuji, and E. Shibata. 2014. "Differential Levels of Amino Acid Transporters System L and ASCT2, and the mTOR Protein in Placenta of Preeclampsia and IUGR." *BMC Pregnancy and Childbirth* 14: 181. doi:10.1186/1471-2393-14-181.

Anonymous. 2010. Strategy for Europe on nutrition, overweight and obesity related health issues. Implementation progress report. Directorate-General for Health and Consumers. European Commission, DG Health and Food Safety, Public Health, Nutrition and Physical Activity Policy. Available at http://ec.europa.eu/health/nutrition_physical_activity/policy/implementation_report_en.htm.

Araújo, J. R., A. Correia-Branco, C. Ramalho, P. Gonçalves, M. J. Pinho, E. Keating, and F. Martel. 2013. "L-Methionine Placental Uptake: Characterization and Modulation in Gestational Diabetes Mellitus." *Reproductive Sciences (Thousand Oaks, Calif.)* 20 (12): 1492–507. doi:10.1177/1933719113488442.

Arends, N. J. T., V. H. Boonstra, H. J. Duivenvoorden, P. L. Hofman, W. S. Cutfield, and A. C. S. Hokken-Koelega. 2005. "Reduced Insulin Sensitivity and the Presence of Cardiovascular Risk Factors in Short Prepubertal Children Born Small for Gestational Age (SGA)." *Clinical Endocrinology* 62 (1): 44–50. doi:10.1111/j.1365-2265.2004.02171.x.

Austin, G. L., L. G. Ogden, and J. O. Hill. 2011. "Trends in Carbohydrate, Fat, and Protein Intakes and Association with Energy Intake in Normal-Weight, Overweight, and Obese Individuals: 1971–2006." *The American Journal of Clinical Nutrition* 93 (4): 836–43. doi:10.3945/ajcn.110.000141.

Avcı, M. E., F. Sanlıkan, M. Celik, A. Avcı, M. Kocaer, and A. Göçmen. 2014. "Effects of Maternal Obesity on Antenatal, Perinatal and Neonatal Outcomes." *The Journal of Maternal–Fetal & Neonatal Medicine: The Official Journal of the European Association of Perinatal Medicine, the Federation of Asia and Oceania Perinatal Societies, the International Society of Perinatal Obstetricians* 1–4. doi:10.3109/14767058.2014.978279.

Belkacemi, L., D. M. Nelson, M. Desai, and M. G. Ross. 2010. "Maternal Undernutrition Influences Placental–Fetal Development." *Biology of Reproduction* 83 (3): 325–31. doi:10.1095/biolreprod.110.084517.

Boney, C. M., A. Verma, R. Tucker, and B. R. Vohr. 2005. "Metabolic Syndrome in Childhood: Association with Birth Weight, Maternal Obesity, and Gestational Diabetes Mellitus." *Pediatrics* 115 (3): e290–6. doi:10.1542/peds.2004-1808.

Bowers, K., S. K. Laughon, M. Kiely, J. Brite, Z. Chen, and C. Zhang. 2013. "Gestational Diabetes, Pre-Pregnancy Obesity and Pregnancy Weight Gain in Relation to Excess Fetal Growth: Variations by Race/ethnicity." *Diabetologia* 56 (6): 1263–71. doi:10.1007/s00125-013-2881-5.

Campbell, M. K., S. Cartier, B. Xie, G. Kouniakis, W. Huang, and V. Han. 2012. "Determinants of Small for Gestational Age Birth at Term." *Paediatric and Perinatal Epidemiology* 26 (6): 525–33. doi:10.1111/j.1365-3016.2012.01319.x.

Catalano, P. M., L. Presley, J. Minium, and S. Hauguel-de Mouzon. 2009. "Fetuses of Obese Mothers Develop Insulin Resistance in Utero." *Diabetes Care* 32 (6): 1076–80. doi:10.2337/dc08-2077.

Cleal, J. K., P. Brownbill, K. M. Godfrey, J. M. Jackson, A. A. Jackson, C. P. Sibley, M. A. Hanson, and R. M. Lewis. 2007. "Modification of Fetal Plasma Amino Acid Composition by Placental Amino Acid Exchangers in Vitro." *The Journal of Physiology* 582 (Pt 2): 871–82. doi:10.1113/jphysiol.2007.130690.

Cleal, J. K., J. D. Glazier, G. Ntani, S. R. Crozier, P. E. Day, N. C. Harvey, S. M. Robinson et al. 2011. "Facilitated Transporters Mediate Net Efflux of Amino Acids to the Fetus across the Basal Membrane of the Placental Syncytiotrophoblast." *The Journal of Physiology* 589 (Pt 4): 987–97. doi:10.1113/jphysiol.2010.198549.

Coan, P. M., O. R. Vaughan, Y. Sekita, S. L. Finn, G. J. Burton, M. Constancia, and A. L. Fowden. 2010. "Adaptations in Placental Phenotype Support Fetal Growth during Undernutrition of Pregnant Mice." *The Journal of Physiology* 588 (Pt 3): 527–38. doi:10.1113/jphysiol.2009.181214.

Coleman-Jensen, A., C. Gregory, and A. Singh. 2014. Household Food Security in the United States in 2013, ERR-173. U.S. Department of Agriculture, Economic Research Service, September 2014.

Desai, M., J. K. Jellyman, G. Han, M. Beall, R. H. Lane, and M. G. Ross. 2014. "Maternal Obesity and High-Fat Diet Program Offspring Metabolic Syndrome." *American Journal of Obstetrics and Gynecology* 211 (3): 237.e1–13. doi:10.1016/j.ajog.2014.03.025.

Desforges, M., H. A. Lacey, J. D. Glazier, S. L. Greenwood, K. J. Mynett, P. F. Speake, and C. P. Sibley. 2006. "SNAT4 Isoform of System A Amino Acid Transporter is Expressed in Human Placenta." *American Journal of Physiology. Cell Physiology* 290 (1): C305–12. doi:10.1152/ajpcell.00258.2005.

Desforges, M., K. J. Mynett, R. L. Jones, S. L. Greenwood, M. Westwood, C. P. Sibley, and J. D. Glazier. 2009. "The SNAT4 Isoform of the System A Amino Acid Transporter is Functional in Human Placental Microvillous Plasma Membrane." *The Journal of Physiology* 587 (Pt 1): 61–72. doi:10.1113/jphysiol.2008.161331.

Ehrenberg, H. M., B. M. Mercer, and P. M. Catalano. 2004. "The Influence of Obesity and Diabetes on the Prevalence of Macrosomia." *American Journal of Obstetrics and Gynecology* 191 (3): 964–8. doi:10.1016/j.ajog.2004.05.052.

Ericsson, A., K. Säljö, E. Sjöstrand, N. Jansson, P. D. Prasad, T. L. Powell, and T. Jansson. 2007. "Brief Hyperglycaemia in the Early Pregnant Rat Increases Fetal Weight at Term by Stimulating Placental Growth and Affecting Placental Nutrient Transport." *The Journal of Physiology* 581 (Pt 3): 1323–32. doi:10.1113/jphysiol.2007.131185.

Eriksson, B., M. Löf, H. Olausson, and E. Forsum. 2010. "Body Fat, Insulin Resistance, Energy Expenditure and Serum Concentrations of Leptin, Adiponectin and Resistin Before, during and after Pregnancy in Healthy Swedish Women." *The British Journal of Nutrition* 103 (1): 50–7. doi:10.1017/S0007114509991371.

FAO, IFAD and WFP. 2014. *The State of Food Insecurity in the World 2014. Strengthening the Enabling Environment for Food Security and Nutrition*. Rome, FAO.

Farley, D., M. E. Tejero, A. G. Comuzzie, P. B. Higgins, L. Cox, S. L. Werner, S. L. Jenkins et al. 2009. "Fetoplacental Adaptations to Maternal Obesity in the Baboon." *Placenta* 30 (9): 752–60. doi:10.1016/j.placenta.2009.06.007.

Farley, D. M., J. Choi, D. J. Dudley, C. Li, S. L. Jenkins, L. Myatt, and P. W. Nathanielsz. 2010. "Placental Amino Acid Transport and Placental Leptin Resistance in Pregnancies Complicated by Maternal Obesity." *Placenta* 31 (8): 718–24. doi:10.1016/j.placenta.2010.06.006.

Flegal, K. M., M. D. Carroll, C. L. Ogden, and L. R. Curtin. 2010. "Prevalence and Trends in Obesity among US Adults, 1999–2008." *JAMA* 303 (3): 235–41. doi:10.1001/jama.2009.2014.

Galtier-Dereure, F., C. Boegner, and J. Bringer. 2000. "Obesity and Pregnancy: Complications and Cost." *The American Journal of Clinical Nutrition* 71 (5 Suppl): 1242S–8S.

Glazier, J. D., I. Cetin, G. Perugino, S. Ronzoni, A. M. Grey, D. Mahendran, A. M. Marconi, G. Pardi, and C. P. Sibley. 1997. "Association between the Activity of the System A Amino Acid Transporter in the Microvillous Plasma Membrane of the Human Placenta and Severity of Fetal Compromise in Intrauterine Growth Restriction." *Pediatric Research* 42 (4): 514–9. doi:10.1203/00006450-199710000-00016.

Jansson, T., V. Scholtbach, and T. L. Powell. 1998. "Placental Transport of Leucine and Lysine is Reduced in Intrauterine Growth Restriction." *Pediatric Research* 44 (4): 532–7. doi:10.1203/00006450-199810000-00011.

Jansson, T., Y. Ekstrand, C. Björn, M. Wennergren, and T. L. Powell. 2002a. "Alterations in the Activity of Placental Amino Acid Transporters in Pregnancies Complicated by Diabetes." *Diabetes* 51 (7): 2214–9.

Jansson, T., K. Ylvén, M. Wennergren, and T. L. Powell. 2002b. "Glucose Transport and System A Activity in Syncytiotrophoblast Microvillous and Basal Plasma Membranes in Intrauterine Growth Restriction." *Placenta* 23 (5): 392–9. doi:10.1053/plac.2002.0826.

Jansson, N., S. L. Greenwood, B. R. Johansson, T. L. Powell, and T. Jansson. 2003. "Leptin Stimulates the Activity of the System A Amino Acid Transporter in Human Placental Villous Fragments." *The Journal of Clinical Endocrinology and Metabolism* 88 (3): 1205–11. doi:10.1210/jc.2002-021332.

Jansson, N., J. Pettersson, A. Haafiz, A. Ericsson, I. Palmberg, M. Tranberg, V. Ganapathy, T. L. Powell, and T. Jansson. 2006. "Down-Regulation of Placental Transport of Amino Acids Precedes the Development of Intrauterine Growth Restriction in Rats Fed a Low Protein Diet." *The Journal of Physiology* 576 (Pt 3): 935–46. doi:10.1113/jphysiol.2006.116509.

Jansson, N., F. J. Rosario, F. Gaccioli, S. Lager, H. N. Jones, S. Roos, T. Jansson, and T. L. Powell. 2013. "Activation of Placental mTOR Signaling and Amino Acid Transporters in Obese Women Giving Birth to Large Babies." *The Journal of Clinical Endocrinology and Metabolism* 98 (1): 105–13. doi:10.1210 /jc.2012-2667.

Jariyapitaksakul, C. and Y. Tannirandorn. 2013. "The Occurrence of Small for Gestational Age Infants and Perinatal and Maternal Outcomes in Normal and Poor Maternal Weight Gain Singleton Pregnancies." *Journal of the Medical Association of Thailand = Chotmaihet Thangphaet* 96 (3): 259–65.

Jones, H. N., C. J. Ashworth, K. R. Page, and H. J. McArdle. 2006. "Expression and Adaptive Regulation of Amino Acid Transport System A in a Placental Cell Line under Amino Acid Restriction." *Reproduction (Cambridge, England)* 131 (5): 951–60. doi:10.1530/rep.1.00808.

Jones, H. N., L. A. Woollett, N. Barbour, P. D. Prasad, T. L. Powell, and T. Jansson. 2009. "High-Fat Diet before and during Pregnancy Causes Marked up-Regulation of Placental Nutrient Transport and Fetal Overgrowth in C57/BL6 Mice." *FASEB Journal: Official Publication of the Federation of American Societies for Experimental Biology* 23 (1): 271–8. doi:10.1096/fj.08-116889.

Jones, H. N., T. Jansson, and T. L. Powell. 2010. "Full-Length Adiponectin Attenuates Insulin Signaling and Inhibits Insulin-Stimulated Amino Acid Transport in Human Primary Trophoblast Cells." *Diabetes* 59 (5): 1161–70. doi:10.2337/db09-0824.

Kavitha, J. V., F. J. Rosario, M. J. Nijland, T. J. McDonald, G. Wu, Y. Kanai, T. L. Powell, P. W. Nathanielsz, and T. Jansson. 2014. "Down-Regulation of Placental mTOR, insulin/IGF-I Signaling, and Nutrient Transporters in Response to Maternal Nutrient Restriction in the Baboon." *FASEB Journal: Official Publication of the Federation of American Societies for Experimental Biology* 28 (3): 1294–1305. doi:10.1096/fj.13-242271.

Kudo, Y. and C. A. Boyd. 2001. "Characterisation of L-Tryptophan Transporters in Human Placenta: A Comparison of Brush Border and Basal Membrane Vesicles." *The Journal of Physiology* 531 (Pt 2): 405–16.

Kuruvilla, A. G., S. W. D'Souza, J. D. Glazier, D. Mahendran, M. J. Maresh, and C. P. Sibley. 1994. "Altered Activity of the System A Amino Acid Transporter in Microvillous Membrane Vesicles from Placentas of Macrosomic Babies Born to Diabetic Women." *The Journal of Clinical Investigation* 94 (2): 689–95. doi:10.1172/JCI117386.

Lager, S. and T. L. Powell. 2012. "Regulation of Nutrient Transport across the Placenta." *Journal of Pregnancy* 2012: 179827. doi:10.1155/2012/179827.

Lager, S., F. Gaccioli, V. I. Ramirez, H. N. Jones, T. Jansson, and T. L. Powell. 2013. "Oleic Acid Stimulates System A Amino Acid Transport in Primary Human Trophoblast Cells Mediated by Toll-like Receptor 4." *Journal of Lipid Research* 54 (3): 725–33. doi:10.1194/jlr.M033050.

Lager, S., T. Jansson, and T. L. Powell. 2014. "Differential Regulation of Placental Amino Acid Transport by Saturated and Unsaturated Fatty Acids." *American Journal of Physiology. Cell Physiology* 307 (8): C738–44. doi:10.1152/ajpcell.00196.2014.

Lin, Y., Y. Zhuo, Z.-F. Fang, L.-Q. Che, and D. Wu. 2012. "Effect of Maternal Dietary Energy Types on Placenta Nutrient Transporter Gene Expressions and Intrauterine Fetal Growth in Rats." *Nutrition (Burbank, Los Angeles County, Calif.)* 28 (10): 1037–43. doi:10.1016/j.nut.2012.01.002.

Mahendran, D., P. Donnai, J. D. Glazier, S. W. D'Souza, R. D. Boyd, and C. P. Sibley. 1993. "Amino Acid (system A) Transporter Activity in Microvillous Membrane Vesicles from the Placentas of Appropriate and Small for Gestational Age Babies." *Pediatric Research* 34 (5): 661–5. doi:10.1203/00006450-199311000-00019.

Malandro, M. S., M. J. Beveridge, M. S. Kilberg, and D. A. Novak. 1996. "Effect of Low-Protein Diet-Induced Intrauterine Growth Retardation on Rat Placental Amino Acid Transport." *The American Journal of Physiology* 271 (1 Pt 1): C295–303.

Mandò, C., S. Tabano, P. Pileri, P. Colapietro, M. A. Marino, L. Avagliano, P. Doi, G. Bulfamante, M. Miozzo, and I. Cetin. 2013. "SNAT2 Expression and Regulation in Human Growth-Restricted Placentas." *Pediatric Research* 74 (2): 104–10. doi:10.1038/pr.2013.83.

Mericq, V., G. Iñiguez, R. Bazaes, C. Bouwman, A. Avila, T. Salazar, and F. Carrasco. 2009. "Differences in Body Composition and Energy Expenditure in Prepubertal Children Born Term or Preterm Appropriate or Small for Gestational Age." *Journal of Pediatric Endocrinology & Metabolism: JPEM* 22 (11): 1041–50.

Misra, V. K. and S. Trudeau. 2011. "The Influence of Overweight and Obesity on Longitudinal Trends in Maternal Serum Leptin Levels during Pregnancy." *Obesity (Silver Spring, Md.)* 19 (2): 416–21. doi:10.1038/oby.2010.172.

Ogden, C. L., M. D. Carroll, B. K. Kit, and K. M. Flegal. 2014. "Prevalence of Childhood and Adult Obesity in the United States, 2011–2012." *JAMA* 311 (8): 806–14. doi:10.1001/jama.2014.732.

Okamoto, Y., M. Sakata, K. Ogura, T. Yamamoto, M. Yamaguchi, K. Tasaka, H. Kurachi, M. Tsurudome, and Y. Murata. 2002. "Expression and Regulation of 4F2hc and hLAT1 in Human Trophoblasts." *American Journal of Physiology. Cell Physiology* 282 (1): C196–204.

Regnault, T. R. H., B. de Vrijer, H. L. Galan, R. B. Wilkening, F. C. Battaglia, and G. Meschia. 2013. "Umbilical Uptakes and Transplacental Concentration Ratios of Amino Acids in Severe Fetal Growth Restriction." *Pediatric Research* 73 (5): 602–11. doi:10.1038/pr.2013.30.

Reinehr, T., M. Kleber, and A. M. Toschke. 2009. "Small for Gestational Age Status is Associated with Metabolic Syndrome in Overweight Children." *European Journal of Endocrinology/European Federation of Endocrine Societies* 160 (4): 579–84. doi:10.1530/EJE-08-0914.

Roos, S., N. Jansson, I. Palmberg, K. Säljö, T. L. Powell, and T. Jansson. 2007. "Mammalian Target of Rapamycin in the Human Placenta Regulates Leucine Transport and is Down-Regulated in Restricted Fetal Growth." *The Journal of Physiology* 582 (Pt 1): 449–59. doi:10.1113/jphysiol.2007.129676.

Roos, S., Y. Kanai, P. D. Prasad, T. L. Powell, and T. Jansson. 2009a. "Regulation of Placental Amino Acid Transporter Activity by Mammalian Target of Rapamycin." *American Journal of Physiology. Cell Physiology* 296 (1): C142–50. doi:10.1152/ajpcell.00330.2008.

Roos, S., O. Lagerlöf, M. Wennergren, T. L. Powell, and T. Jansson. 2009b. "Regulation of Amino Acid Transporters by Glucose and Growth Factors in Cultured Primary Human Trophoblast Cells is Mediated by mTOR Signaling." *American Journal of Physiology. Cell Physiology* 297 (3): C723–31. doi:10.1152/ajpcell.00191.2009.

Rosario, F. J., N. Jansson, Y. Kanai, P. D. Prasad, T. L. Powell, and T. Jansson. 2011. "Maternal Protein Restriction in the Rat Inhibits Placental Insulin, mTOR, and STAT3 Signaling and Down-Regulates Placental Amino Acid Transporters." *Endocrinology* 152 (3): 1119–29. doi:10.1210/en.2010-1153.

Rosario, F. J., M. A. Schumacher, J. Jiang, Y. Kanai, T. L. Powell, and T. Jansson. 2012. "Chronic Maternal Infusion of Full-Length Adiponectin in Pregnant Mice Down-Regulates Placental Amino Acid Transporter Activity and Expression and Decreases Fetal Growth." *The Journal of Physiology* 590 (Pt 6): 1495–509. doi:10.1113/jphysiol.2011.226399.

Rosario, F. J., Y. Kanai, T. L. Powell, and T. Jansson. 2013. "Mammalian Target of Rapamycin Signalling Modulates Amino Acid Uptake by Regulating Transporter Cell Surface Abundance in Primary Human Trophoblast Cells." *The Journal of Physiology* 591 (Pt 3): 609–25. doi:10.1113/jphysiol.2012.238014.

Shin, D. and W. O. Song. 2014. "Prepregnancy Body Mass Index is an Independent Risk Factor for Gestational Hypertension, Gestational Diabetes, Preterm Labor, and Small- and Large-for-Gestational-Age Infants." *The Journal of Maternal–Fetal & Neonatal Medicine: The Official Journal of the European Association of Perinatal Medicine, the Federation of Asia and Oceania Perinatal Societies, the International Society of Perinatal Obstetricians* 29: 1–8. doi:10.3109/14767058.2014.964675.

Sibley, C. P., M. A. Turner, I. Cetin, P. Ayuk, C. A. R. Boyd, S. W. D'Souza, J. D. Glazier, S. L. Greenwood, T. Jansson, and T. Powell. 2005. "Placental Phenotypes of Intrauterine Growth." *Pediatric Research* 58 (5): 827–32. doi:10.1203/01.PDR.0000181381.82856.23.

Starling, A. P., J. T. Brinton, D. H. Glueck, A. L. Shapiro, C. S. Harrod, A. M. Lynch, A. M. Siega-Riz, and D. Dabelea. 2015. "Associations of Maternal BMI and Gestational Weight Gain with Neonatal Adiposity in the Healthy Start Study." *American Journal of Clinical Nutrition* 101: 302–9. doi:10.3945/ajcn.114.094946.

Sun, B., R. H. Purcell, C. E. Terrillion, J. Yan, T. H. Moran, and K. L. K. Tamashiro. 2012. "Maternal High-Fat Diet during Gestation or Suckling Differentially Affects Offspring Leptin Sensitivity and Obesity." *Diabetes* 61 (11): 2833–41. doi:10.2337/db11-0957.

Tarrade, A., D. Rousseau-Ralliard, M.-C. Aubrière, N. Peynot, M. Dahirel, J. Bertrand-Michel, T. Aguirre-Lavin et al. 2013. "Sexual Dimorphism of the Fetoplacental Phenotype in Response to a High Fat and Control Maternal Diets in a Rabbit Model." *PLoS One* 8 (12): e83458. doi:10.1371/journal.pone.0083458.

Verrey, F. 2003. "System L: Heteromeric Exchangers of Large, Neutral Amino Acids Involved in Directional Transport." *Pflügers Archiv: European Journal of Physiology* 445 (5): 529–33. doi:10.1007/s00424 -002-0973-z.

Von Versen-Höynck, F., A. Rajakumar, M. S. Parrott, and R. W. Powers. 2009. "Leptin Affects System A Amino Acid Transport Activity in the Human Placenta: Evidence for STAT3 Dependent Mechanisms." *Placenta* 30 (4): 361–7. doi:10.1016/j.placenta.2009.01.004.

Wallace, J. M., G. W. Horgan, and S. Bhattacharya. 2012. "Placental Weight and Efficiency in Relation to Maternal Body Mass Index and the Risk of Pregnancy Complications in Women Delivering Singleton Babies." *Placenta* 33 (8): 611–8. doi:10.1016/j.placenta.2012.05.006.

Wullschleger, S., R. Loewith, and M. N. Hall. 2006. "TOR Signaling in Growth and Metabolism." *Cell* 124 (3): 471–84. doi:10.1016/j.cell.2006.01.016.

Yu, Z., S. Han, J. Zhu, X. Sun, C. Ji, and X. Guo. 2013. "Pre-Pregnancy Body Mass Index in Relation to Infant Birth Weight and Offspring Overweight/Obesity: A Systematic Review and Meta-Analysis." *PLoS One* 8 (4): e61627. doi:10.1371/journal.pone.0061627.

6 Fatty Acid Uptake and Metabolism in the Human Placenta

Asim K. Duttaroy

CONTENTS

ABSTRACT

In the fetoplacental unit, preferential transport of maternal plasma long-chain polyunsaturated fatty acids (LCPUFAs) across the placenta is of critical importance for fetal growth and development. Fatty acids cross the placental microvillous and basal membranes mainly via plasma membrane fatty acid transport system (fatty acid translocase, fatty acid transport protein, and plasma membrane fatty acid binding protein [p-FABPpm]) and cytoplasmic fatty acid-binding proteins. These indicate that these receptors are potential regulators of placental lipid transfer and homeostasis. Among the fatty acid-binding/transport proteins, p-FABPpm, located exclusively on the maternal-facing membranes of the placenta, may be involved in the sequestration of maternal LCPUFAs by the placenta. This chapter discusses the importance of nuclear receptors and fatty acid-binding/transport proteins in placental fatty acid uptake, transport, and metabolism.

KEY WORDS

Fatty acid uptake, BeWo cells, docosahexaenoic acid, fatty acid-binding proteins, fatty acid transport protein (FATP)-4, lipid droplet protein.

6.1 INTRODUCTION

Fetal growth is dependent on maternal nutrient supply *in utero*, which is determined by placental transport activity. The placenta exhibits specific alterations in the expression and activity of a number of nutrients in pregnancies with altered fetal growth and changes that are important for the development of pregnancy complications. Inappropriate placental supply of these may affect fetal growth and development. Essential fatty acids (EFAs) and their metabolites long-chain polyunsaturated fatty acids (LCPUFAs) are of critical importance in fetoplacental growth and development (Dutta-Roy 2000b; Innis 2007). In fact, fetal brain and retina are very rich in LCPUFA, specially arachidonic acid,

20:4n-6 (ARA), and docosahexaenoic acid, 22:6n-3 (DHA) (Innis 2000). Various studies suggest that learning ability may be impaired if there is a reduction in the accumulation of sufficient DHA during intrauterine life. Premature babies, in particular, born during the last trimester of pregnancy, have been shown to have low levels of DHA in the blood (Whalley et al. 2004). The critical importance of these fatty acids in the fetoplacental unit therefore demands an efficient uptake system for these fatty acids. It is important to understand the mechanisms involved in the placental fatty acid transport and the metabolic relationships between maternal fatty acids and their supply by the placenta to the developing fetus. A growing body of data indicate that placental structural and functional abnormalities can cause numerous adverse pregnancy outcomes. Recent evidence also underscores the importance of placental development in long-term health and disease for both mother and offspring.

6.2 FATTY ACIDS AND THEIR ROLES IN FETAL DEVELOPMENT

Linoleic acid, 18:2n-6 (LA), and α-linolenic acid, 18:3n-3 (ALA), are the two main dietary EFAs that are readily available from dietary sources such as vegetable oils, but their LCPUFA derivatives (ARA, EPA, and DHA) can be consumed in foods of animal origin. Dietary LA and ALA must be converted in the body to their further metabolites, LCPUFA, to exert the full range of biologic actions. Therefore, maternal EFA metabolism (specially in the cases when the dietary intakes of preformed DHA and ARA are low) is crucial for fetal growth and development, as the fetus depends on the maternal supply of LCPUFA such as ARA and DHA. ARA is a precursor for bioactive eicosanoids. These eicosanoids can affect numerous inflammatory responses, including fetal thymic growth, whereas both DHA and ARA are an important structural component of the nervous system.

Human brain growth is at peak velocity during the last trimester and the first few months after birth, leading to the concept that the third-trimester fetus and newborn infant are particularly vulnerable to developmental deficits of DHA. Such an important role of DHA rests on its participation in maintaining membrane fluidity, impulse propagation, synaptic transmission, and its function as a cytosolic signal transducing factor for various gene expressions during the critical period of brain development. The critical role of DHA in neurogenesis, however, suggests that the adverse effects of inadequate DHA in early gestation will be more severe and more difficult to overcome than deficiencies occurring later on. Cohort studies have demonstrated the long-term impact of the deficiency of DHA from infant formula. DHA status at birth was correlated with problem internalizing behaviors in 393 Dutch children at 7 years, an observation that was not present in breastfed infants. Animal studies have demonstrated that DHA deficiency during gestation and soon after birth could not be fully corrected later in life (Krabbendam et al. 2007). At 33 weeks, the hypothalamus glycerophospholipids of young pups had significantly reduced DHA compared with controls (who had received ALA for 3 weeks after birth), even after dietary correction with ALA for 30 weeks. It appeared that the early deficiency of ALA had irreversibly down-regulated the converting enzyme delta-6 desaturase (Li et al. 2006). Optimal maternal to fetal DHA and ARA transfer in gestation is therefore likely to have benefits both before birth and extending into the postnatal period, and thus, mother's physiological adaptation toward this feto–maternal cooperation must be remarkably coordinated. During early pregnancy, LCPUFAs derived from the diet are stored in maternal adipose tissue. During late pregnancy, enhanced lipid catabolism as a consequence of the insulin-resistant condition causes the development of maternal hyperlipidemia, which plays a key role in the availability of LCPUFA to the fetus. Maternal body fat accumulation during early pregnancy allows the accumulation of an important store of LCPUFA derived from both the maternal diet and maternal metabolism. The importance of DHA during pregnancy in fetal development and its postnatal spill-over effect has been studied by examining the relationships between maternal DHA intake during gestation and lactation on cognitive functioning in later childhood. Although interventional studies to inquire into the importance of DHA in pregnancy and fetal development are complicated by different variables, such as food habits, placental functions, and transit to fetal circulation, several epidemiological and interventional studies do suggest that higher maternal intakes of n-6 and n-3 fatty acids, including DHA, increase maternal-to-fetal transfer of the respective fatty acid.

Several studies on fatty acid composition in fetal and maternal plasma have shown that at birth, LA represents about 10% of the total fatty acids in cord plasma compared with 30% in maternal plasma, but surprisingly, ARA concentration in cord plasma is twice (about 10%) that observed in the mother (around 5%). Similarly, ALA concentration in the newborn is half that in the mother (0.3% vs. 0.6%), whereas DHA concentration is double (3% vs. 1.5%) and EPA levels are equally low in fetal and maternal plasma (Dutta-Roy 2000b). Free fatty acids (FFAs) in the maternal circulation are the major source of fatty acids for transport across the placenta. An accelerated breakdown of fat depots occurs during the last trimester of pregnancy. In this late stage of gestation, lipolytic activity in adipose tissue is increased. The fatty acids that are released, as well as fatty acids from dietary lipids and hepatic overproduction of triacylglycerol, are responsible for increasing the amount of triacylglycerol in maternal circulating lipoproteins. Although maternal plasma lipoproteins do not directly cross the placental barrier, hypertriacylglycerolaemia in pregnancy plays a key role in the availability of fatty acids for the fetus. Placental lipase activities were dramatically increased during the last trimester of pregnancy, whereas there was an overall decrease in lipoprotein lipase (LPL) activity, resulting in a subsequent decrease in triacylglycerol storage. Consequently, with decreased triacylglycerol hydrolysis for maternal storage and an increase in placental lipolytic activity, the resulting availability of triacylglycerol is utilized by placental lipase for the provision of FFA for fetal transport. The placental LPL, however, hydrolyses triacyglycerols from posthepatic low-density lipoproteins (LDLs) and very LDLs but not the triacylglycerols present in the chylomicrons (Dutta-Roy 2000b). Placental LPL activity was reduced by 47% in preterm intrauterine growth retardation, whereas in insulin-dependent diabetes mellitus (IDDM) pregnancies, the activity was increased by 39% compared with controls.

6.3 FATTY ACID UPTAKE AND TRANSPORT HUMAN PLACENTAL TROPHOBLASTS

There are several membrane proteins thought to be responsible for tissue fatty acid uptake placenta (Dutta-Roy 2000a; Duttaroy 2009; Glatz and Storch 2001). These include the 40-kDa plasma-membrane-associated fatty acid-binding protein (FABPpm); the heavily glycosylated 88-kDa fatty acid translocase (FAT), also known as CD36; and a family of 63–70-kDa fatty acid transport proteins (FATP-1–FATP-6) (Duttaroy 2009). A 40-kDa protein that binds only long-chain fatty acids was then isolated and purified from human placental membranes (Duttaroy 2009). The human placental (p) FABPpm is different in several aspects, such as pI value and amino acid composition, fatty acid-binding activity, and aspartate aminotransferase (AspAT) activity from the previously described FABPpm from several tissues. This protein is present only in the microvillous membrane of the placenta-facing fetal circulation. Radiolabelled fatty acid binding revealed that p-FABPpm had higher affinities (Kd) and binding capacities (Bmax) for LCPUFAs compared with other fatty acids. The presence of p-FABPpm in the placental membrane-facing maternal circulation may enforce unidirectional flow of the LCPUFA from the mother to the fetus.

FAT/CD36 is a heavily glycosylated FAT (FAT/CD36), the sequence of which was 85% homologous with that of glycoprotein IV (CD36), and is an integral membrane protein (23). This 472-amino-acid (53-kDa) protein is substantially glycosylated (10 predicted N-linked glycolsylated sites). Unlike FABPpm and FATP, FAT is a multifunctional protein and has a number of putative ligands, including FFAs, collagen, thrombospondin, and oxidized LDL. The presence of FAT/CD36 was demonstrated in the human placenta using both pure trophoblast cells and placental membrane preparations. FAT is present in both the placental membranes, microvillous, and basal membranes (Duttaroy 2009). Little is known about the regulation of FAT/CD36 function in placental cells, but several lines point toward a translocational mechanism for increasing long chain fatty acids (LCFAs) uptake by different cells. Caveolin-1 may control FAT/CD36-mediated fatty acid uptake by increasing its surface availability.

FATP is the family of integral transmembrane proteins and consists of six (FATP-1–FATP-6) so far identified members, which show different tissue expression patterns. FATP-1 was first identified in human placental membranes. Later, other isoforms of FATPs were detected in the human placenta. Consistent with the role of FATP-1 in fatty acid internalization, a significant portion of FATP-1 is localized at the plasma membrane. FATPs were classified as FATPs because, when overexpressed, they increase the rate of fatty acid internalization, most notably at low concentrations, when diffusion may not be sufficient. FATP is suggested to act in concert with fatty acyl-coenzyme A (CoA) synthetase, an enzyme that prevents efflux of the incorporated fatty acids by their conversion into acyl-CoA derivatives and hence rendering fatty acid uptake unidirectional. These long-chain fatty acyl-CoA esters act both as substrates and intermediates in various intracellular functions. FATP-mediated uptake of LCFA was diminished in the face of cellular depletion of ATP. Since FATP is likely to be responsible for the increased LCFA necessary to sustain this increased β-oxidation, the tissue-selective effects of various peroxisome proliferator-activated receptors (PPARs) activators and ligands on FATP and ACS provide insight in the relationship between FFA uptake and triglyceride synthesis and β-oxidation of fatty acids. Additionally, whereas FATP-1 possesses ACS activity toward long-chain fatty acids (16–22 carbons), compared with that of Acsl1, the ACS activity of FATP-1 is very low. FATP-1 has only one membrane-spanning region and several membrane-associated regions. Because this arrangement is not typical for a channel or transporter, FATP may increase fatty acid internalization by increasing the rate of "flip-flop," trapping the fatty acids in the inner leaflet of the plasma membrane, or activating the fatty acid to its CoA species. Disruption of the FATP-4 gene in mice established that it performs an essential function in normal mouse development. Surprisingly, little is known on the specificity of FATP enzymes for different fatty acids. Similarly, overexpression of FATP-4 in 293 cells has little effect on ARA internalization. PPAR-γ and retinoid X receptor (RXR) regulate fatty acid transport in primary human trophoblasts. The treatment of human trophoblast cells with both PPAR-γ and RXR agonists resulted in elevated mRNA expression of FATP-1 and FATP-4, but not FATP-2, -3, and -6, in these cells. Similar results were obtained by this group in *in vivo* in mice by using PPAR-γ agonist, reporting also an increase in the placental expression of FABPpm and FAT/CD36. The PPAR/RXR heterodimer may have roles in regulating placental fatty acid uptake. However, exposure to rosiglitazone reduced fetoplacental weight and the thickness of the spongiotrophoblast layer and labyrinthine vasculature.

The presence of cytoplasmic H-fatty acid-binding proteins (FABPs) and L-FABP was demonstrated in human placental trophoblasts. Later, the presence of several other FABPs such as adipose FABP and epidermal FABP subtypes in trophoblasts was reported (Duttaroy 2009). The significance of the presence of several cytoplasmic FABPs in trophoblasts is not known but indicates that complex interactions of these proteins may be essential for effective fatty acid transport and metabolism in the placenta. Exposure to hypoxia markedly increased the expression of L-FABP, H-FABP, and A-FABP with the accumulation of lipid droplet in trophoblasts. Ligands for PPAR-γ enhanced the expression of these proteins in trophoblasts. Hypoxia induced increased expression of FABPs in human trophoblasts, suggesting that FABPs support fat accumulation in the hypoxic placenta.

6.4 PLACENTAL METABOLISM OF FATTY ACIDS

Placental fatty acid metabolism may play a critical role in guiding pregnancy and fetal outcome. A selective cellular metabolism of certain fatty acids may contribute to the placental transfer process, as would the conversion of certain proportion of ARA to prostaglandins, incorporation of some fatty acids into phospholipids and triacylglycerols, and the oxidation and synthesis of fatty acids in the placenta. LCPUFAs can be metabolized to important cell signaling molecules in placenta by several major isoform families, including cyclooxygenases (COXs), lipoxygenases, and cytochrome P450 subfamily 4A (CYP4A). The increased expression of COX-2 is believed to be associated with the PG synthesis at term and parturition. However, there are other enzymes, such as cytosolic phospholipase A_2 (cPLA₂), that are also potential regulating steps in prostaglandin (PG) synthesis in addition to COX. The cPLA₂ catalyzes the release of free ARA, an initial and rate-limiting substrate in PG synthesis, from the sn-2 position of membrane phospholipids. In addition, oxidized lipids, including 9S-hydroxy-octadedienoic acid (HODE), 13S-HODE, and 15S-hydroxy-5Z,11Z,13E-eicosatetraenoic acid (15S-HETE), were shown to activate PPAR-γ in primary human villous trophoblasts. Trophoblast has been shown to oxidize fatty acids in substantial amounts, suggesting that the human placenta utilizes fatty acids as a significant metabolic fuel. In fact, placental oxidation of fatty acids is an important fetal health determinant. Placenta expresses all the enzymes necessary for mitochondrial fatty acid oxidation. Fatty acids are used as a major metabolic fuel by human placentas at all gestational ages, and any defect within this energy-producing pathway may hamper the growth, differentiation, and function of the placenta and thereby may compromise fetal growth and development. More data are required on the relationship between the fatty acid oxidative capacity of placenta and fetal growth and development.

6.5 UPTAKE OF FATTY ACID BY PLACENTAL THIRD-TRIMESTER TROPHOBLAST CELLS, BeWo2

The underlying biochemical mechanisms responsible for the selective concentration of LCPUFA in fetal tissues are not fully understood yet. Evidence on the role of the placenta in preferential accumulation of LCPUFAs in fetal tissues has emerged from studies with the fatty acid-binding characteristics of human placental membranes determined. Placental plasma membrane binding sites have a strong preference for LCPUFAs. When fatty acid uptake was compared between BeWo cells and HepG2 cells, EFAs/LCPUFAs were taken up by BeWo cells preferentially over oleic acid; however, no such discrimination was observed in HepG2 cells (Campbell et al. 1997). Almost 60% of the total DHA taken up by cells was esterified into triacylglycerol, whereas 37% was in phospholipid fractions. The reverse was true for arachidonic acid (AA); 60% of the total uptake was incorporated into phospholipid fractions, whereas <35% was in triacyglycerol fractions (Crabtree et al. 1998).

In addition, involvement of several nuclear transcription factors (PPARs, liver X receptor [LXR], RXR, and sterol regulatory element-binding proteins [SREBP-1]) in the expression of genes responsible for fatty acid uptake, placental trophoblast differentiation, and human chorionic gonadotropin production indicates regulatory roles of fatty acid-activated transcriptions factors in placenta biology (Weedon-Fekjaer, Duttaroy, and Nebb 2005). The presence of several FABPs in the third-trimester human placental trophoblasts and their complex interactions may be essential for effective fatty acid transport and metabolism in the placenta. An increase in the expression of liver type FABP (FABP-1), heart type FABP (FABP-3), and adipose type FABP (FABP-4) with the lipid droplet formation and in hypoxia was observed in human placental last-trimester trophoblasts (Duttaroy 2009). These include the 40-kDa FABPpm; the heavily glycosylated 88-kDa FAT, also known as CD36; and a family of 63–70-kDa FATPs (FATP-1–FATP-6). Placenta-specific membrane fatty acid-binding protein (p-FABPpm) (40 kDa) specifically binds DHA and AA and may be responsible for preferential uptake of these fatty acids from the maternal plasma by the placenta for fetal supply (Dutta-Roy 2000b). Plasma membrane fatty acid-binding protein (p-FABPpm) is exclusively located in the maternal-facing membranes of the placenta. In contrast, FAT and FATP are present on both microvillous and basal membranes of the human placenta (Campbell et al. 1998). The location of FAT and FATP on both sides of the bipolar placental trophoblast cells may favor transport of general FFA pool in both directions, i.e., from the mother to the fetus and vice versa (Figure 6.1). However, p-FABPpm, because of its exclusive location on the microvillous membranes and binding specificity, may favor the unidirectional flow of maternal plasma DHA and AA to the fetal plasma (Duttaroy 2009).

In contrast to the last-trimester trophoblasts, uptake of AA was greater compared with that of EPA and DHA in first-trimester trophoblasts (Basak and Duttaroy 2013). The uptake of individual fatty acids was almost equally inhibited by triacsin C (an inhibitor of CoA formation), indicating that CoA formation step may be involved in the uptake of these fatty acids in the first-trimester human trophoblast cells, HTR8/SVneo. This is again in contrast to what was observed in triacsin C-induced inhibition of the DHA uptake by the last-trimester placental trophoblasts, where DHA uptake was

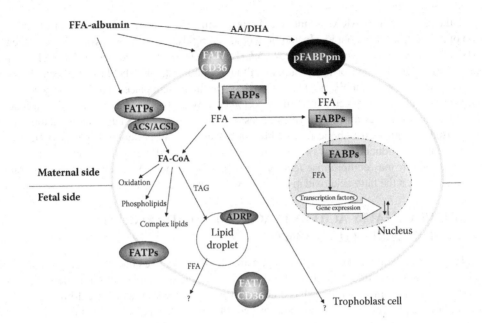

FIGURE 6.1 Schematic overview of proteins involved in fatty acid transport in last trimester trophoblast cells. The location of FAT and FATP on both sides of the bipolar placental cells and the lack of specificity for particular types of FFAs allows transport by all FFAs (nonessential, essential, and long-chain polyunsaturated) bidirectionally, i.e., from the mother to the fetus and vice versa. However, by virtue of its exclusive location on both sides and preference for LCPUFAs, p-FABP$_{pm}$ sequesters maternal plasma LCPUFAs to the placenta. Cytoplasmic FABPs may be responsible for transcytoplasmic movement of FFAs to their sites of esterification, ß-oxidation, or to the fetal circulation via placental basal membranes.

inhibited least by triacsin C compared with other fatty acids (Tobin et al. 2009). DHA, by avoiding CoA formation in the last-trimester trophoblasts, may allow preferential transport across these cells. The first-trimester trophoblast cells are not fatty acid transporting cells like last-trimester placental trophoblast cells are. These extravillous trophoblasts (EVTs) invade the maternal uterine walls and decidua to engraft and remodel uterine spiral arteries, creating the placental blood supply at the end of the first trimester. The local decidual microenvironment is thought to play a key role in regulating trophoblast invasion. Overall, the evidence suggests that in a healthy pregnancy, almost all cell types in the decidua actively promote EVT invasion and further reduced EVT invasion toward the end of the first trimester. Angiogenic activities (as measured by tube formation) of fatty acids were investigated in these cells (Johnsen et al. 2011). Although the underlying mechanisms are yet to be known, DHA stimulated vascular endothelial growth factor (VEGF), the most potent angiogenic factor, whereas other fatty acids stimulated a comparatively weaker angiogenic factor, angiopoietin-like protein 4 (ANGPTL4) (Basak and Duttaroy 2013). ANGPTL4 is also known to regulate lipid metabolism by altering the activity of LPL (Johnsen et al. 2011). However, not much information is available on the metabolism of fatty acids and the roles of ANGPTL4 in these cells. Silencing of ANGPTL4 gene prevented fatty acid-induced tube formation. Thus, gene ablation of ANGPTL4 confirmed that fatty acids mediated their angiogenic action partly via inducing ANGPTL4 expression and secretion in first-trimester trophoblast cells. Triacsin C also inhibited fatty acid-induced tube formation in these cells, indicating that CoA formation of the fatty acids taken up by these cells may be a requisite step for tube formation. In addition, these fatty acids altered the expression of several lipid metabolic genes such as ADRP, FABP4, FABP3, and COX-2. Expression of COX-2 and PGE$_2$ production have been shown to up-regulate the epidermal growth factor receptor (EGFR), phosphoinositide 3-kinase (PI3k), extracellular signal-regulated kinase 1 (Erk1/2) signaling, thereby inducing angiogenesis, cell proliferation, and invasion. Prostaglandin E_2 (PGE_2) also promoted tube formation comparable with VEGF in these cells. PGE_2-induced angiogenesis was inhibited significantly by COX-2 inhibitor, whereas VEGF-induced tube formation was least affected. All these data suggest that PGE_2 may have an independent effect on the tube formation process. Better understanding would be required further on the cross-talk between fatty acids and their modulators such as ANGPTL4 and VEGF in the early placentation process.

6.6 CONCLUSIONS

Fetal nutrition is determined by the mother's diet, the nutrients stored in her body, and, ultimately, the placenta's ability to transport these nutrients from mother to baby. The placenta exhibits specific alterations in the expression and activity of a number of nutrients in pregnancies with altered fetal growth, changes that are important for the development of these pregnancy complications. Human placenta trophoblasts play a crucial role in mobilizing maternal fatty acids and channeling important LCPUFAs to the fetus via multiple mechanisms, including selective uptake by the trophoblast, intracellular metabolic channeling, and selective export to the fetal circulation. Among the fatty acid-binding/transport proteins, p-FABPpm, located exclusively on the maternal-facing membranes of the placenta, may be involved in the sequestration of maternal LCPUFAs by the placenta. Fatty acid uptakes, however, in the first-trimester placental trophoblasts are different from those in last-trimester trophoblasts compared with the third-trimester trophoblasts. Early placental angiogenesis is critical for the establishment of the placental vascularization and, thus, for normal fetal growth and development. DHA and other n-6 fatty acids stimulate angiogenesis in placental first-trimester cells. The dietary fatty acids stimulated the expression of not only major angiogenic factors, such as VEGF and ANGPTL4, but also FABP-4 and FABP-3, which are known to directly modulate angiogenesis. Among all the FABPs, FABP-4 appeared to be the potent regulator of angiogenic process mediated by fatty acids, leptin, or VEGF. A better understanding of fatty acid transport physiology in the fetoplacental unit is needed to have optimum fetoplacental growth and development.

REFERENCES

Basak, S. and A. K. Duttaroy. 2013. "Effects of fatty acids on angiogenic activity in the placental extravillious trophoblast cells." *Prostaglandins Leukot Essent Fatty Acids* 88 (2):155–62. doi:10.1016/j.plefa .2012.10.001.

Campbell, F. M., A. M. Clohessy, M. J. Gordon, K. R. Page, and A. K. Dutta-Roy. 1997. "Uptake of long chain fatty acids by human placental choriocarcinoma (BeWo) cells: Role of plasma membrane fatty acid-binding protein." *J Lipid Res* 38 (12):2558–68.

Campbell, F. M., P. G. Bush, J. H. Veerkamp, and A. K. Dutta-Roy. 1998. "Detection and cellular localization of plasma membrane-associated and cytoplasmic fatty acid-binding proteins in human placenta." *Placenta* 19 (5–6):409–15.

Crabtree, J. T., M. J. Gordon, F. M. Campbell, and A. K. Dutta-Roy. 1998. "Differential distribution and metabolism of arachidonic acid and docosahexaenoic acid by human placental choriocarcinoma (BeWo) cells." *Mol Cell Biochem* 185 (1–2):191–8.

Dutta-Roy, A. K. 2000a. "Cellular uptake of long-chain fatty acids: Role of membrane-associated fatty-acid-binding/transport proteins." *Cell Mol Life Sci* 57 (10):1360–72.

Dutta-Roy, A. K. 2000b. "Transport mechanisms for long-chain polyunsaturated fatty acids in the human placenta." *Am J Clin Nutr* 71 (1 Suppl):315S–22S.

Duttaroy, A. K. 2009. "Transport of fatty acids across the human placenta: A review." *Prog Lipid Res* 48 (1):52–61. doi:10.1016/j.plipres.2008.11.001.

Glatz, J. F. and J. Storch. 2001. "Unravelling the significance of cellular fatty acid-binding proteins." *Curr Opin Lipidol* 12 (3):267–74.

Innis, S. M. 2000. "The role of dietary n-6 and n-3 fatty acids in the developing brain." *Dev Neurosci* 22 (5–6):474–80.

Innis, S. M. 2007. "Fatty acids and early human development." *Early Hum Dev* 83 (12):761–6. doi:10.1016/j .earlhumdev.2007.09.004.

Johnsen, G. M., S. Basak, M. S. Weedon-Fekjaer, A. C. Staff, and A. K. Duttaroy. 2011. "Docosahexaenoic acid stimulates tube formation in first trimester trophoblast cells, HTR8/SVneo." *Placenta* 32:626–632. doi:10.1016/j.placenta.2011.06.009.

Krabbendam, L., E. Bakker, G. Hornstra, and J. van Os. 2007. "Relationship between DHA status at birth and child problem behaviour at 7 years of age." *Prostaglandins Leukot Essent Fatty Acids* 76 (1):29–34. doi:10.1016/j.plefa.2006.09.004.

Li, D., H. S. Weisinger, R. S. Weisinger, M. Mathai, J. A. Armitage, A. J. Vingrys, and A. J. Sinclair. 2006. "Omega 6 to omega 3 fatty acid imbalance early in life leads to persistent reductions in DHA levels in glycerophospholipids in rat hypothalamus even after long-term omega 3 fatty acid repletion." *Prostaglandins Leukot Essent Fatty Acids* 74 (6):391–9. doi:10.1016/j.plefa.2006.03.010.

Tobin, K. A., G. M. Johnsen, A. C. Staff, and A. K. Duttaroy. 2009. "Long-chain polyunsaturated fatty acid transport across human placental choriocarcinoma (BeWo) cells." *Placenta* 30 (1):41–7. doi:10.1016/j .placenta.2008.10.007.

Weedon-Fekjaer, M. S., A. K. Duttaroy, and H. I. Nebb. 2005. "Liver X receptors mediate inhibition of hCG secretion in a human placental trophoblast cell line." *Placenta* 26 (10):721–8. doi:10.1016/j .placenta.2004.10.005.

Whalley, L. J., H. C. Fox, K. W. Wahle, J. M. Starr, and I. J. Deary. 2004. "Cognitive aging, childhood intelligence, and the use of food supplements: Possible involvement of n-3 fatty acids." *Am J Clin Nutr* 80 (6):1650–7.

7 The Roles of Fatty Acids in Fetal Development

Emilio Herrera and Henar Ortega-Senovilla

CONTENTS

ABSTRACT

Polyunsaturated fatty acids (PUFAs) are required by the embryo and oocytes, but until around 25 weeks of gestation, their accumulation by the fetus is relatively small and increases logarithmically with gestational age. Docosahexaenoic acid (DHA) and arachidonic acid (AA) are involved in neurotransmission and retinal function; additionally, AA is of particular importance for growth and development. In humans, mitochondrial fatty acid oxidation plays an important role in placental and fetal metabolism. The sources of PUFA needed to sustain fetal growth are both maternal diet and fat stores and fetal synthesis. In the maternal circulation, PUFAs are carried in their esterified form by plasma lipoproteins; both placental lipoprotein receptors and lipases ensure that they are hydrolyzed before or after their receptor-mediated uptake and fatty acids are released to the fetal circulation. Nonesterified fatty acids in maternal plasma could also be a source of PUFAs for the fetus, crossing the placenta, thanks to the fatty acid-binding proteins and fatty acid transfer proteins. Pregnancy is a state of mild controlled inflammation, and eicosanoids derived from PUFAs can modulate the proinflammatory/anti-inflammatory balance at various points. On the contrary, the role of PUFAs in placental oxidative stress is controversial, with different authors reporting that PUFAs either limit oxidative stress, have no effect, or cause an increase in oxidative stress. Some bioactive proteins called adipokines can be synthesized by the placenta, as is the case of leptin, or have their effect on the placenta by interacting with their receptors, as is the case for adiponectin and others. These adipokines can be also synthesized by the fetus and have different effects on maternal metabolism and fetal development. Supplementation of n-3 PUFA has been shown to modulate the expression of these adipokines in maternal, placental, or fetal tissues, although additional studies are necessary to determine their precise role in fetal growth.

KEY WORDS

Polyunsaturated fatty acids, fetal growth, placenta, adipokines, neurological development, fat depots, inflammation, oxidative stress.

7.1 INTRODUCTION

The fetus needs fatty acids as structural components of tissues; as a source of energy; as precursors of bioactive compounds such as eicosanoids, which include prostacyclins (PCs), prostaglandins (PGs), thromboxanes (TXs), and leukotrienes (LTs); and if metabolic regulation in the fetus is similar to that in the adult, as regulators of transcription factors. Whereas all fatty acids can provide energy, structural and metabolic functions mainly require polyunsaturated fatty acids (PUFAs). These PUFAs have at least two double bonds, one of which is in the third carbon (n-3) or the sixth carbon (n-6) from the terminal methyl group of the hydrocarbon chain and must be obtained from external sources, either in normal dietary sources or by supplementation as a clinical or experimental

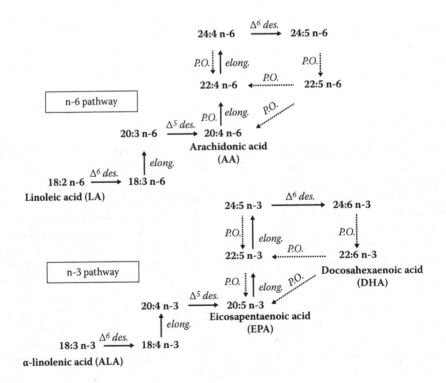

FIGURE 7.1 Schematic n-6 and n-3 pathways for the synthesis of arachidonic acid (AA), eicosapentaenoic acid (EPA), and docosahexaenoic acid (DHA) from dietary essential fatty acids, linoleic acid (LA) and α-linolenic acid (ALA). The process requires a series of common microsomal elongation and desaturase-mediated reactions. The final synthesis of AA and DHA requires additional modifications in peroxisomes. Δ^6 and Δ^5 des., Δ^6- and Δ^5-desaturases; elong., elongase; P.O., peroxisome.

intervention, as α-linolenic acid (ALA, 18:3 n-3) or linoleic acid (LA, 18:2 n-6), known as the essential fatty acids (EFAs), or their long-chain PUFA (LCPUFA) derivatives. ALA and LA are precursors of the LCPUFA of the n-3 and n-6 pathways, respectively, which are produced by the processes of elongation and desaturation (Figure 7.1). Metabolically important n-3 LCPUFAs are eicosapentaenoic acid (EPA, 20:5 n-3) and docosahexaenoic acid (DHA, 22:6 n-3), and arachidonic acid (AA, 20:4 n-6) is the important member of the n-6 family. None of these three acids are absolute requirements of the maternal diet as they can be synthesized from the EFA precursors; however, the conversion of EFA to LCPUFA in term and preterm neonates is very limited, and the tissue and plasma concentrations of these fatty acids depend mainly on the exogenous supply. Thus, since during periods of rapid intrauterine growth, the production of EPA, DHA and AA may be inadequate, they have also been considered as essential for the fetus. The purpose of this chapter is to review the roles of PUFA during pregnancy on fetal development under normal conditions.

7.2 IMPORTANCE OF LCPUFA TO FETAL GROWTH

During the early stages of development, corresponding to the first 8 weeks of intrauterine life, PUFAs are required by the embryo and oocytes (Haggarty et al. 2006). However, from animal studies, it is known that during this stage, the net rate of PUFA utilization by the gametes and embryo is small and does not represent an additional demand on the mother or her diet. During the fetal period, until around 25 weeks of gestation in humans, the accumulation of lipids and of specific fatty acids is relatively small but increases logarithmically with gestational age (Haggarty 2010) and reaches its maximal rate of accretion just before term.

The greatest accretion of individual fatty acids also corresponds to the last 5 weeks of pregnancy, and it has been estimated in Western populations that fetuses have the following order of EFA or LCPUFA tissue accretion: LA (average of 342 mg/day) > AA (average of 95 mg/day) > DHA (average of 42 mg/day) (Kuipers et al. 2012). Despite the fact that AA accumulates more rapidly in the fetus than DHA does, at term, a higher proportion of DHA than AA is found in cerebral tissue (Kuipers et al. 2012). The accretion of DHA during fetal life takes place from around the sixth month of pregnancy and continues during the first 2 years of life, being the predominant fatty acid in phospholipids in the neuronal membranes of the cerebral cortex and in the photoreceptors of the retina (Guesnet and Alessandri 2011). The supply of these fatty acids during pregnancy and the neonatal period is critical for proper function, and both retinal function and learning ability become permanently impaired if the accumulation of DHA during intrauterine life is insufficient (Innis 1991).

DHA is involved in neural membrane fluidity and flexibility as well as neurotransmission; it can regulate ion-channel activity and gene expression and can be metabolized to neuroprotective metabolites. Based on the importance of DHA during fetal development for brain and retina function, several studies have investigated the effects of supplementing the maternal diet. Supplementation of pregnant mothers with LCPUFA improves neonatal LCPUFA status, and supplementation with DHA has been found to increase visual acuity (Smithers et al. 2008).

Preterm infants have lower DHA and AA status than full-term neonates do (Carlson et al. 1993) probably because they do not receive the third-trimester intrauterine supply of EFA and LCPUFA. This is particularly important since the low levels of DHA in premature infants have been shown to affect their eye and brain functions (Carlson et al. 1993; Uauy et al. 1996).

The picture concerning the role of fish-derived LCPUFA as dietary supplement for the pregnant mother is nothing if not confusing and contradictory. During pregnancy, increased intake of seafood and n-3 LCPUFA was shown to promote longer gestation and prevent preterm birth (Olsen and Secher 2002), although there are also studies where no association between higher seafood or n-3 LCPUFA intake and length of gestation was found (Oken et al. 2004). Even in a prospective study with 62,099 participants, it was found that lean fish intake was positively associated with birth weight and head circumference, but fatty fish was not associated with any measures of birth size and supplementary n-3 intake was negatively associated with infant head circumference (Brantsaeter et al. 2012).

In some studies, supplementation with marine oil (around 3 g of n-3 LCPUFA) in the second half of pregnancy resulted in small increases in birth weights and birth lengths compared with controls (Horvath, Koletzko, and Szajewska 2007; Szajewska, Horvath, and Koletzko 2006). However, these effects were commensurate with a small increase in gestation length, and therefore, it seems that the observed increases in birth weight and birth length with n-3 LCPUFA supplementation are a function of the increased duration of pregnancy.

Intervention trials have been conducted also in low-income countries by studying the effect of fish oil (1.2 g DHA and 1.8 g EPA per day) from 25 weeks of gestation until birth (Tofail et al. 2006) or the effect of DHA supplementation only (400 mg/day) from 18 to 22 weeks of gestation until birth (Ramakrishnan et al. 2010). In neither study was there any observable difference in mean birth weight, birth length, or head circumference between the groups. We can conclude, therefore, that low n-3 LCPUFAs are associated with dysfunctional brain and retinal development and possibly with impaired growth.

AA is of particular importance for growth and development, and linear regression analysis between birth weight and any plasma fatty acid in premature infants revealed only a significant correlation with AA and total n-6 LCPUFA (Koletzko and Braun 1991). The growth-promoting effect of AA could be related to its function as a precursor of PGs and other eicosanoids or to its structural roles in membrane phospholipids.

Specific fatty acids can cause competitive inhibition of the Δ^6- and Δ^5-desaturases that control the conversion of EFA into LCPUFA by both the n-3 and n-6 pathways. In this way, an excess of one fatty acid may inhibit the synthesis of another particular LCPUFA that could be essential for fetal growth. Thus, when fish oil is consumed, low plasma levels of AA are found (Amusquivar et al. 2000), the effect being caused by the abundance of EPA and DHA in fish oil, which are known specifically to inhibit the Δ^6-desaturase activity (Raz et al. 1997). The inhibitory effects of an excess of certain dietary fatty acids on the LCPUFA synthetic pathway may become especially important during the perinatal period, when AA status has been correlated to body weight in preterm infants (see above).

Maternal LCPUFA status has also been linked to bone development in children. Data from animal models have suggested a role for LCPUFA in the regulation of bone metabolism, and the major eicosanoid products of AA are known to affect bone turnover in a dose-dependent manner. In human pregnancy, it has been shown that maternal and cord blood LCPUFAs are predictive of bone mass at birth (Weiler et al. 2005).

7.3   LCPUFA AS A SOURCE OF ENERGY FOR THE FETUS

During pregnancy, the fetus is continuously supplied through the placenta with a diet rich in carbohydrates and amino acids and poor in fat, and, based mainly on experiments with rats and other animal species, the fetus has classically been considered to be primarily dependent on glucose oxidation for energy production. However, recently, several laboratories have reevaluated the role of mitochondrial fatty acid oxidation (FAO) in human placental and fetal metabolism (Oey et al. 2003; Strauss 2005). Using different approaches, it has been shown that mRNA expression and activity of FAO enzymes are present in substantial proportions in several human fetal tissues and in placenta (Oey et al. 2003, 2005), indicating that FAO actively contributes to the fetal and placental energy production. In fact, several recessively inherited disorders in several genes of the mitochondrial FAO pathway (Rinaldo, Matern, and Bennett 2002) are associated with prematurity, intrauterine growth retardation (IUGR), fasting-induced hypoketotic hypoglycemia, and hepatic encephalopathy, which may progress to coma and death. These findings suggest that, in contrast to the results obtained in animal studies, FAO plays an important role in the human fetal–placental unit, being the major source of metabolic energy and playing a critical role for placental function and fetal development.

In animal studies, and despite the predominant role of glucose oxidation for energy production, disturbances of enzymes of the FAO pathway are associated with reduced fertility, fetal demise, and fetal growth restriction (Ibdah et al. 2001). Furthermore, inactivation of genes encoding for the transcription factors that regulate the FAO, like the peroxisome proliferator-activated receptors (PPARs), causes embryonic lethality and failure of the syncytiotrophoblast to develop and sustain pregnancy (Barak et al. 1999).

It may therefore be concluded that FAO plays an essential role in the fetal–placental unit, and, although all fatty acids can provide energy by mitochondrial oxidation, it is expected that differences in the proportions of each fatty acid being oxidized will exist; the LCPUFA of maternal origin will probably be the preferred oxidative substrate. The fetus can synthesize saturated and mono-unsaturated fatty acids *de novo* as directly shown in rats (Lorenzo et al. 1981) and deduced in humans from the presence of both fatty acid synthase and stearoyl-CoA desaturase (SCD1) (Kusakabe et al. 2000). Oxidation of newly synthesized fatty acids is probably low. Moreover, although endogenous synthesis of LCPUFA from EFA is likely to be higher in preterm than in term infants, the amount of LCPUFA produced is insufficient to match the accretion rate *in utero*. The primary source of LCPUFA for the fetus is that of maternal origin, which is the preferred substrate for placental transfer when compared with other fatty acids (Haggarty 2010).

7.4 LCPUFA AND NEUROLOGICAL AND VISUAL DEVELOPMENT

LCPUFAs comprise approximately 15% to 30% of brain dry weight and are essential for early brain development. They are involved in both the structure and function of the central nervous system. The brain and retina contain large quantities of n-3 and n-6 LCPUFA, particularly DHA and AA (Crawford 1992). DHA is involved in blood–brain functions and neural membrane fluidity and regulates neurotransmission systems (Kidd 2007); it also has effects on neuronal membrane dynamics and, therefore, on transporter, receptor, and neurotransmitter functions. AA, among other things, helps to maintain hippocampal cell membrane fluidity; protects the brain from oxidative stress by activating PPARγ (Wang et al. 2006); activates syntaxin, a protein involved in the growth and repair of neurons (Darios and Davletov 2006); and is involved in early neurological development (Birch et al. 2000).

Although the fastest stage of neural development is during fetal growth, it also undergoes significant development during the first 5 years of postnatal life. During this period, nutrient intake plays a critical role in the development of the brain's structural and functional maturation.

Examination of intrauterine accretion of n-6 and n-3 LCPUFA has indicated rapid accretion of these fatty acids in the fetal brain. In the third trimester of pregnancy and the 18 months of postnatal life, the brain undergoes an accelerated growth (Darios and Davletov 2006), during which time significant amounts of AA and DHA accumulate in the brain and the physiological demand for these nutrients increases. This requirement is supported by the selective placental transfer of DHA and AA from mother to fetus (Dutta-Roy 2000), the consumption of milk in breastfed infants (Sanders and Naismith 1979), and the synthesis from dietary EFA (Carnielli et al. 1996).

In most tissues, DHA accounts for only a very small proportion of the fatty acid content of the membrane phospholipids, but in the disc membrane of retinal photoreceptors, it contributes 50% of the total fatty acid content of the phospholipids. Furthermore, the abundance of LCPUFA in all the main phospholipids of the disc membrane is believed to play a pivotal role in the conformational change in rhodopsin.

The accretion rates of LCPUFA in the fetal brain and retinal tissues are highest in the third trimester. Thus, preterm delivery, which cuts off the placental supply of LCPUFAs when accretion should still be increasing, will affect their availability and may have consequences for neural and retinal development.

Observational studies have reported that maternal fish consumption during pregnancy has been positively associated with cognitive and visual abilities in the offspring (Daniels et al. 2004) and that pregnant women who consume higher than the recommended quantity of fish have children with higher cognitive scores (Hibbeln et al. 2007). However, these observational studies are unable to establish causality because of the difficulties of adjusting for confounding factors that also influence early childhood development. Therefore, a systematic review of randomized controlled trials (RCTs) has been carried out to determine whether increased n-3 LCPUFA intake during pregnancy improves neurological and visual development in the offspring (Gould, Smithers, and Makrides 2013). A total of 11 RCTs involving 5272 participants were included in the review, and its conclusion was that the evidence neither supports nor refutes the hypothesis that n-3 LCPUFA supplementation in pregnancy improves child cognitive or visual development.

7.5 SOURCES OF PUFAs TO SUSTAIN FETAL GROWTH

7.5.1 MATERNAL DIET

The dietary supply of EFA and LCPUFA may become important during pregnancy. As noted above, during intrauterine development, DHA and AA are of special importance because of their essential function in the brain and retina and the roles of AA and its metabolites in growth and maturation of different organs. Although these LCPUFAs can be synthesized *de novo* from EFA by the fetus, the pathways are not very active, and therefore, the fetus depends on the placental transfer of these two acids from maternal circulation. This transfer appears to occur at a rate that is closely correlated with maternal intake, and maternal plasma percentages of DHA and AA are predictive of their proportions in umbilical cord plasma and red blood cells.

The major n-3 fatty acids present in the diet range from 1.0 to 1.2 g/day in women, corresponding to 0.9 to 1.1 g/day for ALA and 0.052 to 0.069 g/day and 0.004 to 0.093 g/day for its metabolites EPA and DHA, respectively, in US diets. The median intake of n-6 LCPUFA in women ranges from approximately 9 to 11 g/day, of which approximately 85% to 90% corresponds to LA with AA and γ-linolenic acid (18:3 n-6) present only in small amounts (Food and Nutrition Board 2005). ALA is found predominantly in vegetable oils, whereas the major dietary sources of EPA and DHA are fish oils and fatty fish, with smaller amounts present in meat and eggs. LA is found mainly in vegetable oils and represents the most abundant PUFA; AA, however, is not present in plant-derived fats and oils and is present in small amounts in meat, poultry, and eggs, having been formed from dietary LA by animal cells.

During the earliest stages of intrauterine development and until the 25th week of gestation, the net rate of PUFA utilization by the fetus does not make a significant additional demand on the maternal diet. Looking at individual fatty acids, the requirement for DHA until around 25 weeks of gestation is of the order of 100 mg/day and can be met by the normal dietary intake. However, the requirement increases greatly thereafter to reach over 300 mg/day close to term (Haggarty 2010). Although the dietary intake in some populations may be in this range (as it is the case in the northern and other European countries), this is not always the case. Moreover, the exclusion of meat and especially fish from the diet by vegetarians may result in insufficient preformed DHA being consumed to meet the estimated maternal and fetal needs in the later stages of pregnancy (Welch et al. 2010). In any case, a substantial proportion of mothers during the late stages of gestation do not ingest enough preformed DHA to meet maternal and fetal needs. However, adaptive mechanisms involving EFA elongation and desaturation and appropriate synchronization of maternal, placental, and fetal fat metabolism may produce a reduction in maternal dietary needs, sufficient to satisfy the fetal demand.

7.5.2 ENDOGENOUS SYNTHESIS

In human tissues, DHA and AA can be synthesized from their EFA precursors (Figure 7.1), and it has been proposed that this pathway is also active in the fetoplacental unit. There is one study showing the incorporation of ^{14}C-acetate into AA by human placental slices (Zimmermann et al. 1979), and Δ^5 and Δ^6 desaturase mRNA have been detected in the human placenta, although their levels are relatively low compared with other tissues (Cho, Nakamura, and Clarke 1999). Further, no activity in any Δ^5 or Δ^6 desaturase in human placenta has been detected (Chambaz et al. 1985). Thus, it appears that no significant quantities of AA or DHA synthesized by the placenta are supplied to the fetus. However, experimental evidence indicates that endogenous synthesis of LCPUFA does occur in human term and preterm neonates. Evidence of n-6 LCPUFA synthesis from ^{13}C-labelled LA was found in neonates in the first week of life (Szitanyi et al. 1999), and preterm infants born as early as 26 weeks' gestation were able to form AA and DHA from ^{2}H- or ^{13}C-labelled LA and ALA (Carnielli et al. 1996).

In conclusion, experimental evidence in human term and preterm neonates indicates that endogenous synthesis of LCPUFA in the fetus occurs. However, rates of production are very variable, especially in premature infants, and although it is not possible to quantify absolute rates of conversion *in vivo*, its magnitude does not appear sufficient to match the demands of the developing tissues.

7.5.3 MATERNAL FAT DEPOTS

The gross accumulation of fat in human maternal fat depots over a complete pregnancy is approximately equal to the entire weight of the average newborn. Most of this accumulation takes place during the first two thirds of gestation, when fetal growth is still small (Haggarty 2010), and from studies in rats, it is thought to be the result of the combined effects of hyperphagia, enhanced lipogenesis (Palacin et al. 1991), and unmodified or even increased extrahepatic lipoprotein lipase (LPL) (Alvarez et al. 1996; Knopp, Boroush, and O'Sullivan 1975; Martin-Hidalgo et al. 1994). By means of such augmented LPL activity in adipose tissue, dietary-derived LCPUFAs transported in human pregnant plasma in their esterified form (Herrera 2002a,b) in triacylglycerol-rich lipoproteins—very-low-density lipoproteins (VLDL) and chylomicrons—are hydrolyzed, and the released fatty acids are taken up for storage in the subjacent tissue.

The tendency to accumulate fat ceases during late gestation because maternal lipid metabolism becomes catabolic. This is evidenced by increased adipose tissue lipolysis (Elliott 1975) and reduced uptake of circulating triacylglycerols (Herrera, Gomez-Coronado, and Lasuncion 1987) secondary to the reduction in adipose tissue LPL activity (Alvarez et al. 1996). The changes, together with the very active hepatic production of triacylglycerols (Humphrey et al. 1980), are responsible for the marked progressive increase in maternal circulating triacylglycerols occurring during late gestation (Alvarez et al. 1996; Montelongo et al. 1992). The major changes in the maternal lipid metabolism are summarized in Figure 7.2, which depicts the changes in adipose tissue, liver, and intestinal activity that are responsible for the physiological increase in maternal plasma nonesterified fatty acid (NEFA), glycerol, and triacylglycerol-rich lipoproteins (VLDL and chylomicrons).

The net enhanced adipose tissue breakdown taking place during late pregnancy contributes to the dietary fatty acids that were stored in adipose tissue during the first half of gestation, being released into maternal plasma and becoming available to the fetus and the newborn. Although these metabolic interactions have been successfully tested in pregnant sows (Amusquivar et al. 2010) and rats (Fernandes, Tavares do Carmo, and Herrera 2012), they remain to be tested in humans. However, as shown in Table 7.1, in pregnant women at term, there are significant linear correlations of LCPUFA between maternal plasma and adipose tissue and between maternal and cord plasma, suggesting a contribution of those fatty acids previously deposited in adipose tissue to those that become available to the fetus.

7.5.4 PLACENTAL FATTY ACID TRANSFER

Both EFA and LCPUFA derived from maternal diet or released from fat depots as NEFA are taken up by the liver, where a proportion are reesterified and released back into the circulation, where they are transported mainly in their esterified form in maternal plasma lipoproteins, rather than in their NEFA form (Herrera 2002a,b). These must become available to the fetus

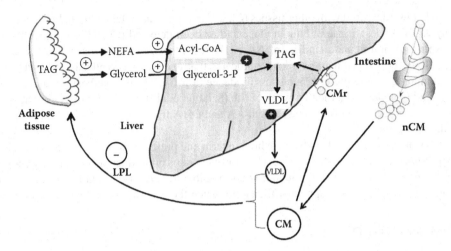

FIGURE 7.2   Major changes in maternal lipid metabolism during late pregnancy. CM, chylomicrons; CMr, chylomicron remnant; LPL, lipoprotein lipase; nCM, nascent chylomicron; NEFA, nonesterified fatty acids; TAG, triacylglycerols; VLDL, very-low-density lipoprotein.

TABLE 7.1

Linear Correlations of LCPUFA in Pregnant Women at Term

Fatty Acid	n	r	p
Between Maternal Plasma and Adipose Tissue			
Arachidonic acid	68	0.3720	<0.01
Eicosapentaenoic acid	68	0.5130	<0.001
Docosahexaenoic acid	68	0.3377	<0.05
Between Maternal and Cord Blood Plasma LCPUFA			
Arachidonic acid	68	0.2741	<0.05
Eicosapentaenoic acid	68	0.2901	<0.05
Docosahexaenoic acid	68	0.4175	<0.001

Source: Values correspond to the study reported in Herrera, E.
   et al., *Eur. J. Clin. Nutr.* 58, 1231–1238, 2004.

despite the lack of a direct placental transfer of maternal lipoproteins. The transfer occurs thanks to the presence of lipoprotein receptors in the placental trophoblast cells that lie at the interface with maternal blood. These cells are therefore positioned to bind maternal lipoproteins and mediate their metabolism and the subsequent transfer of the fatty acids they carry to the fetal circulation. VLDL/apolipoprotein E receptor and low-density lipoproteins, high-density lipoproteins, and scavenger receptors are expressed in human placental tissue (Albrecht et al. 1995; Cummings et al. 1982; Wadsack et al. 2003). In addition, placental tissue expresses LPL activity (Bonet et al. 1992) as well as phospholipase A$_2$ (PLA2) (Varastehpour et al. 2006) and endothelial lipase activities (Gauster et al. 2011). Consequently, esterified fatty acids are hydrolyzed either extracellularly before uptake or intracellularly after receptor-mediated endocytosis. After uptake, they are reesterified before eventual release (see below).

The manner in which placental fatty acids are released into the fetal circulation is not completely understood. One possibility is in the form of NEFA after the intracellular hydrolysis of esterified fatty acids in the placenta. In the fetal circulation, these NEFAs would bind to a specific oncofetal protein, α-fetoprotein, and be rapidly transported to fetal liver, where they can be esterified and released back into circulation in the form of VLDL-triacylglycerols. Another possibility is the release to the fetal circulation in their esterified form associated with specific lipoproteins. This mechanism is consistent with the capacity of the human placenta to secrete lipoproteins containing apolipoprotein B-100 (Madsen et al. 2004). Either of these possibilities is consistent with reports in humans during late gestation of significant and positive correlations between the concentrations of certain PUFAs in maternal plasma triacylglycerols and their concentrations in cord plasma triacylglycerols (Berghaus, Demmelmair, and Koletzko 2000). It is also consistent with the higher amount of esterified ^{13}C-fatty acids than ^{13}C-NEFA in cord blood plasma after oral administration of different ^{13}C-fatty acids to pregnant women at term (Pagan et al. 2013). These relationships may have important implications for newborn weight because positive linear correlations between cord blood triacylglycerols or NEFA and neonatal anthropometric measures (i.e., birth weight and neonatal fat mass) have been found in healthy humans (Schaefer-Graf et al. 2011).

Although most LCPUFAs in maternal circulation are carried in their esterified form in plasma lipoproteins rather than as NEFAs, a certain proportion of maternal NEFAs could be also a source of PUFAs to the fetus. Both a plasma membrane fatty acid-binding protein ($FABP_{pm}$) that would facilitate membrane fatty acid translocation and fatty acid transfer proteins (fatty acid translocase/CD36 and fatty acid transport protein) are present in human placental membranes (Campbell, Gordon, and Dutta-Roy 1996), but the precise way in which membrane-associated FABPs facilitate transmembrane passage of fatty acids is still a matter of speculation (Haggarty 2010).

The combination of all of these processes determines the actual rate of placental fatty acid transfer and its selectivity. The placenta selectively transports AA and DHA from the maternal to the fetal compartment, resulting in a proportional enrichment of these LCPUFAs in the circulating lipids of the fetus (Innis 1991), although their absolute concentrations remain lower than in the maternal site (Sakamoto and Kubota 2004). This permanent maternal–fetal gradient facilitates the transfer of several NEFAs across the placenta, mainly by diffusion. Other factors affecting the fatty acid transfer process are uterine and umbilical blood flow rates and the concentration of fetal serum albumin (Stephenson, Stammers, and Hull 1993). The increase in plasma albumin that occurs during the third trimester in the human fetus may enable the NEFA transport to increase when the fetal demands for neural development and growth are at their greatest.

7.6 ROLE OF PUFAs IN PLACENTAL FUNCTIONS

After implantation, the placenta is responsible for anchoring the fetus in the uterus, forming an anatomical barrier between maternal and fetal circulation, and mediating, as well as regulating, nutrient uptake from the mother by the fetus. In addition, the placenta plays an active role in regulating other aspects of benefit to the fetus, providing a means of mediating hormonal signals and inducing immunological tolerance. Thus, the placenta must control processes like inflammation and oxidative stress that can alter its own metabolism and produce placental disorders with maternal and fetal consequences.

Fatty acids themselves, or their derivatives (eicosanoids), may influence the production of placental hormones and the interaction between hormone and receptor and may regulate placental inflammation and oxidative stress. Maternal dietary supplementation with n-3 PUFAs has demonstrated beneficial effects on human pregnancy outcomes, including increased gestation length, increased fetal growth, and reduced pregnancy risk (Szajewska, Horvath, and Koletzko 2006), although other supplementation studies have not found such benefits (Imhoff-Kunsch et al. 2012), so the subject remains controversial.

7.6.1 INFLAMMATION

The placenta has to maintain a very delicate balance between allowing trophoblast invasion of spiral arteries to take place, on the one hand, and preventing uncontrolled invasion on the other. Maternal immune cells seem to play a key role in this sense, so pregnancy has been described as a state of mild controlled inflammation, with higher circulating levels of proinflammatory mediators in pregnant women than in nonpregnant women (Paulesu et al. 2010). The success of pregnancy is guaranteed by the local secretion of cytokines beneficial to the fetus and pregnancy. Cytokines are part of a complex network of peptide factors, which include interferons (IFNs), interleukins (ILs), tumor necrosis factors (TNFs), colony stimulating factors, and vascular endothelial growth factors, among others. They play a key role in the maternal tolerance of the semiallogeneic embryo and they are also regulators of cell proliferation and differentiation. The cytokines contribute to normal physiological processes in the placenta, which include trophoblast invasion, placental proliferation, and angiogenesis, as well as fetal growth and expansion in the maternal tissues (Forbes and Westwood 2010). Most of these cytokines are produced by cells of normal placentas and by leukocytes infiltrating the placenta. They can exert proinflammatory or anti-inflammatory effects (review in Paulesu et al. 2010). For example, proinflammatory cytokines, like TNFα, IFNγ, IL-1, IL-1β, IL-6, IL-12, and IL-2, among others, are secreted during the early phase of pregnancy, as the same time as blastocyst implantation and placental development during the first trimester of pregnancy (Srivastava et al. 2013), while secretion of anti-inflammatory cytokines like IL-4 and IL-10 begins during the second trimester of gestation (Chatterjee et al. 2014) and continues almost up to term, which allows uterine quiescence and fetal growth and development. Near delivery, a new increase in proinflammatory cytokines occurs, which stimulates the transcription of nuclear factor kappa β, and in turn mediates the transcription of new proinflammatory cytokines. Thus, pregnancy is associated with an evolving balance of cytokines, involving changes in the types or concentrations of cytokines at different phases of pregnancy. Any local or systemic alteration in the maternal immune environment can cause an unexpected pregnancy outcome, such as preeclampsia, preterm labor, or miscarriage. In fact, a decreased production of IL-4 and IL-10 and an increased production of IFNγ and IL-2 have been reported in women with spontaneous miscarriage, as have higher concentrations of placental TNFα, IL-6, and IL-1β in preterm births and in fetuses with intrauterine growth restriction and higher expression and secretion of TNFα and ILs in the placentas of preeclamptic women.

In addition to cytokines, eicosanoids are another important class of immunological mediators, which include PGs, PCs, TXs, and LTs. Most of these bioactive compounds are derived from the LCPUFAs AA and EPA. In response to an inflammatory stimulus, phospholipase enzymes, primarily PLA2, release AA or EPA from the cellular membrane phospholipids. These fatty acids are then metabolized by cyclooxygenase (COX) enzymes to become a PG or TX or by lipoxygenase-5 enzyme to become an LT (Figure 7.3). AA-derived eicosanoids are primarily proinflammatory, acting to enhance local blood flow and increase the production of proinflammatory cytokines and reactive oxygen species (ROS). In contrast, eicosanoids derived from EPA generally have lower inflammatory properties than those derived from AA. This is due, in part, to its synthesis, which occurs at low efficiency, and to their interaction with different membrane and nuclear receptors, which modulate the properties of these derivatives. The activation of PLA2 by cytokines, like TNFα, suggests that this enzyme functions as cellular link between inflammatory pathways and fatty acid metabolism (Varastehpour et al. 2006).

Pregnancy-related inflammation is considered beneficial for a successful pregnancy, but excessive placental inflammation is associated with unfavorable pregnancy outcomes related to placental disturbances, including preterm birth, preeclampsia, and intrauterine growth restriction.

Once the inflammatory response ends, the tissue has to recover its basal condition. Until recently, it was thought that the resolution of inflammation was a passive process that occurred simply as the proinflammatory signals dissipated. However, it is now known that the resolution of inflammation is a highly active process, which is programmed and coordinated by specialized PUFA-derived

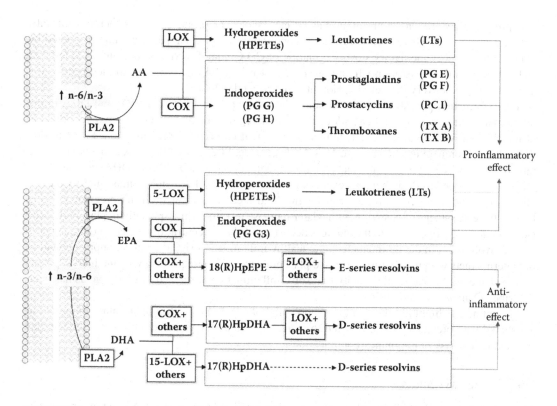

FIGURE 7.3 Schematic synthesis of eicosanoid and proresolving lipid mediators derived from n-6 and n-3 fatty acids. PLA2, phospholipase A2; AA, arachidonic acid; EPA, eicosapentaenoic acid; DHA, docosahexanoic acid; LOX, lipoxygenase; COX, cyclooxygenase.

mediators (Serhan et al. 2002) that are involved in the recovery by the tissue of its basal condition as it was before the development of the immune response. These mediators are directly derived from LCPUFAs via platelet–leucocyte interactions in a complex pathway catalyzed by COX and LOX enzymes (Figure 7.3). Some of these proresolving molecules, like lipoxins, are derived from AA and can decrease the synthesis of TNFα and leucocyte chemotaxis. Most of these molecules, however, are derived from n-3 PUFAs, such as resolvins (RvE, derived from EPA, and RvD derived from DHA), protectins, and maresins, all of them having both proresolving and anti-inflammatory effects. Resolvins control the magnitude and duration of inflammation in animal models (Schwab et al. 2007), inhibit leucocyte infiltration and synthesis of proinflammatory cytokines, and interact directly with cell-surface receptors that induce anti-inflammatory functions (Krishnamoorthy et al. 2010). The presence of resolvins and protectins has been detected in human blood and in murine placental tissues, and both of them were increased by dietary n-3 fatty acids (Jones et al. 2013).

LCPUFAs have an important role in immune responses and can modulate the balance between proinflammatory and anti-inflammatory effects at various points. It has been shown that the decreased production of TNFα was accompanied by a decreased AA/EPA ratio in the membrane phospholipids of mononuclear cells, which indicates the significant contribution of the systemic n-6/n-3 PUFA ratio profile in inflammatory responses (Endres et al. 1989). Also, n-3 PUFAs reduce the gene expression of proinflammatory cytokines IL-6 and IL-1β, preventing pathological preterm birth (Yamashita et al. 2013).

Dietary intake of n-3 PUFAs results in the partial replacement of AA by EPA in cellular membranes; consequently, dietary n-3 PUFA supplementation can reduce inflammation by either disrupting the generation of proinflammatory eicosanoids or promoting the generation of anti-inflammatory forms. Therefore, since uterine contractions that induce parturition are triggered by PG proinflammatory mediators, down-regulation of COX2 may function to prevent preterm labor and delivery. This may explain why a high intake of n-3 PUFAs by pregnant women results in a delayed onset of delivery (Szajewska, Horvath, and Koletzko 2006).

The information presented in this section indicates that the role of AA, EPA, and DHA in the inflammatory process may be the result of signals that regulate the balance between the production of metabolites with inflammatory results and those that can reduce inflammation. Furthermore, these PUFAs compete for enzymes such as Δ^6-desaturase, PLA_2, or COX; thus, a low value of the ratio of AA/n-3 LCPUFA may attenuate the inflammatory reactions by EPA or DHA, competitively inhibiting COX and LOX-5, thereby generating smaller amounts of the highly inflammatory metabolites. The concentrations of these proresolving lipid mediators change during pregnancy, being high in the early stages of gestation with a later increase toward term, especially in placental tissue (Jones et al. 2013), in parallel to the changes occurring in the concentration of eicosanoids, suggesting an involvement in the maintenance of a healthy inflammation signal balance. Supplementation of maternal diets with n-3 PUFAs increased placental levels of these proresolving mediators, potentially enhancing the placental capacity to resolve inflammation at the end of gestation, as has been described (Yamashita et al. 2013).

These findings highlight the therapeutic potential of n-3 PUFAs to limit placental inflammation associated with pregnancy disorders and to increase gestational age avoiding intrauterine retardation and reduce risk of pregnancy complications.

7.6.2 OXIDATIVE STRESS

Measurement of markers of oxidative stress in maternal blood and urine shows that pregnancy per se is a state of oxidative stress due to the high metabolic activity of the placenta. Oxygen is indispensable for the final step of energy metabolism, which is cellular respiration; sometimes in this process, the production of ROS occurs, which can cause severe damage to cellular components, such as membranes, nucleic acids, and proteins, in a process called oxidative stress. To avoid this, the cells have a range of antioxidant defense mechanisms that include (1) antioxidant enzymes (catalase, superoxide dismutase, glutathione peroxidase, thioredoxin system), (2) electron transport inhibitors that limit ROS production, and (3) lipophilic antioxidants (such as vitamin E, vitamin C, and coenzyme Q) that reduce the damage caused by ROS.

The onset of pregnancy takes place in a low-oxygen environment, which indirectly protects the embryo cells from ROS-mediated damage. However, the onset of placental perfusion is accompanied by a rapid influx of ROS, which is paralleled by an increased synthesis of enzymatic antioxidants to limit the ROS-induced cellular damage. Oxidative stress due to excessive ROS and weakened antioxidant defenses is causally associated with an increase both in inflammation and the concentrations of inflammation mediators.

The placenta generates ROS that may contribute to the oxidative stress seen even in normal pregnancies and further increases in placenta-related disorders such as preeclampsia, intrauterine growth restriction, miscarriage, and gestational diabetes (Lappas et al. 2011; Watanabe et al. 2013). Among the ROSs produced by the placenta are superoxide, nitric oxide, and peroxynitrite, with diverse actions on cellular function. One of them is the activation of NFκβ, which then translocates to the nucleus and activates the expression of proinflammatory cytokines such as TNFα, IL-1β, or the proinflammatory enzyme COX2. Also LCPUFAs, proteins, and DNA can be targets for oxidative damage, which is related to a loss of membrane fluidity, loss of enzymes with detoxifying activity, and mutation or aberrant gene expression observed in placental injury.

The role of PUFAs in placental oxidative stress is controversial. n-3 PUFAs could potentially limit oxidative stress by enhancing ROS scavenging capacity or by limiting ROS generation. Some authors have reported that supplementation of maternal diet with n-3 PUFAs reduces the placental concentration of isoprostanes F_2 (Jones et al. 2013), a highly sensitive marker of oxidative stress, and increases the synthesis and activity of antioxidant enzymes in this tissue (Jones et al. 2010). In other studies, however, n-3 PUFA supplementation did not suppress either placental or maternal oxidative stress markers (Stark, Clifton, and Hodyl 2013), and it has even been reported that supplementation with n-3 PUFAs in preterm labor could result in an increase in oxidative stress (Boulis et al. 2014).

7.6.3 ADIPOKINES

Originally, adipokines referred to bioactive proteins synthesized in adipose tissue, which regulate body metabolism and energy homeostasis. Actually, adipokines is a general term that collectively defines bioactive proteins involved in the regulation of energy metabolism, immune response, and the interactions between the two systems. The placenta can express some of these adipokines, suggesting that such molecules can be implicated in placental function and fetal growth (Ahlsson et al. 2013).

Leptin is an adipokine-like hormone, the circulating concentrations of which are proportionally related to adipose tissue amount. Leptin and its receptors are also expressed in placenta, where leptin could be implicated in implantation and placental development and in the process of new placental vessel formation. Moreover, this adipokine and its receptor play a key role in reproductive biology and in the activation of signal transduction pathways in placental cells (review in Maymo et al. 2011). *In vitro*, placental leptin is exported into both the maternal and fetal circulation. Thus, maternal leptin concentrations increase significantly in pregnancy, while human placenta expresses large amounts of leptin mRNA and protein (Laivuori et al. 2006). This suggests that the placenta, rather than maternal adipose tissue, is responsible for the pregnancy-induced rise in leptin. Placental leptin also is correlated with umbilical leptin, and fetal adipose tissue is another source of leptin positively related to both birth weight and fetal adiposity (Tsai et al. 2004). Nevertheless, there is controversy about the role of leptin as a regulator of fetal growth because neonates lacking the leptin gene have a normal birth weight (Montague et al. 1997). The expression of leptin is dysregulated in several pathologies of pregnancy. An increase in the expression of placental leptin and its receptor genes has been found in diabetic (i.e., diabetes mellitus) pregnancies with large for gestational age neonates, compared with small for gestational age diabetic fetuses and controls, suggesting that increased placental leptin and leptin receptor expression may have a role in stimulating fetal overgrowth in type 1 diabetic pregnancy and in gestational diabetes. Recently, it has been reported that methylation of the placental leptin promoter sequence occurred during a specific gestational period and was related with macrosomic infants in normal pregnancy, despite the fact that placental leptin expression was not affected (Xu et al. 2014). In preeclampsia, IUGR, and recurrent miscarriage, higher placental and circulating concentrations of leptin have been described. In contrast, supplementation with n-3 PUFAs is associated with reduced levels of circulating leptin (Hariri et al. 2014), although the effect of n-3 PUFAs on the expression of leptin in placenta is not clear.

Adiponectin is another adipokine that is able to modulate the process of placentation by favoring trophoblast migration and differentiation in early pregnancy (Benaitreau et al. 2010) but inhibits syncytialization in human trophoblasts isolated later in gestation (McDonald and Wolfe 2009). In contrast to leptin, although previous reports suggested that adiponectin is produced and secreted by the placenta, more recent studies failed to confirm this observation (Mazaki-Tovi et al. 2007). However, the placenta does express adiponectin receptors (McDonald and Wolfe 2009), which enables the adiponectin to have its effects on the placenta. Adiponectin cannot be transported across the placenta, meaning that maternal adiponectin and fetal adiponectin are not interchangeable (Qiao et al. 2012). The concentration of adiponectin is higher in cord blood than is found in the maternal circulation at term (Ortega-Senovilla et al. 2011), suggesting that the origin of the high concentration of adiponectin is fetal: although the amount of fetal adipose tissue is small, the cord blood concentration of adiponectin does correlate with neonatal fat mass (Tsai et al. 2004). In addition, at delivery, when fetal adipose tissue experiences an increased rate of lipolysis, the circulating levels of adiponectin, but not of other adipokines such as leptin, increase significantly (Ortega-Senovilla et al. 2013), which suggests that fetal adipose tissue could be the origin of fetal adiponectin. Adiponectin in both maternal and fetal tissues is associated with an increased insulin sensitivity, but not in the placenta, where it has the opposite effect, promoting insulin resistance (Aye, Powell, and Jansson 2013). PUFAs could regulate the concentration of adiponectin through PPARγ, although according to the conclusions of a systematic review (von Frankenberg et al. 2014), only a modest increase in adiponectin concentrations has been observed after supplementation with n-3 PUFAs. More studies are necessary to confirm this relationship, especially in pregnancy.

7.7 CONCLUSIONS

Fatty acids during pregnancy have a key role in fetal development. They are important in fetal growth, and their oxidation plays an essential role as a source of energy for the fetoplacental unit. In particular, LCPUFAs are precursors of bioactive compounds and are involved in the structure and function of the nervous system and retina. The sources of LCPUFA for the fetus are maternal diet, maternal fat depots, and placental transfer, whereas their endogenous synthesis does not seem to match the demands of developing tissues. Placental inflammation and oxidative stress are regulated by fatty acids themselves or by their eicosanoid derivatives, and placental functions are also modulated by the adipokines it produces, with consequences for fetal development, as is the case for leptin, or adipokine receptors, like those for adiponectin, which can also be controlled by PUFA.

ACKNOWLEDGMENTS

The authors thank pp-science-editing.com for editing and linguistic revision of the manuscript. Preparation of this chapter was carried out in part with grants from the Universidad San Pablo–CEU, the Fundación Ramón Areces (CIVP16A1835) of Spain, and the Spanish Ministry of Science and Innovation (SAF2012-39273).

REFERENCES

Ahlsson, F., B. Diderholm, U. Ewald, B. Jonsson, A. Forslund, M. Stridsberg, and J. Gustafsson. 2013. "Adipokines and their relation to maternal energy substrate production, insulin resistance and fetal size." *Eur J Obstet Gynecol Reprod Biol* 168 (1):26–29. doi:10.1016/j.ejogrb.2012.12.009.

Albrecht, E. D., J. S. Babischkin, R. D. Koos, and G. J. Pepe. 1995. "Developmental increase in low density lipoprotein receptor messenger ribonucleic acid levels in placental syncytiotrophoblasts during baboon pregnancy." *Endocrinology* 136 (12):5540–5546. doi:10.1210/endo.136.12.7588306.

Alvarez, J. J., A. Montelongo, A. Iglesias, M. A. Lasuncion, and E. Herrera. 1996. "Longitudinal study on lipoprotein profile, high density lipoprotein subclass, and postheparin lipases during gestation in women." *J Lipid Res* 37 (2):299–308.

Amusquivar, E., F. J. Ruperez, C. Barbas, and E. Herrera. 2000. "Low arachidonic acid rather than alpha-tocopherol is responsible for the delayed postnatal development in offspring of rats fed fish oil instead of olive oil during pregnancy and lactation." *J Nutr* 130 (11):2855–2865.

Amusquivar, E., J. Laws, L. Clarke, and E. Herrera. 2010. "Fatty acid composition of the maternal diet during the first or the second half of gestation influences the fatty acid composition of sows' milk and plasma, and plasma of their piglets." *Lipids* 45 (5):409–418. doi:10.1007/s11745-010-3415-2.

Aye, I. L., T. L. Powell, and T. Jansson. 2013. "Review: Adiponectin—The missing link between maternal adiposity, placental transport and fetal growth?" *Placenta* 34 Suppl:S40–S45. doi:10.1016/j.placenta.2012.11.024.

Barak, Y., M. C. Nelson, E. S. Ong, Y. Z. Jones, P. Ruiz-Lozano, K. R. Chien, A. Koder, and R. M. Evans. 1999. "PPAR gamma is required for placental, cardiac, and adipose tissue development." *Mol Cell* 4 (4):585–595.

Benaitreau, D., E. Dos Santos, M. C. Leneveu, N. Alfaidy, J. J. Feige, P. de Mazancourt, R. Pecquery, and M. N. Dieudonne. 2010. "Effects of adiponectin on human trophoblast invasion." *J Endocrinol* 207 (1):45–53. doi:10.1677/JOE-10-0170.

Berghaus, T. M., H. Demmelmair, and B. Koletzko. 2000. "Essential fatty acids and their long-chain polyunsaturated metabolites in maternal and cord plasma triglycerides during late gestation." *Biol Neonate* 77 (2):96–100.

Birch, E. E., S. Garfield, D. R. Hoffman, R. Uauy, and D. G. Birch. 2000. "A randomized controlled trial of early dietary supply of long-chain polyunsaturated fatty acids and mental development in term infants." *Dev Med Child Neurol* 42 (3):174–181.

Bonet, B., J. D. Brunzell, A. M. Gown, and R. H. Knopp. 1992. "Metabolism of very-low-density lipoprotein triglyceride by human placental cells: The role of lipoprotein lipase." *Metabolism* 41 (6):596–603.

Boulis, T. S., B. Rochelson, O. Novick, X. Xue, P. K. Chatterjee, M. Gupta, M. H. Solanki, M. Akerman, and C. N. Metz. 2014. "Omega-3 polyunsaturated fatty acids enhance cytokine production and oxidative stress in a mouse model of preterm labor." *J Perinat Med* 42 (6):693–698. doi:10.1515/jpm-2014-0243.

Brantsaeter, A. L., B. E. Birgisdottir, H. M. Meltzer, H. E. Kvalem, J. Alexander, P. Magnus, and M. Haugen. 2012. "Maternal seafood consumption and infant birth weight, length and head circumference in the Norwegian Mother and Child Cohort Study." *Br J Nutr* 107 (3):436–444. doi:10.1017/S0007114511003047.

Campbell, F. M., M. J. Gordon, and A. K. Dutta-Roy. 1996. "Preferential uptake of long chain polyunsaturated fatty acids by isolated human placental membranes." *Mol Cell Biochem* 155 (1):77–83.

Carlson, S. E., S. H. Werkman, P. G. Rhodes, and E. A. Tolley. 1993. "Visual-acuity development in healthy preterm infants: Effect of marine-oil supplementation." *Am J Clin Nutr* 58 (1):35–42.

Carnielli, V. P., D. J. Wattimena, I. H. Luijendijk, A. Boerlage, H. J. Degenhart, and P. J. Sauer. 1996. "The very low birth weight premature infant is capable of synthesizing arachidonic and docosahexaenoic acids from linoleic and linolenic acids." *Pediatr Res* 40 (1):169–174. doi:10.1203/00006450-199607000-00030.

Chambaz, J., D. Ravel, M. C. Manier, D. Pepin, N. Mulliez, and G. Bereziat. 1985. "Essential fatty acids interconversion in the human fetal liver." *Biol Neonate* 47 (3):136–140.

Chatterjee, P., V. L. Chiasson, K. R. Bounds, and B. M. Mitchell. 2014. "Regulation of the Anti-Inflammatory Cytokines Interleukin-4 and Interleukin-10 during Pregnancy." *Front Immunol* 5:253. doi:10.3389/fimmu.2014.00253.

Cho, H. P., M. Nakamura, and S. D. Clarke. 1999. "Cloning, expression, and fatty acid regulation of the human delta-5 desaturase." *J Biol Chem* 274 (52):37335–37339.

Crawford, M. A. 1992. "The role of dietary fatty acids in biology: Their place in the evolution of the human brain." *Nutr Rev* 50 (4 Pt 2):3–11.

Cummings, S. W., W. Hatley, E. R. Simpson, and M. Ohashi. 1982. "The binding of high and low density lipoproteins to human placental membrane fractions." *J Clin Endocrinol Metab* 54 (5):903–908. doi:10.1210/jcem-54-5-903.

Daniels, J. L., M. P. Longnecker, A. S. Rowland, J. Golding, and Alspac Study Team. University of Bristol Institute of Child Health. 2004. "Fish intake during pregnancy and early cognitive development of offspring." *Epidemiology* 15 (4):394–402.

Darios, F. and B. Davletov. 2006. "Omega-3 and omega-6 fatty acids stimulate cell membrane expansion by acting on syntaxin 3." *Nature* 440 (7085):813–817. doi:10.1038/nature04598.

Dutta-Roy, A. K. 2000. "Transport mechanisms for long-chain polyunsaturated fatty acids in the human placenta." *Am J Clin Nutr* 71 (1 Suppl):315S–322S.

Elliott, J. A. 1975. "The effect of pregnancy on the control of lipolysis in fat cells isolated from human adipose tissue." *Eur J Clin Invest* 5 (2):159–163.

Endres, S., R. Ghorbani, V. E. Kelley, K. Georgilis, G. Lonnemann, J. W. van der Meer, J. G. Cannon, T. S. Rogers, M. S. Klempner, P. C. Weber et al. 1989. "The effect of dietary supplementation with n-3 polyunsaturated fatty acids on the synthesis of interleukin-1 and tumor necrosis factor by mononuclear cells." *N Engl J Med* 320 (5):265–271. doi:10.1056/NEJM198902023200501.

Fernandes, F. S., Md Tavares do Carmo, and E. Herrera. 2012. "Influence of maternal diet during early pregnancy on the fatty acid profile in the fetus at late pregnancy in rats." *Lipids* 47 (5):505–517. doi:10.1007/s11745-012-3660-7.

Food and Nutrition Board. 2005. *Dietary Reference Intakes for Energy, Carbohydrate, Fiber, Fat, Fatty Acids, Cholesterol, Protein and Amino Acids.* Washington, DC: The National Academies Press.

Forbes, K. and M. Westwood. 2010. "Maternal growth factor regulation of human placental development and fetal growth." *J Endocrinol* 207 (1):1–16. doi:10.1677/JOE-10-0174.

Gauster, M., U. Hiden, M. van Poppel, S. Frank, C. Wadsack, S. Hauguel-de Mouzon, and G. Desoye. 2011. "Dysregulation of placental endothelial lipase in obese women with gestational diabetes mellitus." *Diabetes* 60 (10):2457–2464. doi:10.2337/db10-1434.

Gould, J. F., L. G. Smithers, and M. Makrides. 2013. "The effect of maternal omega-3 (n-3) LCPUFA supplementation during pregnancy on early childhood cognitive and visual development: A systematic review and meta-analysis of randomized controlled trials." *Am J Clin Nutr* 97 (3):531–544. doi:10.3945/ajcn.112.045781.

Guesnet, P. and J. M. Alessandri. 2011. "Docosahexaenoic acid (DHA) and the developing central nervous system (CNS)—Implications for dietary recommendations." *Biochimie* 93 (1):7–12. doi:10.1016/j.biochi.2010.05.005.

Haggarty, P. 2010. "Fatty acid supply to the human fetus." *Annu Rev Nutr* 30:237–255. doi:10.1146/annurev.nutr.012809.104742.

Haggarty, P., M. Wood, E. Ferguson, G. Hoad, A. Srikantharajah, E. Milne, M. Hamilton, and S. Bhattacharya. 2006. "Fatty acid metabolism in human preimplantation embryos." *Hum Reprod* 21 (3):766–773. doi:10.1093/humrep/dei385.

Hariri, M., R. Ghiasvand, A. Shiranian, G. Askari, B. Iraj, and A. Salehi-Abargouei. 2014. "Does omega-3 fatty acids supplementation affect circulating leptin levels? A systematic review and meta-analysis on randomized controlled clinical trials." *Clin Endocrinol (Oxf)*. 80 (2):221–228. doi:10.1111/cen.12508.

Herrera, E. 2002a. "Implications of dietary fatty acids during pregnancy on placental, fetal and postnatal development—A review." *Placenta* 23 Suppl A:S9–S19. doi:10.1053/plac.2002.0771.

Herrera, E. 2002b. "Lipid metabolism in pregnancy and its consequences in the fetus and newborn." *Endocrine* 19 (1):43–55. doi:10.1385/ENDO:19:1:43.

Herrera, E., D. Gomez-Coronado, and M. A. Lasuncion. 1987. "Lipid metabolism in pregnancy." *Biol Neonate* 51 (2):70–77.

Hibbeln, J. R., J. M. Davis, C. Steer, P. Emmett, I. Rogers, C. Williams, and J. Golding. 2007. "Maternal seafood consumption in pregnancy and neurodevelopmental outcomes in childhood (ALSPAC study): An observational cohort study." *Lancet* 369 (9561):578–585. doi:10.1016/S0140-6736(07)60277-3.

Horvath, A., B. Koletzko, and H. Szajewska. 2007. "Effect of supplementation of women in high-risk pregnancies with long-chain polyunsaturated fatty acids on pregnancy outcomes and growth measures at birth: A meta-analysis of randomized controlled trials." *Br J Nutr* 98 (2):253–259. doi:10.1017/S0007114507709078.

Humphrey, J. L., M. T. Childs, A. Montes, and R. H. Knopp. 1980. "Lipid metabolism in pregnancy. VII. Kinetics of chylomicron triglyceride removal in fed pregnant rat." *Am J Physiol* 239 (1):E81–E87.

Ibdah, J. A., H. Paul, Y. Zhao, S. Binford, K. Salleng, M. Cline, D. Matern, M. J. Bennett, P. Rinaldo, and A. W. Strauss. 2001. "Lack of mitochondrial trifunctional protein in mice causes neonatal hypoglycemia and sudden death." *J Clin Invest* 107 (11):1403–1409. doi:10.1172/JCI12590.

Imhoff-Kunsch, B., V. Briggs, T. Goldenberg, and U. Ramakrishnan. 2012. "Effect of n-3 long-chain polyunsaturated fatty acid intake during pregnancy on maternal, infant, and child health outcomes: A systematic review." *Paediatr Perinat Epidemiol* 26 Suppl 1:91–107. doi:10.1111/j.1365-3016.2012.01292.x.

Innis, S. M. 1991. "Essential fatty acids in growth and development." *Prog Lipid Res* 30 (1):39–103.

Jones, M. L., P. J. Mark, J. L. Lewis, T. A. Mori, J. A. Keelan, and B. J. Waddell. 2010. "Antioxidant defenses in the rat placenta in late gestation: Increased labyrinthine expression of superoxide dismutases, glutathione peroxidase 3, and uncoupling protein 2." *Biol Reprod* 83 (2):254–260. doi:10.1095/biolreprod.110.083907.

Jones, M. L., P. J. Mark, T. A. Mori, J. A. Keelan, and B. J. Waddell. 2013. "Maternal dietary omega-3 fatty acid supplementation reduces placental oxidative stress and increases fetal and placental growth in the rat." *Biol Reprod* 88 (2):37. doi:10.1095/biolreprod.112.103754.

Kidd, P. M. 2007. "Omega-3 DHA and EPA for cognition, behavior, and mood: Clinical findings and structural-functional synergies with cell membrane phospholipids." *Altern Med Rev* 12 (3):207–227.

Knopp, R. H., M. A. Boroush, and J. B. O'Sullivan. 1975. "Lipid metabolism in pregnancy. II. Postheparin lipolytic activity and hypertriglyceridemia in the pregnant rat." *Metabolism* 24 (4):481–493.

Koletzko, B. and M. Braun. 1991. "Arachidonic acid and early human growth: Is there a relation?" *Ann Nutr Metab* 35 (3):128–131.

Krishnamoorthy, S., A. Recchiuti, N. Chiang, S. Yacoubian, C. H. Lee, R. Yang, N. A. Petasis, and C. N. Serhan. 2010. "Resolvin D1 binds human phagocytes with evidence for proresolving receptors." *Proc Natl Acad Sci U S A* 107 (4):1660–1665. doi:10.1073/pnas.0907342107.

Kuipers, R. S., M. F. Luxwolda, P. J. Offringa, E. R. Boersma, D. A. Dijck-Brouwer, and F. A. Muskiet. 2012. "Fetal intrauterine whole body linoleic, arachidonic and docosahexaenoic acid contents and accretion rates." *Prostaglandins Leukot Essent Fatty Acids* 86 (1–2):13–20. doi:10.1016/j.plefa.2011.10.012.

Kusakabe, T., M. Maeda, N. Hoshi, T. Sugino, K. Watanabe, T. Fukuda, and T. Suzuki. 2000. "Fatty acid synthase is expressed mainly in adult hormone-sensitive cells or cells with high lipid metabolism and in proliferating fetal cells." *J Histochem Cytochem* 48 (5):613–622.

Laivuori, H., M. J. Gallaher, L. Collura, W. R. Crombleholme, N. Markovic, A. Rajakumar, C. A. Hubel, J. M. Roberts, and R. W. Powers. 2006. "Relationships between maternal plasma leptin, placental leptin mRNA and protein in normal pregnancy, pre-eclampsia and intrauterine growth restriction without pre-eclampsia." *Mol Hum Reprod* 12 (9):551–556. doi:10.1093/molehr/gal064.

Lappas, M., U. Hiden, G. Desoye, J. Froehlich, S. Hauguel-de Mouzon, and A. Jawerbaum. 2011. "The role of oxidative stress in the pathophysiology of gestational diabetes mellitus." *Antioxid Redox Signal* 15 (12):3061–3100. doi:10.1089/ars.2010.3765.

Lorenzo, M., T. Caldes, M. Benito, and J. M. Medina. 1981. "Lipogenesis *in vivo* in maternal and foetal tissues during late gestation in the rat." *Biochem J* 198 (2):425–428.

Madsen, E. M., M. L. Lindegaard, C. B. Andersen, P. Damm, and L. B. Nielsen. 2004. "Human placenta secretes apolipoprotein B-100-containing lipoproteins." *J Biol Chem* 279 (53):55271–55276. doi:10.1074/jbc.M411404200.

Martin-Hidalgo, A., C. Holm, P. Belfrage, M. C. Schotz, and E. Herrera. 1994. "Lipoprotein lipase and hormone-sensitive lipase activity and mRNA in rat adipose tissue during pregnancy." *Am J Physiol* 266 (6 Pt 1):E930–E935.

Maymo, J. L., A. Perez Perez, Y. Gambino, J. C. Calvo, V. Sanchez-Margalet, and C. L. Varone. 2011. "Review: Leptin gene expression in the placenta—Regulation of a key hormone in trophoblast proliferation and survival." *Placenta* 32 Suppl 2:S146–S153. doi:10.1016/j.placenta.2011.01.004.

Mazaki-Tovi, S., H. Kanety, C. Pariente, R. Hemi, Y. Efraty, E. Schiff, A. Shoham, and E. Sivan. 2007. "Determining the source of fetal adiponectin." *J Reprod Med* 52 (9):774–778.

McDonald, E. A. and M. W. Wolfe. 2009. "Adiponectin attenuation of endocrine function within human term trophoblast cells." *Endocrinology* 150 (9):4358–4465. doi:10.1210/en.2009-0058.

Montague, C. T., I. S. Farooqi, J. P. Whitehead, M. A. Soos, H. Rau, N. J. Wareham, C. P. Sewter, J. E. Digby, S. N. Mohammed, J. A. Hurst, C. H. Cheetham, A. R. Earley, A. H. Barnett, J. B. Prins, and S. O'Rahilly. 1997. "Congenital leptin deficiency is associated with severe early-onset obesity in humans." *Nature* 387 (6636):903–908. doi:10.1038/43185.

Montelongo, A., M. A. Lasuncion, L. F. Pallardo, and E. Herrera. 1992. "Longitudinal study of plasma lipoproteins and hormones during pregnancy in normal and diabetic women." *Diabetes* 41 (12):1651–1659.

Oey, N. A., M. E. den Boer, J. P. Ruiter, R. J. Wanders, M. Duran, H. R. Waterham, K. Boer, J. A. van der Post, and F. A. Wijburg. 2003. "High activity of fatty acid oxidation enzymes in human placenta: Implications for fetal-maternal disease." *J Inherit Metab Dis* 26 (4):385–392.

Oey, N. A., M. E. den Boer, F. A. Wijburg, M. Vekemans, J. Auge, C. Steiner, R. J. Wanders, H. R. Waterham, J. P. Ruiter, and T. Attie-Bitach. 2005. "Long-chain fatty acid oxidation during early human development." *Pediatr Res* 57 (6):755–759. doi:10.1203/01.PDR.0000161413.42874.74.

Oken, E., K. P. Kleinman, S. F. Olsen, J. W. Rich-Edwards, and M. W. Gillman. 2004. "Associations of seafood and elongated n-3 fatty acid intake with fetal growth and length of gestation: Results from a US pregnancy cohort." *Am J Epidemiol* 160 (8):774–783. doi:10.1093/aje/kwh282.

Olsen, S. F. and N. J. Secher. 2002. "Low consumption of seafood in early pregnancy as a risk factor for preterm delivery: Prospective cohort study." *BMJ* 324 (7335):447.

Ortega-Senovilla, H., U. Schaefer-Graf, K. Meitzner, M. Abou-Dakn, K. Graf, U. Kintscher, and E. Herrera. 2011. "Gestational diabetes mellitus causes changes in the concentrations of adipocyte fatty acid-binding protein and other adipocytokines in cord blood." *Diabetes Care* 34 (4):2061–2066. doi:10.1016/j.beem.2010.05.006.

Ortega-Senovilla, H., U. Schaefer-Graf, K. Meitzner, K. Graf, M. Abou-Dakn, and E. Herrera. 2013. "Lack of relationship between cord serum angiopoietin-like protein 4 (ANGPTL4) and lipolytic activity in human neonates born by spontaneous delivery." *PLoS One* 8 (12):e81201. doi:10.1371/journal.pone.0081201.

Pagan, A., M. T. Prieto-Sanchez, J. E. Blanco-Carnero, A. Gil-Sanchez, J. J. Parrilla, H. Demmelmair, B. Koletzko, and E. Larque. 2013. "Materno–fetal transfer of docosahexaenoic acid is impaired by gestational diabetes mellitus." *Am J Physiol Endocrinol Metab* 305 (7):E826–E833. doi:10.1152/ajpendo.00291.2013.

Palacin, M., M. A. Lasuncion, M. Asuncion, and E. Herrera. 1991. "Circulating metabolite utilization by periuterine adipose tissue in situ in the pregnant rat." *Metabolism* 40 (5):534–539.

Paulesu, L., J. Bhattacharjee, N. Bechi, R. Romagnoli, S. Jantra, and F. Ietta. 2010. "Pro-inflammatory cytokines in animal and human gestation." *Curr Pharm Des* 16 (32):3601–3615.

Qiao, L., H. S. Yoo, A. Madon, B. Kinney, W. W. Hay, Jr., and J. Shao. 2012. "Adiponectin enhances mouse fetal fat deposition." *Diabetes* 61 (12):3199–3207. doi:10.2337/db12-0055.

Ramakrishnan, U., A. D. Stein, S. Parra-Cabrera, M. Wang, B. Imhoff-Kunsch, S. Juarez-Marquez, J. Rivera, and R. Martorell. 2010. "Effects of docosahexaenoic acid supplementation during pregnancy on gestational age and size at birth: Randomized, double-blind, placebo-controlled trial in Mexico." *Food Nutr Bull* 31 (2 Suppl):S108–S116.

Raz, A., N. K. Belsky, F. Przedecki, and M. G. Obukowicz. 1997. "Fish oil inhibits Δ6 desaturase activity *in vivo*: Utility in a dietary paradigm to obtain mice depleted of arachidonic acid." *J Nutr Biochem* 8:558–565.

Rinaldo, P., D. Matern, and M. J. Bennett. 2002. "Fatty acid oxidation disorders." *Annu Rev Physiol* 64:477–502. doi:10.1146/annurev.physiol.64.082201.154705.

Sakamoto, M. and M. Kubota. 2004. "Plasma fatty acid profiles in 37 pairs of maternal and umbilical cord blood samples." *Environ Health Prev Med* 9 (2):67–69. doi:10.1007/BF02897935.

Sanders, T. A. and D. J. Naismith. 1979. "A comparison of the influence of breast-feeding and bottle-feeding on the fatty acid composition of the erythrocytes." *Br J Nutr* 41 (3):619–623.

Schaefer-Graf, U. M., K. Meitzner, H. Ortega-Senovilla, K. Graf, K. Vetter, M. Abou-Dakn, and E. Herrera. 2011. "Differences in the implications of maternal lipids on fetal metabolism and growth between gestational diabetes mellitus and control pregnancies." *Diabet Med* 28 (9):1053–1059. doi:10.1111/j.1464-5491.2011.03346.x.

Schwab, J. M., N. Chiang, M. Arita, and C. N. Serhan. 2007. "Resolvin E1 and protectin D1 activate inflammation-resolution programmes." *Nature* 447 (7146):869–874. doi:10.1038/nature05877.

Serhan, C. N., S. Hong, K. Gronert, S. P. Colgan, P. R. Devchand, G. Mirick, and R. L. Moussignac. 2002. "Resolvins: A family of bioactive products of omega-3 fatty acid transformation circuits initiated by aspirin treatment that counter proinflammation signals." *J Exp Med* 196 (8):1025–1037.

Smithers, L. G., R. A. Gibson, A. McPhee, and M. Makrides. 2008. "Higher dose of docosahexaenoic acid in the neonatal period improves visual acuity of preterm infants: Results of a randomized controlled trial." *Am J Clin Nutr* 88 (4):1049–1056.

Srivastava, A., J. Sengupta, A. Kriplani, K. K. Roy, and D. Ghosh. 2013. "Profiles of cytokines secreted by isolated human endometrial cells under the influence of chorionic gonadotropin during the window of embryo implantation." *Reprod Biol Endocrinol* 11:116. doi:10.1186/1477-7827-11-116.

Stark, M. J., V. L. Clifton, and N. A. Hodyl. 2013. "Differential effects of docosahexaenoic acid on preterm and term placental pro-oxidant/antioxidant balance." *Reproduction* 146 (3):243–251. doi:10.1530/REP-13-0239.

Stephenson, T., J. Stammers, and D. Hull. 1993. "Placental transfer of free fatty acids: Importance of fetal albumin concentration and acid-base status." *Biol Neonate* 63 (5):273–280.

Strauss, A. W. 2005. "Surprising? Perhaps not. Long-chain fatty acid oxidation during human fetal development." *Pediatr Res* 57 (6):753–754. doi:10.1203/01.PDR.0000161412.24792.55.

Szajewska, H., A. Horvath, and B. Koletzko. 2006. "Effect of n-3 long-chain polyunsaturated fatty acid supplementation of women with low-risk pregnancies on pregnancy outcomes and growth measures at birth: A meta-analysis of randomized controlled trials." *Am J Clin Nutr* 83 (6):1337–1344.

Szitanyi, P., B. Koletzko, A. Mydlilova, and H. Demmelmair. 1999. "Metabolism of 13C-labeled linoleic acid in newborn infants during the first week of life." *Pediatr Res* 45 (5 Pt 1):669–673. doi:10.1203/00006450-199905010-00010.

Tofail, F., I. Kabir, J. D. Hamadani, F. Chowdhury, S. Yesmin, F. Mehreen, and S. N. Huda. 2006. "Supplementation of fish-oil and soy-oil during pregnancy and psychomotor development of infants." *J Health Popul Nutr* 24 (1):48–56.

Tsai, P. J., C. H. Yu, S. P. Hsu, Y. H. Lee, C. H. Chiou, Y. W. Hsu, S. C. Ho, and C. H. Chu. 2004. "Cord plasma concentrations of adiponectin and leptin in healthy term neonates: Positive correlation with birthweight and neonatal adiposity." *Clin Endocrinol (Oxf)* 61 (1):88–93. doi:10.1111/j.1365-2265.2004.02057.x.

Uauy, R., P. Peirano, D. Hoffman, P. Mena, D. Birch, and E. Birch. 1996. "Role of essential fatty acids in the function of the developing nervous system." *Lipids* 31 Suppl:S167–S176.

Varastehpour, A., T. Radaelli, J. Minium, H. Ortega, E. Herrera, P. Catalano, and S. Hauguel-de Mouzon. 2006. "Activation of phospholipase A2 is associated with generation of placental lipid signals and fetal obesity." *J Clin Endocrinol Metab* 91 (1):248–255. doi:10.1210/jc.2005-0873.

von Frankenberg, A. D., F. M. Silva, J. C. de Almeida, V. Piccoli, F. V. do Nascimento, M. M. Sost, C. B. Leitao, L. L. Remonti, D. Umpierre, A. F. Reis, L. H. Canani, M. J. de Azevedo, and F. Gerchman. 2014. "Effect of dietary lipids on circulating adiponectin: A systematic review with meta-analysis of randomised controlled trials." *Br J Nutr* 112 (8):1235–1250. doi:10.1017/S0007114514002013.

Wadsack, C., A. Hammer, S. Levak-Frank, G. Desoye, K. F. Kozarsky, B. Hirschmugl, W. Sattler, and E. Malle. 2003. "Selective cholesteryl ester uptake from high density lipoprotein by human first trimester and term villous trophoblast cells." *Placenta* 24 (2–3):131–143.

Wang, Z. J., C. L. Liang, G. M. Li, C. Y. Yu, and M. Yin. 2006. "Neuroprotective effects of arachidonic acid against oxidative stress on rat hippocampal slices." *Chem Biol Interact* 163 (3):207–217. doi:10.1016/j .cbi.2006.08.005.

Watanabe, K., T. Mori, A. Iwasaki, C. Kimura, H. Matsushita, K. Shinohara, and A. Wakatsuki. 2013. "Increased oxygen free radical production during pregnancy may impair vascular reactivity in pre-eclamptic women." *Hypertens Res* 36 (4):356–360. doi:10.1038/hr.2012.208.

Weiler, H., S. Fitzpatrick-Wong, J. Schellenberg, U. McCloy, R. Veitch, H. Kovacs, J. Kohut, and C. Kin Yuen. 2005. "Maternal and cord blood long-chain polyunsaturated fatty acids are predictive of bone mass at birth in healthy term-born infants." *Pediatr Res* 58 (6):1254–1258. doi:10.1203/01.pdr.0000185129.73971.74.

Welch, A. A., S. Shakya-Shrestha, M. A. Lentjes, N. J. Wareham, and K. T. Khaw. 2010. "Dietary intake and status of n-3 polyunsaturated fatty acids in a population of fish-eating and non-fish-eating meat-eaters, vegetarians, and vegans and the product–precursor ratio [corrected] of alpha-linolenic acid to long-chain n-3 polyunsaturated fatty acids: Results from the EPIC-Norfolk cohort." *Am J Clin Nutr* 92 (5):1040–1051. doi:10.3945/ajcn.2010.29457.

Xu, X., X. Yang, Z. Liu, K. Wu, C. Lin, Y. Wang, and H. Yan. 2014. "Placental leptin gene methylation and macrosomia during normal pregnancy." *Mol Med Rep* 9 (3):1013–1018. doi:10.3892/mmr.2014.1913.

Yamashita, A., K. Kawana, K. Tomio, A. Taguchi, Y. Isobe, R. Iwamoto, K. Masuda, H. Furuya, T. Nagamatsu, K. Nagasaka, T. Arimoto, K. Oda, O. Wada-Hiraike, T. Yamashita, Y. Taketani, J. X. Kang, S. Kozuma, H. Arai, M. Arita, Y. Osuga, and T. Fujii. 2013. "Increased tissue levels of omega-3 polyunsaturated fatty acids prevents pathological preterm birth." *Sci Rep* 3:3113. doi:10.1038/srep03113.

Zimmermann, T., L. Winkler, U. Moller, H. Schubert, and E. Goetze. 1979. "Synthesis of arachidonic acid in the human placenta *in vitro.*" *Biol Neonate* 35 (3–4):209–212.

8 Role of Maternal Long-Chain Polyunsaturated Fatty Acids in Placental Development and Function

Alka Rani, Akshaya Meher,
Nisha Wadhwani, and Sadhana Joshi

CONTENTS

ABSTRACT

During pregnancy, maternal long-chain polyunsaturated fatty acids (LCPUFAs) are preferentially transferred by the placenta to meet the requirements of the developing fetus. These LCPUFAs are essentially required by the trophoblast cells right from early gestation for several physiological processes involved in optimum placental growth and activity. They are structural constituents of the cell membrane, stimulate angiogenesis, and are metabolized into various eicosanoids, which modulate inflammation in the placenta. LCPUFAs and their metabolites also act as ligands for transcription factors like peroxisome proliferator-activated receptors, which regulate the expression of various physiologically important genes. Several pregnancy complications like preeclampsia are associated with increased placental inflammation and oxidative stress, and omega-3 LCPUFAs are known to reduce excess inflammation and oxidative damage in the trophoblast cells. This chapter describes the multiple roles of maternal LCPUFAs in placental development and function, reducing the risk of adverse pregnancy outcomes.

KEY WORDS

Polyunsaturated fatty acids, placenta, trophoblast, inflammation, oxidative stress, epigenetics, angiogenesis, omega-3 fatty acids, pregnancy.

8.1 MATERNAL NUTRITION AND PREGNANCY OUTCOME

During pregnancy, nutrition is known to play a major role in optimizing the health and well-being of both the mother and the baby. Epidemiological evidence suggests that maternal nutritional status is associated with adverse pregnancy outcomes (Bawadi et al. 2010). Maternal nutrition has been reported to be associated with pregnancy complications like preeclampsia and also results in preterm deliveries (Scholl 2008).

The development of the conceptus depends on an adequate and balanced supply of both macronutrients and micronutrients. Macronutrients are majorly required as sources of energy, while micronutrients play a role in the metabolism of macronutrients and are involved in various structural and cellular processes (Rao, Padmavathi, and Raghunath 2012). The period during pregnancy is considered the most vulnerable period in the human life cycle, and maternal nutrients are known to influence embryonic development and intrauterine fetal growth (Symonds et al. 2006).

During early pregnancy, development and differentiation of various fetal organs take place, and an inadequate supply of nutrients forces the fetus to adapt, down-regulate growth, and prioritize the development of essential organs (Fall et al. 2003). Furthermore, it is also known that deficiency of essential nutrients during pregnancy leads to congenital defects, intrauterine growth restriction (IUGR), and low birth weight (LBW) of the fetus (Wu, Imhoff-Kunsch, and Girard 2012). Pregnancy complications are reported to lead to high rates of maternal and infant morbidity and mortality.

It is well established that fetal growth and development have a unique requirement for the supply of dietary lipids from the mother (Herrera 2002). Lipids are esters of moderate to long-chain fatty acids, which are carboxylic acids with a long aliphatic hydrocarbon tail, either saturated or unsaturated. Dietary essential fatty acids (EFAs) are polyunsaturated fatty acids (PUFAs) that cannot be synthesized endogenously by the human body. Their longer chain derivatives, called long-chain PUFAs (LCPUFAs; ≥20 C-atoms), are indispensable for growth, development, and maintenance of good health of the fetus (Muskiet 2010).

8.1.1 LONG-CHAIN POLYUNSATURATED FATTY ACIDS

LCPUFAs are classified into two important families, omega-6 and omega-3 fatty acids, depending on the position of the first double bond in the hydrocarbon chain from the methyl end. The simplest members of omega-6 and omega-3 family traditionally recognized are linoleic acid (LA; 18:2, n-6) and α-linolenic acid (ALA; 18:3, n-3), respectively. LA and ALA are EFAs, which get converted into LCPUFA, i.e., arachidonic acid (AA; 20:4, n-6) and docosahexaenoic acid (DHA; 22:6, n-3), after going through further desaturation and elongation of the hydrocarbon chain. Along with AA and DHA, dihomo-γ-linolenic acid (20:3, n-6) and eicosapentaenoic acid (EPA; 20:5, n-3) are also functionally important intermediate LCPUFAs. The biosynthetic pathway of LCPUFA requires sequential activities of Δ6-desaturase, Δ5-desaturase, and elongases for the conversion of 18-carbon (LA and ALA) to 20-carbon (AA and EPA) to final 24-carbon LCPUFA (Leonard et al. 2002). However, peroxisomal β-oxidation of 24-carbon LCPUFA is required to form 22-carbon DHA as the product called Sprecher's pathway (Ferdinandusse et al. 2001) (Figure 8.1). There exists a competition between precursors of both the omega-6 and omega-3 families (LA and ALA) for desaturation, and the ratio of LA:ALA in the diet can affect the biosynthesis of omega-6 and omega-3 LCPUFAs. The activities of Δ6- and Δ5-desaturases and the production of AA and DHA are thus regulated by nutritional status, hormones, and feedback inhibition by the end products (Calder 2012).

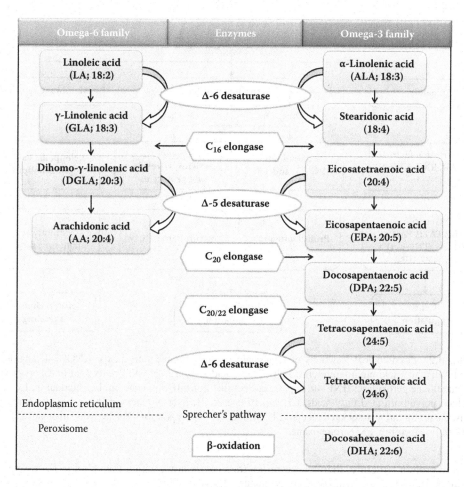

FIGURE 8.1 Biosynthesis pathway of long-chain polyunsaturated fatty acids.

LCPUFAs are a family of biologically active fatty acids involved in multiple mechanisms that connect the cell membrane, the cytosol, and the nucleus. They are of particular relevance because of their numerous physiological functions, i.e., storing energy, signaling, and acting as structural components (Cetin, Alvino, and Cardellicchio 2009). Even though both the families of LCPUFAs are important, the omega-3 fatty acids have been found to be more beneficial due to its various protective functions inside the cell.

LCPUFAs further metabolize to their respective eicosanoids (prostaglandins, thromboxanes, and leukotrienes), eicosanoid-like mediators, resolvins, and protectins, which have modulatory properties in inflammation, immunity, platelet aggregation, smooth muscle contraction, and renal function (Calder 2013). AA, an omega-6 fatty acid, is known to generate proinflammatory lipid mediators, while the fatty acids of the omega-3 family, i.e., EPA and DHA, lead to the formation of anti-inflammatory, proresolving, and cytoprotective lipid mediators (Patterson et al. 2012).

LCPUFAs also regulate the expression of vital genes through changes in the activity or abundance of various transcription factors (Pegorier, Le May, and Girard 2004). LCPUFAs and their derivatives are natural ligands for transcription factors, such as peroxisome proliferator-activated receptors (PPARα, β, and γ), liver X receptors, retinoid X receptor (RXR), and hepatic nuclear factor-4α, or indirectly affect the activity of sterol regulatory element binding proteins and nuclear factor-κB (NF-κB) (Jump et al. 2008). These ligand-activated transcription factors undergo a conformational

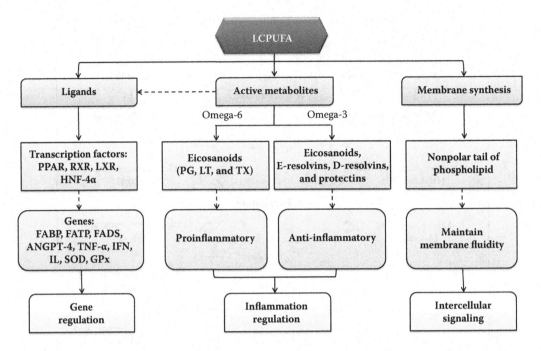

FIGURE 8.2 Physiological functions of long-chain polyunsaturated fatty acids. ANGPT-4, angiopoetin like 4; FABP, fatty acid-binding proteins; FADS, fatty acid desaturases; FATP, fatty acid transport proteins; GPx, glutathione peroxidase; HNF-4α, hepatic nuclear factor-4α; IFN, interferon; IL, interleukin; LCPUFA, long-chain polyunsaturated fatty acids; LT, leukotriene; LXR, liver X receptor; PG, prostaglandin; PPAR, peroxisome proliferation associated receptor; RXR, retinoid X receptor; SOD, superoxide dismutase; TNF-α, tumor necrosis factor-α; TX, thromboxane.

change in protein structure, thereby recruiting the coactivators, which then bind to the target gene and initiate the process of transcription (Schwabe 1996).

LCPUFAs maintain membrane fluidity of the cells and influence membrane function. The composition of plasma membrane is influenced by the availability of different LCPUFAs. With the omega-3 fatty acids being functionally more important, the incorporation of EPA and DHA is preferred to that of AA (Calder 2012). Changing the structure and composition of cell membrane and lipid rafts can, in turn, affect membrane fluidity and alter intracellular signaling pathways inside the cell by displacing receptors and signaling proteins. Further, membrane phospholipids also act as substrates for the release of LCPUFAs for the biosynthesis of lipid mediators or ligands for transcription factors (Eyster 2007).

Therefore, as discussed above, LCPUFAs are associated with membrane synthesis and production of eicosanoids and ligands for transcription factors and act as signaling molecules, all of which are obligatory for normal physiological processes (Figure 8.2).

8.1.2 ROLE OF LCPUFA DURING PREGNANCY

During pregnancy, the fatty acid levels in maternal blood influences its availability and transport to the fetus. The first trimester of the pregnancy is considered an anabolic period, during which the net body weight increases and fats are stored in maternal adipose tissue (Herrera 2002). During the third trimester of pregnancy, the maternal lipid metabolism switches from anabolic to a catabolic condition as the fetus intensifies its nutrient demands to support exponential tissue growth (Cetin, Alvino, and Cardellicchio 2009). An intense decline in maternal fatty acid levels makes the mother susceptible to various kinds of complications during pregnancy. Therefore, it is crucial that maternal dietary intake must be sufficient right from early pregnancy to satisfy her requirements as well as those of her growing fetus for a better pregnancy outcome.

A number of studies have emphasized the importance of LCPUFAs in improving pregnancy outcome. Studies have shown that maternal omega-3 fatty acid supplementation during pregnancy results in modest increases in birth size and length of gestation, reducing the risk of early preterm and LBW (Coletta, Bell, and Roman 2010; De Giuseppe, Roggi, and Cena 2014). This finding has been recently confirmed in a study that examined the effect of DHA supplementation (600 mg/day) in the last half of gestation and found an increase in the length of gestation and infant size (Carlson et al. 2013).

8.1.3 Fetal Development

As discussed above, the fetus exponentially accumulates a relatively large amount of lipids after 25 weeks of gestation (Haggarty 2010). This is because during the third trimester of pregnancy, considerable amounts of fatty acids are directed toward the renal cortex tissue of the brain and the retinal membrane synapses of the eyes of the fetus (De Giuseppe, Roggi, and Cena 2014). The lipid constitution of the human brain is approximately 50%–60% of dry weight, of which 35% is composed of LCPUFAs, especially AA and DHA (Zeman et al. 2012). Concentrations of AA in the brain of the fetus are higher than DHA in the first half of pregnancy, whereas in the later stage, DHA predominates (Simpson et al. 2011). DHA is involved in the formation of photoreceptor membranes and affects rhodopsin activation, development of rod and cone cells, and functional maturation of the central nervous system (Uauy et al. 2001). Hence, an adequate amount of LCPUFA must be available to the fetus, which ultimately depends on the maternal LCPUFA status. Deficiency of LCPUFA during this critical period of fetal development leads to neurological or neurodegenerative diseases later in life (Heaton et al. 2013).

Further, fatty acids are also required by the developing conceptus as a source of energy, to maintain the fluidity, permeability, and conformation of membranes and as precursors of important bioactive compounds such as the prostacyclins, prostaglandins, thromboxanes, and leukotrienes (Haggarty 2010).

Although LCPUFAs are critical for fetal growth and development, the fetus has a limited capacity to synthesize these fatty acids and is dependent on the maternal transfer through the placenta. Thus, the placenta, with its nutrient transport function, plays a crucial role in mediating the effects of maternal nutrition on the lifelong health consequences in the offspring (Lager and Powell 2012).

8.2 PLACENTA

The placenta is a highly specialized temporary organ that connects the mother and the developing embryo/fetus. It requires a constant and abundant source of energy for its own rapid growth and maturation and for the transport of essential nutrients, ions, vitamins, waste, and other molecules for fetal growth and homeostasis (Duttaroy 2009). The placental transfer capacity increases as the size of the conceptus and nutrient requirements increase. To meet these requirements, there is an increase in placental surface area for nutrient transfer, thinning of the cellular barrier, an increase in fetal capillary surface area, an increase in placental nutrient transporter abundance, and modulation of placental blood flow (Sandovici et al. 2012). Thus, the development and establishment of the placenta and its circulatory system play a pivotal role in the successful maintenance of maternal health and also facilitate the development of the embryo and fetus.

8.2.1 Development of the Placenta

After fertilization, the first specialized cells of the placenta form the outer layer of the blastocyst and are called trophoblast cells (Myllynen and Vahakangas 2013). After the embryo implants on the endometrial wall of the uterus, the trophoblast cells proliferate and differentiate along two pathways, i.e., villous and extravillous. The villous cytotrophoblast cells fuse to form the multinucleated syncytiotrophoblast, which forms the outer epithelial layer of the placental villi, the placental membrane barrier between maternal and fetal circulations. Extravillous trophoblast cells invade into the maternal decidua and remodel uterine arteries to facilitate blood flow to the placenta (Gude et al. 2004). During this process of establishment of vascular network in the placenta, several growth factors and their receptors involved in angiogenesis are known to play a key role (Castellucci et al. 2000).

The invasion of trophoblast cells is progressively completed at the beginning of the second trimester, which allows maternal blood flow to the placenta. This leads to hemodynamic changes within the placenta for structural changes in the uteroplacental arteries that get transformed into low-resistance vessels (Jauniaux et al. 2003). Once fetal viability is attained, the existing capillaries progressively transform into intermediate and then terminal villi, ultimately forming the "villous tree." The villous trees are grouped to form functional units of placenta called as lobules or cotyledons (Kingdom et al. 2000).

Along with hemodynamic changes within the placenta, the onset of maternal blood flow also shoots up the oxygen tension threefold within the intervillous space. This oxidative tension gets normalized as the pregnancy progresses and the placenta becomes fully functional (Jauniaux et al. 2000). After 20 weeks of gestation, the villous membrane fully expresses several nutrient transporters that are regulated by fetal, maternal, and placental signals (Lager and Powell 2012).

In addition to the above, pregnancy also induces inflammation that plays a key role in maternal tolerance of the semiallogenic fetus. A mild inflammatory response is suggested to be beneficial for a successful and normal pregnancy (Paulesu et al. 2010). Both proinflammatory as well as anti-inflammatory cytokines are secreted in the placenta, where they play critical roles in several processes, including trophoblast invasion, differentiation, proliferation, and regulation of placental inflammation and angiogenesis (Szukiewicz 2012).

Thus, fetoplacental and uteroplacental circulations necessitate the regulation of placental angiogenesis, oxidative stress, and inflammation. LCPUFAs, being physiologically potent molecules, are involved in all the above processes of placental growth and development and are discussed later in this chapter.

8.2.2 FUNCTIONS OF THE PLACENTA

The placental trophoblast cells protect the fetus from maternal infections and also ensure appropriate bidirectional nutrient/waste flow required for growth and maturation of the embryo/fetus. It releases metabolic products and hormones into maternal and/or fetal circulations, which influence fetal growth (Gude et al. 2004).

8.2.2.1 Transport of LCPUFA

Fatty acids can cross lipid bilayers of the placental syncytiotrophoblast membrane by simple diffusion. Nonesterified fatty acids are available at the microvillous membrane for transport; these are derived from both maternal stored and circulating lipids, free fatty acids bound to albumin, or from triglycerides (Haggarty 2010). In tissues where demand for fatty acids is high, uptake of fatty acids by simple diffusion may be insufficient to meet minimum requirements (Kazantzis and Stahl 2012). Therefore, the placental transport of fatty acids involves complex and multistep pathways. They are up taken by plasma membrane-integrated fatty acid transport proteins (FATPs), fatty acid translocases (CD36), membrane-bound fatty acid-binding proteins (FABPpm), and intracellular trafficking by cytosolic fatty acid-binding proteins (FABP) (Dube et al. 2012). Among the various types of FABP, only five have been identified in trophoblasts (FABP-1, 3–5, and 7) (Cunningham and McDermott 2009). The FATP family contains six members, among which five are expressed in human placenta (FATP-1–FATP-4 and FATP-6) (Lager and Powell 2012). These proteins are present on both the microvillous and basal membranes of the trophoblast cells, where the binding of LCPUFAs is highly reversible and specific from mother to the fetal side (Duttaroy 2000).

Reports indicate higher AA and DHA concentrations in fetal blood than in the maternal circulation (Al et al. 1995; Berghaus, Demmelmair, and Koletzko 1998). Studies show that the placenta preferentially transports AA and DHA than other LCPUFAs to the fetal side. FATP-1 and FATP-4 are directly correlated with DHA, and FABP-1 and FABP-3 have greater affinity for AA and DHA, suggesting that in the placenta, they are specifically involved in LCPUFA transfer (Larque et al. 2006). Placenta-specific FABPpm (p-FABPpm), being exclusively on the microvillous membrane of syncytiotrophoblast, is directly involved in the uptake of AA and DHA from maternal circulation (Cunningham and McDermott 2009).

In conditions of increased cellular fatty acid metabolism, these proteins are up-regulated and facilitate transfer across membranes and intracellular channeling of fatty acids (Haggarty 2004). In primary human trophoblast, expressions of various FATPs and FABPs are up-regulated in hypoxia through PPARγ and RXR signaling (Biron-Shental et al. 2007). Reports suggest that p-FABPpm binds directly with various FABPs in the nucleus to deliver specific ligands to transcription factors, like PPAR (Velkov 2013). However, the mechanism underlying trophoblast fatty acid uptake and trafficking is still a matter of speculation.

8.3 ROLE OF LCPUFA IN PLACENTAL DEVELOPMENT AND FUNCTION

Poor placental development has been associated with many pregnancy complications, and numerous reports indicate its association with altered LCPUFA levels (Dhobale et al. 2011; Kulkarni Mehendale et al. 2011b; Wadhwani et al. 2014). In addition, a positive association of placental DHA with placental weight was reported in preterm pregnancy, suggesting a role of LCPUFA in placental development and function (Dhobale et al. 2011). The various functions in which LCPUFA are involved in a syncytiotrophoblast cell are illustrated in Figure 8.3.

8.3.1 BUILDING BLOCKS OF GROWING PLACENTA

Fatty acids are important for the growth and development of placenta right from early pregnancy. During implantation, PUFAs play a critical role in the growth of the embryo at the implantation site (Chirala et al. 2003; McKeegan and Sturmey 2011). Reports indicate that from implantation until the onset of maternal blood flow in the placenta, the trophoblast cells are supported by secretion from the endometrial gland delivered into the placenta. This secretion contains numerous lipid droplets, which regulate placental cell proliferation and differentiation (Burton, Jauniaux, and Charnock-Jones 2007).

Early implantation and placentation processes are regulated by transcription factors, among which PPARγ has been extensively studied (Fournier et al. 2011). PPARγ ligands are known to increase the uptake and accumulation of fatty acids in human placenta (Borel et al. 2008). A series of animal studies have shown that inactivation of PPARγ leads to an irreversible arrest of trophoblast differentiation, early embryonic lethality, and severe developmental placental damage (Barak et al. 2002; Yessoufou et al. 2006).

Thus, the coordination between LCPUFA and PPAR plays a very important role during implantation and early placentation. As mentioned earlier, after implantation, the placental extravillous trophoblast cells migrate toward deciduas to form the adequate vascular network, which is the most important part of placental development.

8.3.2 INDUCERS OF PLACENTAL ANGIOGENESIS

Angiogenesis and vascularization in the placenta require various growth factors, including the vascular endothelial growth factor (VEGF) family, placental growth factor, the transforming growth factor β family, and angiopoietins (ANGPTs) (Carmeliet 2003). Among the various angiogenic

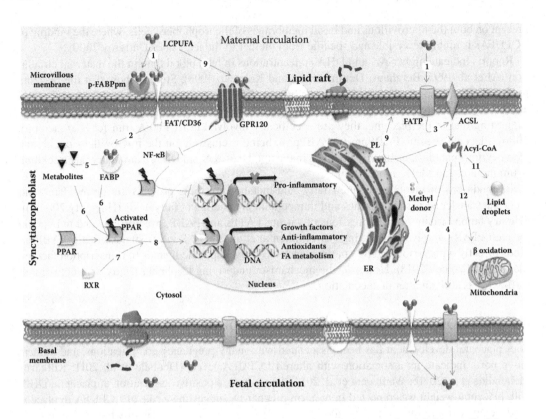

FIGURE 8.3 Multiple roles of long-chain polyunsaturated fatty acids in syncytiotrophoblast cell of the placenta. (1) LCPUFAs are uptaken by various fatty acid transporters (FATP, p-FABPpm, FAT/CD36) on microvillous membrane; (2) intracellular trafficking by FABP; (3) LCPUFA activation by ACSL to form long-chain acyl-CoA; either of long-chain acyl-CoA or FABP-bound LCPUFA is diverted to further processes; (4) transport to fetal circulation through FATP and FAT/CD36 present on the basal membrane; (5) conversion into physiologically active metabolites; (6) LCPUFA or its metabolites activate transcription factor PPAR; (7) activated PPAR binds to RXR; (8) heterodimer of PPAR and RXR initiates transcription of the gene required for various physiological processes; (9) binding to GPR120 blocking the activation of NF-κB, which transcribes pro-inflammatory genes; (10) phospholipid formation in the ER for the synthesis of membrane; (11) storage as lipid droplets; (12) transport to mitochondria for β-oxidation. ACSL, acyl-CoA synthetase; ER, endoplasmic reticulum; FABP, fatty acid-binding protein; FAT/CD36, fatty acid translocase; FATP, fatty acid transport protein; GPR120, G-protein receptor 120; LCPUFA, long-chain polyunsaturated fatty acid; NF-κB, nuclear factor kappa B; p-FABPpm, placenta-specific plasma membrane fatty acid-binding protein; PL, phospholipid; PPAR, peroxisome proliferation associated receptor; RXR, retinoid X receptor.

factors, the family of VEGF has been extensively studied. Angiogenic activities of LCPUFAs are reported on the first-trimester placental trophoblast cell line and have been shown to be highest for DHA followed by EPA and AA (Basak and Duttaroy 2013).

Reports have demonstrated that DHA stimulates the expression of VEGF-A, while EPA and AA stimulate ANGPT like 4. It has been observed that DHA induces maximum tube (capillary-like structures) formation by stimulating cell proliferation in the placenta as compared with other fatty acids (Johnsen et al. 2011). Studies have reported that prostaglandins synthesized from AA are also involved in the process of angiogenesis along with VEGF, associated with enhanced tubular network formation (Chung et al. 2000; Cooper et al. 1995; Finetti et al. 2008). Further, it has been reported that PPARγ regulates the process of placental angiogenesis (Nadra et al. 2010). However, the mechanism involving LCPUFAs in inducing angiogenesis through PPAR signaling is not completely understood.

Dietary fatty acids are also known to regulate fatty acid transferring proteins such as FABP-4 and FABP-3, which further modulate several angiogenic pathways (Basak, Das, and Duttaroy 2013). Hence, it is evident that LCPUFAs are involved in the process of angiogenesis, thereby playing a critical role in the placental vascular development. Altered angiogenesis is responsible for poor development of placental network, making it vulnerable to the upcoming oxidative stress.

8.3.3 COMBATING PLACENTAL OXIDATIVE STRESS

Once the vascular network is primarily established, maternal blood flow is initiated in the placenta at the end of the first trimester (Jauniaux et al. 2003). The early stages of human embryonic development take place in a low-oxygen environment, but the placenta becomes increasingly oxygenated with onset of maternal blood flow, leading to the production of free radicals like reactive oxygen species (ROS) in the trophoblast cells (Burton, Hempstock, and Jauniaux 2003). A range of antioxidant enzymes, including the superoxide dismutases (SODs), catalase, glutathione peroxidase (GPx), and/or the thioredoxin system, are reported to be present within the placenta (Jones et al. 2010). Oxidative stress occurs if there is an imbalance between the levels of prooxidants and antioxidants in the cell. Excessive production of ROS may occur physiologically during certain periods of placental development (Luo et al. 2006). It becomes adverse when excess ROS start attacking PUFAs in the cell membranes, forming lipid peroxides. Lipid peroxides are involved in endothelial cell injury, vasoconstriction, and imbalance between thromboxane and prostacyclin (Madazli et al. 1999). This is further responsible for placenta-originated pregnancy complications like preeclampsia.

Several experimental and clinical studies report prooxidant as well as antioxidant activities of omega-3 fatty acids, especially DHA, in a dose-dependent manner (Assies et al. 2004; Palozza et al. 1996; Richard et al. 2008). Omega-3 fatty acids are known to modulate the production of either ROS or ROS scavenging antioxidants (Gorjão et al. 2009; Wang et al. 2005). Studies have reported that omega-3 fatty acids enhance the activities and expression of antioxidant enzymes, such as GPx and SOD (Lluís et al. 2013; Takahashi et al. 2002; Wang et al. 2004). Animal studies have demonstrated that placental oxidative damage is reduced with maternal dietary omega-3 fatty acid supplementation (Jones et al. 2013a,b). Further, a study on placental trophoblast cell line indicates that oxidative DNA damage was reduced in the presence of modest levels of DHA (Shoji et al. 2009). Similarly, in a placental explant culture study, lower DHA doses were sufficient to inhibit lipopolysaccharide (LPS)-induced oxidative stress and increase the total antioxidant capacity (Stark, Clifton, and Hodyl 2013).

These studies indicate that omega-3 fatty acids are involved in combating oxidative stress in the trophoblast cells right from early gestation. However, the actual underlying mechanism through which omega-3 fatty acids regulate oxidative stress requires further research. A recent review suggests that maternal dietary omega-3 fatty acid supplementation may limit placental oxidative stress associated with several pregnancy disorders (Jones, Mark, and Waddell 2014).

8.3.4 REGULATION OF PLACENTAL INFLAMMATION

Reports indicate that excessive inflammation in the trophoblast is responsible for the development of several pregnancy complications like preeclampsia, preterm delivery, and IUGR (Kovo et al. 2014). Different proinflammatory cytokines, such as interleukins (IL-1, -2, and -8), tumor necrosis factor-α (TNF-α), and interferon-γ, and anti-inflammatory cytokines, such as IL-4 and IL-10, are known to be expressed in the placenta (Raghupathy, Al-Azemi, and Azizieh 2012).

LCPUFAs and their derivatives are known to influence several processes involved in the inflammatory responses. Reports have demonstrated that omega-3 fatty acids like DHA and EPA can reduce excessive inflammation, and therefore, high levels of tissue omega-3 fatty acids are considered to be beneficial (Mori and Beilin 2004; Simopoulos 2002). Animal studies have demonstrated that increased placental inflammatory cytokine levels of IL-6 and TNF-α as a consequence of an imbalance in the maternal micronutrients could be normalized by supplementation of omega-3 fatty acids (Meher, Joshi, and Joshi 2014).

Several mechanisms have been proposed for the anti-inflammatory activity possessed by omega-3 fatty acids. One of the mechanisms is possibly by influencing the activity of LCPUFA receptor GPR120, which is predominantly expressed in the microvillous membrane of the trophoblast (Lager et al. 2014).

AA-produced eicosanoids are known to act as mediators of inflammation, while omega-3 fatty acids are the precursors of resolvins and protectins that exert anti-inflammatory and protective activities (Pietrantoni et al. 2014). Studies have reported that maternal omega-3 fatty acid supplementation enhances placental levels of the specialized proresolving mediators and their precursors and reduces maternal systemic levels of TNF-α (Jones et al. 2013a). Omega-3 fatty acids are also known to inhibit cytokine production and NF-κB activity possibly by interrupting the production of proinflammatory eicosanoids through competition for active sites of cyclooxygenase and lipoxygenase enzymes (Calder 2003). Another mechanism through which omega-3 fatty acids modulate inflammatory responses is through PPAR signaling (Kong et al. 2010). PPARs are known to be involved in the regulation of different anti-inflammatory genes like cytokines and adhesion molecules (Jawerbaum and Capobianco 2011).

8.3.5 Influences Placental Epigenome

Epigenetics is defined as mitotically or meiotically heritable functional modifications to genes without the underlying change in the nucleotide sequence. This involves an important mechanism, i.e., DNA methylation, where elevated methylation is associated with gene inactivation, whereas lack of methylation activates gene expression (Novakovic and Saffery 2012). DNA demethylation, followed by remethylation process, occurs during the period of embryogenesis and early placentation (Gheorghe et al. 2010). The epigenome of the placenta is known to regulate the expression of genes involved in the proliferation and differentiation of placental trophoblast cells (Hemberger 2007). Any alteration in the expression of vital genes leads to altered placental development and complications during pregnancy (Gheorghe et al. 2010).

Studies indicate that placental epigenetic modifications are influenced by environmental factors and nutrients (Myatt 2006). Animal studies report that an imbalance in maternal nutrients during pregnancy can alter global DNA methylation patterns in the placenta (Kulkarni et al. 2011a). The focus shifted to fatty acids when a high-fat diet fed to mice during gestation showed epigenetic alterations throughout the placental genome (Gallou-Kabani et al. 2010). Recent studies support the relationship between LCPUFA and epigenetics wherein supplementation of omega-3 fatty acids altered methylation patterns of specific Cytosine-phosphate-Guanine dinucleotide (CpG) loci of fatty acid synthesizing enzyme (Δ6-desaturase) in the adult human (Burdge and Lillycrop 2014; Hoile et al. 2014).

Studies have suggested that inadequate levels of maternal LCPUFA containing phospholipids, one of the major methyl group acceptors, may cause diversion of methyl groups toward DNA, eventually resulting in aberrant DNA methylation patterns (Kale et al. 2009; Khot, Chavan-Gautam, and Joshi 2014; Kulkarni et al. 2011b). Altered LCPUFA levels as well as altered methylation of specific genes involved in placental angiogenesis have been reported in preeclampsia (Kulkarni et al. 2011b; Sundrani et al. 2013, 2014). Studies indicate that epigenetic variation is influenced by the interaction between fatty acid and the genome, increasing the risk for disease (Burdge, Hoile, and Lillycrop 2012; Burdge and Lillycrop 2014). However, there is a need for rigorous investigations to understand the epigenetic modifications induced by fatty acids on placental gene function and metabolism.

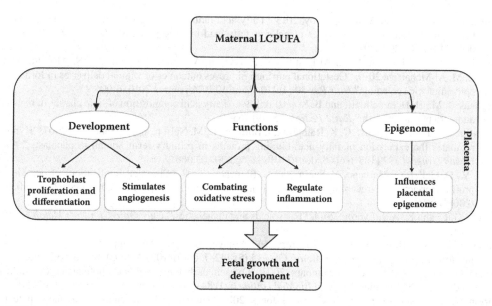

FIGURE 8.4 Overview of the roles of maternal long-chain polyunsaturated fatty acids in placental development and function.

8.4 CONCLUSION

To summarize, maternal LCPUFA metabolism influences placental growth and development (Figure 8.4). Appropriate placental development is critical since it plays a key role in the transport and metabolism of nutrients, acts as an interface between the mother and the fetus, and is a source of various hormones that influence fetal growth and development. LCPUFAs and their metabolites are involved in various processes in the placenta, e.g., growth of the trophoblast cells and angiogenesis. They are also involved in counteracting oxidative stress and regulating inflammation in the placenta. LCPUFAs affect the expression of placental genes by either influencing the signaling of transcription factors or through changes in the placental epigenome. However, more research is required to elucidate the different molecular mechanisms through which LCPUFA influences placental growth and function across gestation. Further, it is also necessary to examine the potential of dietary LCPUFA for therapeutic intervention in the prevention of placental disorders like preeclampsia.

REFERENCES

Al, M. D., A. C. van Houwelingen, A. D. Kester, T. H. Hasaart, A. E. de Jong, and G. Hornstra. 1995. "Maternal essential fatty acid patterns during normal pregnancy and their relationship to the neonatal essential fatty acid status." *Br J Nutr* 74 (1):55–68.

Assies, J., A. Lok, C. L. Bockting, G. J. Weverling, R. Lieverse, I. Visser, N. G. Abeling, M. Duran, and A. H. Schene. 2004. "Fatty acids and homocysteine levels in patients with recurrent depression: An explorative pilot study." *Prostaglandins Leukot Essent Fatty Acids* 70 (4):349–56. doi:10.1016/j.plefa.2003.12.009.

Barak, Y., D. Liao, W. He, E. S. Ong, M. C. Nelson, J. M. Olefsky, R. Boland, and R. M. Evans. 2002. "Effects of peroxisome proliferator-activated receptor delta on placentation, adiposity, and colorectal cancer." *Proc Natl Acad Sci U S A* 99 (1):303–8. doi:10.1073/pnas.012610299.

Basak, S. and A. K. Duttaroy. 2013. "Effects of fatty acids on angiogenic activity in the placental extravillious trophoblast cells." *Prostaglandins Leukot Essent Fatty Acids* 88 (2):155–62. doi:10.1016/j.plefa.2012.10.001.

Basak, S., M. K. Das, and A. K. Duttaroy. 2013. "Fatty acid-induced angiogenesis in first trimester placental trophoblast cells: Possible roles of cellular fatty acid-binding proteins." *Life Sci* 93 (21):755–62. doi:10.1016/j.lfs.2013.09.024.

Bawadi, H. A., O. Al-Kuran, L. A. Al-Bastoni, R. F. Tayyem, A. Jaradat, G. Tuuri, S. N. Al-Beitawi, and L. M. Al-Mehaisen. 2010. "Gestational nutrition improves outcomes of vaginal deliveries in Jordan: An epidemiologic screening." *Nutr Res* 30 (2):110–7. doi:10.1016/j.nutres.2010.01.005.

Berghaus, T. M., H. Demmelmair, and B. Koletzko. 1998. "Fatty acid composition of lipid classes in maternal and cord plasma at birth." *Eur J Pediatr* 157 (9):763–8.

Biron-Shental, T., W. T. Schaiff, C. K. Ratajczak, I. Bildirici, D. M. Nelson, and Y. Sadovsky. 2007. "Hypoxia regulates the expression of fatty acid-binding proteins in primary term human trophoblasts." *Am J Obstet Gynecol* 197 (5):516.e1–6. doi:10.1016/j.ajog.2007.03.066.

Borel, V., D. Gallot, G. Marceau, V. Sapin, and L. Blanchon. 2008. "Placental implications of peroxisome proliferator-activated receptors in gestation and parturition." *PPAR Res* 2008:758562. doi:10.1155/2008/758562.

Burdge, G. C. and K. A. Lillycrop. 2014. "Fatty acids and epigenetics." *Curr Opin Clin Nutr Metab Care* 17 (2):156–61.

Burdge, G. C., S. P. Hoile, and K. A. Lillycrop. 2012. "Epigenetics: Are there implications for personalised nutrition?" *Curr Opin Clin Nutr Metab Care* 15 (5):442–7. doi:10.1097/MCO.0b013e3283567dd2.

Burton, G. J., J. Hempstock, and E. Jauniaux. 2003. "Oxygen, early embryonic metabolism and free radical-mediated embryopathies." *Reprod BioMed Online* 6 (1):84–96. doi:10.1016/S1472-6483(10)62060-3.

Burton, G. J., E. Jauniaux, and D. S. Charnock-Jones. 2007. "Human early placental development: potential roles of the endometrial glands." *Placenta* 28 Suppl A:S64–9. doi:10.1016/j.placenta.2007.01.007.

Calder, P. C. 2003. "n–3 Polyunsaturated fatty acids and inflammation: From molecular biology to the clinic." *Lipids* 38 (4):343–52.

Calder, P. C. 2012. "Mechanisms of action of (n-3) fatty acids." *J Nutr* 142 (3):592S–9S. doi:10.3945/jn.111.155259.

Calder, P. C. 2013. "Omega-3 polyunsaturated fatty acids and inflammatory processes: Nutrition or pharmacology?" *Br J Clin Pharmacol* 75 (3):645–62. doi:10.1111/j.1365-2125.2012.04374.x.

Carlson, S. E., J. Colombo, B. J. Gajewski, K. M. Gustafson, D. Mundy, J. Yeast, M. K. Georgieff, L. A. Markley, E. H. Kerling, and D. J. Shaddy. 2013. "DHA supplementation and pregnancy outcomes." *Am J Clin Nutr* 97 (4):808–15. doi:10.3945/ajcn.112.050021.

Carmeliet, P. 2003. "Angiogenesis in health and disease." *Nat Med* 9 (6):653–60.

Castellucci, M., G. Kosanke, F. Verdenelli, B. Huppertz, and P. Kaufmann. 2000. "Villous sprouting: Fundamental mechanisms of human placental development." *Hum Reprod Update* 6 (5):485–94.

Cetin, I., G. Alvino, and M. Cardellicchio. 2009. "Long chain fatty acids and dietary fats in fetal nutrition." *J Physiol* 587 (Pt 14):3441–51. doi:10.1113/jphysiol.2009.173062.

Chirala, S. S., H. Chang, M. Matzuk, L. Abu-Elheiga, J. Mao, K. Mahon, M. Finegold, and S. J. Wakil. 2003. "Fatty acid synthesis is essential in embryonic development: fatty acid synthase null mutants and most of the heterozygotes die in utero." *Proc Natl Acad Sci U S A* 100 (11):6358–63. doi:10.1073/pnas.0931394100.

Chung, I. B., F. D. Yelian, F. M. Zaher, B. Gonik, M. I. Evans, M. P. Diamond, and D. M. Svinarich. 2000. "Expression and regulation of vascular endothelial growth factor in a first trimester trophoblast cell line." *Placenta* 21 (4):320–4. doi:10.1053/plac.1999.0481.

Coletta, J. M., S. J. Bell, and A. S. Roman. 2010. "Omega-3 fatty acids and pregnancy." *Rev Obstet Gynecol* 3 (4):163–71.

Cooper, J. C., A. M. Sharkey, J. McLaren, D. S. Charnock-Jones, and S. K. Smith. 1995. "Localization of vascular endothelial growth factor and its receptor, flt, in human placenta and decidua by immunohistochemistry." *J Reprod Fertil* 105 (2):205–13.

Cunningham, P. and L. McDermott. 2009. "Long chain PUFA transport in human term placenta." *J Nutr* 139 (4):636–9. doi:10.3945/jn.108.098608.

De Giuseppe, R., C. Roggi, and H. Cena. 2014. "n-3 LC-PUFA supplementation: Effects on infant and maternal outcomes." *Eur J Nutr* 53 (5):1147–54. doi:10.1007/s00394-014-0660-9.

Dhobale, M. V., N. Wadhwani, S. S. Mehendale, H. R. Pisal, and S. R. Joshi. 2011. "Reduced levels of placental long chain polyunsaturated fatty acids in preterm deliveries." *Prostaglandins Leukot Essent Fatty Acids* 85 (3–4):149–53. doi:10.1016/j.plefa.2011.06.003.

Dube, E., A. Gravel, C. Martin, G. Desparois, I. Moussa, M. Ethier-Chiasson, J. C. Forest, Y. Giguere, A. Masse, and J. Lafond. 2012. "Modulation of fatty acid transport and metabolism by maternal obesity in the human full-term placenta." *Biol Reprod* 87 (1):14, 1–11. doi:10.1095/biolreprod.111.098095.

Duttaroy, A. K. 2000. "Transport mechanisms for long-chain polyunsaturated fatty acids in the human placenta." *Am J Clin Nutr* 71 (1 Suppl):315S–22S.

Duttaroy, A. K. 2009. "Transport of fatty acids across the human placenta: A review." *Prog Lipid Res* 48 (1):52–61. doi:10.1016/j.plipres.2008.11.001.

Eyster, K. M. 2007. "The membrane and lipids as integral participants in signal transduction: Lipid signal transduction for the non-lipid biochemist." *Adv Physiol Educ* 31 (1):5–16. doi:10.1152/advan.00088.2006.

Fall, C. H. D., C. S. Yajnik, S. Rao, A. A. Davies, N. Brown, and H. J. W. Farrant. 2003. "Micronutrients and fetal growth." *J Nutr* 133 (5):1747S–56S.

Ferdinandusse, S., S. Denis, P. A. W. Mooijer, Z. Zhang, J. K. Reddy, A. A. Spector, and R. J. A. Wanders. 2001. "Identification of the peroxisomal β-oxidation enzymes involved in the biosynthesis of docosahexaenoic acid." *J Lipid Res* 42 (12):1987–95.

Finetti, F., R. Solito, L. Morbidelli, A. Giachetti, M. Ziche, and S. Donnini. 2008. "Prostaglandin E2 regulates angiogenesis via activation of fibroblast growth factor receptor-1." *J Biol Chem* 283 (4):2139–46. doi:10.1074/jbc.M703090200.

Fournier, T., J. Guibourdenche, K. Handschuh, V. Tsatsaris, B. Rauwel, C. Davrinche, and D. Evain-Brion. 2011. "PPARγ and human trophoblast differentiation." *J Reprod Immunol* 90 (1):41–9. doi:10.1016/j.jri.2011.05.003.

Gallou-Kabani, C., A. Gabory, J. Tost, M. Karimi, S. Mayeur, J. Lesage, E. Boudadi, M. S. Gross, J. Taurelle, A. Vige, C. Breton, B. Reusens, C. Remacle, D. Vieau, T. J. Ekstrom, J. P. Jais, and C. Junien. 2010. "Sex- and diet-specific changes of imprinted gene expression and DNA methylation in mouse placenta under a high-fat diet." *PLoS One* 5 (12):e14398. doi:10.1371/journal.pone.0014398.

Gheorghe, C. P., R. Goyal, A. Mittal, and L. D. Longo. 2010. "Gene expression in the placenta: Maternal stress and epigenetic responses." *Int J Dev Biol* 54 (2–3):507.

Gorjão, R., A. K. Azevedo-Martins, H. G. Rodrigues, F. Abdulkader, M. Arcisio-Miranda, J. Procopio, and R. Curi. 2009. "Comparative effects of DHA and EPA on cell function." *Pharmacol Ther* 122 (1):56–64.

Gude, N. M., C. T. Roberts, B. Kalionis, and R. G. King. 2004. "Growth and function of the normal human placenta." *Thromb Res* 114 (5–6):397–407. doi:10.1016/j.thromres.2004.06.038.

Haggarty, P. 2004. "Effect of placental function on fatty acid requirements during pregnancy." *Eur J Clin Nutr* 58 (12):1559–70. doi:10.1038/sj.ejcn.1602016.

Haggarty, P. 2010. "Fatty acid supply to the human fetus." *Annu Rev Nutr* 30:237–55. doi:10.1146/annurev.nutr.012809.104742.

Heaton, A. E., S. J. Meldrum, J. K. Foster, S. L. Prescott, and K. Simmer. 2013. "Does docosahexaenoic acid supplementation in term infants enhance neurocognitive functioning in infancy?" *Front Hum Neurosci* 7:774. doi:10.3389/fnhum.2013.00774.

Hemberger, M. 2007. "Epigenetic landscape required for placental development." *Cell Mol Life Sci* 64 (18):2422–36.

Herrera, E. 2002. "Implications of dietary fatty acids during pregnancy on placental, fetal and postnatal development—A review." *Placenta* 23 Suppl A:S9–19. doi:10.1053/plac.2002.0771.

Hoile, S. P., R. Clarke-Harris, R. C. Huang, P. C. Calder, T. A. Mori, L. J. Beilin, K. A. Lillycrop, and G. C. Burdge. 2014. "Supplementation with n-3 long-chain polyunsaturated fatty acids or olive oil in men and women with renal disease induces differential changes in the DNA methylation of FADS2 and ELOVL5 in peripheral blood mononuclear cells." *PLoS One* 9 (10):e109896. doi:10.1371/journal.pone.0109896.

Jauniaux, E., A. L. Watson, J. Hempstock, Y. P. Bao, J. N. Skepper, and G. J. Burton. 2000. "Onset of maternal arterial blood flow and placental oxidative stress. A possible factor in human early pregnancy failure." *Am J Pathol* 157 (6):2111–22. doi:10.1016/S0002-9440(10)64849-3.

Jauniaux, E., J. Hempstock, N. Greenwold, and G. J. Burton. 2003. "Trophoblastic oxidative stress in relation to temporal and regional differences in maternal placental blood flow in normal and abnormal early pregnancies." *Am J Pathol* 162 (1):115–25. doi:10.1016/s0002-9440(10)63803-5.

Jawerbaum, A. and E. Capobianco. 2011. "Review: Effects of PPAR activation in the placenta and the fetus: Implications in maternal diabetes." *Placenta* 32:S212–7.

Johnsen, G. M., S. Basak, M. S. Weedon-Fekjaer, A. C. Staff, and A. K. Duttaroy. 2011. "Docosahexaenoic acid stimulates tube formation in first trimester trophoblast cells, HTR8/SVneo." *Placenta* 32 (9):626–32. doi:10.1016/j.placenta.2011.06.009.

Jones, M. L., P. J. Mark, J. L. Lewis, T. A. Mori, J. A. Keelan, and B. J. Waddell. 2010. "Antioxidant defenses in the rat placenta in late gestation: Increased labyrinthine expression of superoxide dismutases, glutathione peroxidase 3, and uncoupling protein 2." *Biol Reprod* 83 (2):254–60. doi:10.1095/biolreprod.110.083907.

Jones, M. L., P. J. Mark, J. A. Keelan, A. Barden, E. Mas, T. A. Mori, and B. J. Waddell. 2013a. "Maternal dietary omega-3 fatty acid intake increases resolvin and protectin levels in the rat placenta." *J Lipid Res* 54 (8):2247–54. doi:10.1194/jlr.M039842.

Jones, M. L., P. J. Mark, T. A. Mori, J. A. Keelan, and B. J. Waddell. 2013b. "Maternal dietary omega-3 fatty acid supplementation reduces placental oxidative stress and increases fetal and placental growth in the rat." *Biol Reprod* 88 (2):37. doi:10.1095/biolreprod.112.103754.

Jones, M. L., P. J. Mark, and B. J. Waddell. 2014. "Maternal dietary omega-3 fatty acids and placental function." *Reproduction* 147 (5):R143–52. doi:10.1530/REP-13-0376.

Jump, D. B., D. Botolin, Y. Wang, J. Xu, O. Demeure, and B. Christian. 2008. "Docosahexaenoic acid (DHA) and hepatic gene transcription." *Chem Phys Lipids* 153 (1):3–13. doi:10.1016/j.chemphyslip.2008.02.007.

Kale, A., S. Joshi, A. Pillai, N. Naphade, M. Raju, H. Nasrallah, and S. P. Mahadik. 2009. "Reduced cerebrospinal fluid and plasma nerve growth factor in drug-naive psychotic patients." *Schizophr Res* 115 (2–3):209–14. doi:10.1016/j.schres.2009.07.022.

Kazantzis, M. and A. Stahl. 2012. "Fatty acid transport proteins, implications in physiology and disease." *Biochim Biophys Acta* 1821 (5):852–7. doi:10.1016/j.bbalip.2011.09.010.

Khot, V., P. Chavan-Gautam, and S. Joshi. 2014. "Proposing interactions between maternal phospholipids and the one carbon cycle: A novel mechanism influencing the risk for cardiovascular diseases in the offspring in later life." *Life Sci.* 129 (0):16–21. doi:10.1016/j.lfs.2014.09.026.

Kingdom, J., B. Huppertz, G. Seaward, and P. Kaufmann. 2000. "Development of the placental villous tree and its consequences for fetal growth." *Eur J Obstet Gynecol Reprod Biol* 92 (1):35–43.

Kong, W., J. H. Yen, E. Vassiliou, S. Adhikary, M. G. Toscano, and D. Ganea. 2010. "Docosahexaenoic acid prevents dendritic cell maturation and in vitro and in vivo expression of the IL-12 cytokine family." *Lipids Health Dis* 9:12. doi:10.1186/1476-511x-9-12.

Kovo, M., L. Schreiber, O. Elyashiv, A. Ben-Haroush, G. Abraham, and J. Bar. 2014. "Pregnancy outcome and placental findings in pregnancies complicated by fetal growth restriction with and without preeclampsia." *Reprod Sci.* 2 (3):316–21. doi:10.1177/1933719114542024.

Kulkarni, A., K. Dangat, A. Kale, P. Sable, P. Chavan-Gautam, and S. Joshi. 2011a. "Effects of altered maternal folic acid, vitamin B12 and docosahexaenoic acid on placental global DNA methylation patterns in Wistar rats." *PLoS One* 6 (3):e17706. doi:10.1371/journal.pone.0017706.

Kulkarni, A. V., S. S. Mehendale, H. R. Yadav, and S. R. Joshi. 2011b. "Reduced placental docosahexaenoic acid levels associated with increased levels of sFlt-1 in preeclampsia." *Prostaglandins Leukot Essent Fatty Acids* 84 (1–2):51–5. doi:10.1016/j.plefa.2010.09.005.

Lager, S. and T. L. Powell. 2012. "Regulation of nutrient transport across the placenta." *J Pregnancy* 2012:179827. doi:10.1155/2012/179827.

Lager, S., V. I. Ramirez, F. Gaccioli, T. Jansson, and T. L. Powell. 2014. "Expression and localization of the omega-3 fatty acid receptor GPR120 in human term placenta." *Placenta* 35 (7):523–5. doi:10.1016/j.placenta.2014.04.017.

Larque, E., S. Krauss-Etschmann, C. Campoy, D. Hartl, J. Linde, M. Klingler, H. Demmelmair, A. Cano, A. Gil, B. Bondy, and B. Koletzko. 2006. "Docosahexaenoic acid supply in pregnancy affects placental expression of fatty acid transport proteins." *Am J Clin Nutr* 84 (4):853–61.

Leonard, A. E., B. Kelder, E. G. Bobik, L.-T. Chuang, C. J. Lewis, J. J. Kopchick, P. Mukerji, and Y.-S. Huang. 2002. "Identification and expression of mammalian long-chain PUFA elongation enzymes." *Lipids* 37 (8):733–40. doi:10.1007/s11745-002-0955-6.

Lluís, L., N. Taltavull, M. Muñoz-Cortés, V. Sánchez-Martos, M. Romeu, M. Giralt, E. Molinar-Toribio, J. L. Torres, J. Pérez-Jiménez, M. Pazos, L. Méndez, J. M. Gallardo, I. Medina, and M. R. Nogués. 2013. "Protective effect of the omega-3 polyunsaturated fatty acids: Eicosapentaenoic acid/Docosahexaenoic acid 1:1 ratio on cardiovascular disease risk markers in rats." *Lipids Health Dis* 12 (1):1–8. doi:10.1186/1476-511X-12-140.

Luo, Z. C., W. D. Fraser, P. Julien, C. L. Deal, F. Audibert, G. N. Smith, X. Xiong, and M. Walker. 2006. "Tracing the origins of "fetal origins" of adult diseases: Programming by oxidative stress?" *Med Hypotheses* 66 (1):38–44.

Madazli, R., A. Benian, K. Gümüştaş, H. Uzun, V. Ocak, and F. Aksu. 1999. "Lipid peroxidation and antioxidants in preeclampsia." *Eur J Obstet Gynecol Reprod Biol* 85 (2):205–8.

McKeegan, P. J. and R. G. Sturmey. 2011. "The role of fatty acids in oocyte and early embryo development." *Reprod Fertil Dev* 24 (1):59–67. doi:10.1071/RD11907.

Meher, A. P., A. A. Joshi, and S. R. Joshi. 2014. "Maternal micronutrients, omega-3 fatty acids, and placental PPARγ expression." *Appl Physiol Nutr Metab* 39 (7):793–800. doi:10.1139/apnm-2013-0518.

Mori, T. A. and L. J. Beilin. 2004. "Omega-3 fatty acids and inflammation." *Curr Atheroscler Rep* 6 (6):461–7. doi:10.1007/s11883-004-0087-5.

Muskiet, F. A. J. 2010. "Pathophysiology and evolutionary aspects of dietary fats and long-chain polyunsaturated fatty acids across the life cycle." In *Fat Detection: Taste, Texture, and Post Ingestive Effects*, edited by J. P. Montmayeur and J. le Coutre. Taylor & Francis Group, LLC. Boca Raton, FL.

Myatt, L. 2006. "Placental adaptive responses and fetal programming." *J Physiol* 572 (1):25–30.

Myllynen, P. and K. Vahakangas. 2013. "Placental transfer and metabolism: An overview of the experimental models utilizing human placental tissue." *Toxicol In Vitro* 27 (1):507–12. doi:10.1016/j.tiv.2012.08.027.

Nadra, K., L. Quignodon, C. Sardella, E. Joye, A. Mucciolo, R. Chrast, and B. Desvergne. 2010. "PPARgamma in placental angiogenesis." *Endocrinology* 151 (10):4969–81. doi:10.1210/en.2010-0131.

Novakovic, B. and R. Saffery. 2012. "The ever growing complexity of placental epigenetics—Role in adverse pregnancy outcomes and fetal programming." *Placenta* 33 (12):959–70. doi:10.1016/j.placenta .2012.10.003.

Palozza, P., E. Sgarlata, C. Luberto, E. Piccioni, M. Anti, G. Marra, F. Armelao, P. Franceschelli, and G. M. Bartoli. 1996. "n-3 fatty acids induce oxidative modifications in human erythrocytes depending on dose and duration of dietary supplementation." *Am J Clin Nutr* 64 (3):297–304.

Patterson, E., R. Wall, G. F. Fitzgerald, R. P. Ross, and C. Stanton. 2012. "Health implications of high dietary omega-6 polyunsaturated fatty acids." *J Nutr Metab* 2012:539426. doi:10.1155/2012/539426.

Paulesu, L., J. Bhattacharjee, N. Bechi, R. Romagnoli, S. Jantra, and F. Ietta. 2010. "Pro-inflammatory cytokines in animal and human gestation." *Curr Pharm Des* 16 (32):3601–15.

Pegorier, J. P., C. Le May, and J. Girard. 2004. "Control of gene expression by fatty acids." *J Nutr* 134 (9):2444S–9S.

Pietrantoni, E., F. Del Chierico, G. Rigon, P. Vernocchi, G. Salvatori, M. Manco, F. Signore, and L. Putignani. 2014. "Docosahexaenoic acid supplementation during pregnancy: A potential tool to prevent membrane rupture and preterm labor." *Int J Mol Sci* 15 (5):8024–36.

Raghupathy, R., M. Al-Azemi, and F. Azizieh. 2012. "Intrauterine growth restriction: Cytokine profiles of trophoblast antigen-stimulated maternal lymphocytes." *Clin Dev Immunol* 2012:734865. doi:10.1155/2012/734865.

Rao, K. R., I. J. Padmavathi, and M. Raghunath. 2012. "Maternal micronutrient restriction programs the body adiposity, adipocyte function and lipid metabolism in offspring: A review." *Rev Endocr Metab Disord* 13 (2):103–8. doi:10.1007/s11154-012-9211-y.

Richard, D., K. Kefi, U. Barbe, P. Bausero, and F. Visioli. 2008. "Polyunsaturated fatty acids as antioxidants." *Pharmacol Res* 57 (6):451–5. doi:10.1016/j.phrs.2008.05.002.

Sandovici, I., K. Hoelle, E. Angiolini, and M. Constancia. 2012. "Placental adaptations to the maternal-fetal environment: implications for fetal growth and developmental programming." *Reprod Biomed Online* 25 (1):68–89. doi:10.1016/j.rbmo.2012.03.017.

Scholl, T. O. 2008. "Maternal nutrition before and during pregnancy." *Nestle Nutr Workshop Ser Pediatr Program* 61:79–89. doi:10.1159/0000113172.

Schwabe, J. W. R. 1996. "Transcriptional control: How nuclear receptors get turned on." *Curr Biol* 6 (4):372–4. doi:10.1016/S0960-9822(02)00498-0.

Shoji, H., C. Franke, H. Demmelmair, and B. Koletzko. 2009. "Effect of docosahexaenoic acid on oxidative stress in placental trophoblast cells." *Early Hum Dev* 85 (7):433–7. doi:10.1016/j.earlhumdev.2009.02.003.

Simopoulos, A. P. 2002. "Omega-3 fatty acids in inflammation and autoimmune diseases." *J Am Coll Nutr* 21 (6):495–505.

Simpson, J. L., L. B. Bailey, K. Pietrzik, B. Shane, and W. Holzgreve. 2011. "Micronutrients and women of reproductive potential: Required dietary intake and consequences of dietary deficiency or excess. Part II—vitamin D, vitamin A, iron, zinc, iodine, essential fatty acids." *J Matern Fetal Neonatal Med* 24 (1):1–24. doi:10.3109/14767051003678226.

Stark, M. J., V. L. Clifton, and N. A. Hodyl. 2013. "Differential effects of docosahexaenoic acid on preterm and term placental pro-oxidant/antioxidant balance." *Reproduction* 146 (3):243–51. doi:10.1530/REP-13-0239.

Sundrani, D. P., U. S. Reddy, A. A. Joshi, S. S. Mehendale, P. M. Chavan-Gautam, A. A. Hardikar, G. R. Chandak, and S. R. Joshi. 2013. "Differential placental methylation and expression of VEGF, FLT-1 and KDR genes in human term and preterm preeclampsia." *Clin Epigenetics* 5 (1):6. doi:10.1186/1868-7083-5-6.

Sundrani, D. P., U. S. Reddy, P. M. Chavan-Gautam, S. S. Mehendale, G. R. Chandak, and S. R. Joshi. 2014. "Altered methylation and expression patterns of genes regulating placental angiogenesis in preterm pregnancy." *Reprod Sci* 21 (12):1508–17. doi:10.1177/1933719114532838.

Symonds, M. E., T. Stephenson, D. S. Gardner, and H. Budge. 2006. "Long-term effects of nutritional programming of the embryo and fetus: mechanisms and critical windows." *Reprod Fertil Dev* 19 (1):53–63.

Szukiewicz, D. 2012. "Cytokines in placental physiology and disease." *Mediators Inflamm* 2012:640823. doi:10.1155/2012/640823.

Takahashi, M., N. Tsuboyama-Kasaoka, T. Nakatani, M. Ishii, S. Tsutsumi, H. Aburatani, and O. Ezaki. 2002. "Fish oil feeding alters liver gene expressions to defend against PPARα activation and ROS production." *Am J Physiol Gastrointest Liver Physiol* 282:G338–48.

Uauy, R., D. R. Hoffman, P. Peirano, D. G. Birch, and E. E. Birch. 2001. "Essential fatty acids in visual and brain development." *Lipids* 36 (9):885–95.

Velkov, T. 2013. "Interactions between human liver fatty acid binding protein and peroxisome proliferator activated receptor selective drugs." *PPAR Res* 2013:938401. doi:10.1155/2013/938401.

Wadhwani, N., V. Patil, H. Pisal, A. Joshi, S. Mehendale, S. Gupte, G. Wagh, and S. Joshi. 2014. "Altered maternal proportions of long chain polyunsaturated fatty acids and their transport leads to disturbed fetal stores in preeclampsia." *Prostaglandins Leukot Essent Fatty Acids.* 91 (1–2):21–30. doi:10.1016/j.plefa.2014.05.006.

Wang, H.-H., T.-M. Hung, J. Wei, and A.-N. Chiang. 2004. "Fish oil increases antioxidant enzyme activities in macrophages and reduces atherosclerotic lesions in apoE-knockout mice." *Cardiovasc Res* 61 (1):169–76.

Wang, G., Y. Gong, J. Anderson, D. Sun, G. Minuk, M. S. Roberts, and F. J. Burczynski. 2005. "Antioxidative function of L-FABP in L-FABP stably transfected Chang liver cells." *Hepatology* 42 (4):871–9. doi:10.1002/hep.20857.

Wu, G., B. Imhoff-Kunsch, and A. W. Girard. 2012. "Biological mechanisms for nutritional regulation of maternal health and fetal development." *Paediatr Perinat Epidemiol* 26 Suppl 1:4–26. doi:10.1111/j.1365-3016.2012.01291.x.

Yessoufou, A., A. Hichami, P. Besnard, K. Moutairou, and N. A. Khan. 2006. "Peroxisome proliferator-activated receptor alpha deficiency increases the risk of maternal abortion and neonatal mortality in murine pregnancy with or without diabetes mellitus: Modulation of T cell differentiation." *Endocrinology* 147 (9):4410–8. doi:10.1210/en.2006-0067.

Zeman, M., R. Jirak, M. Vecka, J. Raboch, and A. Zak. 2012. "N-3 polyunsaturated fatty acids in psychiatric diseases: Mechanisms and clinical data." *Neuro Endocrinol Lett* 33 (8):736–48.

9 Importance of Cholesterol and Cholesterol Transporters in the Placental Trophoblast during Pregnancy

Arjun Jain and Christiane Albrecht

CONTENTS

ABSTRACT

Membrane transporters are essential during pregnancy, being a core component of the exchange of nutrients, gases, and metabolic products between the mother and the developing fetus. Important compounds to be transported include vitamins and minerals, amino acids, glucose, as well as cholesterol. Cholesterol transport across the plasma membrane is mediated mainly by members of the ATP-binding cassette (ABC) transporter family. Cholesterol is present in every cell of the body, where it helps maintain the integrity of cell membranes and also plays an important role in cell signaling events. Cholesterol also acts as a precursor for the biosynthesis of steroids that include sex hormones, glucocorticoids, mineralcorticoids, as well as bile acids and oxysterols. Cholesterol transport is therefore crucial for a host of different physiological processes. The following chapter addresses the involvement and importance of ABC transporters in these different processes. The critical role that ABC transporters play for a successful pregnancy outcome is highlighted by pathological processes that result from malfunction of cholesterol transport during pregnancy. Avenues of future research are also described, which may help to further delineate the function and mechanism of action of ABC transporters.

KEY WORDS

Cholesterol, placenta, trophoblast, ABCA1, ABCG1, JAK/STAT signaling, Ca^{2+} signaling, angiogenesis, endothelial dysfunction, oxysterols, sonic hedgehog pathway, dual placenta perfusion, Transwell® model.

9.1 INTRODUCTION

Cholesterol plays an important role in many aspects of mammalian development. From the very beginning, during early embryogenesis, cholesterol is required for the maturation of the sonic hedgehog protein, which is a secreted molecule necessary for morphogenesis (Ming et al. 1998). Cholesterol also acts as a precursor for the biosynthesis of steroids, which include sex hormones, glucocorticoids, mineralcorticoids, as well as bile acids and oxysterols. For example, large amounts of cholesterol are utilized by the placenta for steroidogenesis, particularly progesterone synthesis (Conley and Mason 1990). Therefore, any disruptions in cholesterol supply can alter the synthesis of important steroidal hormones and their metabolites. At the subcellular level, cholesterol is a structural lipid component of membranes and also participates in the formation of lipid rafts, which serve as platforms for intracellular signaling events (Pike 2004).

Given this wide array of functions, materno–fetal cholesterol transport across the placental trophoblast is a very important event during pregnancy.

9.2 PLACENTA AND TROPHOBLAST

Trophoblasts are cells forming the outer layer of a blastocyst, which provides nutrients to the embryo and develop into a large part of the placenta. During pregnancy, maternal and fetal blood does not mix but is separated by the placenta. The placenta is a multifunctional organ that provides hormonal equilibrium for the maintenance of pregnancy. It is also involved in nutrient exchange/ transport and oxygen supply from mother to fetus and in the removal of metabolites from the fetal to maternal circulation. The placenta, therefore, is essential in pregnancy. The placental bed, the area of the uterus underlying the placenta, plays a key role in supporting placental function by supplying oxygenated blood to the intervillous space (Lyall 2005). In the second two trimesters of pregnancy, the placenta requires increasing access to the maternal blood supply. This is achieved by extensive remodeling of the maternal spiral arteries (Figure 9.1), which are the end arteries of the uteroplacental circulation that deliver blood directly into the placental intervillous space (Pijnenborg et al. 2006). Remodeling depends on one of the subtypes of the trophoblasts, which differentiates into tumor-like cells (extravillous cytotrophoblasts) that invade the lining of the pregnant uterus from 6 to 18 weeks of gestation (Red-Horse et al. 2004). From 12 weeks on, the trophoblasts penetrate the maternal decidual tissue and extensively remodel the spiral arteries, including their distal myometrial segments, such that they lose their smooth muscle and become greatly dilated (Pijnenborg et al. 2006). This process completes by around 20 weeks, such that the maternal circulation can supply the expanding intervillous space of the placenta. Trophoblast invasion of the uterus is tightly controlled by a number of different factors, expressed within the decidua, as well as on the trophoblasts themselves. These include cell adhesion molecules and the extracellular matrix, proteinases and their inhibitors, growth factors, and cytokines (Knofler 2010). Therefore, it is at this very early stage in pregnancy that trophoblasts (and factors expressed by the trophoblasts) are already implicated in ensuring a smooth and successful development of the intrauterine environment required

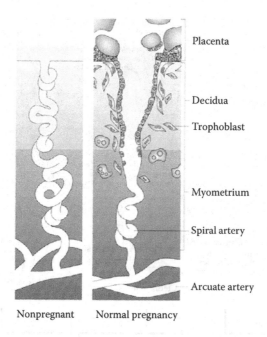

Placenta

Decidua

Trophoblast

Myometrium

Spiral artery

Arcuate artery

Nonpregnant   Normal pregnancy

FIGURE 9.1 Schematic representation of the placenta showing the endometrial spiral arteries. A comparison between uninvaded arteries in the nonpregnant state and differentiated arteries during pregnancy is shown. The placenta is supplied by the maternal spiral arteries that undergo major modifications during pregnancy to accommodate the increase in uterine blood flow from 45 ml/min in the nonpregnant state to 750 ml/min at term (Burton et al. 2009). In normal pregnancy, the maternal spiral arteries supplying the placenta undergo physiological conversion, where they lose their smooth muscle and elastic coats and become transformed into dilated flaccid conduits. These changes usually extend as far as the inner third of the myometrium. (Adapted from Moffett-King, A. *Nat. Rev. Immunol.*, 2, 656–663, 2002.)

for a successful pregnancy. Upon completion of trophoblast invasion and development of appropriate blood supply to the placenta, membrane transport proteins in the placental trophoblast become important in delivering/transporting essential nutrients across the placenta to the developing fetus and also removing waste substances from the fetal circulation (Figure 9.2a). There are different modes of transport across the placenta (Figure 9.2b), which include adenosine triphosphate (ATP)-dependent nutrient transporters. Of these, cholesterol transporters are an important class of transporters that play a critical role in fetal development.

9.3 CHOLESTEROL TRANSPORTERS

Cholesterol is present in every cell of the body, where it helps maintain the integrity of cell membranes and also plays an important role in cell signaling (Baardman et al. 2013). ATP-binding cassette (ABC) transporters have been shown to carry out cholesterol efflux from placental endothelial cells, providing evidence of a mechanism for the delivery of placental cholesterol to the fetal circulation (Stefulj et al. 2009).

9.3.1 ABC Transporter A1

The ABC transporter A1 (ABCA1), a member of the ABC-transporter superfamily, is a transmembrane protein that mediates the transport of cholesterol, phospholipids, and other lipophilic molecules across cellular membranes. It removes excess cellular cholesterol from peripheral cells by transferring it to lipid-poor apolipoprotein (apo) A1 (Neufeld et al. 2001). Hereby, it plays a key role

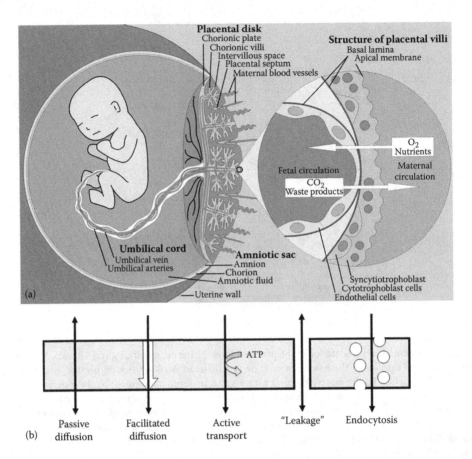

FIGURE 9.2 Maternal–fetal transport across the placenta. (a) Schematic representation of the materno–fetal barrier and cells involved in the transfer of nutrients, gases, and waste products. (b) Different placental transport mechanisms. Transfer across the placenta can occur via passive or facilitated diffusion, active transport mechanisms based on ATP hydrolysis, or endocytotic processes. Under specific physiological or pathophysiological conditions, paracellular transfer or "leakage" may take place.

in a crucial physiological process called "reverse cholesterol transport," a mechanism by which cholesterol from peripheral tissues is transported to the liver in the form of high-density lipoproteins (HDLs), where it can be eliminated into the bile (Figure 9.3). The importance of ABCA1 in this process was revealed when mutant ABCA1 was identified as the causative gene of Tangier disease (Bodzioch et al. 1999; Brooks-Wilson et al. 1999; Rust et al. 1999) and familial HDL deficiency (Marcil et al. 2003). These diseases are characterized by low levels of HDL, cholesteryl ester accumulation in tissue macrophages, and an increased risk of atherosclerotic cardiovascular disease. Recently, there has also been a role suggested for ABCA1 in normal and pathological pregnancies at the placenta level (see below).

ABCA1 is highly expressed in rodent and human placental tissues (Langmann et al. 2003; Albrecht et al. 2007; Albrecht and Viturro 2007; Bhattacharjee et al. 2010). Its importance in the normal development of gestation and the conceptus was recognized by the dramatic pathologic changes occurring during pregnancy in ABCA1 knockout mice (Christiansen-Weber et al. 2000). Functional loss of ABCA1 resulted in severe placental perturbations such as placental malformation with structural abnormalities, hemorrhage, and cell debris in the spongiotrophoblast and labyrinthine trophoblast. These abnormalities were associated with intrauterine growth restriction (IUGR) and increased rates of neonatal death (Christiansen-Weber et al. 2000; McNeish et al. 2000).

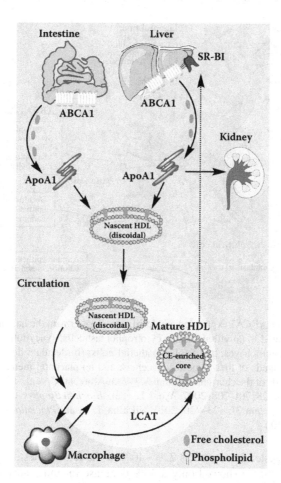

FIGURE 9.3 Role of ABCA1 in HDL formation and reverse cholesterol transport. Apolipoprotein (apo) A1 secreted from liver and intestine is lipidated via its interaction with ABCA1, producing nascent HDL. After entering the circulation, nascent HDLs acquire free cholesterol from macrophages and other cell types in the periphery and become cholesteryl ester (CE)-enriched mature HDL by the action of lecithin–cholesterol acyltransferase (LCAT). Mature HDLs are mainly taken up by the liver through scavenger receptor type B, class I (SR-BI). Apo A1 entering the circulation rapidly associates with plasma HDL or is catabolized by the kidney. (Adapted from Lee, J.Y., Parks, J.S., *Curr. Opin. Lipidol.* 16, 19–25, 2005.)

An essential function of ABCA1 in the human placenta is cholesterol transport from mother to fetus, an aspect extensively discussed in the literature (Albrecht et al. 2007; Stefulj et al. 2009; Aye et al. 2010; Bhattacharjee et al. 2010). Whether, how, and in which placental cell type ABCA1 contributes to transplacental cholesterol transport in humans is not fully clear yet. However, it is clear that the actual physical barrier between the maternal and fetal circulation in term placentas is made up of the villous syncytiotrophoblast, a multinucleated cell layer originating from precursor cytotrophoblast cells, and fetal villous endothelial cells (Schneider 1991). Previous research has shown that ABCA1 is expressed in cytotrophoblast cells in early and term placental tissues and variably also in syncytiotrophoblast cells, among other cell types (Figure 9.4).

In humans, the significance of ABCA1-induced cholesterol efflux for transplacental cholesterol transport is still unclear. Both placental tissue and fetal organs have the capacity for de novo cholesterol synthesis. However, a significantly higher cholesterol concentration in the umbilical cord vein (which delivers blood to the fetus) compared with the umbilical arteries (Parker et al. 1983) suggests transfer from maternal or placental sources to the fetus. In the third trimester of gestation,

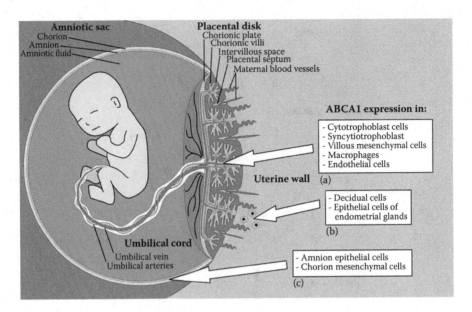

FIGURE 9.4 Summary of ABCA1 expression and localization patterns in the human placenta. Localization of ABCA1 was demonstrated in (a) villous tissue: cytotrophoblast cells, syncytiotrophoblast, villous mesenchymal cells, placental macrophages, and fetal endothelial cells; (b) decidua: decidual cells and epithelial cells of the endometrial glands of first-trimester placentas; and (c) placental membranes: amnion epithelial cells and mesenchymal cells of the chorion membranes. (From Albrecht, C. et al., *Placenta* 31, 741–742, 2010; Albrecht, C. et al., *Placenta* 28, 701–708, 2007; Aye, I. L. et al., *Biochim Biophys Acta* 1801, 1013–1024, 2010; Bhattacharjee, J. et al., *Placenta* 31, 423–430, 2010; Nikitina, L. et al., *Placenta*, in press; Plosch, T. et al., *Placenta* 31, 910–918, 2010.)

maternally derived cholesterol contributes 22%–40% to the fetal cholesterol pool. However, studies of ABCA1 knockout mice showed only a 30% decrease in transplacental cholesterol transfer in ABCA1$^{-/-}$ embryos (Lindegaard et al. 2008). In primary trophoblast cells, inhibition of ABCA1 reduced cholesterol efflux up to 45%, but ABCA1 upregulation resulted in much lower changes in cholesterol efflux than expected by the increased protein and mRNA expression levels (Aye et al. 2010). This could be because there is no concomitant increase in the levels of the acceptor (apoA1), leading to a saturation and plateau in the levels of cholesterol efflux. In addition, it should also be considered that ABCA1-dependent cholesterol efflux is not the only mechanism of cholesterol export in the placenta (Aye et al. 2010). Several transporters are expressed in the placenta, and some of them have been reported to be involved in cellular lipid transport (e.g., ABCA7, ABC transporter G [ABCG] 5, and ABCG8), in facilitating the efflux of cholesterol from macrophages (e.g., ABCG1), or generally in cellular lipid homeostasis (e.g., NCP1, NCP1L1). While ABCA1 mediates the transport of cholesterol and phospholipids from cells to lipid-poor apoA1, ABCG1 and ABCG4 mediate the transport of cholesterol from cells to lipidated lipoproteins (Vaughan and Oram 2006). It has also recently been demonstrated that ABCA1 and ABCG1 synergize to mediate cholesterol export to apoA1 (Gelissen et al. 2006). Moreover, it has been suggested that ABCG1 and ABCG4 act in concert with ABCA1 to maximize the removal of excess cholesterol from cells and to generate cholesterol-rich lipoprotein particles (Vaughan and Oram 2006).

9.3.2 ABC TRANSPORTER G1

ABCG1 is another transporter responsible for cellular cholesterol efflux. However, unlike ABCA1, ABCG1 promotes efflux of cholesterol and oxysterols to HDLs, whereas ABCA1 predominantly mediates efflux to apoA1. Accordingly, silencing of ABCA1 expression in primary trophoblasts in

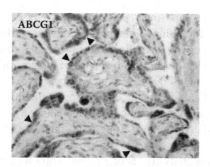

FIGURE 9.5 Immunohistochemical staining of ABCG1. ABCG1 expression was detected in the villous syncytiotrophoblast (black arrowheads). In contrast to ABCA1, stromal cells were negative for ABCG1.

culture, or pharmacological antagonism by glyburide, has been shown to decrease cholesterol efflux to apoA-I compared with controls, while ABCG1 silencing decreases cholesterol efflux to HDL. In contrast, treatment with endogenous or synthetic liver X receptor α/β ligands, such as T0901317, increases ABCA1 and ABCG1 expression and enhances cholesterol efflux to apoA-I and HDL, respectively (Aye et al. 2010).

ABCG1 is highly expressed in the placenta. However, unlike ABCA1, which shows also abundant expression in cell types not directly involved in materno–fetal transport processes, ABCG1 expression seems to be restricted to fetal capillaries and the syncytiotrophoblast of the placenta (Figure 9.5) (Stefulj et al. 2009; Baumann et al. 2013).

9.4 CELLULAR PATHWAYS ASSOCIATED WITH CHOLESTEROL TRANSPORT

9.4.1 ABCA1 AND JAK/STAT SIGNALING

As introduced earlier, cholesterol and, hence, cholesterol transporters are implicated in a host of different cellular processes, including important signaling mechanisms essential for fetal development and a successful pregnancy. Recent investigations revealed an association between ABCA1 and the janus kinase/signal transducer and activator of transcription (JAK/STAT) signaling pathway (Tang et al. 2009). Tang et al. (2009) reported that apoA1 binding ABCA1 leads to autophosphorylation and activation of JAK2. This in turn leads to activation of STAT3. It has been found that this activation of the JAK2/STAT3 pathway via interaction of apoA-I with ABCA1 can have an anti-inflammatory effect. Whereas the JAK2/STAT3 pathway is oncogenic and proinflammatory in many cell types (Bromberg et al. 1999), it has an anti-inflammatory effect in macrophages. Constitutive expression of active STAT3 in cultured macrophages greatly reduces LPS-induced inflammatory cytokine production, as evinced by an ~60% reduction in tumor necrosis factor-α and interleukin-6 production in these cells (Williams et al. 2007; Tang et al. 2009).

Given that inflammation is a key component of the pathophysiology of pregnancy disorders, such as preeclampsia (Redman and Sargent 2004), further research is warranted to shed light on whether ABCA1-mediated cholesterol efflux would confer a protective effect against inflammation in the placenta (trophoblast).

9.4.2 EFFECTS ON CA²⁺ SIGNALING

Annexins are a family of structurally related calcium and membrane-binding proteins. They contain a conserved core that is responsible for Ca^{2+} and phospholipid binding. Therefore, although synthesized as cytosolic proteins, annexins are predominantly associated with different intracellular membranes as well as the plasma membrane primarily because of their ability to bind negatively charged phospholipids in a Ca^{2+}-dependent manner. This provides a connection between Ca^{2+} signaling and membrane functions and enables annexins to participate in the organization of membrane domains or signaling platforms and the formation of complex protein networks (Enrich et al. 2011). Hence, there is an important link between Ca^{2+} signaling and cholesterol transport, as cholesterol and phospholipids transported by the ABC transporters make up an integral part of cell membranes.

Ca^{2+} signaling has important consequences in pregnancy. For example, a disruption in cell Ca^{2+} homeostasis can affect organelles, such as the endoplasmic reticulum (ER). Loss of Ca^{2+} from the ER induces ER stress responses that are implicated in the pathophysiology of pregnancy disorders, such as IUGR and preeclampsia (Burton and Yung 2011; Jain et al. 2012). Without getting into the intricacies of ER stress response pathways, ER stress relates to many of the clinical manifestations of preeclampsia and IUGR through its effects on protein synthesis inhibition and induction of proinflammatory responses, which contribute to a smaller placental size (and growth restricted fetus) as well as endothelial dysfunction and ensuing hypertension and proteinuria (in preeclampsia). Furthermore, during placental development, trophoblast cells develop along cell lineages, forming the villous cytotrophoblast with the overlaying syncytiotrophoblast (Benirschke et al. 2006). Imbalances in the intrauterine environment around the time of implantation and invasion can lead to abnormal trophoblast development associated with complicated pregnancies (Bowen et al. 2002). ER stress can also potentially contribute to a disruption in normal placental development through its effects on protein synthesis inhibition and induction of proinflammatory cytokines (Zhang and Kaufman 2008). This would compound the direct effects that cholesterol efflux may have during pregnancy on angiogenesis and endothelial dysfunction.

9.4.3 EFFECTS ON ANGIOGENESIS AND ENDOTHELIAL DYSFUNCTION

As earlier explained, ABCA1 mediates cholesterol efflux from cells by transferring cholesterol to apoA-I, which leads to the formation of HDL. The apoA-I binding protein (AIBP) accelerates cholesterol efflux from endothelial cells to HDL, and this process is found to effect angiogenesis. Previous research has shown that AIBP- and HDL-mediated cholesterol depletion from endothelial cells reduces lipid rafts, interferes with vascular endothelial growth factor receptor-2 (VEGFR2) dimerization (and signalling), and inhibits vascular endothelial growth factor-induced angiogenesis (Fang et al. 2013). The role of AIBP in promoting cholesterol efflux from endothelial cells to HDL and the importance of this mechanism in regulation of angiogenesis would have important implications during pregnancy and the physiological conversion of the spiral arteries to accommodate the increase in uterine blood flow.

The role of cholesterol efflux mechanisms in protecting cells against endothelial dysfunction has also been previously reported (Terasaka et al. 2008; Whetzel et al. 2010). Endothelial dysfunction is of course a key component of the pathophysiology of preeclampsia (Redman et al. 1999; Shamshirsaz et al. 2012). In addition, given that spiral artery conversion is such an essential event in laying the foundation for a successful pregnancy, the effects of cholesterol transport on angiogenesis, as well as endothelial dysfunction, are important issues that remain to be further explored during pregnancy and in the placental trophoblast.

9.4.4 CHOLESTEROL EFFLUX PROTECTS TROPHOBLASTS FROM OXYSTEROL-INDUCED TOXICITY

Another critical role of cholesterol efflux is the protection of placental trophoblasts from oxysterol-induced toxicity (Aye et al. 2010). Oxysterols are oxidized metabolites of cholesterol, which are formed by enzymatic or catalytic (nonenzymatic) oxidation of cholesterol, obtained either from de novo synthesis or from various dietary sources (Brown and Jessup 1999).

As already described, ABCA1 and ABCG1 are expressed in placental trophoblasts, where they are thought to be involved in the initial stages of delivering maternal cholesterol to the fetal circulation. In addition, depending on their subcellular orientation, these transporters are also involved in the efflux of sterol metabolites from the placenta as part of a cytoprotective role. Placental trophoblasts are exposed to oxysterols, such as 25-hydroxycholesterol (25-OHC) and 7-ketocholesterol (7-ketoC), that may either be present in the maternal circulation or generated by the placenta under oxidative stress. Placental ABCA1 and ABCG1 have been found to confer a protective effect in the placenta against oxysterols. A study by Aye et al. (2010) demonstrated that trophoblast cells with increased expression of ABCA1 and ABCG1 were less sensitive to 25-OHC and 7-ketoC (Aye et al. 2010). Furthermore, cells were more sensitive to the toxic effect of these oxysterols when ABCA1/G1 expression was inhibited, presumably because of the increase in accumulation of oxysterols in these cells. Therefore, in addition to cholesterol efflux, ABCA1 and ABCG1 appear to also play a protective role against toxic oxysterols. It remains to be investigated how these processes fit into the pathophysiology of placenta-related pregnancy disorders, such as preeclampsia.

9.4.5 EFFECTS ON SONIC HEDGEHOG PATHWAY

Sonic hedgehog (Shh) is a morphogen that is crucial for normal development of a variety of organ systems, including the brain and spinal cord, the eye, craniofacial structures, and the limbs (Ming et al. 1998). The Shh protein undergoes autocatalytic cleavage into a 19-kDa N-terminal (Shh-N) and a 25-kDa C-terminal (Shh-C) domain (Hammerschmidt et al. 1997). This cleavage is mediated by enzymatic activity present in the Shh-C domain. The N-terminal peptide remains tightly associated with the surface of the cell in which it was synthesized. Cleavage of Shh occurs through formation of an internal thioester intermediate that is cleaved by a nucleophilic substitution, with cholesterol acting as the nucleophile (Porter et al. 1996). In addition, the C terminus of Shh-N undergoes covalent cholesterol modification, and this process is thought to be required for the correct spatial restriction of the actions of Shh. Therefore, cholesterol clearly plays an important role in the processing and functioning of the Shh protein. The importance of cholesterol in this process is evinced by studies that found that developmental disorders dependent on the Shh pathway are related to a malfunction in cholesterol transport and biosynthesis. For example, the Smith–Lemli–Opitz (SLO) syndrome, which is an autosomal-recessive, multiple congenital anomaly syndrome with craniofacial, limb, and genital anomalies, is associated with dysfunctional cholesterol biosynthesis (Ming et al. 1998). SLO syndrome results from mutations in the gene encoding Δ-7-sterol reductase, the final step of cholesterol biosynthesis, which leads to hypocholesterolemia and, thus, an inability to modify Shh (Kelley et al. 1996).

Another developmental disorder, human brain malformation holoprosencephaly (HPE), is characterized by a defect in the midline of the embryonic forebrain. Mutations in the *SHH* gene or other genes, either part of the Shh pathway itself or which affect Shh function, have been associated with HPE. This includes failure of Shh to undergo cholesterol modification. A previous study found that rodent embryos developed HPE-like features if, early in gestation, the mothers were administered agents that induce hypocholesterolemia (Roessler and Muenke 1998). The lack of cholesterol would significantly perturb cholesterol modification of Shh. Furthermore, HPE is also associated with severe cases of SLO syndrome, which, as described above, is associated with defective cholesterol biosynthesis that leads to impaired cholesterol modification of Shh (Kelley et al. 1996). In addition, in mouse homozygous-null mutants of megalin, a protein involved in cholesterol transport, HPE-like features are also observed (Willnow et al. 1996). Lack of cholesterol modification might result in perturbed concentration gradients of Shh in crucial tissues. It has therefore been previously suggested that the level of maternal cholesterol early in gestation might be one of the factors that contribute to the variable phenotype associated with human HPE caused by *SHH* mutations (Ming et al. 1998).

9.5 PATHOPHYSIOLOGICAL PROCESSES ASSOCIATED WITH MALFUNCTION OF CHOLESTEROL TRANSPORT

As the placenta is responsible for nutrient and waste exchange between mother and fetus, placental transport and metabolism of lipids are critical events for fetal development and survival. Biochemical abnormalities in lipid metabolism may account for the disrupted transport across the syncytiotrophoblast in preeclampsia. Indeed, previous studies have found impaired transport systems across the placenta in pathological pregnancies (Myatt 2010; Krishna and Bhalerao 2011). Accordingly, as already described above, functional loss of ABCA1 in ABCA1 null mice results in dramatic effects on the development of the placenta and the embryo (Christiansen-Weber et al. 2000).

Recent studies have demonstrated differential ABCA1 mRNA and protein expression in placentas obtained from patients with preeclampsia, where ABCA1 was specifically down-regulated in syncytiotrophoblasts and fetal endothelial cells, i.e., particularly at the sites of maternal–fetal cholesterol exchange, compared with in control placentas (Körner et al. 2012).

There are only minimal data on ABCG1 expression levels in gestational disease. Recently, there have been reported reduced ABCG1 levels in the villous syncytiotrophoblast of placentas from preeclamptic pregnancies compared with placentas from normotensive controls, as revealed by immunohistochemical staining (Körner et al. 2012).

Cholesterol can modulate the physical state of the phospholipid bilayer by decreasing fatty acyl chain mobility and thereby lowering membrane fluidity (Sen et al. 1998). Previous studies have found that there is an increased cholesterol content found in preeclamptic placental tissue that is reflective of an increase in cholesterol in the syncytiotrophoblast basal cell membrane (Huang et al. 2013). It was proposed that this increased cholesterol content may affect membrane fluidity and compromise transport across the placenta. A potential increase in the cholesterol content of the syncytiotrophoblast basal cell membrane can be masked when whole placental tissue is examined and may be one reason why some groups do not observe a significant increase in cholesterol in preeclamptic versus control placentas. As already described, cholesterol and phospholipid efflux from various tissues is mediated via ABC transporters, in particular ABCA1 and ABCG1, which are highly expressed in the placenta. Given that recent studies demonstrate reduced ABCA1 and ABCG1 expression in the syncytiotrophoblast of preeclamptic placental tissue as compared with controls (Körner et al. 2012), the increased phospholipid (and cholesterol) content found in preeclamptic samples (Huang et al. 2013) may be attributed to impaired ABCA1/G1 transporter function, resulting in compromised cholesterol and phospholipid efflux from the placenta.

Reduced trophoblast invasion, resulting in deficient conversion of the uterine spiral arteries, is widely accepted as a key feature in the pathophysiology of both preeclampsia and IUGR. Deficient spiral artery conversion is associated with reduced placental perfusion. Another factor that can further contribute to malperfusion of the placenta is the acute atherotic changes that can be associated with already deficient spiral artery conversion. These changes are characterized by the presence of lipid-laden mononuclear cells that form intimal plaques (Brosens 1964; Sheppard and Bonnar 1976). The plaques project into the vessel lumen and thus may restrict uteroplacental blood flow depending on their size. Reduced ABC transporter expression levels found in preeclampsia can contribute to the increased accumulation of cholesterol and phospholipids in the placenta, which could be a source of the acute atherotic lesions evident in the maternal spiral arteries in preeclampsia and IUGR.

As already discussed above, there is also a link between Ca^{2+} signaling and cholesterol transport, which has implications for different physiological and pathological processes during pregnancy. This includes induction of ER stress responses that are an important factor in the pathophysiology of pregnancy disorders, such as IUGR and preeclampsia. In addition, ER stress can also have an effect back on cholesterol transport by affecting ABC transporter expression and function. Under ER stress, there is inhibition of nonessential protein synthesis through phosphorylation of the translation initiation factor eIF2α (Jain et al. 2012). As membrane proteins are synthesized in the ER, the expression levels of membrane transport proteins, including the ABC transporters, may also be affected (down-regulated) under ER stress. This is supported by a recent study that found that ABCG2 expression and function are compromised under inflammation-driven ER dysfunction in inflammatory bowel disease (Deuring et al. 2012). The effects of ER stress on membrane transporters in the placental trophoblast remains to be further explored.

In summary, evidence that aberrant cholesterol transport is associated with pregnancy disorders, including IUGR and preeclampsia, highlights the importance of cholesterol transporters in the placenta/placental trophoblast during pregnancy. Further studies on the precise mechanism of action of these transporters and dysfunction in gestational disease will shed more light on their precise contribution to a successful pregnancy.

9.6 AVENUES OF FURTHER RESEARCH

9.6.1 METHODS TO STUDY TRANSPLACENTAL CHOLESTEROL TRANSPORT

The predominant expression of ABCG1 in the placenta has been found to be in the basolateral membrane, which suggests that the transporter transfers its substrates primarily to the fetus via the placental endothelium, via interaction with a donor (HDL). On the other hand, ABCA1 immunostaining data indicate expression in the microvillous/apical membrane, implying that this transporter effluxes cholesterol in the maternal direction (Aye et al. 2010). However, various studies indicate that ABCA1 is likely to be involved in transporting cholesterol to both the fetal and maternal circulations. To conclusively demonstrate the role of ABCA1- or ABCG1-dependent cholesterol efflux in either the maternal or fetal direction, there now exist in vitro/ex vivo techniques that would allow for a detailed investigation into the directionality of ABCA1- and ABCG1-mediated cholesterol efflux.

9.6.2 DUAL PLACENTAL PERFUSION TECHNIQUE

The ex vivo dual placental perfusion of an isolated human placental cotyledon is a powerful technique to study transport systems during pregnancy. This technique allows retention of a high level of structural organization of placental tissue and therefore more closely mimics the in vivo state (Dancis 1985).

The method of perfusion is generally performed as previously described by Schneider et al. (1972). In brief, the technique involves cannulating a branch of both the umbilical artery and vein of an isolated cotyledon of the human placenta. This comprises the fetal circulation. On the maternal side of the placenta, the intervillous space is perfused by cannulae piercing the basal plate. The perfusion media is supplemented with glucose and the entire system is gassed with normoxia appropriate conditions (Figure 9.6). In general, the system allows simulation of physiological conditions at term pregnancy and, of course, study of the transport of any selected substrate (including cholesterol) across a "live" human placenta.

In addition, a recent study by Jain et al. (2014) has demonstrated that hypoxic treatment of the dual placental perfusion system stimulates a preeclampsia-like inflammatory response in the perfused placental cotyledon. This technique therefore provides a valuable tool to study cholesterol transport, as well as the directionality of ABCA1- and ABCG1-mediated cholesterol efflux under both physiological and pathological conditions.

9.6.3 TRANSWELL® SYSTEM USING PRIMARY TROPHOBLAST CELLS

A study of the directionality of the ABC transporters using the placenta perfusion technique will require the use of specific inhibitors of ABCA1 or ABCG1, and unfortunately, no such inhibitors are currently available. Glyburide, which has been used in previous studies, is a nonselective ABC inhibitor (Payen et al. 2001), and there are no known ABCG1 antagonists. To resolve this issue, some groups have employed Transwell assays using the placental cell line BeWo to examine transcellular transport of nutrients and drugs (Bode et al. 2006). However, ABCA1 and ABCG1 are expressed at much lower levels in BeWo cells compared with primary trophoblasts (Aye et al.,

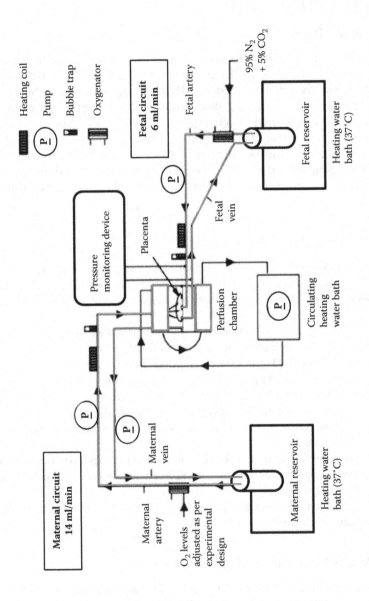

FIGURE 9.6   Dual placental perfusion model. Schematic representation of the placental perfusion model, showing maternal- and fetal-side perfusions. The perfused cotyledon is connected by artery–vein pairs of tubing (on both the maternal and fetal sides) to the respective reservoirs. The gas concentration is set for each circuit. On the maternal side, previous groups have either used "air" or achieved an oxygen tension in the intervillous space of 5%–7% for normoxia and <3% for hypoxia. The fetal side is gassed with 95% N_2 and 5% CO_2.

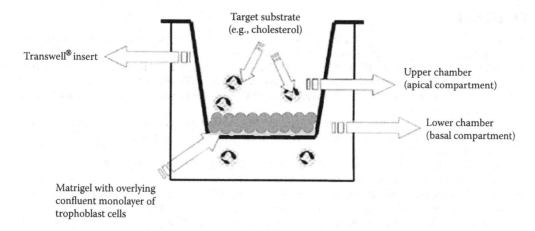

FIGURE 9.7 Transwell® model using primary trophoblast cells. Freshly isolated primary trophoblast cells are loaded on Matrigel-coated Transwell inserts. Transepithelial electrical resistance is continuously monitored to assess and confirm confluency of the monolayer. Using this model allows studies on the directional transport of diverse compounds (e.g., cholesterol, amino acids, glucose) between the apical and basal compartment.

unpublished observations), and the relevance of these cells to in vivo placental transport has been questioned (Evseenko et al. 2006; Aye et al. 2010).

Our research team has recently developed a confluent monolayer in vitro model using primary trophoblast cells from human term placenta, which morphologically and functionally highly resembles the microvilli structure found in vivo. Highly purified cytotrophoblast cells were isolated and selectively cultured on Matrigel-coated Transwell® inserts to exhibit a distinctive apical–basal (maternal–fetal) axis of polarity (Figure 9.7). The cell morphology, transepithelial electrical resistance, and permeability properties of specific markers were monitored and revealed the formation of a trophoblast monolayer in culture. The syncytialization progress was characterized by a gradually increased level of fusogen gene expression assessed by quantitative real time polymerase chain reaction. The formation of a tightly packed monolayer studded by microvilli was further confirmed using confocal and electron microscopy. In pilot studies, this model has already been successfully used to study the bidirectional transport of glucose. The newly devised strategy provides a novel innovative tool to investigate the trans-trophoblast barrier function in physiological and pathophysiological conditions. In this context, cholesterol (as well as other) transporter function can be studied in an ex vivo setting of the placenta. Once a confluent monolayer is obtained, the apical side of the monolayer can be radiolabeled with free cholesterol (Figure 9.7) and the cellular cholesterol efflux induced with cholesterol acceptors added to the basolateral chamber. ABCA1-dependent cholesterol efflux can be determined by addition of lipid-poor apoA1 as a cholesterol acceptor. Applying the cholesterol and cholesterol acceptors on the reverse sides, respectively, would allow an assessment of the directionality of selected ABC transporter activity.

In all, such tools will help to further increase our understanding of the precise mechanism of actions and functions of cholesterol transporters in the placental trophoblast, such that we may eventually be able to define the ABCs of transplacental cholesterol transport.

ACKNOWLEDGMENTS

C.A. was supported by grants from the Swiss National Science Foundation (310030_149958) and the Swiss National Center of Competence in Research, NCCR TransCure. We thank Xiao Huang and Sampada Kallol for help with the figures.

REFERENCES

Albrecht, C. and E. Viturro (2007). "The ABCA subfamily—Gene and protein structures, functions and associated hereditary diseases." *Pflugers Arch* 453 (5): 581–589.

Albrecht, C., S. Soumian et al. (2007). "Placental ABCA1 expression is reduced in primary antiphospholipid syndrome compared to pre-eclampsia and controls." *Placenta* 28 (7): 701–708.

Albrecht, C., L. Nikitina et al. (2010). "Localization of ABCA1 in first trimester and term placental tissues." *Placenta* 31 (8): 741–742.

Aye, I. L. M. H., B. J. Waddell et al. (2010). "Placental ABCA1 and ABCG1 transporters efflux cholesterol and protect trophoblasts from oxysterol induced toxicity." *Biochim Biophys Acta-Mol Cell Biol Lipids* 1801 (9): 1013–1024.

Baardman, M. E., W. S. Kerstjens-Frederikse et al. (2013). "The role of maternal-fetal cholesterol transport in early fetal life: Current insights." *Biol Reprod* 88 (1): 24.

Baumann, M., M. Korner et al. (2013). "Placental ABCA1 and ABCG1 expression in gestational disease: Preeclampsia affects ABCA1 levels in syncytiotrophoblasts." *Placenta* 34 (11): 1079–1086.

Benirschke, K., P. Kaufmann, and R. N. Baergen. (2006). *Pathology of the Human Placenta*. New York, Springer Verlag.

Bhattacharjee, J., F. Ietta et al. (2010). "Expression and localization of ATP binding cassette transporter A1 (ABCA1) in first trimester and term human placenta." *Placenta* 31 (5): 423–430.

Bode, C. J., H. Jin et al. (2006). "In vitro models for studying trophoblast transcellular transport." *Methods Mol Med* 122: 225–239.

Bodzioch, M., E. Orso et al. (1999). "The gene encoding ATP-binding cassette transporter 1 is mutated in Tangier disease." *Nat Genet* 22 (4): 347–351.

Bowen, J. M., L. Chamley et al. (2002). "Cytokines of the placenta and extra-placental membranes: Biosynthesis, secretion and roles in establishment of pregnancy in women." *Placenta* 23 (4): 239–256.

Bromberg, J. F., M. H. Wrzeszczynska et al. (1999). "Stat3 as an oncogene." *Cell* 98 (3): 295–303.

Brooks-Wilson, A., M. Marcil et al. (1999). "Mutations in ABC1 in Tangier disease and familial high-density lipoprotein deficiency." *Nat Genet* 22 (4): 336–345.

Brosens, I. (1964). "A study of the spiral arteries of the decidua basalis in normotensive and hypertensive pregnancies." *J Obstet Gynaecol Br Commonw* 71: 222–230.

Brown, A. J. and W. Jessup (1999). "Oxysterols and atherosclerosis." *Atherosclerosis* 142 (1): 1–28.

Burton, G. J., A. W. Woods et al. (2009). "Rheological and physiological consequences of conversion of the maternal spiral arteries for uteroplacental blood flow during human pregnancy." *Placenta* 30 (6): 473–482.

Burton, G. J. and H. W. Yung (2011). "Endoplasmic reticulum stress in the pathogenesis of early-onset preeclampsia." *Pregnancy Hypertens* 1 (1–2): 72–78.

Christiansen-Weber, T. A., J. R. Voland et al. (2000). "Functional loss of ABCA1 in mice causes severe placental malformation, aberrant lipid distribution, and kidney glomerulonephritis as well as high-density lipoprotein cholesterol deficiency." *Am J Pathol* 157 (3): 1017–1029.

Conley, A. J. and J. I. Mason (1990). "Placental steroid hormones." *Baillieres Clin Endocrinol Metab* 4 (2): 249–272.

Dancis, J. (1985). "Why perfuse the human placenta." *Contrib Gynecol Obstet* 13: 1–4.

Deuring, J. J., C. de Haar et al. (2012). "Absence of ABCG2-mediated mucosal detoxification in patients with active inflammatory bowel disease is due to impeded protein folding." *Biochem J* 441 (1): 87–93.

Enrich, C., C. Rentero et al. (2011). "Annexin A6-Linking Ca(2+) signaling with cholesterol transport." *Biochim Biophys Acta* 1813 (5): 935–947.

Evseenko, D. A., J. W. Paxton et al. (2006). "ABC drug transporter expression and functional activity in trophoblast-like cell lines and differentiating primary trophoblast." *Am J Physiol Regul Integr Comp Physiol* 290 (5): R1357–R1365.

Fang, L., S. H. Choi et al. (2013). "Control of angiogenesis by AIBP-mediated cholesterol efflux." *Nature* 498 (7452): 118–122.

Gelissen, I. C., M. Harris et al. (2006). "ABCA1 and ABCG1 synergize to mediate cholesterol export to apoA-I." *Arterioscler Thromb Vasc Biol* 26 (3): 534–540.

Hammerschmidt, M., A. Brook et al. (1997). "The world according to hedgehog." *Trends Genet* 13 (1): 14–21.

Huang, X., A. Jain et al. (2013). "Increased placental phospholipid levels in pre-eclamptic pregnancies." *Int J Mol Sci* 14 (2): 3487–3499.

Jain, A., M. Olovsson et al. (2012). "Endothelin-1 induces endoplasmic reticulum stress by activating the PLC-IP(3) pathway: Implications for placental pathophysiology in preeclampsia." *Am J Pathol* 180 (6): 2309–2320.

Jain, A., H. Schneider et al. (2014). "Hypoxic treatment of human dual placental perfusion induces a preeclampsia-like inflammatory response." *Lab Invest* 94 (8): 873–880.

Kelley, R. L., E. Roessler et al. (1996). "Holoprosencephaly in RSH/Smith–Lemli–Opitz syndrome: Does abnormal cholesterol metabolism affect the function of Sonic Hedgehog?" *Am J Med Genet* 66 (4): 478–484.

Knofler, M. (2010). "Critical growth factors and signalling pathways controlling human trophoblast invasion." *Int J Dev Biol* 54 (2–3): 269–280.

Körner, M., F. Wenger et al. (2012). "PP141. The lipid transporters ABCA1 and ABCG1 are differentially expressed in preeclamptic and IUGR placentas." *Pregnancy Hypertens* 2 (3): 315–316.

Krishna, U. and S. Bhalerao (2011). "Placental insufficiency and fetal growth restriction." *J Obstet Gynaecol India* 61 (5): 505–511.

Langmann, T., R. Mauerer et al. (2003). "Real-time reverse transcription-PCR expression profiling of the complete human ATP-binding cassette transporter superfamily in various tissues." *Clin Chem* 49 (2): 230–238.

Lee, J. Y. and J. S. Parks (2005). "ATP-binding cassette transporter AI and its role in HDL formation." *Curr Opin Lipidol* 16 (1): 19–25.

Lindegaard, M. L., C. A. Wassif et al. (2008). "Characterization of placental cholesterol transport: ABCA1 is a potential target for in utero therapy of Smith–Lemli–Opitz syndrome." *Hum Mol Genet* 17 (23): 3806–3813.

Lyall, F. (2005). "Priming and remodelling of human placental bed spiral arteries during pregnancy—A review." *Placenta* 26 Suppl A: S31–S36.

Marcil, M., R. Bissonnette et al. (2003). "Cellular phospholipid and cholesterol efflux in high-density lipoprotein deficiency." *Circulation* 107 (10): 1366–1371.

McNeish, J., R. J. Aiello et al. (2000). "High density lipoprotein deficiency and foam cell accumulation in mice with targeted disruption of ATP-binding cassette transporter-1." *Proc Natl Acad Sci U S A* 97 (8): 4245–4250.

Ming, J. E., E. Roessler et al. (1998). "Human developmental disorders and the Sonic hedgehog pathway." *Mol Med Today* 4 (8): 343–349.

Moffett-King, A. (2002). "Natural killer cells and pregnancy." *Nat Rev Immunol* 2 (9): 656–663.

Myatt, L. (2010). "Review: Reactive oxygen and nitrogen species and functional adaptation of the placenta." *Placenta* 31 Suppl: S66–S69.

Neufeld, E. B., A. T. Remaley et al. (2001). "Cellular localization and trafficking of the human ABCA1 transporter." *J Biol Chem* 276 (29): 27584–27590.

Nikitina, L., F. Wenger et al. (2011). "Expression and localization pattern of ABCA1 in diverse human placental primary cells and tissues." *Placenta* 32 (6): 420–30.

Parker, C. R., Jr., T. Deahl et al. (1983). "Analysis of the potential for transfer of lipoprotein-cholesterol across the human placenta." *Early Hum Dev* 8 (3–4): 289–295.

Payen, L., L. Delugin et al. (2001). "The sulphonylurea glibenclamide inhibits multidrug resistance protein (MRP1) activity in human lung cancer cells." *Br J Pharmacol* 132 (3): 778–784.

Pijnenborg, R., L. Vercruysse et al. (2006). "The uterine spiral arteries in human pregnancy: Facts and controversies." *Placenta* 27 (9–10): 939–958.

Pike, L. J. (2004). "Lipid rafts: Heterogeneity on the high seas." *Biochem J* 378 (Pt 2): 281–292.

Plosch, T., A. Gellhaus et al. (2010). "The liver X receptor (LXR) and its target gene ABCA1 are regulated upon low oxygen in human trophoblast cells: A reason for alterations in preeclampsia?" *Placenta* 31 (10): 910–918.

Porter, J. A., K. E. Young et al. (1996). "Cholesterol modification of hedgehog signaling proteins in animal development." *Science* 274 (5285): 255–259.

Red-Horse, K., Y. Zhou et al. (2004). "Trophoblast differentiation during embryo implantation and formation of the maternal–fetal interface." *J Clin Invest* 114 (6): 744–754.

Redman, C. W. and I. L. Sargent (2004). "Preeclampsia and the systemic inflammatory response." *Semin Nephrol* 24 (6): 565–570.

Redman, C. W., G. P. Sacks et al. (1999). "Preeclampsia: An excessive maternal inflammatory response to pregnancy." *Am J Obstet Gynecol* 180 (2 Pt 1): 499–506.

Roessler, E. and M. Muenke (1998). "Holoprosencephaly: A paradigm for the complex genetics of brain development." *J Inherit Metab Dis* 21 (5): 481–497.

Rust, S., M. Rosier et al. (1999). "Tangier disease is caused by mutations in the gene encoding ATP-binding cassette transporter 1." *Nat Genet* 22 (4): 352–355.

Schneider, H. (1991). "The role of the placenta in nutrition of the human fetus." *Am J Obstet Gynecol* 164 (4): 967–973.

Schneider, H., M. Panigel et al. (1972). "Transfer across the perfused human placenta of antipyrine, sodium and leucine." *Am J Obstet Gynecol* 114 (6): 822–828.

Sen, A., P. K. Ghosh et al. (1998). "Changes in lipid composition and fluidity of human placental basal membrane and modulation of bilayer protein functions with progress of gestation." *Mol Cell Biochem* 187 (1–2): 183–190.

Shamshirsaz, A. A., M. Paidas et al. (2012). "Preeclampsia, hypoxia, thrombosis, and inflammation." *J Pregnancy* 2012: 374047.

Sheppard, B. L. and J. Bonnar (1976). "The ultrastructure of the arterial supply of the human placenta in pregnancy complicated by fetal growth retardation." *Br J Obstet Gynaecol* 83 (12): 948–959.

Stefulj, J., U. Panzenboeck et al. (2009). "Human endothelial cells of the placental barrier efficiently deliver cholesterol to the fetal circulation via ABCA1 and ABCG1." *Circ Res* 104 (5): 600–608.

Tang, C., Y. Liu et al. (2009). "The macrophage cholesterol exporter ABCA1 functions as an anti-inflammatory receptor." *J Biol Chem* 284 (47): 32336–32343.

Terasaka, N., S. Yu et al. (2008). "ABCG1 and HDL protect against endothelial dysfunction in mice fed a high-cholesterol diet." *J Clin Invest* 118 (11): 3701–3713.

Vaughan, A. M. and J. F. Oram (2006). "ABCA1 and ABCG1 or ABCG4 act sequentially to remove cellular cholesterol and generate cholesterol-rich HDL." *J Lipid Res* 47 (11): 2433–2443.

Whetzel, A. M., J. M. Sturek et al. (2010). "ABCG1 deficiency in mice promotes endothelial activation and monocyte–endothelial interactions." *Arterioscler Thromb Vasc Biol* 30 (4): 809–817.

Williams, L. M., U. Sarma et al. (2007). "Expression of constitutively active STAT3 can replicate the cytokine-suppressive activity of interleukin-10 in human primary macrophages." *J Biol Chem* 282 (10): 6965–6975.

Willnow, T. E., J. Hilpert et al. (1996). "Defective forebrain development in mice lacking gp330/megalin." *Proc Natl Acad Sci U S A* 93 (16): 8460–8464.

Zhang, K. and R. J. Kaufman (2008). "From endoplasmic-reticulum stress to the inflammatory response." *Nature* 454 (7203): 455–462.

10 Maternal Fatty Acids and Their Effects on Placentation

Sanjay Basak and Asim K. Duttaroy

CONTENTS

ABSTRACT

During intrauterine life, the human placenta plays a functional role in transferring long-chain fatty acids (LCFAs) selectively from the maternal circulation to the fetus. Although the indispensible requirements of LCFAs for brain and retina development is well established, only recent have data highlighted their importance in early fetoplacental development. Recent data indicate the importance of LCFA in the process of early placentation. Angiogenesis is a critical step involving several other cellular processes in placentation. This chapter will highlight hitherto the unknown role of LCFAs on the growth and development of the placenta.

KEY WORDS

Angiogenic growth factors, docosahexaenoic acid (DHA), vascular endothelium growth factors, first trimester pregnancy, n-3 fatty acids, angiopoietin 4, fatty acid binding protein 4, placentation, maternal fatty acids.

10.1 INTRODUCTION

The angiogenic process is a highly complex, dynamic process regulated at every stage by several proangiogenic and antiangiogenic molecules. Several growth factors such as vascular endothelial growth factor (VEGF), angiopoietin-like 4 (ANGPTL4), platelet-derived growth factor (PDGF), fibroblast growth factor (FGF), and placental growth factor are involved in angiogenesis (Folkman and Klagsbrun 1987; Aiello and Wong 2000; Gealekman et al. 2008). These factors are responsible for promoting and sustaining angiogenesis. VEGF causes dilation of blood vessels and endothelial cell proliferation/migration. PDGF recruits smooth muscle cells to stabilize new vessels, whereas FGF promotes endothelial cell proliferation and the physical organization of endothelial cells into tube-like structures. Matrix metalloproteinase (MMP) causes breakdown of the basement membrane, and angiopoietin mediates vascular remodeling and maintains vascular integrity (Morisada et al. 2006). In general, n-3 fatty acids have anti-inflammatory and anticancer effects, whereas n-6 fatty acids promote inflammation and carcinogenesis (Dutta-Roy 2000; Sterescu et al. 2006; Sapieha et al. 2011). N-3 long-chain polyunsaturated fatty acids (LCPUFAs), such as eicosapentaenoic acid, 20:5n-3 (EPA), and docosahexaenoic acid, 22:6n-3 (DHA), inhibit angiogenesis, whereas n-6 LCPUFA, such as arachidonic acid, 20:4n-6 (AA), promotes angiogenesis (Belury 2002; Sterescu et al. 2006; Spencer et al. 2009; Chen 2010; Sapieha et al. 2011). These fatty acids influence angiogenesis via several mechanisms, such as the expression of angiogenic factors, VEGF, ANGPTL4, and other modulators such as eicosanoids, cyclooxygenase (COX), fatty acid-binding proteins (FABPs), and nitric oxide (NO) (Spencer et al. 2009).

Since supplementation of n-3 fatty acids is recommended in pregnancy for optimal fetoplacental growth and development (Innis 1991; Uauy et al. 2001), it is therefore important to investigate the effects of these fatty acids in placental angiogenesis. With the recent spate of clinical work on regulators of angiogenesis, these observations lead us to believe that regulation of placental angiogenesis could become a novel and powerful method for ensuring positive outcomes for most pregnancies. This chapter deals with effects of fatty acids on placental angiogenesis.

10.2 ESSENTIAL FATTY ACIDS AND THEIR METABOLITES

Essential fatty acids (EFAs) belong to the n-6 (omega-6) and n-3 (omega-3) families, starting with the precursors linoleic acid, 18:2n-6 (LA), and alpha-linolenic acid, 18:3n-3 (ALA). The n-6 series of EFAs contain two or more double bonds, with the first double bond on the sixth carbon from the methyl end of the molecule; the n-3 EFAs contain three or more double bonds, with the first double bond on the third carbon atom from the methyl end. N-3 and n-6 fatty acids play crucial biological roles that include altering the properties of cell membranes, providing substrates for the production of signaling molecules or functioning mediators, and modulating gene expression (Smith 1989; Innis 1991; Dutta-Roy 1994). The primary n-6 fatty acid is LA, which can be converted to AA. The three main n-3 fatty acids are ALA, DHA, and EPA. Through the same desaturase and elongase enzymes, ALA can be converted into EPA and DHA. The enzymes responsible for the metabolism of both n-6 and n-3 fatty acids are COX, lipooxygenase (LOX), and cytochrome P450 (CYP 450). Several eicosanoids derived from the n-6 fatty acids promote tumor angiogenesis, such as prostaglandins (PGH_2, PGE_2, PGI_2), leukotrienes (4-series LTs), thromboxanes (TXA_2), and hydroxyeicosatraenoic acids (12-HETE, 15-HETE) (Smith 1989; Nie et al. 2000; Hoagland et al. 2001; Pai et al. 2001; Bagga et al. 2003; Pola et al. 2004; Kamiyama et al. 2006; Jin et al. 2009). These eicosanoids make the tumor microenvironment more favorable for neoplasms and metastasis by encouraging the transcription of angiogenic growth factors, increasing the rate of endothelial cell migration and proliferation, and increasing the rate of vascularization. In contrast, n-3 fatty acid metabolism produces leukotrienes and prostaglandins that attenuate excess vascularization. N-3 and n-6 fatty acids compete with each other for incorporation into the cell membrane in addition to enzymes for eicosanoid production, including COX-2 and 5-LOX. Thus, high levels of tissue n-3 fatty acids can reduce angiogenesis through decreased production of proangiogenic AA-derived eicosanoids, membrane receptor–ligand interactions, and n-3 fatty acid's intrinsic antitumor properties (Nie et al. 2000; Pai et al. 2001; Bagga et al. 2003; Pola et al. 2004; Kamiyama et al. 2006; Yuan et al. 2009). Furthermore, n-3 fatty acids have been found to down-regulate the expression of angiogenic growth factors such as VEGF, PDGF, interleukin (IL)-6, and MMP-2 (Kang and Weylandt 2008; Spencer et al. 2009). N-3 fatty acids are found only in marine fish and certain vegetables and nuts, whereas corn and soybean oils, processed foods, and grain-fed meat contain high levels of n-6 fatty acids. Now, the ratio of n-6/-3 fatty acids is approximately 15:1 or higher; our bodies may not be accustomed to utilizing such high levels of n-6 fatty acids. This is considered to be one of many factors responsible for the relatively recent rise in chronic diseases, predominantly those associated with inflammation, including cancer, heart disease, arthritis, and diabetes (Simopoulos 2002). The maternal, fetal, and neonatal EFA/LCPUFA status is an important determinant of health and disease in infancy and later life (Innis 1991; Uauy et al. 2001). In fact, fetal brain and retina are very rich in AA and DHA (Innis 2007). Numerous studies have demonstrated a positive effect of supplementation with DHA in pregnant women in terms of less premature birth and in the child; complex brain performance, like visual acuity, attention spans, and intelligence; and mother's overall health. In addition, DHA may reduce the incidence of preeclampisia and postapartum depression by stimulating placental angiogenesis.

10.3 FETOPLACENTAL GROWTH AND DEVELOPMENT: ROLE OF ANGIOGENESIS

Most research on the developmental origins of health and disease has implicated poor nutrition in the fetus, most often conferred by deficiencies in maternal nutrition, as an important causal factor that programs offspring physiology susceptible to adult disease (Ganu et al. 2012). However, it is underappreciated that the placenta, particularly trophoblast invasion, is the key to the health of both the mother and child in both the short- and long-term. Inappropriate angiogenesis may lead to several pregnancy-related disorders, including preeclampsia, preterm birth, and gestational diabetes, as well as intrauterine growth restriction (IUGR). Although gene polymorphism is important and is responsible for placental invasion, dietary and environmental factors may also contribute to inadequate placental angiogenesis (Abajo et al. 2012). Angiogenesis is critical for successful fetal outcome as the placental blood flow is dependent on placental vascularization (Carmeliet and Jain 2011). Lack of placental vascular development may contribute to inadequate cytotrophoblast invasion, as evident in preeclampsia (Chaiworapongsa et al. 2011). There are similarities between the invasiveness of tumor cells and placental first-trimester trophoblast cells during embryo implantation, placentation, as well as vascularization (Torry and Rongish 1992; Murray and Lessey 1999). Abnormal spiral arterial remodeling due to insufficient angiogenesis is a key pathological feature observed in preeclampsia and in IUGR. Studies have shown that preeclampsia features a shift in angiogenesis and antiangiogenic factors toward an insufficient placental blood circulation (Torry et al. 1998).

10.4 MODULATION OF ANGIOGENESIS BY LONG-CHAIN FATTY ACIDS

Both n-3 and n-6 fatty acids are involved directly or indirectly in angiogenesis (Hardman 2004; Spencer et al. 2009; Salvado et al. 2012). Eicosanoids produced from AA stimulate angiogenesis, whereas those produced from EPA and DHA inhibit angiogenesis and tumorigenesis (Hardman 2004; Spencer et al. 2009; Salvado et al. 2012). In marked contrast to the effects observed with n-3 LCPUFAs, n-6 LCPUFAs have stimulatory or neutral effects on angiogenic processes such as tube formation, cell migration, or cell proliferation (Hardman 2004; Szymczak, Murray, and Petrovic 2008). The expression of enzymes involved in the biosynthesis of eicosanoids, notably COX-2, 5-LOX (lipoxygenase), and 12-LOX, is up-regulated during tumor initiation and progression. COX-2 contributes to neovascularization, which is essential for tumor development. Overexpression of COX-2 in colon carcinoma cells increases their angiogenicity, as shown by an increased ability to stimulate endothelial cell migration and tube formation by producing prostaglandins and inducing proangiogenic factors such as VEGF and basic FGF (bFGF). In addition, inflammatory cells infiltrating the tumor tissue (e.g., macrophages and neutrophils) may release proinflammatory cytokines such as IL-1β or tumor necrosis-α (TNF-α) that can induce angiogenesis, an effect partially attributable to increased COX-2 expression in tumor, stromal, and vascular endothelial cells. The antiangiogenic activity of n-3 LCPUFAs is mediated usually via inhibition of production of AA-derived eicosanoids. LCPUFAs and their derivatives are reported to modulate several angiogenic factors such as VEGF, ANGPTL4, PDGF, leptin, and TNF-α (Spencer et al. 2009; Salvado et al. 2012). Numerous studies have demonstrated that VEGF or its receptors are up-regulated in many tumors (Takahashi 2011). N-3 fatty acids affect the expression of proangiogenic factors (Massaro et al. 2010; Scoditti et al. 2010). EPA and DHA significantly suppress endothelial cell proliferation, migration, and tubule formation (Kanayasu et al. 1991; Yang, Morita, and Murota 1998; Murota, Onodera, and Morita 2000; Kim et al. 2005; Spencer et al. 2009). Down-regulation of VEGF receptors by EPA is mediated via suppression of nuclear factor-κB activation (Ghosh-Choudhury et al. 2009). In addition, EPA down-regulates the expression of Flk-1 receptors in a dose-dependent manner and up-regulates the expression of Flt-1 receptors (Yang, Morita, and Murota 1998). The tube formation induced by VEGF was suppressed by n-3 LCPUFAs via down-regulation of VEGF receptor in the endothelial cells (Tsuji, Murota, and Morita 2003; Calviello et al. 2004; Szymczak, Murray, and Petrovic 2008; Spencer et al. 2009). EPA and DHA have shown to have potent antiangiogenic effects in cancer cells by inhibiting the production of many important angiogenic mediators such as VEGF, PDGF, COX-2, PGE$_2$, and NO. 4-Hydroxy-DHA, a 5-lipoxygenase product of DHA, was reported to inhibit endothelial cell proliferation and sprouting angiogenesis via peroxisome proliferator-activated receptor-γ (PPARγ) (Sapieha et al. 2011). In addition, both EPA and DHA decrease the levels of O$_2^-$ and thereby reduce reactive oxygen species-mediated angiogenesis (Maraldi et al. 2010; Matesanz et al. 2010). N-3 LCPUFAs can increase NO production by displacing endothelial nitric oxide synthase (eNOS) from the caveolar fraction (Li et al. 2007). Increased NO levels by these fatty acids may decrease VEGFR signal-mediated angiogenesis (Matesanz et al. 2010). Indeed, a high ratio of O$_2^-$/NO is implicated as a contributory factor in disturbed angiogenesis in diabetes (Matesanz et al. 2010; Hamed et al. 2011). All these reports summarized that n-6 fatty acids increase whereas n-3 fatty acids decrease angiogenesis. Since tumor progression and metastasis depend on angiogenesis, reducing the tissue n-6/n-3 fatty acids may be beneficial in cancers.

10.5 FABPs AND THEIR ROLES IN ANGIOGENESIS

FABPs, ubiquitously expressed in tissues, including the placenta, may play a role in intracellular fatty acid transport and metabolism (Campbell et al. 1998; Duttaroy 2009). The transport properties of FABPs are governed, in part, by specific protein–protein and protein–membrane interactions, and the helix–turn–helix domain of FABPs is critical, although likely not exclusive, in specifying these interactions (Storch and Thumser 2010). Several FABPs have been shown to deliver their ligands to nuclear transcription factors, thus modulating gene expression in a tissue-specific manner. FABPs may be envisioned as central regulators of lipid disposition at the cell and tissue levels that have a profound impact on any processes involving fatty acid-induced angiogenesis. Recent data have suggested that certain FABPs have a role in angiogenesis. In fact, FABP expression is widely regulated by various proangiogenic mediators (Mousiolis et al. 2012). Among FABPs, FABP-4, originally identified as an adipocyte-specific protein, promotes proliferation of endothelial cells. FABP-4 mRNA and protein levels were significantly induced in cultured endothelial cells by VEGF and bFGF treatment. The effect of VEGF-A on FABP-4 expression was inhibited by siRNA-mediated knockdown of VEGFR2, whereas the VEGFR1 agonists, placental growth factor (PlGF)1 and 2, had no such effect. Thus, FABP-4 emerged as a novel target of the VEGF/VEGFR2 pathway and a positive regulator of cell proliferation and angiogenesis in endothelial cells (Elmasri et al. 2009, 2012; Cataltepe et al. 2012; Ghelfi et al. 2013). FABP-4 was expressed in an angiogenesis-dependent pathology, infantile hemangioma, being the most common tumor of infancy and endothelial cells (Fishman and Mulliken 1993). FABP-4 has a role in the activation of several mitogenic pathways and expression of several key mediators of angiogenesis (Elmasri et al. 2012). The expression of FABPs was regulated by fatty acids and leptin in first-trimester trophoblastic cells, HTR8/SVneo. c9,t11-CLA, an isomer of conjugated LA (CLA), specifically increased FABP-4 expression by 10-fold compared with t10,c12-CLA. The c9,t11-CLA-induced FABP-4 expression was associated with tube formation and increased amount of ANGPTL4 secretion (Basak and Duttaroy 2013a). Leptin, a potent angiogenic growth factor, stimulates mRNA expression of FABP-4 along with several proangiogenic factors in first-trimester placental cells (Basak and Duttaroy 2012). FABP-3 and its expression correlate with inhibition of α1-integrin activity, cell adhesion, and invasion in breast cancer cells (Kusakari et al. 2006; Nevo et al. 2010). Further, expression of FABP-5 has been shown to modulate MMP-9 production and regulates invasive property of oral cancer cells (Fang et al. 2010). Despite similar ligand binding characteristics and highly homologous tertiary structures, each FABP appears to have unique functions in specific tissues (Storch and Thumser 2010). Recent data demonstrated that maternal serum FABP-4 is independently associated with the subsequent development of preeclampsia. Elevated maternal serum FABP-4 levels may also play a role in the pathogenesis of preeclampsia through pathways related to insulin resistance, inflammation, and abnormal lipid metabolism. Increasing evidence suggests the angiogenic role of fatty acid transport/binding proteins in different cell systems, including first-trimester placental trophoblast (Basak and Duttaroy 2013a,b; Ghelfi et al. 2013).

10.6 POSSIBLE MECHANISMS FOR FATTY ACID-MEDIATED ANGIOGENESIS IN HUMAN PLACENTAL FIRST-TRIMESTER TROPHOBLAST CELLS

During the third trimester of pregnancy, DHA requirements increase to support fetal growth, particularly of the brain and eyes (Innis 1991). DHA was taken up preferentially compared with other fatty acids by last-trimester placental trophoblasts (see Chapter 6). DHA was also taken up by first-trimester placental trophoblasts (Basak and Duttaroy 2013b). DHA increased tube formation to the greatest extent as compared with other long-chain fatty acids (LCFAs) by increasing capillary tube length and tube numbers of extravillous trophoblast cells, HTR8/SVneo (Figure 10.1). DHA stimulated tube formation via expression of the most potent angiogenic factor, VEGF, in extravillous trophoblast cells (Johnsen et al. 2011). DHA may also help early placentation process by increasing angiogenesis (Johnsen et al. 2011). This is in contrast with the generally observed inhibitory effects of n-3 LCPUFAs on angiogenesis in many cell types, including tumors (Spencer et al. 2009). The mechanism responsible for the increased expression of VEGF in placental trophoblast cells by DHA is not known at present. Expression of VEGF by DHA, however, is very unique as its mRNA is induced by a variety of growth factors and cytokines, including PDGF, EGF, TNF-α, transforming growth factor (TGF)-β1, and IL-1β, but not by any fatty acids. DHA-induced VEGF expression was not accompanied with the expression of COX-2 and HIF1α genes in these cells (Johnsen et al. 2011), indicating that DHA metabolites per se may not be involved in the VEGF expression. Since the PPARγ ligand did not stimulate VEGF expression in these cells, it is

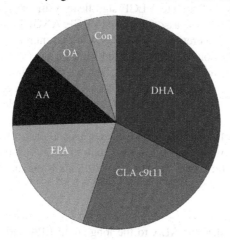

FIGURE 10.1 Comparative effect of fatty acids on capillary tube elongation of the HTR8/SVneo cells. Tube networks were measured by tube length (pixel), and percentage of tube network formation was calculated considering control as 100%.

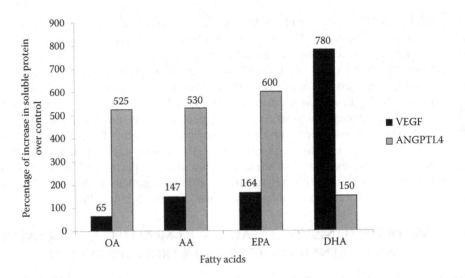

FIGURE 10.2 Effects of fatty acids on the secretion of angiogenic growth factors, VEGF, and ANGPTL4 in first-trimester trophoblast cells, HT8/SVneo. Soluble protein secretion was measured by enzyme linked immunosorbent assay (ELISA) and calculated as the percentage of control. Percentage of increase over control labeled for respective fatty acids is shown.

unlikely that DHA stimulation of VEGF expression involves PPARγ (Gottlicher et al. 1993). DHA may also alter phosphorylation events in native mRNA processing, mRNA transport and stabilization, and mRNA degradation rates (Salem et al. 2001; Uauy et al. 2001). DHA stimulates VEGF expression and secretion, whereas other fatty acids such as EPA, arachidonic acid (AA), and oleic acid (OA) promote ANGPTL4 secretion without affecting VEGF synthesis in placental trophoblast cells (Figure 10.2). These data indicate the different mechanisms of action of DHA compared with other fatty acids in the angiogenic process (Johnsen et al. 2011). The mechanisms that determine the angiogenic capacity of DHA compared with other fatty acids may underlie important differences in the mechanism of actions of these structurally different fatty acids. On the basis of available data, we postulate that free fatty acids such as c9t11-CLA, EPA, DHA, and leptin stimulate the expression of FABP-4, which has been demonstrated as a target protein for VEGF. First-trimester trophoblast cells, HTR8/SVneo, express and secrete VEGF significantly in the presence of fatty acids, and FABP-4 could be a mediator of these associations of VEGF, ANGPTL4, and FABP-4. The mechanism responsible for increased secretion of ANGPTL4 in placental trophoblast cells by fatty acids other than DHA is yet to be resolved. More detailed work is, however, required for understanding the mechanisms involved in fatty acid-stimulated angiogenesis. Future work should explore the roles of ANGPTL4, VEGF, and FABP-4 in first-trimester human placental trophoblasts and their involvement in angiogenesis. cis-9,trans-11(c9t11)-CLA increased tubule formation (as a measure of angiogenesis) in first-trimester human placental cells mediated via ANGPTL4 (Johnsen et al. 2011; Basak and Duttaroy 2013a). In placental first-trimester trophoblast cells, the effects of fatty acids were quite opposite to what was observed in case tumors: LCFAs induce VEGF and ANGPTL4 expression (Johnsen et al. 2011; Basak and Duttaroy 2013a,b; Kang and Liu 2013).

10.7 DHA, 22:6n-3

The conversion of the plant-derived ALA to the long-chain EPA and DHA can be increased by supplementing ALA-sufficient diets. Humans in most countries consume ≥1 g/day of ALA (Plourde and Cunnane 2007). ALA intakes, however, do not result in a net increase in plasma DHA in humans (Plourde and Cunnane 2007; Neff et al. 2011). Even ALA intakes of as much as 30–40 g/day do not result in a net increase in plasma DHA in humans (Plourde and Cunnane 2007) but should still lead to some DHA synthesis. Furthermore, in vegetarians, ALA supplementation was demonstrated to increase the proportion of EPA but not DHA. When given as preformed DHA, however, there are consistent and dramatic increases in DHA in membrane phospholipids. For instance, when DHA was administered to vegetarians for 8 weeks, there was a significant increase in the proportion of DHA in membrane phospholipids (Plourde and Cunnane 2007). It seems that only supplementation with preformed DHA reliably increases tissue DHA (Cunnane et al. 2013). Indeed, there is evidence that small amounts of only EPA and DHA can reverse omega-3 deficiency (Cunnane et al. 2013). While EPA is required for eicosanoid synthesis, the widespread presence and preferential retention of cell membrane phospholipids for DHA, particularly in the brain, indicate that DHA may be conditionally essential (Horrocks and Yeo 1999; Bradbury 2011).

The n-3 and n-6 fatty acids compete with each other for the same enzymes, notably delta-6 desaturase; an excess of n-6 dominates the enzyme, thus further inhibiting the synthesis of n-3 fatty acids, specially DHA. Over the past century, the balance between n-3 and n-6 fatty acids has been dramatically shifted in favor of omega-6 fatty acids. The domestication of livestock and poultry resulted in a shift in livestock feed from an n-3-rich plant-based diet to an n-6-rich seed-based diet (Horrocks and Yeo 1999). The underlying factor for the increases in the incidences of these diseases may be attributable to an inadequate proportion of DHA in membrane phospholipids, driven largely by excessive consumption of n-6 fatty acids.

10.8 DHA IN FETOPLACENTAL DEVELOPMENT

The perinatal supply of DHA is of great importance for pregnancy outcomes and for fetoplacental growth and development (Innis 1991; Dutta-Roy 2000). A preferential active materno–fetal DHA transport across the placenta has been demonstrated, which is likely mediated by a complex interplay of fatty acid binding/transport proteins (Duttaroy 2004). Because of limited fetal capacity to synthesize DHA, the fetus depends on DHA transfer across the placenta (Dutta-Roy 2000). Molecular mechanisms of placental DHA uptake and transport are not fully understood, but it has been clearly demonstrated that there is a preferential DHA transfer. Thus, the placenta is of pivotal importance for the selective channeling of DHA from maternal diet and body stores to the fetus. Several studies have associated various fatty acid transport and binding proteins with the preferential DHA transfer, but also the importance of the different enzymes has been shown (Duttaroy 2009).

Several studies confirmed the benefit of omega-3 supplementation during pregnancy in terms of proper development of the brain and retina (Innis and Friesen 2008). Of the two most important long-chain omega-3 fatty acids, EPA and DHA, DHA is more important for proper cell membrane function and is vital to the development of the fetal brain and retina (Innis and Friesen 2008). During the third trimester, vast amounts of DHA accumulate in fetal tissue (Innis 2007). The two most infiltrated fetal areas include the retina and brain (Ramakrishnan et al. 2010), which may correlate with normal eyesight and brain function (Innis 2007). The results on higher birth weight and length of gestation were also confirmed in different meta-analyses about the effects of n-3 LCPUFA supplementation during pregnancy (Larque et al. 2012). The effects of n-3 LCPUFA supplementation in high-risk pregnancies are controversial (Imhoff-Kunsch et al. 2012). In a European multicenter trial involving women with a preterm delivery history, those randomly assigned to receive an n-3 LCPUFA supplement had significantly lower rate of recurrent preterm delivery before 37 weeks and before 34 weeks (Larque et al. 2012). Moreover, in a prospective cohort study in Denmark with 8729 pregnant women, low consumption of fish was a strong risk factor for preterm delivery and low birth weight (Olsen and Secher 2002). In addition, daily intake of either 3 g EPA or placebo did not prevent the recurrence of intrauterine growth retardation or pregnancy-induced hypertension in 63 subjects with high-risk pregnancies (Rogers et al. 2004). The results of the meta-analyses showed no clear difference in the relative risk of birth before 37 completed weeks in high-risk pregnancies. Thus, the efficacy of n-3 LCPUFA supplements to reduce the risk of preterm birth and low birth weight needs further work.

10.9 DHA AND EARLY PLACENTATION PROCESS: IMPORTANCE OF DHA SUPPLEMENTATION AT THE PRECONCEPTION STAGE

DHA, which is critical for fetal brain and retinal development, may also be involved in the placentation process by stimulating tube formation in first-trimester placental trophoblast cells (Innis 1991; Johnsen et al. 2011). Invasive extravillous trophoblasts of the human placenta are critically involved in successful pregnancy outcome. They remodel the uterine spiral arteries to increase blood flow and oxygen delivery to the placenta and the developing fetus. This invasive behavior of extravillous trophoblasts follows a precise chronology of vascular events during the first trimester of gestation. Defective invasion of the uterine spiral arteries is directly involved in preeclampsia, a major and frequent complication of human pregnancy with serious fetal and maternal consequences. Several factors are involved in this angiogenic process, including VEGF, ANGPTL4, PDGF, and platelet-activating factor. DHA-induced tube formation may be mediated, in part, via increased expression and secretion of VEGF. DHA increased tube formation maximally in serum-starved HTR8/SVneo cells after 16 hours of incubation compared with other fatty acids. DHA stimulated the expression of VEGF mRNA and its protein secretion but did not increase mRNA expression and protein release of ANGPTL4 in placental first-trimester placental trophoblast cells, HTR8/SVneo. Impaired placental development due to reduced trophoblast invasion and angiogenesis are associated with preeclampsia and IUFR. Maternal supply of dietary DHA therefore not only is important for fetal growth and development but may also play an important role in placental angiogenic processes and vascular remodeling during early pregnancy. During pregnancy, the placenta transfers nutrients, including DHA, from the mother to the fetus (Duttaroy 2009). The amount of omega-3 fatty acid in the fetus is correlated with the amount ingested by the mother, so it is essential that the mother has adequate nutrition (Helland et al. 2008). Several studies showed that maternal intake of n-3 LCPUFA during pregnancy resulted in a slightly longer gestation period and somewhat higher birth weight (Mantzioris et al. 1994; Larque et al. 2012). The sample size is critical for identifying differences in these variables, and large studies found differences in birth outcomes as a result of n-3 supplementation during pregnancy (Makrides et al. 2010; Ramakrishnan et al. 2010). It is important to consider that the higher birth weight reported for n-3 LCPUFA supplementation during pregnancy was probably a result of the greater gestational length of these pregnancies, since the differences in birth weight disappeared when using the gestational age as covariable (Olsen et al. 1992).

10.10 SUMMARY

Early placental angiogenesis is critical for the establishment of placental vascularization and, thus, for normal fetal growth and development. Inadequate placental vascular development may compromise fetoplacental growth and development. It seems reasonable to suggest that placental vascular defects and placental dysfunction may be an important cause of infertility to the mother and fetal growth retardation. With the recent spate of studies on regulators of angiogenesis, these observations lead us to believe that regulation of placental angiogenesis could become a novel and powerful way for ensuring positive outcomes for most pregnancies. DHA and other n-6 fatty acids, including CLA, stimulate angiogenesis in placental first-trimester cells. These dietary fatty acids stimulated the expression not only of major angiogenic factors such as VEGF and ANGPTL4 but also of FABP-4 and FABP-3, which are known to directly modulate angiogenesis. Among all the FABPs, FABP-4 appeared to be the potent regulator of angiogenic process mediated by fatty acids, leptin, or VEGF.

ACKNOWLEDGMENTS

This study was supported by the Thune Holst Foundation, Norway, and the BOYSCAST visiting fellowship program, India.

REFERENCES

Abajo, A., N. Bitarte, R. Zarate, V. Boni, I. Lopez, M. Gonzalez-Huarriz, J. Rodriguez, E. Bandres, and J. Garcia-Foncillas. 2012. "Identification of colorectal cancer metastasis markers by an angiogenesis-related cytokine-antibody array." *World J Gastroenterol* 18 (7):637–45. doi:10.3748/wjg.v18.i7.637.

Aiello, L. P. and J. S. Wong. 2000. "Role of vascular endothelial growth factor in diabetic vascular complications." *Kidney Int Suppl* 77:S113–9.

Bagga, D., L. Wang, R. Farias-Eisner, J. A. Glaspy, and S. T. Reddy. 2003. "Differential effects of prostaglandin derived from omega-6 and omega-3 polyunsaturated fatty acids on COX-2 expression and IL-6 secretion." *Proc Natl Acad Sci U S A* 100 (4):1751–6. doi:10.1073/pnas.0334211100.

Basak, S. and A. K. Duttaroy. 2012. "Leptin induces tube formation in first-trimester extravillous trophoblast cells." *Eur J Obstet Gynecol Reprod Biol.* 164 (1):24–9. doi:10.1016/j.ejogrb.2012.05.033.

Basak, S. and A. K. Duttaroy. 2013a. "cis-9,trans-11 conjugated linoleic acid stimulates expression of angiopoietin like-4 in the placental extravillous trophoblast cells." *Biochim Biophys Acta* 1831 (4):834–43. doi:10.1016/j.bbalip.2013.01.012.

Basak, S. and A. K. Duttaroy. 2013b. "Effects of fatty acids on angiogenic activity in the placental extravillous trophoblast cells." *Prostaglandins Leukot Essent Fatty Acids* 88 (2):155–62. doi:10.1016/j.plefa.2012.10.001.

Belury, M. A. 2002. "Dietary conjugated linoleic acid in health: Physiological effects and mechanisms of action." *Annu Rev Nutr* 22:505–31. doi:10.1146/annurev.nutr.22.021302.121842.

Bradbury, J. 2011. "Docosahexaenoic acid (DHA): An ancient nutrient for the modern human brain." *Nutrients* 3 (5):529–54. doi:10.3390/nu3050529.

Calviello, G., F. Di Nicuolo, S. Gragnoli, E. Piccioni, S. Serini, N. Maggiano, G. Tringali, P. Navarra, F. O. Ranelletti, and P. Palozza. 2004. "n-3 PUFAs reduce VEGF expression in human colon cancer cells modulating the COX-2/PGE2 induced ERK-1 and -2 and HIF-1alpha induction pathway." *Carcinogenesis* 25 (12):2303–10. doi:10.1093/carcin/bgh265.

Campbell, F. M., P. G. Bush, J. H. Veerkamp, and A. K. Dutta-Roy. 1998. "Detection and cellular localization of plasma membrane-associated and cytoplasmic fatty acid-binding proteins in human placenta." *Placenta* 19 (5–6):409–15.

Carmeliet, P. and R. K. Jain. 2011. "Molecular mechanisms and clinical applications of angiogenesis." *Nature* 473 (7347):298–307. doi:10.1038/nature10144.

Cataltepe, O., M. C. Arikan, E. Ghelfi, C. Karaaslan, Y. Ozsurekci, K. Dresser, Y. Li, T. W. Smith, and S. Cataltepe. 2012. "Fatty acid binding protein 4 is expressed in distinct endothelial and nonendothelial cell populations in glioblastoma." *Neuropathol Appl Neurobiol.* 38 (5):400–10. doi:10.1111/j.1365-2990.2011.01237.x.

Chaiworapongsa, T., R. Romero, Z. A. Savasan, J. P. Kusanovic, G. Ogge, E. Soto, Z. Dong, A. Tarca, B. Gaurav, and S. S. Hassan. 2011. "Maternal plasma concentrations of angiogenic/anti-angiogenic factors are of prognostic value in patients presenting to the obstetrical triage area with the suspicion of preeclampsia." *J Matern Fetal Neonatal Med* 24 (10):1187–207. doi:10.3109/14767058.2011.589932.

Chen, J. 2010. "Src may be involved in the anti-cancer effect of conjugated linoleic acid. Comment on: CLA reduces breast cancer cell growth and invasion through ER and PI3K/Akt pathways." *Chem Biol Interact* 186 (2):250–1; author reply 252–3. doi:10.1016/j.cbi.2010.03.052.

Cunnane, S. C., R. Chouinard-Watkins, C. A. Castellano, and P. Barberger-Gateau. 2013. "Docosahexaenoic acid homeostasis, brain aging and Alzheimer's disease: Can we reconcile the evidence?" *Prostaglandins Leukot Essent Fatty Acids* 88 (1):61–70. doi:10.1016/j.plefa.2012.04.006.

Dutta-Roy, A. K. 1994. "Insulin mediated processes in platelets, erythrocytes and monocytes/macrophages: Effects of essential fatty acid metabolism." *Prostaglandins Leukot Essent Fatty Acids* 51 (6):385–99.

Dutta-Roy, A. K. 2000. "Transport mechanisms for long-chain polyunsaturated fatty acids in the human placenta." *Am J Clin Nutr* 71 (1 Suppl):315S–22S.

Duttaroy, A. K. 2004. "Fetal growth and development: Roles of fatty acid transport proteins and nuclear transcription factors in human placenta." *Indian J Exp Biol* 42 (8):747–57.

Duttaroy, A. K. 2009. "Transport of fatty acids across the human placenta: A review." *Prog Lipid Res* 48 (1):52–61. doi:10.1016/j.plipres.2008.11.001.

Elmasri, H., C. Karaaslan, Y. Teper, E. Ghelfi, M. Weng, T. A. Ince, H. Kozakewich, J. Bischoff, and S. Cataltepe. 2009. "Fatty acid binding protein 4 is a target of VEGF and a regulator of cell proliferation in endothelial cells." *FASEB J* 23 (11):3865–73. doi:10.1096/fj.09-134882.

Elmasri, H., E. Ghelfi, C. W. Yu, S. Traphagen, M. Cernadas, H. Cao, G. P. Shi, J. Plutzky, M. Sahin, G. Hotamisligil, and S. Cataltepe. 2012. "Endothelial cell–fatty acid binding protein 4 promotes angiogenesis: Role of stem cell factor/c-kit pathway." *Angiogenesis* 15 (3):457–68. doi:10.1007/s10456-012-9274-0.

Fang, L. Y., T. Y. Wong, W. F. Chiang, and Y. L. Chen. 2010. "Fatty-acid-binding protein 5 promotes cell proliferation and invasion in oral squamous cell carcinoma." *J Oral Pathol Med* 39 (4):342–8. doi:10.1111/j.1600-0714.2009.00836.x.

Fishman, S. J. and J. B. Mulliken. 1993. "Hemangiomas and vascular malformations of infancy and childhood." *Pediatr Clin North Am* 40 (6):1177–200.

Folkman, J. and M. Klagsbrun. 1987. "Angiogenic factors." *Science* 235 (4787):442–7.

Ganu, R. S., R. A. Harris, K. Collins, and K. M. Aagaard. 2012. "Early origins of adult disease: Approaches for investigating the programmable epigenome in humans, nonhuman primates, and rodents." *ILAR J* 53 (3–4):306–21. doi:10.1093/ilar.53.3-4.306.

Gealekman, O., A. Burkart, M. Chouinard, S. M. Nicoloro, J. Straubhaar, and S. Corvera. 2008. "Enhanced angiogenesis in obesity and in response to PPARgamma activators through adipocyte VEGF and ANGPTL4 production." *Am J Physiol Endocrinol Metab* 295 (5):E1056–64. doi:10.1152/ajpendo.90345.2008.

Ghelfi, E., C. W. Yu, H. Elmasri, M. Terwelp, C. G. Lee, V. Bhandari, S. A. Comhair, S. C. Erzurum, G. S. Hotamisligil, J. A. Elias, and S. Cataltepe. 2013. "Fatty acid binding protein 4 regulates VEGF-induced airway angiogenesis and inflammation in a transgenic mouse model: Implications for asthma." *Am J Pathol* 182 (4):1425–33. doi:10.1016/j.ajpath.2012.12.009.

Ghosh-Choudhury, T., C. C. Mandal, K. Woodruff, P. St Clair, G. Fernandes, G. G. Choudhury, and N. Ghosh-Choudhury. 2009. "Fish oil targets PTEN to regulate NFkappaB for downregulation of anti-apoptotic genes in breast tumor growth." *Breast Cancer Res Treat* 118 (1):213–28. doi:10.1007/s10549-008-0227-7.

Gottlicher, M., A. Demoz, D. Svensson, P. Tollet, R. K. Berge, and J. A. Gustafsson. 1993. "Structural and metabolic requirements for activators of the peroxisome proliferator-activated receptor." *Biochem Pharmacol* 46 (12):2177–84.

Hamed, E. A., M. M. Zakary, R. M. Abdelal, and E. M. Abdel Moneim. 2011. "Vasculopathy in type 2 diabetes mellitus: Role of specific angiogenic modulators." *J Physiol Biochem* 67 (3):339–49. doi:10.1007/s13105-011-0080-8.

Hardman, W. E. 2004. "(n-3) fatty acids and cancer therapy." *J Nutr* 134 (12 Suppl):3427S–30S.

Helland, I. B., L. Smith, B. Blomen, K. Saarem, O. D. Saugstad, and C. A. Drevon. 2008. "Effect of supplementing pregnant and lactating mothers with n-3 very-long-chain fatty acids on children's IQ and body mass index at 7 years of age." *Pediatrics* 122 (2):e472–9. doi:10.1542/peds.2007-2762.

Hoagland, K. M., K. G. Maier, C. Moreno, M. Yu, and R. J. Roman. 2001. "Cytochrome P450 metabolites of arachidonic acid: Novel regulators of renal function." *Nephrol Dial Transplant* 16 (12):2283–5.

Horrocks, L. A. and Y. K. Yeo. 1999. "Health benefits of docosahexaenoic acid (DHA)." *Pharmacol Res* 40 (3):211–25. doi:10.1006/phrs.1999.0495.

Imhoff-Kunsch, B., V. Briggs, T. Goldenberg, and U. Ramakrishnan. 2012. "Effect of n-3 long-chain polyunsaturated fatty acid intake during pregnancy on maternal, infant, and child health outcomes: A systematic review." *Paediatr Perinat Epidemiol* 26 Suppl 1:91–107. doi:10.1111/j.1365-3016.2012.01292.x.

Innis, S. M. 1991. "Essential fatty acids in growth and development." *Prog Lipid Res* 30 (1):39–103.

Innis, S. M. 2007. "Fatty acids and early human development." *Early Hum Dev* 83 (12):761–6. doi:10.1016/j.earlhumdev.2007.09.004.

Innis, S. M. and R. W. Friesen. 2008. "Essential n-3 fatty acids in pregnant women and early visual acuity maturation in term infants." *Am J Clin Nutr* 87 (3):548–57.

Jin, Y., M. Arita, Q. Zhang, D. R. Saban, S. K. Chauhan, N. Chiang, C. N. Serhan, and R. Dana. 2009. "Anti-angiogenesis effect of the novel anti-inflammatory and pro-resolving lipid mediators." *Invest Ophthalmol Vis Sci* 50 (10):4743–52. doi:10.1167/iovs.08-2462.

Johnsen, G. M., S. Basak, M. S. Weedon-Fekjaer, A. C. Staff, and A. K. Duttaroy. 2011. "Docosahexaenoic acid stimulates tube formation in first trimester trophoblast cells, HTR8/SVneo." *Placenta* 32:626–32. doi:10.1016/j.placenta.2011.06.009.

Kamiyama, M., A. Pozzi, L. Yang, L. M. DeBusk, R. M. Breyer, and P. C. Lin. 2006. "EP2, a receptor for PGE2, regulates tumor angiogenesis through direct effects on endothelial cell motility and survival." *Oncogene* 25 (53):7019–28. doi:10.1038/sj.onc.1209694.

Kanayasu, T., I. Morita, J. Nakao-Hayashi, N. Asuwa, N. Fujisawa, T. Ishii, H. Ito, and S. Murota. 1991. "Eicosapentaenoic acid inhibits tube formation of vascular endothelial cells in vitro." *Lipids* 26 (4):271–6.

Kang, J. X. and K. H. Weylandt. 2008. "Modulation of inflammatory cytokines by omega-3 fatty acids." *Subcell Biochem* 49:133–43. doi:10.1007/978-1-4020-8831-5_5.

Kang, J. X. and A. Liu. 2013. "The role of the tissue omega-6/omega-3 fatty acid ratio in regulating tumor angiogenesis." *Cancer Metastasis Rev* 32 (1–2):201–10. doi:10.1007/s10555-012-9401-9.

Kim, H. J., C. A. Vosseler, P. C. Weber, and W. Erl. 2005. "Docosahexaenoic acid induces apoptosis in proliferating human endothelial cells." *J Cell Physiol* 204 (3):881–8. doi:10.1002/jcp.20351.

Kusakari, Y., E. Ogawa, Y. Owada, N. Kitanaka, H. Watanabe, M. Kimura, H. Tagami, H. Kondo, S. Aiba, and R. Okuyama. 2006. "Decreased keratinocyte motility in skin wound on mice lacking the epidermal fatty acid binding protein gene." *Mol Cell Biochem* 284 (1–2):183–8. doi:10.1007/s11010-005-9048-8.

Larque, E., A. Gil-Sanchez, M. T. Prieto-Sanchez, and B. Koletzko. 2012. "Omega 3 fatty acids, gestation and pregnancy outcomes." *Br J Nutr* 107 Suppl 2:S77–84. doi:10.1017/S0007114512001481.

Li, Q., Q. Zhang, M. Wang, S. Zhao, J. Ma, N. Luo, N. Li, Y. Li, G. Xu, and J. Li. 2007. "Eicosapentaenoic acid modifies lipid composition in caveolae and induces translocation of endothelial nitric oxide synthase." *Biochimie* 89 (1):169–77. doi:10.1016/j.biochi.2006.10.009.

Makrides, M., R. A. Gibson, A. J. McPhee, L. Yelland, J. Quinlivan, and P. Ryan. 2010. "Effect of DHA supplementation during pregnancy on maternal depression and neurodevelopment of young children: A randomized controlled trial." *JAMA* 304 (15):1675–83. doi:10.1001/jama.2010.1507.

Mantzioris, E., M. J. James, R. A. Gibson, and L. G. Cleland. 1994. "Dietary substitution with an alpha-linolenic acid-rich vegetable oil increases eicosapentaenoic acid concentrations in tissues." *Am J Clin Nutr* 59 (6):1304–9.

Maraldi, T., C. Prata, C. Caliceti, F. Vieceli Dalla Sega, L. Zambonin, D. Fiorentini, and G. Hakim. 2010. "VEGF-induced ROS generation from NAD(P)H oxidases protects human leukemic cells from apoptosis." *Int J Oncol* 36 (6):1581–9.

Massaro, M., E. Scoditti, M. A. Carluccio, M. C. Campana, and R. De Caterina. 2010. "Omega-3 fatty acids, inflammation and angiogenesis: Basic mechanisms behind the cardioprotective effects of fish and fish oils." *Cell Mol Biol* 56 (1):59–82.

Matesanz, N., G. Park, H. McAllister, W. Leahey, A. Devine, G. E. McVeigh, T. A. Gardiner, and D. M. McDonald. 2010. "Docosahexaenoic acid improves the nitroso-redox balance and reduces VEGF-mediated angiogenic signaling in microvascular endothelial cells." *Invest Ophthalmol Vis Sci* 51 (12):6815–25. doi:10.1167/iovs.10-5339.

Morisada, T., Y. Kubota, T. Urano, T. Suda, and Y. Oike. 2006. "Angiopoietins and angiopoietin-like proteins in angiogenesis." *Endothelium* 13 (2):71–9. doi:10.1080/10623320600697989.

Mousiolis, A. V., P. Kollia, C. Skentou, and I. E. Messinis. 2012. "Effects of leptin on the expression of fatty acid-binding proteins in human placental cell cultures." *Mol Med Report* 5 (2):497–502. doi:10.3892/mmr.2011.686.

Murota, S. I., M. Onodera, and I. Morita. 2000. "Regulation of angiogenesis by controlling VEGF receptor." *Ann N Y Acad Sci* 902:208–12; discussion 212–3.

Murray, M. J. and B. A. Lessey. 1999. "Embryo implantation and tumor metastasis: Common pathways of invasion and angiogenesis." *Semin Reprod Endocrinol* 17 (3):275–90. doi:10.1055/s-2007-1016235.

Neff, L. M., J. Culiner, S. Cunningham-Rundles, C. Seidman, D. Meehan, J. Maturi, K. M. Wittkowski, B. Levine, and J. L. Breslow. 2011. "Algal docosahexaenoic acid affects plasma lipoprotein particle size distribution in overweight and obese adults." *J Nutr* 141 (2):207–13. doi:10.3945/jn.110.130021.

Nevo, J., A. Mai, S. Tuomi, T. Pellinen, O. T. Pentikainen, P. Heikkila, J. Lundin, H. Joensuu, P. Bono, and J. Ivaska. 2010. "Mammary-derived growth inhibitor (MDGI) interacts with integrin alpha-subunits and suppresses integrin activity and invasion." *Oncogene* 29 (49):6452–63. doi:10.1038/onc.2010.376.

Nie, D., M. Lamberti, A. Zacharek, L. Li, K. Szekeres, K. Tang, Y. Chen, and K. V. Honn. 2000. "Thromboxane A(2) regulation of endothelial cell migration, angiogenesis, and tumor metastasis." *Biochem Biophys Res Commun* 267 (1):245–51. doi:10.1006/bbrc.1999.1840.

Olsen, S. F. and N. J. Secher. 2002. "Low consumption of seafood in early pregnancy as a risk factor for preterm delivery: Prospective cohort study." *BMJ* 324 (7335):447.

Olsen, S. F., J. D. Sorensen, N. J. Secher, M. Hedegaard, T. B. Henriksen, H. S. Hansen, and A. Grant. 1992. "Randomised controlled trial of effect of fish-oil supplementation on pregnancy duration." *Lancet* 339 (8800):1003–7.

Pai, R., I. L. Szabo, B. A. Soreghan, S. Atay, H. Kawanaka, and A. S. Tarnawski. 2001. "PGE(2) stimulates VEGF expression in endothelial cells via ERK2/JNK1 signaling pathways." *Biochem Biophys Res Commun* 286 (5):923–8. doi:10.1006/bbrc.2001.5494.

Plourde, M. and S. C. Cunnane. 2007. "Extremely limited synthesis of long chain polyunsaturates in adults: Implications for their dietary essentiality and use as supplements." *Appl Physiol Nutr Metab* 32 (4):619–34. doi:10.1139/H07-034.

Pola, R., E. Gaetani, A. Flex, T. R. Aprahamian, M. Bosch-Marce, D. W. Losordo, R. C. Smith, and P. Pola. 2004. "Comparative analysis of the in vivo angiogenic properties of stable prostacyclin analogs: A possible role for peroxisome proliferator-activated receptors." *J Mol Cell Cardiol* 36 (3):363–70. doi:10.1016/j.yjmcc.2003.10.016.

Ramakrishnan, U., A. D. Stein, S. Parra-Cabrera, M. Wang, B. Imhoff-Kunsch, S. Juarez-Marquez, J. Rivera, and R. Martorell. 2010. "Effects of docosahexaenoic acid supplementation during pregnancy on gestational age and size at birth: Randomized, double-blind, placebo-controlled trial in Mexico." *Food Nutr Bull* 31 (2 Suppl):S108–16.

Rogers, I., P. Emmett, A. Ness, and J. Golding. 2004. "Maternal fish intake in late pregnancy and the frequency of low birth weight and intrauterine growth retardation in a cohort of British infants." *J Epidemiol Community Health* 58 (6):486–92.

Salem, N., Jr., B. Litman, H. Y. Kim, and K. Gawrisch. 2001. "Mechanisms of action of docosahexaenoic acid in the nervous system." *Lipids* 36 (9):945–59.

Salvado, M. D., A. Alfranca, J. Z. Haeggstrom, and J. M. Redondo. 2012. "Prostanoids in tumor angiogenesis: Therapeutic intervention beyond COX-2." *Trends Mol Med* 18 (4):233–43. doi:10.1016/j.molmed.2012.02.002.

Sapieha, P., A. Stahl, J. Chen, M. R. Seaward, K. L. Willett, N. M. Krah, R. J. Dennison, K. M. Connor, C. M. Aderman, E. Liclican, A. Carughi, D. Perelman, Y. Kanaoka, J. P. Sangiovanni, K. Gronert, and L. E. Smith. 2011. "5-Lipoxygenase metabolite 4-HDHA is a mediator of the antiangiogenic effect of omega-3 polyunsaturated fatty acids." *Sci Transl Med* 3 (69):69ra12. doi:10.1126/scitranslmed.3001571.

Scoditti, E., M. Massaro, M. A. Carluccio, A. Distante, C. Storelli, and R. De Caterina. 2010. "PPARgamma agonists inhibit angiogenesis by suppressing PKCalpha- and CREB-mediated COX-2 expression in the human endothelium." *Cardiovasc Res* 86 (2):302–10. doi:10.1093/cvr/cvp400.

Simopoulos, A. P. 2002. "Omega-3 fatty acids in inflammation and autoimmune diseases." *J Am Coll Nutr* 21 (6):495–505.

Smith, W. L. 1989. "The eicosanoids and their biochemical mechanisms of action." *Biochem J* 259 (2):315–24.

Spencer, L., C. Mann, M. Metcalfe, M. Webb, C. Pollard, D. Spencer, D. Berry, W. Steward, and A. Dennison. 2009. "The effect of omega-3 FAs on tumour angiogenesis and their therapeutic potential." *Eur J Cancer* 45 (12):2077–86. doi:10.1016/j.ejca.2009.04.026.

Sterescu, A. E., E. Rousseau-Harsany, C. Farrell, J. Powell, M. David, and J. Dubois. 2006. "The potential efficacy of omega-3 fatty acids as anti-angiogenic agents in benign vascular tumors of infancy." *Med Hypotheses* 66 (6):1121–4. doi:10.1016/j.mehy.2005.12.040.

Storch, J. and A. E. Thumser. 2010. "Tissue-specific functions in the fatty acid-binding protein family." *J Biol Chem* 285 (43):32679–83. doi:10.1074/jbc.R110.135210.

Szymczak, M., M. Murray, and N. Petrovic. 2008. "Modulation of angiogenesis by omega-3 polyunsaturated fatty acids is mediated by cyclooxygenases." *Blood* 111 (7):3514–21. doi:10.1182/blood-2007-08-109934.

Takahashi, S. 2011. "Vascular endothelial growth factor (VEGF), VEGF receptors and their inhibitors for antiangiogenic tumor therapy." *Biol Pharm Bull* 34 (12):1785–8.

Torry, R. J. and B. J. Rongish. 1992. "Angiogenesis in the uterus: Potential regulation and relation to tumor angiogenesis." *Am J Reprod Immunol* 27 (3–4):171–9.

Torry, D. S., H. S. Wang, T. H. Wang, M. R. Caudle, and R. J. Torry. 1998. "Preeclampsia is associated with reduced serum levels of placenta growth factor." *Am J Obstet Gynecol* 179 (6 Pt 1):1539–44.

Tsuji, M., S. I. Murota, and I. Morita. 2003. "Docosapentaenoic acid (22:5, n-3) suppressed tube-forming activity in endothelial cells induced by vascular endothelial growth factor." *Prostaglandins Leukot Essent Fatty Acids* 68 (5):337–42.

Uauy, R., D. R. Hoffman, P. Peirano, D. G. Birch, and E. E. Birch. 2001. "Essential fatty acids in visual and brain development." *Lipids* 36 (9):885–95.

Yang, S. P., I. Morita, and S. I. Murota. 1998. "Eicosapentaenoic acid attenuates vascular endothelial growth factor-induced proliferation via inhibiting Flk-1 receptor expression in bovine carotid artery endothelial cells." *J Cell Physiol* 176 (2):342–9. doi:10.1002/(SICI)1097-4652(199808)176:2<342::AID-JCP12>3.0.CO;2-5.

Yuan, Y. M., S. H. Fang, X. D. Qian, L. Y. Liu, L. H. Xu, W. Z. Shi, L. H. Zhang, Y. B. Lu, W. P. Zhang, and E. Q. Wei. 2009. "Leukotriene D4 stimulates the migration but not proliferation of endothelial cells mediated by the cysteinyl leukotriene cyslt(1) receptor via the extracellular signal-regulated kinase pathway." *J Pharmacol Sci* 109 (2):285–92.

Section III

Vitamins, Minerals, and Placentation

11 Maternal Micronutrients, Placental Growth, and Fetal Outcome

Irene Cetin, Chiara Mandò, and Manuela Cardellicchio

CONTENTS

ABSTRACT

Pregnancy can be regarded as a three-compartment model, with the mother, placenta, and fetus interacting to ensure proper fetal growth and development. Maternal health, along with maternal diet, body composition, metabolism, and placental nutrient supply, is the main factor that can negatively or positively influence fetal development. Before reaching the fetus, nutrients from maternal diet are used by the placenta for its own metabolism. The quality and quantity of nutrients that reach the fetus are indeed influenced by placental shape, size, and characteristics. Placental growth and development are influenced by the maternal diet itself.

This chapter aims to show how fetal and postnatal growth and development are strictly dependent on proper maternal nutritional intake before and during pregnancy and how oversupply, deficiency, or poor quality of nutrients may influence placental development and adversely affect pregnancy outcome and expression of fetal genetic potential.

KEY WORDS

Micronutrients, placenta, pregnancy, supplementation.

11.1 INTRODUCTION

Pregnancy requires a limited increase in daily caloric intake: from 100 kcal/day in the first trimester to 300 kcal/day in the second and third trimester (Rasmussen and Yaktine 2009). The increase in caloric requirements is easily reached by increasing macronutrient consumption, with a correct balance between carbohydrates (40%–50%), fats (25%–30%), and proteins (15%–20%).

Micronutrients include vitamins (vitamin A, B, C, D, E, and K), minerals (calcium and phosphorus), and the so-called trace elements (iron, zinc, selenium, and manganese), which are requested only in small amounts. However, they play a crucial role in the production of enzymes, hormones, and other substances necessary for the proper functioning of the body. During pregnancy, micronutrient requirement increases much more than macronutrients, in some cases even doubling the prepregnancy requirement.

Malnutrition can result from a diet that does not allow an adequate caloric intake (undernutrition), but it may also follow from a diet based on poor-quality nutrients with reduced amounts of micronutrients. This is typical in nowadays obese "western" diets.

Here, we will present possible effects of a nutritionally unbalanced diet and the role of individual micronutrients on pregnancy outcome (Table 11.1).

11.2 EFFECTS OF MALNUTRITION

The effects of maternal undernutrition are well documented by the Dutch famine during the second world war, when pro capita food availability was progressively reduced because of German embargo to 1300 kcal/day. This condition immediately affected pregnancy and fetal outcomes, and led also to impaired health in later life.

TABLE 11.1
Fetal Outcomes Related to Single Micronutrient Deficiencies and Their Biological Activity

Micronutrient Deficiency	Biological Activity	Fetal Outcome
Folate	Regulate nucleic acid and DNA synthesis	Increased risk of neural tubal defects and congenital heart disease
Iron	Regulate oxygen transport Essential for cells' catalytic pathways	Increased risk of low birth weight, preterm delivery, and maternal postpartum hemorrhage
Iodine	Essential for thyroid hormones production	Increased risk of iodine deficiency disorders (abortion, cretinism, neurocognitive delay)
Calcium	Acts like a secondary cell messenger	Increased risk of developing hypertensive disorders
Vitamin D	Essential for calcium homeostasis and bone mineralization Regulation of immune function	Increased risk of preeclampsia, gestational diabetes mellitus, impaired fetal skeletal development
Selenium	Antioxidant activity Support thyroid function	Association with preterm deliveries, miscarriages, and preeclampsia
Copper	Antioxidant activity Involved in iron metabolism	Sever deficiency linked to miscarriage, structural abnormalities, low birth weight, and elevated risk of cardiovascular disease and reduced fertility
Zinc	Antioxidant activity Implicated in nucleic acid synthesis, cellular division, and differentiation	Subadequate maternal intakes associated with prolonged labor, fetal growth restriction, and embryonic or fetal death

The effects of famine depended on the stage of gestation in which it occurred. Famine during mid or late gestation reduced placental length and area and was associated with smaller babies as a result of reduced placental efficiency. Babies in early gestation during the famine, or conceived after the famine ended, had higher birth weights, suggesting increased placental efficiency due to compensatory mechanisms (Roseboom, de Rooij, and Painter 2006; Ruager-Martin, Hyde, and Modi 2010; Roseboom et al. 2011).

Moreover, exposure to undernutrition during any stage of gestation was associated with higher risk of later glucose intolerance. Interestingly, exposure only during early gestation increased risk of obesity, coronary heart disease, schizophrenia, and depression (Roseboom, de Rooij, and Painter 2006). In summary, famine showed that not only early gestation is a pregnancy vulnerable period but also that preconceptional and periconceptional nutrition may have negative consequences on the offspring's health, probably based on abnormal placentation occurring early in pregnancy.

The global transition toward diets enriched in processed foods, refined sugars, refined fats, oils and meat has contributed to the rapid increase in obesity all over the world. In western countries the prevalence of overweight and obese women (body mass index >30 kg/m^2) in fertile ages is now 44% (Linné 2004).

Obese women have a higher risk of amenorrhea and infertility, with decreased success of infertility treatments (Ruager-Martin, Hyde, and Modi 2010).

Moreover, when obese women become pregnant, they have a higher risk of miscarriage, gestational diabetes, fetal growth restriction, fetal overweight, and preeclampsia. Placental-to-fetal weight ratio has been shown to be increased in obese pregnancies, suggesting that the placentas of obese women are less efficient (Calabrese and Mandò 2014). Similar changes in placental biometric parameters have been associated with increased risks of cardiovascular disease in later life (Barker et al. 1993). Similarly, offspring of obese mother have higher prevalence of obesity and type II diabetes mellitus later in life (Szostak-Wegierek 2014).

A number of studies have investigated the relationship between type of nutrition and unfavorable obstetric outcomes. However, identifying the potential influence of single substances is difficult. The usual diet contains thousands of nutrients, and the same substance is present in different foods and foods are not consumed independently of each other. To avoid these methodological limitations, more recent studies have investigated dietary patterns that reflect overall dietary behavior; these studies are population specific and are influenced by geographic and sociocultural factors. The so-called prudent dietary pattern is based on raw and cooked vegetables, salad, onion, garlic, fruit and berries, nuts, vegetable oils, water as beverage, whole grain cereals, poultry, and fiber-rich bread. This dietary pattern has been recently associated with a lower risk of preterm delivery (Englund-Ogge et al. 2014). Similarly, the greater the adherence to the New Nordic Diet, based on consumption of Nordic fruits, root vegetables, cabbages, potatoes, oatmeal porridge, whole grains, wild fish, game, berries, milk, and water, the lower is the risk of developing preeclampsia (Ruager-Martin, Hyde, and Modi 2010; Englund-Ogge et al. 2014; Hillesund et al. 2014).

It is therefore well recognized that unhealthy lifestyle and preconceptional diet significantly contribute to impaired reproduction and pregnancy outcome (Cetin, Berti, and Calabrese 2010). Most women during reproductive age, and above all pregnant women, do not get enough trace elements in their diet, representing an important topic of public health not only in developing countries but also in industrialized countries, where dietary patterns, typified by snacking, breakfast skipping, fast foods, soft drinks, and convenience foods, are nutritionally unbalanced and fail to meet recommended daily allowance for micronutrients (Blumfield, Hure, Macdonald-Wicks, Smith, and Collins 2013). This situation is further exacerbated by the reduction of minerals, vitamins, and protein in fruits and vegetables because of environmental dilution effects (Tilman and Clark 2014).

It is likely that dietary patterns with better micronutrient intakes positively influence placental development, thus decreasing the risk of developing pathologies related to abnormal placentation, such as preeclampsia and intrauterine growth restriction (IUGR), and to an abnormal maternal–placental interface, like premature delivery.

11.3   ROLE OF SPECIFIC DIETARY MICRONUTRIENTS

11.3.1   FOLIC ACID

Folate is a water-soluble B-complex vitamin (B9) that plays a crucial role in the one-carbon metabolism for nucleic acid and DNA synthesis, cell replication, regulation of gene expression, amino acid metabolism, and neurotransmitter synthesis. Folate is widely distributed in foods (green-leafy vegetables, fruits, liver, bread, etc.), and its inadequate intake can cause anemia, leucopenia, and thrombocytopenia. Folate is also implicated in methionine metabolism, and its deficiency leads to hyperhomocysteinemia, a possible cause of endothelial dysfunction. Moreover, folate also acts as an antioxidant, protecting cell membranes and DNA from free radical damage (Solanky, Requena Jimenez, D'Souza, Sibley, and Glazier 2010).

During pregnancy, increased folate intake is required for rapid cell proliferation and tissue growth of the fetoplacental unit and for expansion of maternal blood volume. Pregnant women may thus be at risk for folate deficiency. The diet alone is not adequate to obtain concentrations required periconceptionally, so supplementing dietary intake with folic acid has been recommended. In particular, maternal folic acid supplementation protects against neural tube defects (NTDs), with a reduction in the incidence between 35% and 70%, and may reduce the risk and severity of congenital heart disease (Burdge and Lillycrop 2012). The current recommended daily intake for folic acid is 400 to 800 µg for women at least 2 months before conception. The optimal maternal folate status to reduce as low as possible NTDs risk should be at least 906 nmol/L (Daly, Kirke, Molloy, Weir, and Scott 1995). The recommended dose is higher (4000 µg) for women who have had an infant with an NTD or who have increased needs.

Unfortunately, despite recommendations, the incidence of NTDs was not reduced as expected because about 50% of pregnancies are unplanned and many women do not follow health guidelines. Folate may also have a key role in the regulation of extravillous trophoblast (EVT) invasion, which is a crucial part of placental development, and could be of benefit in preventing pregnancy disorders associated with inadequate EVT invasion (Williams, Bulmer, Innes, and Broughton Pipkin 2011).

The use of folic acid supplements during pregnancy is generally considered safe. Nevertheless, recent data postulate that it may have additional, unforeseen persistent effects in the offspring throughout epigenetic mechanism like a short-term increased incidence of allergy-related respiratory impairment in children or an increased risk of mammary tumors in rats (Burdge and Lillycrop 2012). Indeed, folic acid is a donor of methyl groups, thus contributing to the regulation of DNA methylation and consequent gene expression. However, studies are still limited and insufficient to suggest the need to change current recommendations for folic acid intake in pregnancy.

11.3.1.1   Folate Placental Transport

Maternal-to-fetal transport of folates at the level of the placental syncytiotrophoblast is crucial for both placental and fetal development and growth because neither the placenta nor the fetus can synthesize this vitamin (Table 11.2). The human placenta expresses the reduced folate carrier (RFC1), the proton-coupled folate transporter, and the folate receptor (FR) isoforms α and β. FR α is located at the apical membrane of the syncytiotrophoblast, the outermost layer of the placental villi in direct contact with the maternal blood. FR binds folate with high affinity and accomplishes its internalization through receptor-mediated endocytosis. All these transporters are believed to act coordinately to ensure the vectorial transfer of folate from maternal to fetal circulation (Solanky, Requena Jimenez, D'Souza, Sibley, and Glazier 2010).

11.3.2   IRON

Iron (Fe) is a microelement essential for the normal functioning of many cell catalytic pathways, in particular those involved in redox processes (Cetin, Berti, Mando, and Parisi 2011). It also plays an important role in oxygen transport by forming complexes with molecular oxygen in hemoglobin and myoglobin.

TABLE 11.2

Micronutrient Placenta Transport Systems

Micronutrients	Placental Transport Systems	References
Folate	Reduced folate carrier (RFC1)	Solanky, Requena Jimenez, D'Souza, Sibley,
	Proton-coupled folate transporter (PCFT)	and Glazier (2010)
	Folate receptor α and β (FR)	
Iron	Transferrin receptor 1 (TFRC)	Cetin, Berti, Mando, and Parisi (2011)
	Divalent metal transporter-1 (DMT1)	
	Ferroportin	
Iodine	Sodium iodide symporter (NIS)	Burns, O'Herlihy, and Smyth (2013)
	Pendrin (PDS)	
Calcium	Ca^{2+}-ATPase pump	Forestier, Daffos, Rainaut, Bruneau, and
	Na^+/Ca^{2+} exchanger	Trivin (1987)
Vitamin D	Placenta express vitamin D receptor (VDR) and	Shin, Choi, Longtine, and Nelson (2010)
	numbers of hydroxilases, but transplacental	
	transport is still unknown	
Selenium	Anion exchange pathway shared with sulphate	Shennan (1988)
	(passive diffusion under a concentration gradient)	
Copper	Copper transporter (CTR1) (related to iron	McArdle, Andersen, Jones, and Gambling
	transport, unclear mechanism)	(2008)
Zinc	Unknown—probably involves placental zinc	Donangelo and King (2012)
	transporters and metallothionein	
Vitamin C	Unknown	
Vitamin E	Unknown	

Fe demand markedly increases during pregnancy; this need is less evident early in pregnancy (because of the cessation of menstruation) and reaches a maximum of 3–8 mg of iron per day during the third trimester of pregnancy. The net Fe cost of pregnancy has been estimated from 480 mg to 1.15 g. Among these, nearly 300 mg is deposited in the fetus and 90 mg in the placenta at term (Bothwell 2000).

Iron deficiency, with or without anemia, represents the most common nutritional deficit worldwide. Anemia (defined by the World Health Organization [WHO] as hemoglobin levels of ≤11 g/dL) is one of the world's leading causes of disability and, thus, one of the most serious global public health problems. Iron (Fe) deficiency during pregnancy alters embryonic growth and development and strongly increases the risk of low birth weight and preterm delivery (Allen 2000; McArdle, Andersen, Jones, and Gambling 2008), as well as the risk of altered newborn development and cardiovascular disease in the adult (Godfrey and Barker 1995; Malhotra et al. 2002; Gambling et al. 2003; Zimmermann and Hurrell 2007; Kidanto, Mogren, Lindmark, Massawe, and Nystrom 2009). Data on human infants are consistent with altered myelination of white matter, changes in monoamine metabolism in striatum, and functioning of the hippocampus. Iron deficiency is also associated with a higher risk of postpartum hemorrhage in the mother. At a molecular level, changes in enzyme functions and signaling pathways and alterations in oxidative stress are possible effects of Fe imbalance (Cetin, Berti, Mando, and Parisi 2011). The prevalence of anemia in pregnancy varies considerably worldwide because of differences in socioeconomic conditions, lifestyle, and health-seeking behaviors across different cultures. Anemia affects nearly 52% of pregnant women in developing countries compared with 23% in the developed world.

The large numbers of reproductive-aged women with preexisting anemia, coupled with the elevated iron requirements of pregnancy, make pregnant women particularly vulnerable to iron deficiency anemia.

For this reason, the Centers for Disease Control and Prevention recommends 27 mg/day for all pregnant women. In the last guidelines (2012), the WHO advised supplementation from 30 to 60 mg of elemental Fe per day during pregnancy.

Iron supplementation is recommended to reduce the risk of low birth weight and preterm delivery. However, excessive supplements might expose women to increased oxidative stress, lipid peroxidation, altered glucose metabolism, and pregnancy-induced hypertensive disorders.

11.3.2.1 Iron Placental Transport

Iron required for fetal growth and development is actively transported from the mother to the fetus by the placenta, by complex transport mechanisms (Cetin, Berti, Mando, and Parisi 2011).

Maternal Fe is stored in maternal liver as ferritin; after it is released from ferritin in the maternal serum as Fe^{2+}, iron is oxidized by ceruloplasmin to Fe^{3+} and binds two sites in the transferrin protein (Table 11.2). The diferric transferrin strongly binds the transferrin receptor 1 (TFRC) located in the placental microvillous membrane surface that is internalized into the placental cell endosome via clathrin-coated vesicles (Gambling, Lang, and McArdle 2011). A significant reduction in TFRC gene and protein expression has been shown in human IUGR placentas (Mando et al. 2011). The reduced pH in the endosome leads to the release of iron. The divalent metal transporter-1 is probably involved in iron transport from the endosome to the cell cytoplasm. Iron is consequently transferred outside the cell through the fetal side by ferroportin, and it is immediately oxidized to Fe^{3+} by the copper ferroxidase zyklopen (Zp). Fe^{3+} can be stored by ferritin in the placental stroma, or it can bind transferrin and be transported to the fetal circulation through the endothelium of fetal capillaries by still unknown mechanisms (Gambling, Lang, and McArdle 2011).

Hepcidin is another important protein involved both in inflammation processes and in Fe homeostasis. Up-regulation of maternal hepcidin leads to decreased iron absorption from maternal gut and vice versa. Moreover, iron levels in the fetal liver are related to the expression of maternal liver transferrin receptors and hepcidin, giving rise to fetal control of the mobilization of the mother's iron stores. Furthermore, hepcidin produced by the fetal liver negatively regulates iron placental absorption.

11.3.3 IODINE

Iodine is a chemical element contained in rocks. Rainfall and erosion transport iodine in sea water, where it partially accumulates in seaweed, fish, and shellfish and partially evaporates back into the atmosphere and again on the earth's surface with rain. The amount of iodine existing in edible plants depends on the type of their growing soil, while the amount of iodine in meat depends on animal feeding.

Iodine is essential both for mother and fetus thyroid hormone production and for normal fetal neurodevelopment. During pregnancy, requirements of iodine increase by about 50% for a physiological increase in maternal thyroid hormone production, an increase in renal iodine clearance, and for fetal iodine needs (Perez-Lopez 2007).

Iodine deficiency affects 2 billion people worldwide; thus, the WHO (2004) considers iodine deficiency "the single most important preventable cause of brain damage" worldwide.

Although iodine deficiency afflicts mostly developing countries, industrialized nations are not immune, and even moderate iodine deficiency is becoming a public health problem (Bath, Steer, Golding, Emmett, and Rayman 2013).

The most common method to assess iodine status in pregnant women is the evaluation of urinary iodine concentration because more than 90% of iodine has a kidney excretion. A median urinary iodine concentration of over 150 µg/L is required to define a population that has an adequate iodine intake.

A daily iodine intake of 250 µg for all pregnant and lactating women to avoid deficiency is currently recommended by the WHO (2004).

Hypothyroidism is the first effect of inadequate iodine intake and is primarily responsible for damage to the developing brain and other harmful effects known as "iodine deficiency disorders" (IDDs). IDDs cover a wide spectrum of clinical manifestations ranging from abortion to congenital anomalies, deafness, neurological cretinism (most extreme form), neurocognitive delay, mental retardation, as well as attention deficit hyperactivity disorders (Delange 1994). The severity of neurodevelopmental damage depends on the period affected by this condition and on its severity. The most critical period is from the second trimester of pregnancy to the third year after birth.

In 1994, a joint WHO-UNICEF Commission recommended the use of iodized salt as the best cost-effective strategy to ensure adequate intake of iodine in the population. Iodine supplementation reduces of 73% the incidence of cretinism in severe iodine deficiency areas and increases neurocognitive scores in children of mothers supplemented preconceptionally and until the end of the first trimester (WHO, UNICEF, and ICCIDD 2007).

11.3.3.1 Iodine Placental Transport

The amount of iodine that the fetus receives depends not only on maternal intake but also on the ability of the placenta to carry it to the fetal compartment. Deiodinases D3 and D2, expressed by the placenta, dissociate iodine from maternal thyroxine (Table 11.2). Iodine is taken up by the sodium iodide symporter (NIS) and released to the fetal circulation by pendrin. The up-regulation of NIS has been demonstrated in placental tissues of rats subjected to a low-iodine diet, suggesting the existence of a compensatory system to ensure a normal fetal development (Burns, O'Herlihy, and Smyth 2013).

11.3.4 CALCIUM

Calcium (Ca^{2+}) is a micronutrient contained primarily in milk and dairy products that is essential for fetal bone mineralization. The absorption of Ca^{2+} from foods depends on different factors, such as vitamin D status and the consumption of dietary components that enhance (orange juice) or inhibit (antiacids) Ca^{2+} absorption.

Ca^{2+} ion is an important mineral for fetal development that also acts like a powerful secondary cell messenger. Maternal calcium requirement increases markedly during pregnancy and lactation: the fetal demand ranges from 50 mg/day at midgestation up to 330 mg/day at term. This need could be met through skeleton Ca^{2+} mobilization, increased intestinal absorption efficiency, and enhanced renal Ca^{2+} retention mainly during breastfeeding (Olausson et al. 2012).

Recently, a large prospective cohort study reported that maternal calcium or vitamin D deficiencies able to cause parathyroid hormone (PTH) increases, rather than low calcium intake or insufficient vitamin D alone, has an adverse influence on fetal growth (Scholl, Chen, and Stein 2014).

Nutrition policy and dietary guidelines with respect to Ca^{2+} in pregnancy and lactation differ among countries: the WHO recommends 1.5–2.0 g elemental calcium per day from 20 weeks' gestation until the end of pregnancy for all pregnant women, particularly those at higher risk of gestational hypertension. The IOM recommends 1.0 g/day in adult pregnant women and 1.3 g/day in pregnant adolescents.

Two Cochrane systematic reviews state that calcium supplementation reduces the risk of developing hypertensive disorders (gestational hypertension and preeclampsia) but significantly increases the risk of developing HELLP (hemolysis, elevated liver enzymes, and low platelet count) syndrome. Higher-birth-weight babies, a reduced risk of preterm delivery, and lower infant blood pressure have all been linked with a high calcium intake during pregnancy (Imdad, Jabeen, and Bhutta 2011; Hofmeyr, Lawrie, Atallah, Duley, and Torloni 2014).

11.3.4.1 Calcium Placental Transport

Calcium concentration is lower in syncytiotrophoblast cells, compared with maternal blood, to favor passive and fast transfer of Ca^{2+} across the epithelial layer (Table 11.2). On the basal membrane of the trophoblast layer, a number of pumps and exchangers, such as Ca^{2+}-ATPase and Na^+/Ca^{2+} exchanger, actively extrude calcium into the fetal circulation, so that fetal Ca^{2+} is maintained at a higher level than in maternal serum by active transport across the placenta from approximately 20 weeks' gestation (Forestier, Daffos, Rainaut, Bruneau, and Trivin 1987). In the third trimester, the placenta up-regulates Ca^{2+} transport to promote the increasing demands of the growing fetus.

11.3.5 VITAMIN D

Vitamin D refers to a family of fat-soluble pro hormones that can be synthesized from steroid precursors or introduced by diet. Humans produce vitamin D_3 (cholecalciferol) from skin dehydrocholesterol by means of ultraviolet B light. The predominant form in maternal circulation is $25OHD_3$ obtained from liver hydroxilation of vitamin D_3. Subsequently, $25OHD_3$ is hydroxylated by kidney enzymes in the biologically active form $1,25(OH)_2D_3$.

Vitamin D is well known for its essential role in calcium homeostasis and bone mineralization (Curtis, Moon, Dennison, and Harvey 2014). However, recently, a number of further biological activities have been ascribed to vitamin D, including the regulation of immune function, cell proliferation, differentiation, and gene expression. These actions are mediated through the binding to the vitamin D nuclear receptor (VDR), expressed in many tissues like in placenta, pancreatic b-cells, cardiovascular system, and brain (Shin, Choi, Longtine, and Nelson 2010).

Placenta in particular expresses VDR and several kinds of hydroxilases (Table 11.2). Kidney synthesis of $1,25(OH)_2D$ increases during pregnancy, and its serum concentration is higher in the maternal compared with the fetal circulation, to facilitate the transfer from the mother to the fetus.

Furthermore, decidua and placenta produce a large amount of $1,25(OH)_2D$ by their own enzyme activity (Shin, Choi, Longtine, and Nelson 2010).

In early gestation, vitamin D has an immunomodulatory effect, inhibiting the release of Th1 cytokines and increasing the release of Th2 cytokines to prevent rejection of the implanted embryo (Adams and Hewison 2008).

Vitamin D also acts in an autocrine manner, regulating the secretion of several hormones (human chorionic gonadotropin [hCG], hormone placental lactogen [hPL], estradiol, and progesterone) in syncytiotrophoblast cells (Shin, Choi, Longtine, and Nelson 2010).

Vitamin D deficiency during pregnancy (values below 30 ng/mL) is very common even in sunny countries (Jani, Palekar, Munipally, Ghugre, and Udipi 2014) and is associated with a higher risk for the mother of developing preeclampsia and gestational diabetes mellitus (Robinson, Alanis, Wagner, Hollis, and Johnson 2010). Inadequate intake is also associated with low birth weight, craniotabes, impaired skeletal development in utero, and health problems later in childhood like asthma and schizophrenia (Mulligan, Felton, Riek, and Bernal-Mizrachi 2010; Jani, Palekar, Munipally, Ghugre, and Udipi 2014).

Despite these data, supplementation is not recommended during pregnancy as part of routine antenatal care because of the limited evidence currently available to directly assess the benefits and harms of the use of vitamin D. In cases of documented deficiency, vitamin D supplements may be given at the current reference nutrient intake (RNI) (200 IU) per day as recommended by the WHO/ Food and Agriculture Organization (FAO) or according to national guidelines.

11.3.6 ANTIOXIDANTS

Free radical production is a physiological event; however, when an imbalance occurs between prooxidants and antioxidant capacity, cells become vulnerable to oxidative stress attack.

The human body is able to control free radical activity through specific endogenous (glutathione, ceruloplasmin, and metallothionein) and exogenous (vitamin E, tocopherols, vitamin C, and β-carotene) antioxidants.

Oxidative stress can damage the reproductive system from the earliest stages of development to labor and delivery and has been widely implicated in infertility, miscarriage, congenital malformations, and preeclampsia (Mistry and Williams 2011).

11.3.6.1 Vitamin C and E

Both these vitamins are obtained from the diet. Vitamin E is a tocopherol that protects polyunsaturated fatty acids, the principal constituents of cellular membranes, from auto-oxidation. The major food sources of vitamin E are vegetable oils, such as sunflower oil and olive oil; moreover, almonds, hazelnuts, peanuts, whole grains, and eggs are equally rich, as well as spinach, asparagus, peas, and tomatoes.

Vitamin C or L-ascorbic acid is present mainly in fruits like citrus and pineapple and in vegetables as lettuce and spinach; it acts as a reducing agent protecting against free-radical-induced oxidative damage.

Vitamin C is commonly included in low doses (<200 mg/day) within multivitamin preparations for pregnancy alone or in combination with vitamin E.

Several studies have described elevated markers of oxidative stress in placental tissue from women with preeclampsia and IUGR (Mikhail et al. 1994). Further recent observations suggested that vitamin C and E supplements could prevent or ameliorate preeclampsia (Conde-Agudelo, Romero, Kusanovic, and Hassan 2011). However, although the concentrations of these vitamins are significantly reduced in women with preeclampsia, supplementation in most large randomized clinical trials have failed to show any benefit (Poston et al. 2011).

11.3.6.2 Selenium

Selenium is a trace element that acts primarily as a component of the antioxidant enzyme glutathione peroxidase in preventing the damage caused by free radicals on cell membranes and is also an essential component of the enzyme system (thioredoxin reductases and iodothyronine deionases) that converts thyroxine (T4) to triiodothyronine (T3), playing a prominent role in supporting thyroid function (Rayman 2000). Lastly, selenium seems to play an antagonistic role against heavy metals, such as mercury, cadmium, and silver. Plant foods are the major dietary sources of selenium in most countries.

During pregnancy, maternal selenium concentrations and glutathione peroxidase activity fall (Zachara, Wardak, Didkowski, Maciag, and Marchaluk 1993). Selenium intake recommendations during pregnancy differ worldwide, ranging from 60 µg/day for the IOM to 75 µg/day for the Department of Health.

Selenium is transported across the placenta by passive diffusion under a concentration gradient via an anion exchange pathway shared with sulphate (Table 11.2) (Shennan 1988).

Selenium deficiency has been associated with a number of adverse pregnancy outcomes such as preterm deliveries, miscarriages, and preeclampsia (Mistry, Wilson, Ramsay, Symonds, and Broughton Pipkin 2008). The hypothesis is that selenium deficiency causes reduced activity of glutathione peroxidase and consequently exposes the cell membranes to oxidative damage during placentation and in the early stages of embryonic development.

To date, only a small number of selenium supplementation trials during pregnancy have been carried out, and results on the effect of optimization of selenium status in women at risk of adverse pregnancy outcomes are still controversial.

11.3.6.3 Zinc

Zinc is a key element essential for the synthesis of a great number of enzymes. Zinc has antioxidant activities and is involved in carbohydrate and protein metabolism, nucleic acid synthesis, cellular division, and differentiation. Consequently, zinc plays a crucial role during embryogenesis, fetal growth, and development. The WHO estimated in 2002 that suboptimal zinc nutrition affects nearly half the world's population.

During pregnancy, zinc requirement increases, and in the third trimester, it is approximately doubled compared with that for nonpregnant women (Izquierdo Alvarez et al. 2007). Depending on zinc bioavailability in the habitual diet of the pregnant woman, about 2 to 4 mg of additional dietary zinc is needed daily to meet these additional needs. Studies have shown that the fetus has notably higher zinc concentrations compared with the mother, but the specific mechanism of placental zinc transport is unknown; it probably involves placental zinc transporters and metallothionein (Donangelo and King 2012).

Subadequate maternal zinc intakes may affect pregnancy outcomes, including prolonged labor, fetal growth restriction, embryonic or fetal death, and infant development. In developing countries, where zinc deficiency is severe, maternal zinc supplementation seems to positively correlate with birth weights and reduced incidence of pregnancy-induced hypertension. On the contrary, in developed countries, zinc supplementation has consistently shown limited benefits (Donangelo and King 2012; Mori et al. 2012).

11.3.6.4 Copper

Despite copper being present in very small amounts in the human body, it is an essential element for several physiological functions. Copper acts primarily as a cofactor for many enzymes functioning as antioxidants and as oxido-reductases; it is also present in ceruloplasmin, which catalyzes the conversion of ferric ion to its ferrous form and promotes the absorption of iron from the gastrointestinal tract (Izquierdo Alvarez et al. 2007). It has been involved in connective tissue formation, iron metabolism, cardiac function, immune function, and central nervous system development. The richest dietary sources of copper include shellfish, nuts, seeds, legumes, grains' bran and germ, liver, and organ meats.

Copper deficiency is rare, and a number of studies have shown that copper concentration progressively rises during pregnancy, being associated with increases in blood estrogens, increased synthesis of ceruloplasmin, and decreased biliary excretion (McArdle, Andersen, Jones, and Gambling 2008). These evidences led to the recommendation by the IOM that copper supplementation should not be undertaken during normal pregnancy.

Maternal severe copper deficiency, occurring in developing countries, can result in short-term consequences like miscarriage, structural abnormalities, and low birth weight and long-term consequences such as elevated risk of cardiovascular disease and reduced fertility. Further evidence showed lower level of copper in preeclamptic patients when compared with control subjects (Sarwar et al. 2013).

Copper is transferred across the placenta by a copper transporter expressed early in pregnancy. Placental copper transport is also related to iron transport, but the specific mechanism is still unclear (Gambling et al. 2003; McArdle, Andersen, Jones, and Gambling 2008). Iron supplementation in pregnant women has been shown to significantly reduce serum copper concentrations; moreover, anemic pregnant women have higher serum copper concentrations compared with nonanemic ones. These data support the hypothesis that iron has the ability to decrease copper concentrations and/or to limit its bioavailability in pregnancy.

11.4 MULTIPLE-MICRONUTRIENT SUPPLEMENTATION

Maternal anemia is a widespread problem. For this reason, the WHO strongly recommends daily oral iron and folic acid supplementation as part of antenatal care to reduce the risk of low birth weight and maternal anemia and improve pregnancy outcomes. However, in low- and middle-income countries, pregnant women are affected by several micronutrient deficiencies, and they could benefit from multiple micronutrient supplementation. A recent Cochrane review reported that multiple-micronutrient supplementation reduced the number of low-birth-weight and small-for-gestational age babies when compared with iron-folate supplements (Haider and Bhutta 2012). Despite these proven benefits, more evidence is needed to guide a universal policy change and to suggest replacement of routine iron and folate supplementation with a multiple-micronutrient advice.

In industrialized countries, although a balanced diet is generally accessible, a switch to a high-fat and low-quality diet has led to inadequate vitamin and mineral intake during pregnancy. Recent data show that micronutrient intake is lower than recommended, in particular for iron, folate, calcium, and vitamin D (Haider and Bhutta 2012; Blumfield, Hure, Macdonald-Wicks, Smith, and Collins 2013). These data are, however, insufficient to support a routine multiple supplementation but underline the importance of an individualized approach to recognize nutritional deficiencies of individuals, thus leading to healthful dietary practices before conception and, eventually, to a targeted supplementation.

11.5 CONCLUSIONS

As attested by evidence reported both for macronutrient and micronutrient unbalanced intake, maternal nutrition is clearly able to influence individual health even before birth. A healthy, balanced maternal diet before conception reduces the risk of complications during pregnancy and later in life. While undernutrition is an issue mainly of developing countries, malnutrition is becoming a global problem. The role of micronutrients is particularly relevant in determining the formation of a normal placenta at the beginning of pregnancy and is fundamental later on in the developing fetus. The regulation of placental transport of micronutrients is only partially known and needs further research. Spreading awareness of the importance of maternal nutrition before and during pregnancy and stimulating a cultural change in favor of a balanced healthy diet and high-quality food consumption are necessary for improving future global health. Looking forward to these significant changes, single or multiple micronutrient supplementation, together with food fortification, remains the only effective strategy.

REFERENCES

Adams, J. S. and M. Hewison (2008). "Unexpected actions of vitamin D: New perspectives on the regulation of innate and adaptive immunity." *Nat Clin Pract Endocrinol Metab* 4(2): 80–90.

Allen, L. H. (2000). "Anemia and iron deficiency: Effects on pregnancy outcome." *Am J Clin Nutr* 71(5 Suppl): 1280S–1284S.

Barker, D. J., P. D. Gluckman, K. M. Godfrey, J. E. Harding, J. A. Owens, and J. S. Robinson (1993). "Fetal nutrition and cardiovascular disease in adult life." *Lancet* 341(8850): 938–941.

Bath, S. C., C. D. Steer, J. Golding, P. Emmett, and M. P. Rayman (2013). "Effect of inadequate iodine status in UK pregnant women on cognitive outcomes in their children: Results from the Avon Longitudinal Study of Parents and Children (ALSPAC)." *Lancet* 382(9889): 331–337.

Blumfield, M. L., A. J. Hure, L. Macdonald-Wicks, R. Smith, and C. E. Collins (2013). "A systematic review and meta-analysis of micronutrient intakes during pregnancy in developed countries." *Nutr Rev* 71(2): 118–132.

Bothwell, T. H. (2000). "Iron requirements in pregnancy and strategies to meet them." *Am J Clin Nutr* 72(1 Suppl): 257S–264S.

Burdge, G. C. and K. A. Lillycrop (2012). "Folic acid supplementation in pregnancy: Are there devils in the detail?" *Br J Nutr* 108(11): 1924–1930.

Burns, R., C. O'Herlihy, and P. P. Smyth (2013). "Regulation of iodide uptake in placental primary cultures." *Eur Thyroid J* 2(4): 243–251.

Calabrese, S. and C. Mandò (2014). "Placental biometry in male and female fetuses of obese and normal weight women." *Reprod Sci* 21: 71A–418A.

Cetin, I., C. Berti, and S. Calabrese (2010). "Role of micronutrients in periconceptional period." *Hum Reprod Update* 216(1): 80–95.

Cetin, I., C. Berti, C. Mando, and F. Parisi (2011). "Placental iron transport and maternal absorption." *Ann Nutr Metab* 59(1): 55–58.

Conde-Agudelo, A., R. Romero, J. P. Kusanovic, and S. S. Hassan (2011). "Supplementation with vitamins C and E during pregnancy for the prevention of preeclampsia and other adverse maternal and perinatal outcomes: A systematic review and metaanalysis." *Am J Obstet Gynecol* 204(6): 503.e501–e512.

Curtis, E. M., R. J. Moon, E. M. Dennison, and N. C. Harvey (2014). "Prenatal calcium and vitamin D intake, and bone mass in later life." *Curr Osteoporos Rep* 12(2): 194–204.

Daly, L. E., P. N. Kirke, A. Molloy, D. G. Weir, and J. M. Scott (1995). "Folate levels and neural tube defects. Implications for prevention." *JAMA* 274(21): 1698–1702.

Delange, F. (1994). "The disorders induced by iodine deficiency." *Thyroid* 4(1): 107–128.

Donangelo, C. M. and J. C. King (2012). "Maternal zinc intakes and homeostatic adjustments during pregnancy and lactation." *Nutrients* 4(7): 782–798.

Englund-Ogge, L., A. L. Brantsaeter, V. Sengpiel, M. Haugen, B. E. Birgisdottir, R. Myhre, H. M. Meltzer, and B. Jacobsson (2014). "Maternal dietary patterns and preterm delivery: Results from large prospective cohort study." *BMJ* 348: g1446.

Forestier, F., F. Daffos, M. Rainaut, M. Bruneau, and F. Trivin (1987). "Blood chemistry of normal human fetuses at midtrimester of pregnancy." *Pediatr Res* 21(6): 579–583.

Gambling, L., S. Dunford, D. I. Wallace, G. Zuur, N. Solanky, S. K. Srai, and H. J. McArdle (2003). "Iron deficiency during pregnancy affects postnatal blood pressure in the rat." *J Physiol* 552(Pt 2): 603–610.

Gambling, L., C. Lang, and H. J. McArdle (2011). "Fetal regulation of iron transport during pregnancy." *Am J Clin Nutr* 94(6 Suppl): 1903S–1907S.

Godfrey, K. M. and D. J. Barker (1995). "Maternal nutrition in relation to fetal and placental growth." *Eur J Obstet Gynecol Reprod Biol* 61(1): 15–22.

Haider, B. A. and Z. A. Bhutta (2012). "Multiple-micronutrient supplementation for women during pregnancy." *Cochrane Database Syst Rev* 11: CD004905.

Hillesund, E. R., N. C. Overby, S. M. Engel, K. Klungsoyr, Q. E. Harmon, M. Haugen, and E. Bere (2014). "Associations of adherence to the New Nordic Diet with risk of preeclampsia and preterm delivery in the Norwegian Mother and Child Cohort Study (MoBa)." *Eur J Epidemiol* 29(10): 753–765.

Hofmeyr, G. J., T. A. Lawrie, A. N. Atallah, L. Duley, and M. R. Torloni (2014). "Calcium supplementation during pregnancy for preventing hypertensive disorders and related problems." *Cochrane Database Syst Rev* 6: CD001059.

Imdad, A., A. Jabeen, and Z. A. Bhutta (2011). "Role of calcium supplementation during pregnancy in reducing risk of developing gestational hypertensive disorders: A meta-analysis of studies from developing countries." *BMC Public Health* 11 Suppl 3: S18.

Izquierdo Alvarez, S., S. G. Castanon, M. L. Ruata, E. F. Aragues, P. B. Terraz, Y. G. Irazabal, E. G. Gonzalez, and B. G. Rodriguez (2007). "Updating of normal levels of copper, zinc and selenium in serum of pregnant women." *J Trace Elem Med Biol* 21 Suppl 1: 49–52.

Jani, R., S. Palekar, T. Munipally, P. Ghugre, and S. Udipi (2014). "Widespread 25-hydroxyvitamin D deficiency in affluent and nonaffluent pregnant Indian women." *Biomed Res Int* 2014: 892162.

Kidanto, H. L., I. Mogren, G. Lindmark, S. Massawe, and L. Nystrom (2009). "Risks for preterm delivery and low birth weight are independently increased by severity of maternal anaemia." *S Afr Med J* 99(2): 98–102.

Linnè, Y. (2004). "Effects of obesity on women's reproduction and complication during pregnancy" *Obes Rev.* 5(3): 137–143.

Malhotra, M., J. B. Sharma, S. Batra, S. Sharma, N. S. Murthy, and R. Arora (2002). "Maternal and perinatal outcome in varying degrees of anemia." *Int J Gynaecol Obstet* 79(2): 93–100.

Mando, C., S. Tabano, P. Colapietro, P. Pileri, F. Colleoni, L. Avagliano, P. Doi, G. Bulfamante, M. Miozzo, and I. Cetin (2011). "Transferrin receptor gene and protein expression and localization in human IUGR and normal term placentas." *Placenta* 32(1): 44–50.

McArdle, H. J., H. S. Andersen, H. Jones, and L. Gambling (2008). "Copper and iron transport across the placenta: Regulation and interactions." *J Neuroendocrinol* 20(4): 427–431.

Mikhail, M. S., A. Anyaegbunam, D. Garfinkel, P. R. Palan, J. Basu, and S. L. Romney (1994). "Preeclampsia and antioxidant nutrients: Decreased plasma levels of reduced ascorbic acid, alpha-tocopherol, and beta-carotene in women with preeclampsia." *Am J Obstet Gynecol* 171(1): 150–157.

Mistry, H. D. and P. J. Williams (2011). "The importance of antioxidant micronutrients in pregnancy." *Oxid Med Cell Longev* 2011: 841749.

Mistry, H. D., V. Wilson, M. M. Ramsay, M. E. Symonds, and F. Broughton Pipkin (2008). "Reduced selenium concentrations and glutathione peroxidase activity in preeclamptic pregnancies." *Hypertension* 52(5): 881–888.

Mori, R., E. Ota, P. Middleton, R. Tobe-Gai, K. Mahomed, and Z. A. Bhutta (2012). "Zinc supplementation for improving pregnancy and infant outcome." *Cochrane Database Syst Rev* 7: CD000230.

Mulligan, M. L., S. K. Felton, A. E. Riek, and C. Bernal-Mizrachi (2010). "Implications of vitamin D deficiency in pregnancy and lactation." *Am J Obstet Gynecol* 202(5): 429.e421–e429.

Olausson, H., G. R. Goldberg, M. A. Laskey, I. Schoenmakers, L. M. Jarjou, and A. Prentice (2012). "Calcium economy in human pregnancy and lactation." *Nutr Res Rev* 25(1): 40–67.

Perez-Lopez, F. R. (2007). "Iodine and thyroid hormones during pregnancy and postpartum." *Gynecol Endocrinol* 23(7): 414–428.

Poston, L., N. Igosheva, H. D. Mistry, P. T. Seed, A. H. Shennan, S. Rana, S. A. Karumanchi, and L. C. Chappell (2011). "Role of oxidative stress and antioxidant supplementation in pregnancy disorders." *Am J Clin Nutr* 94(6 Suppl): 1980S–1985S.

Rasmussen, K. M. and A. L. Yaktine, ed. (2009). *Weight Gain During Pregnancy: Reexamining the Guidelines.* National Academies Press, Washington, DC, 324 pp.

Rayman, M. P. (2000). "The importance of selenium to human health." *Lancet* 356(9225): 233–241.

Robinson, C. J., M. C. Alanis, C. L. Wagner, B. W. Hollis, and D. D. Johnson (2010). "Plasma 25-hydroxyvitamin D levels in early-onset severe preeclampsia." *Am J Obstet Gynecol* 203(4): 366.e361–e366.

Roseboom, T., S. de Rooij, and R. Painter (2006). "The Dutch famine and its long-term consequences for adult health." *Early Hum Dev* 82(8): 485–491.

Roseboom, T. J., R. C. Painter, S. R. de Rooij, A. F. van Abeelen, M. V. Veenendaal, C. Osmond, and D. J. Barker (2011). "Effects of famine on placental size and efficiency." *Placenta* 32(5): 395–399.

Ruager-Martin, R., M. J. Hyde, and N. Modi (2010). "Maternal obesity and infant outcomes." *Early Hum Dev* 86(11): 715–722.

Sarwar, M. S., S. Ahmed, M. S. Ullah, H. Kabir, G. K. Rahman, A. Hasnat, and M. S. Islam (2013). "Comparative study of serum zinc, copper, manganese, and iron in preeclamptic pregnant women." *Biol Trace Elem Res* 154(1): 14–20.

Scholl, T. O., X. Chen, and T. P. Stein (2014). "Maternal calcium metabolic stress and fetal growth." *Am J Clin Nutr* 99(4): 918–925.

Shennan, D. B. (1988). "Selenium (selenate) transport by human placental brush border membrane vesicles." *Br J Nutr* 59(1): 13–19.

Shin, J. S., M. Y. Choi, M. S. Longtine, and D. M. Nelson (2010). "Vitamin D effects on pregnancy and the placenta." *Placenta* 31(12): 1027–1034.

Solanky, N., A. Requena Jimenez, S. W. D'Souza, C. P. Sibley, and J. D. Glazier (2010). "Expression of folate transporters in human placenta and implications for homocysteine metabolism." *Placenta* 31(2): 134–143.

Szostak-Wegierek, D. (2014). "Intrauterine nutrition: Long-term consequences for vascular health." *Int J Womens Health* 6: 647–656.

Tilman, D. and M. Clark (2014). "Global diets link environmental sustainability and human health." *Nature* 515(7528): 518–522.

WHO, UNICEF, and ICCIDD (2007). *Assessment of Iodine Deficiency Disorders and Monitoring Their Elimination*, 3rd edn. Geneva: World Health Organisation.

Williams, P. J., J. N. Bulmer, B. A. Innes, and F. Broughton Pipkin (2011). "Possible roles for folic acid in the regulation of trophoblast invasion and placental development in normal early human pregnancy." *Biol Reprod* 84(6): 1148–1153.

World Health Organization (WHO) (2004). *World Health Organisation Global Database on Iodine Deficiency.* Iodine Status Worldwide. Geneva: World Health Organization.

Zachara, B. A., C. Wardak, W. Didkowski, A. Maciag, and E. Marchaluk (1993). "Changes in blood selenium and glutathione concentrations and glutathione peroxidase activity in human pregnancy." *Gynecol Obstet Invest* 35(1): 12–17.

Zimmermann, M. B. and R. F. Hurrell (2007). "Nutritional iron deficiency." *Lancet* 370(9586): 511–520.

12 Folic Acid Uptake and Its Regulation in the Placenta

Elisa Keating, João R. Araújo, and Fátima Martel

CONTENTS

ABSTRACT

Folates are crucial nutrients to the developing fetus, and being nutritionally essential, they must be obtained from the maternal blood through placental transport. The strict importance of folates to fetal and pregnancy health is well demonstrated by the fact that an inverse relationship is known to exist between folate status in pregnancy and the risk of neural tube defects. However, given the present policies of folate supplementation during pregnancy, there is an actual concern on the possible implications of excessive exposure to folates during pregnancy for the future health.

The placental transport of folates is a complex process involving three different transport systems (folate receptor α, reduced folate carrier 1, and proton-coupled folate transporter) functioning in a coordinate manner to ensure the vectorial transfer of folates from maternal to fetal circulation. Current and emerging research on the molecular mechanisms of placental transport of folates and its regulation support the conclusion that the placental transport of folates may be compromised by several dietary substances, therapeutic agents, drugs of abuse, and markers of pathological conditions, which may in turn threaten, to some degree, the normal development and growth of the fetus.

KEY WORDS

Folates, placenta, transport, modulation, folate receptor α, reduced folate carrier, proton-coupled folate transporter.

12.1 FOLATE IN PREGNANCY: RELEVANCE, POLICY, AND IMPLICATIONS IN FUTURE HEALTH

12.1.1 FOLATE STRUCTURE AND METABOLISM

Folate is the generic term used to designate a family of hydrosoluble B vitamins that comprises folic acid (FA; pteroyl-L-monoglutamic acid), as well as the naturally occurring reduced folates (Figure 12.1) (Office of Dietary Supplements 2012). Folate structure comprises a pteridine ring and a p-aminobenzoate moiety, which is linked through an amide bond to up to eight glutamate residues (Figure 12.1).

FA is the synthetic, fully oxidized structure that contains only one glutamate residue. It is not encountered in nature, but given its low price and greater chemical stability when compared with reduced folates, it is the form used in food fortification and in vitamin pills. Moreover, its bioavailability is greater than that of reduced folates because, in contrast to the polyglutaminated naturally occurring folates, it is attached to only one glutamate residue, which enhances its rate of intestinal absorption (Winkels et al. 2007). As such, in countries with implemented policies for FA food fortification, flour-containing staple foods, such as bread, pastas, as well as breakfast cereals, and other grain products are rich sources of synthetic FA.

Reduced folates, the bioactive coenzyme members of the folate family, include dihydrofolate and tetrahydrofolates carrying one-carbon units such as 5-methyl-tetrahydrofolate (5-MTHF), formyl-tetrahydrofolates (5-formyl-tetrahydrofolate [5-FTHF] and 10-formyltetrahydrofolate [10-FTHF]), and 5,10-methylene-tetrahydrofolate (Figure 12.1). Of these, polyglutaminated 5-MTHF and FTHFs are the most abundant forms naturally found in food (Jagerstad and Jastrebova 2013; Lucock 2000). Dark green leafy vegetables, specially spinach and Brussels sprouts, liver, yeast, and asparagus are rich sources of reduced folates (Office of Dietary Supplements 2012).

Folates, after ingestion as polyglutamates, are hydrolysed by γ-glutamyl hydrolase in the intestine and absorbed and systemically delivered as monoglutamates (Ohrvik and Witthoft 2011). After entering the cells by a transporter-mediated process (see Section 12.2), folates are sequentially conjugated with glutamate units by folylpolyglutamate synthase, forming folylpolyglutamates (Assaraf 2006; Lucock 2000), such as 5-methyl-tetrahydrofolate polyglutamate (Figure 12.2). This mechanism is responsible for the cellular retention and accumulation of folates because (a) polyglutamates cannot cross lipid bilayers, (b) polyglutamination ensures the formation of a downhill concentration gradient for folates, and (c) folates conjugated with four or more glutamate residues are no longer recognized by folate transport systems (Assaraf 2006).

Physiologically, folates are critical for (a) the metabolism of amino acids such as serine, glycine, and methionine, (b) the synthesis of S-adenosyl methionine (SAM), a major cellular methyl donor and substrate of DNA methyltransferases (Dnmts), and (c) the synthesis of purines and thymidylate (Figure 12.2). As such, cellular folate retention and availability affect cellular methylation reactions, including DNA methylation (and thus epigenetic regulation of gene expression) and is also critical for the provision of the building blocks of DNA that will enable normal cell division.

12.1.2 FOLATE AND PREGNANCY OUTCOME: FOCUS ON NEURAL TUBE DEFECTS

Given the above-referred cellular functions of folate, it is not surprising that folate requirements increase in stages of life such as pregnancy and child development and growth, which are known to be associated with increased rates of cell division. Indeed, folate deficiency, one of the most prevalent vitamin deficiencies in the Western world, may precipitate in pregnancy and manifest as megaloblastic anemia, with obvious implications in pregnancy outcome (Molloy et al. 2008). Besides megaloblastic anemia, the important role played by folate during pregnancy is made evident by the inverse relationship known to exist between folate status in pregnancy and the risk of neural tube defects (NTDs).

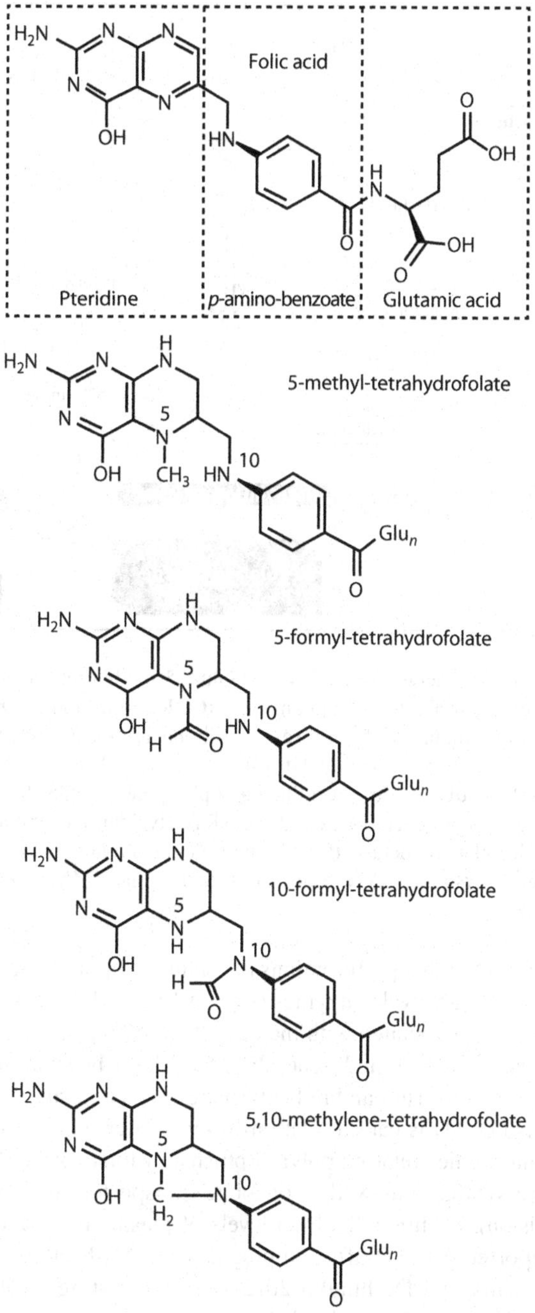

FIGURE 12.1 Chemical structures of folic acid (FA), 5-methyl-tetrahydrofolate (5-MTHF), 5-formyl-tetrahydrofolate (5-FTHF), 10-formyl-tetrahydrofolate (10-FTHF), and 5,10-methylene-tetrahydrofolate.

NTDs are among the most prevalent congenital anomalies worldwide, affecting 1 in 1000 live births (Denny et al. 2013). They arise from defects in the process of neural tube formation (neurulation), which occurs early during the fourth week of pregnancy and that will give rise to the brain and spinal cord of the baby (Czeizel et al. 2013). During neurulation, neural tube may fail to close in its anterior region, resulting in anencephaly, or in its posterior region, resulting in spina bifida (Denny

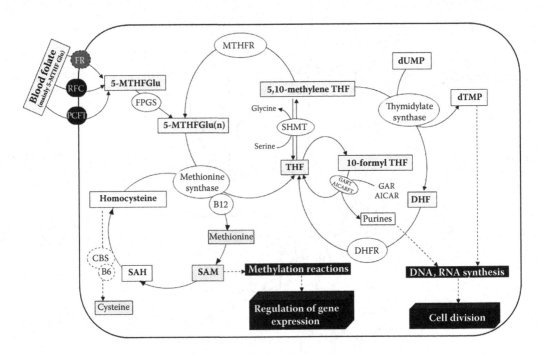

FIGURE 12.2 Cellular folate metabolism. 5-MTHFGlu, 5-methyl-tetrahydrofolate monoglutamate; 5-MTHFGlu(n), 5-methyl-tetrahydrofolate polyglutamate; AICAR, 5-aminoimidazole-4-carboxamide ribonucleotide; AICARFT, 5-aminoimidazole-4-carboxamide ribonucleotide transformylase; B6, vitamin B_6; B12, vitamin B_{12}; CBS, cystathionine b-synthase; DHF, dihydrofolate; DHFR, dihydrofolate reductase; dTMP, deoxythymidine monophosphate; dUMP, deoxyuridine monophosphate; FPGS, folylpolyglutamate synthase; FR, folate receptor; GAR, glycinamide ribonucleotide; GART, glycinamide ribonucleotide transformylase; MTHFR, methylenetetrahydrofolate reductase; PCFT, proton-coupled folate transporter; RFC, reduced folate carrier; SAH, *S*-adenosyl homocysteine; SAM, *S*-adenosyl methionine; SHMT, serine hydroxymethyltransferase; THF, tetrahydrofolate.

et al. 2013). It is widely accepted that perturbations of folate metabolism, resulting from folate deficiency or polymorphisms in folate cycle enzymes (Figure 12.2), which normally precipitate a state of hyperhomocysteinemia, are associated with increased risk of NTDs.

In the 1970s, Smithells, Sheppard, and Schorah (1976) described that mothers giving birth to NTD-affected infants had lower serum and red cell folate levels and suggested folate deficiency as an etiological factor for NTDs. This causal relationship was later reinforced by Daly et al. (1995). There are also innumerous studies relating polymorphisms of folate cycle enzymes (e.g., 5-MTHF reductase and methionine synthase) as well as of folate transporters with NTDs (see Tamura and Picciano 2006 for a revision). Additionally, high levels of plasma or amniotic fluid homocysteine have recurrently been reported in NTD-affected pregnancies (Mills et al. 1995; Ratan et al. 2008; Wenstrom et al. 2000; Yajnik and Deshmukh 2012), also suggesting a causal effect of hyperhomocysteinemia in NTDs. However, it should also be noted that an important amount of scientific data questions this *folate dysmetabolism hypothesis* for the etiology of NTDs, as several authors have reported that women with an NTD-affected pregnancy do not have signs of folate deficiency (Denny et al. 2013; Yajnik and Deshmukh 2012) and that many polymorphisms of folate cycle enzymes or of folate transporters do not associate with folate deficiency (Denny et al. 2013) or with NTDs (Wallingford et al. 2013; Yajnik and Deshmukh 2012). Despite this still unsolved paradox, it is nowadays consensual that supplementation of maternal diet with FA decreases the incidence of NTDs (De-Regil et al. 2010; Wolff et al. 2009).

The first striking demonstration of the protective effect of FA supplementation on NTDs was made in 1991, with a randomized clinical trial that included 1817 high-risk (with a previous

NTD-affected pregnancy) women (MRC 1991). In this study, daily administration of 4 mg FA was demonstrated to exert a 72% protective effect in NTD recurrence. Shortly after, in 1992, Czeizel and Dudas (1992) conducted another randomized trial involving 4753 women and showed that periconceptional clinical administration of a multivitamin supplement containing FA (0.8 mg/day) reduced the incidence of first occurrence of NTDs. This is in fact a clear demonstration of folate's relevance for pregnancy health, posing this vitamin more as a corrective rather than as an etiologic factor in NTDs, as wisely suggested by Denny et al. (2013).

Additionally, supplementation with FA has been described to prevent other poor pregnancy outcomes such as small-for-gestational age newborns (Hodgetts et al. 2014; Kim et al. 2014), preterm birth (Bukowski et al. 2009; Mantovani et al. 2014), preeclampsia (Kim et al. 2014), acute lymphoblastic leukemia, and acute myeloid leukemia (Metayer et al. 2014). Reinforcing this, low folate levels late in pregnancy are associated with increased risk of preterm birth (Siega-Riz et al. 2004). Importantly, the relationship between FA supplementation and the risk of preeclampsia is about to be further explored in a trial with more than 3500 women with increased risk of preeclampsia (Wen et al. 2013).

While there is strong and growing scientific evidence that folate plays an essential role in pregnancy health, it is also true that some studies have failed to prove its protective effects against specific pregnancy outcomes (e.g., Sengpiel et al. 2014; Vollset et al. 2013). Controversy in this field is most probably related with the variability in the period of FA administration and the dose administered or ingested among observational studies. Indeed, guidelines for the timing of pregnancy and dose of FA administration vary not only with the country but also with the hospital where the recruitment is performed. Also important, the molecular mechanisms underlying the protective effects of this vitamin are still largely unknown and await further investigation.

12.1.3 Folate Policy and Concerns

In the late 1990s, shortly after the publication of the randomized clinical trials demonstrating that FA administration was effective in preventing NTDs recurrence (MRC 1991) and occurrence (Czeizel and Dudas 1992), the Food and Drug Administration mandated the fortification of all grain products with FA in the United States. Knowledge that a very low compliance to FA supplementation by women expecting a pregnancy existed was also an important incitement to the implementation of this policy. After this implementation, FA fortification of food was demonstrated to associate negatively with the prevalence of NTDs (Honein et al. 2001) and to produce a general increase in serum folate levels (with concomitant decrease in homocysteine levels) in a US representative population sample (Pfeiffer et al. 2005).

Ten years later, in 2009, 52 countries worldwide had also implemented mandatory fortification of food with FA. At that time, several European Union countries permitted voluntary fortification, although none had implemented mandatory fortification (Reilly et al. 2009), given the uncertainty about potential health hazards.

At present, the World Health Organization (2012) recommends providing a daily supplementation with 400 μg FA to women throughout pregnancy. However, given the globalization of these public nutrition policies and the lack of knowledge about the side effects of high FA exposure, there is the concern that FA intake may be exceeding the recommended upper levels, as already demonstrated (Bailey et al. 2010; Hoyo et al. 2011), with a consequent increase in folate blood levels (Brown et al. 2011) with possible health implications.

The fact that the long-term effects of exposure to high doses of FA are still largely unexplored makes the concern even more severe. Several studies report this serious concern, much of them referring that the risks may be particularly associated to the amount of unmetabolized synthetic FA that may accumulate in blood (Lucock and Yates 2009; Sauer, Mason, and Choi 2009; Ulrich and Potter 2006). In fact, FA is easily metabolized in human body to 5-MTHF, but this process is saturated at doses near 400 μg (Kelly et al. 1997). At higher doses, synthetic FA may indeed accumulate in blood or in organs and exert deleterious effects.

One of the deleterious effects of excess FA relates to cancer, a disease in which FA plays a dual role. Indeed, on one hand, it prevents the development of early neoplastic lesions, thereby exerting a protective effect; on the other hand, it increases the progression of established neoplasms, thereby increasing cancer incidence (Ulrich and Potter 2006). Thus, excessive FA ingestion may increase the incidence of cancer, as demonstrated in several studies in which a positive association was found between FA blood levels and breast (Charles et al. 2004; Stolzenberg-Solomon et al. 2006) or colorectal (Hirsch et al. 2009; Mason et al. 2007) cancer risk. Nevertheless, one meta-analysis recently concluded that FA supplementation did not modulate (increase or decrease) site-specific cancer incidence during the first 5 years of supplementation (Vollset et al. 2013).

12.1.4 FOLATE AND FETAL PROGRAMMING: FOCUS ON METABOLIC HEALTH

The Barker hypothesis states that adverse influences early in development, particularly during intra-uterine life, can result in permanent changes in physiology and metabolism, resulting in increased disease risk in adulthood (Barker and Osmond 1986). The succeeding fetal programming hypothesis proposes that environmental and nutritional stimuli acting during early life induce changes in DNA methylation that will adversely and permanently affect health in later life (Burdge and Lillycrop 2010).

Folates are recognized as important players in fetal programming (Kim, Friso, and Choi 2009) as they enable the production of SAM (Figure 12.2), a major substrate of Dnmts, the enzymes that catalyze DNA methylation reactions. Indeed, a direct role of folate in placental DNA methylation has been demonstrated (Kim et al. 2009).

Many animal studies have clearly shown that methyl-rich diets can restore "healthy" epigeno-types. As such, there is now a good amount of scientific work on the programming effects of mater-nal FA supplementation over the offspring's health, with a focus on autism (Castro et al. 2014), asthma, cancer, and insulin resistance (see Burdge and Lillycrop 2012 for a review). For instance, Cooney, Dave, and Wolff (2002) demonstrated in the agouti mouse model that maternal methyl supplements, including FA, increased DNA methylation in the A^{vy} allele, inducing in the progeny a change in coat color and a decrease in the propensity to develop obesity and diabetes. Also, FA supplementation during pregnancy has been demonstrated to prevent cardiovascular dysfunction (Torrens et al. 2006) and altered feeding behavior (Engeham, Haase, and Langley-Evans 2010) in the offspring of mothers exposed to protein restriction.

However, some recent studies have investigated the putative relationship between FA supple-mentation and the development of metabolic syndrome (MetS) later in life. MetS comprises a constellation of risk factors, such as central obesity, glucose intolerance, insulin resistance, dyslip-idemia, and hypertension, for cardiovascular disease and type 2 diabetes. It is highly and increas-ingly prevalent, and it is suggested to be determined during fetal development due to nutritional, hormonal, or metabolic inputs from the mother (Sinclair et al. 2007; Xita and Tsatsoulis 2010). Specifically, Yajnik and coworkers studied the relationship between folate and fetal programming of metabolic dysfunction in human subjects, and they have shown that high maternal erythrocyte folate concentrations were associated with higher adiposity and higher insulin resistance in the offspring (Krishnaveni et al. 2014; Yajnik et al. 2008). These findings were corroborated by two very recent animal studies. In one of these studies, it was shown that supplementation of the diet of pregnant mice with high FA doses (corresponding to 20 times the recommended dose for pregnancy) worsens the metabolic response to a high-fat diet stimulus in adult offspring (Huang et al. 2014). In the other study, using the same high dose of FA as Huang's work, our group dem-onstrated that perigestational exposure of dams to high FA worsens the metabolic phenotype of female offspring, predisposing them to an insulin resistant state and rendering them more sus-ceptible to dysmetabolism after fructose feeding (Keating et al. 2015). Importantly, it was also apparent that high FA exposure was able to induce later-in-life dysmetabolism in exposed mothers (Keating et al. 2015).

Thus, we truly believe that a U-shaped curve describes the relationship between the effect of FA exposure in early stages of development and health. As such, further research is needed to find a safe upper dose of FA.

12.2 FOLATE PLACENTAL TRANSPORT

The human placenta is a specialized organ of fetal origin that performs the exchange of nutrients and metabolic waste between maternal and fetal blood, synthesizes peptide and steroid hormones, and protects the fetus from immunological rejection. Good development of the placenta is critical for normal fetal growth and development and for maintenance of a healthy pregnancy.

The syncytiotrophoblast (STB), the functional unit of the placenta, is a polarized structure composed of a brush border membrane (BBM) with numerous microvilli, which greatly increase its surface area and directly contacts maternal blood, and a basal membrane (BM) that faces fetal circulation (Figure 12.3). As a highly differentiated epithelium, the STB is able to mediate and to regulate the transport of nutrients and gases from maternal to fetal blood and to clear waste metabolites from fetal blood. As such, the STB constitutes the rate-limiting barrier for permeation across the placenta (Audus 1999), and a complex network of membrane transporters, which are differentially distributed on the BBM and the BM of the STB, elicits the vectorial transcellular transport of substances (e.g., macronutrients and vitamins) between maternal and fetal circulations.

Neither the placenta nor the fetus is able to synthesize folates, so this vitamin must be obtained from the maternal circulation through placental transport (Giugliani, Jorge, and Gonçalves 1985; Hutson et al. 2012). The human placenta expresses three folate transport systems that act coordinately to ensure the vectorial transfer of folates from maternal to fetal circulation (Keating, Gonçalves, Campos et al. 2009; Solanky et al. 2010; Zhao, Matherly, and Goldman 2009). These transporters, which are not exclusive

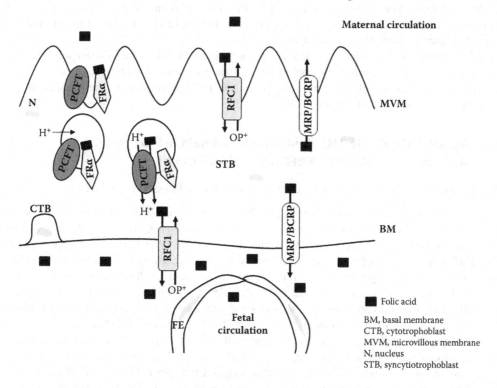

FIGURE 12.3 Main folic acid transporters present at the human syncytiotrophoblast. BCRP, breast cancer resistance protein; FE, fetal endothelium; FRα, folate receptor α; MRP, multidrug resistance-associated protein; PCFT, proton-coupled folate transporter; RFC1, reduced folate carrier 1.

to the placenta rather having a wide tissue distribution, are the reduced folate carrier (RFC1), the alpha isoform of the folate receptor (FRα), and the proton-coupled folate transporter (PCFT) (Figure 12.3).

RFC1 is a folate:organic phosphate exchanger that utilizes the transmembrane organic phosphate gradient to mediate transport of folates into cells against their concentration gradients (Zhao, Matherly, and Goldman 2009; Zhao et al. 2011). This bidirectional transporter is expressed in both microvillous membrane (MVM) and BM of the STB (Solanky et al. 2010) (Figure 12.3) and has a maximal activity at physiological pH and a higher affinity for reduced folates (such as 5-MTHF) over FA (Zhao, Matherly, and Goldman 2009; Zhao et al. 2011).

FRα is a high-affinity folate-binding protein selectively expressed in the MVM of the STB (Figure 12.3). This transporter is embedded in the membrane by a glycosylphosphoinositol anchor (Solanky et al. 2010; Zhao, Matherly, and Goldman 2009; Zhao et al. 2011) and mediates the unidirectional uptake of folates at neutral to mildly acidic pH. FRα has a higher affinity for FA over reduced folates (Zhao, Matherly, and Goldman 2009; Zhao et al. 2011).

Finally, PCFT is a high-affinity folate:H^+ symporter, with an optimal activity at acidic pH (5.5–6.0), and it utilizes the transmembrane H^+ gradient to achieve the transport of folates into cells against their concentration gradients (Keating et al. 2009; Zhao, Matherly, and Goldman 2009; Zhao et al. 2011). PCFT has similar affinities for FA and reduced folates (Hou and Matherly 2014), and it is predominantly present at the MVM, where it colocalizes with FRα (Solanky et al. 2010) (Figure 12.3).

Maternal-to-fetal transport of folates through the STB is believed to involve all the above-mentioned transport systems. Specifically, folates bind to FRα at the MVM of human STB. Since FRα colocalizes with PCFT, FA:FRα complex and PCFT are both internalized into an endosome. During cytoplasmic transit, this endosome is acidified (pH 6.0–6.5) due to an influx of protons, which promotes the dissociation of folates from FRα and establishes a favorable H^+ gradient that allows PCFT-mediated folate efflux into the cytoplasm. After this process, FRα and PCFT are recycled back to the MVM surface. At the MVM, RFC1 provides an alternative pathway for folate uptake. Efflux across the BM toward fetal circulation is believed to involve RFC1 rather than FRα or PCFT (Figure 12.3) (Solanky et al. 2010).

Other potential folate transporters localized at the BM and MVM of the STB (namely, the ATP-binding cassette efflux transporters: multidrug resistance-associated proteins and breast cancer resistance protein; Zhao et al. 2011) may also play a role in FA transport, but their exact contribution is still poorly understood (Figure 12.3).

12.3 MODULATION OF THE PLACENTAL TRANSPORT OF FOLATES AND IMPLICATIONS IN PREGNANCY OUTCOME

12.3.1 IMPACT OF PREGNANCY PATHOLOGIES ON PLACENTAL TRANSPORT OF FOLATES

The placental transport of folates has been studied in common pregnancy pathologies such as fetal growth restriction (FGR) (Bisseling et al. 2004; Keating, Gonçalves, Costa et al. 2009), gestational diabetes mellitus (GDM) (Araújo et al. 2013), and obesity (Table 12.1). FGR affects approximately 10% of all pregnancies and is characterized by the fetus not reaching its predetermined growth potential (i.e., a fetal weight below the 10th percentile) (Brett et al. 2014; Lausman et al. 2013). Although low birth weight and maternal folate deficiency are believed to be intimately associated, FGR pregnancies do not appear to be associated with a decrease in folate placental transport (Bisseling et al. 2004; Keating, Gonçalves, Costa et al. 2009). Instead, using primary cultures of human cytotrophoblasts (CT cells), which spontaneously differentiate into a functional and polarized STB-like structure (Bischof and Irminger-Finger 2005; Bloxam, Bax, and Bax 1997), we reported an increase in folate transport. This observation suggests that placentas from FGR pregnancies may exhibit a compensation for the weakness, i.e., an upregulation of folate transport in an effort to sustain normal fetal growth (Keating, Gonçalves, Costa et al. 2009). Of note, a similar compensatory behavior of the placenta was observed in maternal and paternal folate deficiency. Indeed, both

TABLE 12.1

Effect of Pregnancy-Associated Pathologies on Placental Folate Transport

Pregnancy Condition	Folate Transport	Substrate Model	Experimental Model	Reference
Fetal growth restriction	↑ / =	FA	Human primary cultured cytotrophoblasts	Keating et al. (2009)
		5-MTHF	Human placental cotyledons	Bisseling et al. (2004)
Gestational diabetes	=	FA	Human primary cultured cytotrophoblasts	Araújo et al. (2013)
Obesity	=	5-MTHF	Human placental tissue	Carter et al. (2011)

Note: ↓, decrease; ↑, increase; =, not changed. 5-MTHF, 5-methyltetrahydrofolate; FA, folic acid.

in female rats fed a folate-depleted diet before and during pregnancy and in male rats fed a folate-depleted diet before mating, the placental expression of FRα was upregulated in comparison with females or males fed a folate-repleted diet, respectively (Kim et al. 2011, Xiao et al. 2005).

GDM and obesity constitute the two most prevalent metabolic diseases affecting pregnant women (Herring and Oken 2011; Lappas et al. 2011; Sacks et al. 2012). Each one of them has been estimated to occur in at least 20% of all pregnancies (Herring and Oken 2011; Sacks et al. 2012). GDM is defined as any degree of glucose intolerance with onset or first recognition during pregnancy (American Diabetes Association [ADA] 2013). This condition is associated with fetal macrosomia (Metzger et al. 2008) and cardiovascular and metabolic diseases later in life in the offspring (Boney et al. 2005; Gluckman et al. 2008; Lee et al. 2007). Despite the recognized negative effects of GDM on fetal growth and development, knowledge about the impact of this disease on placental transport of folates is limited to only one study (Araújo et al. 2013) (Table 12.1). In that study, we verified that FA uptake depended more on the activity of PCFT than of RFC1 in CT cells isolated from GDM pregnancies compared with CT cells isolated from normal pregnancies, although, as a whole, uptake was quantitatively similar in both cells. The good metabolic control of diabetic women after diagnosis might have prevented the appearance of quantitative differences in FA transport (Araújo et al. 2013). It would be interesting to analyze in future studies the placental transport of folates in GDM women with poor metabolic control.

Insulin resistance, hyperglycemia (ADA 2014), and hyperinsulinemia (Lepercq et al. 1998) are the main hallmarks of GDM. Although not exclusive, hyperleptinemia (Ategbo et al. 2006; Guvener et al. 2012) and elevated levels of proinflammatory cytokines, such as tumor necrosis factor-α (TNF-α) and interleukin 6 (Ategbo et al. 2006; Plomgaard et al. 2007), are also associated with this disease. The modulation of FA placental transport by GDM-associated conditions has been studied in BeWo cells (Araújo et al. 2013), a well-characterized human trophoblast cell model that exhibits morphological, hormonal, enzymatic, and FA transport characteristics similar to CT cells (Bode et al. 2006; Keating et al. 2006; Liu, Soares, and Audus 1997) (Table 12.2). A reduction in FA uptake was observed after short-term (4 hours) and particularly long-term (24 hours) exposure to high levels of leptin and after short-term (4 hours) exposure to lipopolysaccharide (in concentrations known to induce interleukin-6 and TNF-α secretion by trophoblasts; Torricelli et al. 2009) or high levels of TNF-α. On the other hand, elevated concentrations of glucose and insulin had no effect on FA uptake. The long-term inhibitory effect of leptin on FA uptake was found to be independent of janus kinase/signal transducer and activator of transcription, phosphoinositide 3-kinase, protein kinase A and C, and mitogen-activated protein kinases (p38, extracellular signal-regulated kinase and c-Jun N-terminal kinase) (Araújo et al. 2013). As a whole, these results suggest that GDM-associated conditions do not seem to regulate the placental transport of FA in the same manner as GDM (Table 12.2).

Maternal obesity is defined as a pregravid body mass index greater than 30 kg/m^2 (Chu et al. 2007) and is associated with perinatal and complications later in life similar to those described for GDM

TABLE 12.2

Effect of Conditions Associated With Some Pregnancy Pathologies on Placental Folate Transport

Condition	Folate Transport	Experimental Model	Substrate Model	Reference
Elevated levels of leptin	↓	BeWo cells	FA	Araújo et al. (2013)
Elevated levels of proinflammatory mediators	↓	BeWo cells	FA	Araújo et al. (2013)
Elevated levels of insulin	=	BeWo cells	FA	Araújo et al. (2013)
Elevated levels of glucose	=	BeWo cells	FA	Araújo et al. (2013)
Elevated levels of serotonin	=	Human primary cultured cytotrophoblasts	FA	Keating et al. (2009)

Note: ↓, decrease; ↑, increase; =, not changed. FA, folic acid.

(Herring and Oken 2011). Concerning the impact of this disease on folate placental transport, Carter et al. (2011) found that neither the activity nor the protein expression levels of FRα, PCFT, and RFC1 were altered in placental tissue from obese pregnant women compared with normoponderal pregnant women. In accordance, they also reported that fetal blood concentrations of folates were similar in both groups (Carter et al. 2011). However, since in this study blood levels of folates in both obese and normoponderal mothers were higher than those usually found in pregnant women (Zhang et al. 2009), the authors suggested that a higher maternal folate status might have prevented changes in folate placental transport to occur in obese mothers. In fact, after adjustment for dietary folate intake (particularly FA-fortified foods), Kim et al. (2012) demonstrated that a higher maternal body mass index was associated with lower maternal serum folate levels. Therefore, it is possible that a decrease in the availability of folates to the fetus might occur in maternal obesity (Kim et al. 2012). Further studies adjusted for potential confounders are needed to better understand the role of obesity on folate placental transport and metabolism.

Preeclampsia, a placenta-mediated disease characterized by hypertension and proteinuria, is also prevalent among pregnant women (2% to 8% of all pregnancies) (Brett et al. 2014). However, to the best of our knowledge, the effect of this pathology on the placental transport of folates has never been studied. The only information on this subject is that high levels of serotonin—a hallmark of preeclampsia—does not alter FA uptake in CT cells (Keating, Gonçalves, Campos et al. 2009).

Collectively, the data reviewed in this section suggest that FGR, GDM, and obesity do not seem to impair the placental transport of folates (Table 12.1), which could indicate that the placenta might be able to adapt folate transport in response to disease.

12.3.2 IMPACT OF PHARMACOTHERAPY AND DRUGS OF ABUSE ON PLACENTAL TRANSPORT OF FOLATES

Pregnant women—and, consequently, the placenta and the fetus—are frequently exposed to several xenobiotics because of pharmacotherapy of maternal or fetal disease and lifestyle factors such as smoking, alcohol, and drugs of abuse (McHugh, Wigderson, and Greenfield 2014). Indeed, the need of pregnant women to consume therapeutic drugs is well demonstrated by the elevated prevalence of GDM, maternal obesity, and hypertensive disorders, such as preeclampsia (see Section 12.3.1). Moreover, it has been estimated that 16% of pregnant women smoke cigarettes, 8.5% consume alcohol, and 9%–16% use illicit drugs (with marijuana, cocaine, and amphetamines the most commonly used) (Friguls et al. 2012; McHugh, Wigderson, and Greenfield 2014). These substances, most of which are able to cross the placenta, have negative consequences for fetal and postnatal development, including FGR, low birth weight, preterm delivery, and lower cognitive performance later in life in the offspring (McHugh, Wigderson, and Greenfield 2014). Taking this into consideration, knowledge about the impact of therapeutic drugs commonly prescribed to pregnant women and of drugs of abuse on folates placental transport is of major importance.

Using CT cells, we reported a decrease in FA uptake after a short-term (20 minutes) and long-term (48 hours) exposure to the antihypertensive drugs labetalol and atenolol, respectively (Keating, Gonçalves, Campos et al. 2009). On the contrary, other antihypertensive drugs, clonidine and α-methyldopa, and the antidiabetic insulin did not alter FA uptake. Moreover, an increase in placental transport of FA was observed in female rats exposed during days 15–19 of pregnancy to the glucocorticoid dexamethasone (Wyrwoll et al. 2012), which is used to accelerate fetal lung maturation and prevent preterm delivery (Miracle et al. 2008; Wyrwoll et al. 2012).

Concerning drugs of abuse, both short-term (20 minutes) and long-term (48 hours) exposure to amphetamine or its derivative 3,4-methylenedioxymethamphetamine (ecstasy) and long-term exposure (48 hours) to nicotine or tetrahydrocannabinol (THC; the main psychoactive cannabinoid present in marijuana) decreased FA uptake in CT cells (Keating, Gonçalves, Campos et al. 2009). Interestingly enough, the decrease in FA uptake induced by atenolol and THC was associated with a decrease (in the same order of magnitude) in RFC1 mRNA levels (Keating, Gonçalves, Campos et al. 2009). Moreover, cannabinoid receptor agonists and antagonists were also able to alter FA uptake in BeWo cells (Araújo, Gonçalves, and Martel 2009).

Altogether, and considering that all these substances were tested in concentrations comprising their known therapeutic or recreational blood levels, these data suggest that inhibition of FA placental uptake may constitute one possible mechanism for the fetotoxicity of amphetamine, ecstasy, nicotine, and THC, reinforcing the harmfulness of their consumption, particularly during pregnancy. On the other hand, these data seem to reinforce the harmlessness of clonidine, α-methyldopa, insulin, and glucocorticoids but not of atenolol use during pregnancy (Table 12.3).

TABLE 12.3
Effect of Therapeutic Drugs, Drugs of Abuse, or Dietary Compounds on Placental Folate Transport

Compound	Folate Transport	Experimental Model	Substrate Model	Reference
Antihypertensive drugs	↓ / =	Human primary cultured cytotrophoblasts	FA	Keating et al. (2009)
Insulin	=	Human primary cultured cytotrophoblasts	FA	Keating et al. (2009)
Glucocorticoids	↑	Pregnant rats (*in vivo*)	FA	Wyrwoll et al. (2012)
Amphetamine, MDMA, nicotine and THC	↓	Human primary cultured cytotrophoblasts	FA	Keating et al. (2009)
Ethanol	↓	BeWo cells	FA	Keating et al. (2009)
		Human primary cultured cytotrophoblasts		Keating et al. (2008)
Xanthohumol, quercetin	↑	BeWo cells	FA	Keating et al. (2008)
Epicatechin, theophylline	↓	BeWo cells	FA	Keating et al. (2008)
Isoxanthohumol	↑ / ↓	BeWo cells	FA	Keating et al. (2008)
Catechin, chrysin, epigallocatechin-3-gallate, myricetin, resveratrol, rutin, caffeine	=	BeWo cells	FA	Keating et al. (2008)

Note: ↓, decrease; ↑, increase; =, not changed. FA, folic acid; MDMA, 3,4-methylenedioxymethamphetamine; THC, tetrahydrocannabinol.

Alcohol abuse during pregnancy is known to cause fetal alcohol spectrum disorders, of which fetal alcohol syndrome is the most common and severe disorder of this spectrum (McHugh, Wigderson, and Greenfield 2014). Fetal alcohol syndrome is estimated to occur in 2%–5% of all pregnancies and is characterized by the appearance of physical and mental defects in the off-spring such as growth deficits, abnormal facial features, and central nervous system abnormalities (McHugh, Wigderson, and Greenfield 2014). A possible explanation for these adverse consequences of alcohol ingestion might be related with its ability to reduce fetal levels of folates (Hutson et al. 2012; Keating, Gonçalves, Campos et al. 2009). In fact, in pregnant women chronically exposed to alcohol, folate levels were shown to be decreased in fetal cord blood, which suggests that alcohol might impair folate transport to the fetus (Hutson et al. 2012). Furthermore, Keating et al., using both CT and BeWo cells, demonstrated that chronic exposure (48 hours) to ethanol (the main alcohol found in alcoholic beverages) induced a decrease in FA uptake and, in a quantitatively similar way, a down-regulation in RFC1 and FRα mRNA expression levels (Keating, Gonçalves, Campos et al. 2009; Keating et al. 2008). These results suggest that impairment in FA placental uptake with a consequent decrease in the fetal levels of this vitamin may constitute one of the mechanisms involved in alcohol fetotoxicity.

Collectively, the data reviewed in this section suggest that placental transport of folates is impaired by some drugs of abuse and ethanol (Table 12.3), and this could be an explanation to the fetal and placental toxicity associated with exposure to these xenobiotics during pregnancy.

12.3.3 IMPACT OF DIETARY BIOACTIVE COMPOUNDS ON PLACENTAL TRANSPORT OF FOLATES

Knowing that folates are ingested together with other nutrients and bioactive substances, it seems of major importance to know if these are able to interfere with the placental transport of folates. Currently, polyphenols—a group of bioactive phytochemicals present in fruits, vegetables, and beverages (e.g., green tea, red wine and beer) (Landete 2012)—and methylxanthines—pharmacologically active compounds present in coffee, black tea and cocoa (Franco, Onatibia-Astibia, and Martinez-Pinilla 2013)—are receiving much attention because of their antioxidant, anti-inflammatory, cardio-protective, and neuroprotective properties (Andriantsitohaina et al. 2012; Franco, Onatibia-Astibia, and Martinez-Pinilla 2013; Landete 2012). Taking this into consideration, the effect of some poly-phenols and methylxanthines upon FA uptake was studied in BeWo cells (Keating et al. 2008). Short-term exposure (26 minutes) to the polyphenols epicatechin or isoxanthohumol or to the meth-ylxanthine theophylline inhibited FA uptake (Keating et al. 2008). Isoxanthohumol, but not epicat-echin, seemed to act as a competitive inhibitor of FA uptake, by reducing the transporter's affinity for FA (Keating et al. 2008). On the other hand, long-term exposure (48 hours) to the polyphenols xanthohumol, isoxanthohumol, or quercetin stimulated FA uptake in BeWo cells, but this increase was not associated with an up-regulation of FA transporters mRNA levels. So, these chronic effects may eventually be the result of a direct interaction of polyphenols with FA transporters, leading to an increase in their activity (Keating et al. 2008). Other polyphenols such as catechin, chrysin, epigallocatechin-3-gallate, myricetin, resveratrol, and rutin and the methylxanthine caffeine were not able to alter FA uptake.

As a whole, these data indicate that distinct classes of polyphenols might possess different effects upon placental uptake of folates (Table 12.3). Also, importantly, although beer, red wine, tea, and coffee constitute the main dietary sources of the dietary bioactive compounds that alter FA uptake, care should be taken when speculating about the effect of a beverage based on the effect of a single polyphenol (Martel, Monteiro, and Calhau 2010).

12.4 CONCLUSIONS

Placental folate transport is a complex process that seems to involve several different transport systems (FRα, RFC1, and PCFT), functioning coordinately to ensure the vectorial transfer of folates from maternal to fetal circulation. This functional redundancy is likely to contribute to an efficient transfer of this vitamin through the placenta, ensuring an adequate supply of folates to the developing fetus even in cases of maternal marginal vitamin status.

The placental transport of folates may be compromised by several dietary substances, therapeutic agents, drugs of abuse, and markers of pathological conditions, and this may, in some degree, threaten the normal development and growth of the fetus. Of note, the involvement of folates in epigenetic regulation, particularly DNA methylation, which plays a crucial role in gene expression imprinting processes and embryonic development (Jansson and Powell 2007), suggests that changes in its placental transport may have an important role in the fetal programming.

REFERENCES

American Diabetes Association. 2013. "Diagnosis and classification of diabetes mellitus." *Diabetes Care* 36:S67–74. doi:10.2337/dc13-S067.

Andriantsitohaina, R., C. Auger, T. Chataigneau, N. Étienne-Selloum, H. Li, M. C. Martínez, V. B. Schini-Kerth, and I. Laher. 2012. "Molecular mechanisms of the cardiovascular protective effects of polyphenols." *Br J Nutr* 108 (9):1532–49. doi:10.1017/S0007114512003406.

Araújo, J. R., A. Correia-Branco, L. Moreira, C. Ramalho, F. Martel, and E. Keating. 2013. "Folic acid uptake by the human syncytiotrophoblast is affected by gestational diabetes, hyperleptinemia, and TNF-α." *Pediatr Res* 73 (4 Pt 1):388–94. doi:10.1038/pr.2013.14.

Araújo, J. R., P. Gonçalves, and F. Martel. 2009. "Effect of cannabinoids upon the uptake of folic acid by BeWo cells." *Pharmacology* 83 (3):170–6. doi:10.1159/000192587.

Assaraf, Y. G. 2006. "The role of multidrug resistance efflux transporters in antifolate resistance and folate homeostasis." *Drug Resist Update* 9 (4–5):227–46. doi:10.1016/j.drup.2006.09.001.

Ategbo, J. M., O. Grissa, A. Yessoufou, A. Hichami, K. L. Dramane, K. Moutairou, A. Miled, A. Grissa, M. Jerbi, Z. Tabka, and N. A. Khan. 2006. "Modulation of adipokines and cytokines in gestational diabetes and macrosomia." *J Clin Endocrinol Metab* 91:4137–43. doi:10.1210/jc.2006-0980.

Audus, K. L. 1999. "Controlling drug delivery across the placenta." *Eur J Pharm Sci* 8 (3):161–5.

Bailey, R. L., M. A. McDowell, K. W. Dodd, J. J. Gahche, J. T. Dwyer, and M. F. Picciano. 2010. "Total folate and folic acid intakes from foods and dietary supplements of US children aged 1–13 y." *Am J Clin Nutr* 92 (2):353–8. doi:10.3945/ajcn.2010.29652.

Barker, D. J. and C. Osmond. 1986. "Infant mortality, childhood nutrition, and ischaemic heart disease in England and Wales." *Lancet* 1 (8489):1077–81.

Bischof, P. and I. Irminger-Finger. 2005. "The human cytotrophoblastic cell, a mononuclear chameleon." *Int J Biochem Cell Biol* 37 (1):1–16.

Bisseling, T. M., E. A. Steegers, J. J. van den Heuvel, H. L. Siero, F. M. van de Water, A. J. Walker, R. P. Steegers-Theunissen, P. Smits, and F. G. Russel. 2004. "Placental folate transport and binding are not impaired in pregnancies complicated by fetal growth restriction." *Placenta* 25 (6):588–93.

Bloxam, D. L., B. E. Bax, and C. M. Bax. 1997. "Culture of syncytiotrophoblast for the study of human placental transfer. Part II: Production, culture and use of syncytiotrophoblast." *Placenta* 18 (2–3):99–108.

Bode, C. J., H. Jin, E. Rytting, P. S. Silverstein, A. M. Young, and K. L. Audus. 2006. "In vitro models for studying trophoblast transcellular transport." *Methods Mol Med* 122:225–39. doi:10.1385/1-59259-989-3:225.

Boney, C. M., A. Verma, R. Tucker, and B. R. Vohr. 2005. "Metabolic syndrome in childhood: Association with birth weight, maternal obesity, and gestational diabetes mellitus." *Pediatrics* 115:e290–6. doi:10.1542/peds.2004-1808.

Brett, K. E., Z. M. Ferraro, J. Yockell-Lelievre, A. Gruslin, and K. B. Adamo. 2014. "Maternal-fetal nutrient transport in pregnancy pathologies: The role of the placenta." *Int J Mol Sci* 15 (9):16153–85. doi:10.3390/ijms150916153.

Brown, R. D., M. R. Langshaw, E. J. Uhr, J. N. Gibson, and D. E. Joshua. 2011. "The impact of mandatory fortification of flour with folic acid on the blood folate levels of an Australian population." *Med J Aust* 194 (2):65–7.

Bukowski, R., F. D. Malone, F. T. Porter, D. A. Nyberg, C. H. Comstock, G. D. V. Hankins, K. Eddleman, S. J. Gross, L. Dugoff, S. D. Craigo, I. E. Timor-Tritsch, S. R. Carr, H. M. Wolfe, and M. E. D'Alton. 2009. "Preconceptional folate supplementation and the risk of spontaneous preterm birth: A cohort study." *PLoS Med* 6 (5):e1000061. doi:10.1371/journal.pmed.1000061.

Burdge, G. C. and K. A. Lillycrop. 2010. "Nutrition, epigenetics, and developmental plasticity: Implications for understanding human disease." *Annu Rev Nutr* 30:315–39. doi:10.1146/annurev.nutr.012809.104751.

Burdge, G. C. and K. A. Lillycrop. 2012. "Folic acid supplementation in pregnancy: Are there devils in the detail?" *Br J Nutr* 108 (11):1924–30. doi:10.1017/s0007114512003765.

Carter, M. F., T. L. Powell, C. Li, L. Myatt, D. Dudley, P. Nathanielsz, and T. Jansson. 2011. "Fetal serum folate concentrations and placental folate transport in obese women." *Am J Obstet Gynecol* 205 (1):83.e17–25. doi:10.1016/j.ajog.2011.02.053.

Castro, K., L. D. Klein, D. Baronio, C. Gottfried, R. Riesgo, and I. S. Perry. 2014. "Folic acid and autism: What do we know?" *Nutr Neurosci.* doi:10.1179/1476830514y.0000000142.

Charles, D., A. R. Ness, D. Campbell, G. Davey Smith, and M. H. Hall. 2004. "Taking folate in pregnancy and risk of maternal breast cancer." *BMJ* 329 (7479):1375–6. doi:10.1136/bmj.329.7479.1375.

Chu, S. Y., W. M. Callaghan, S. Y. Kim, C. H. Schmid, J. Lau, L. J. England, and P. M. Dietz. 2007. "Maternal obesity and risk of gestational diabetes mellitus." *Diabetes Care* 30 (8):2070–6.

Cooney, C. A., A. A. Dave, and G. L. Wolff. 2002. "Maternal methyl supplements in mice affect epigenetic variation and DNA methylation of offspring." *J Nutr* 132 (8):2393S–400S.

Czeizel, A. E. and I. Dudas. 1992. "Prevention of the first occurrence of neural-tube defects by periconceptional vitamin supplementation." *N Engl J Med* 327 (26):1832–5. doi:10.1056/NEJM199212243272602.

Czeizel, A. E., I. Dudas, A. Vereczkey, and F. Banhidy. 2013. "Folate deficiency and folic acid supplementation: The prevention of neural-tube defects and congenital heart defects." *Nutrients* 5 (11):4760–75. doi:10.3390/nu5114760.

Daly, L. E., P. N. Kirke, A. Molloy, D. G. Weir, and J. M. Scott. 1995. "Folate levels and neural tube defects. Implications for prevention." *JAMA* 274 (21):1698–702.

Denny, K. J., A. Jeanes, K. Fathe, R. H. Finnell, S. M. Taylor, and T. M. Woodruff. 2013. "Neural tube defects, folate, and immune modulation." *Birth Defects Res A Clin Mol Teratol* 97 (9):602–9. doi:10.1002/bdra.23177.

De-Regil, L. M., A. C. Fernandez-Gaxiola, T. Dowswell, and J. P. Pena-Rosas. 2010. "Effects and safety of periconceptional folate supplementation for preventing birth defects." *Cochrane Database Syst Rev* (10):CD007950. doi:10.1002/14651858.CD007950.pub2.

Engeham, S. F., A. Haase, and S. C. Langley-Evans. 2010. "Supplementation of a maternal low-protein diet in rat pregnancy with folic acid ameliorates programming effects upon feeding behaviour in the absence of disturbances to the methionine–homocysteine cycle." *Br J Nutr* 103 (7):996–1007. doi:10.1017/S0007114509992662.

Franco, R., A. Oñatibia-Astibia, and E. Martínez-Pinilla. 2013. "Health benefits of methylxanthines in cacao and chocolate." *Nutrients* 5 (10):4159–73. doi:10.3390/nu5104159.

Friguls, B., X. Joya, J. Garcia-Serra, M. Gómez-Culebras, S. Pichini, S. Martinez, O. Vall, and O. Garcia-Algar. 2012. "Assessment of exposure to drugs of abuse during pregnancy by hair analysis in a Mediterranean island." *Addiction* 107 (8):1471–9. doi:10.1111/j.1360-0443.2012.03828.x.

Giugliani, E. R., S. M. Jorge, and A. L. Gonçalves. 1985. "Serum and red blood cell folate levels in parturients, in the intervillous space of the placenta and in full-term newborns." *J Perinat Med* 13 (2):55–9.

Gluckman, P. D., M. A. Hanson, C. Cooper, and K. L. Thornburg. 2008. "Effect of in utero and early-life conditions on adult health and disease." *N Engl J Med* 359:61–73. doi:10.1056/NEJMra0708473.

Guvener, M., H. I. Ucar, M. Oc, and A. Pinar. 2012. "Plasma leptin levels increase to a greater extent following on-pump coronary artery surgery in type 2 diabetic patients than in nondiabetic patients." *Diabetes Res Clin Pract* 96:371–8. doi:10.1016/j.diabres.2012.01.008.

Herring, S. J. and E. Oken. 2011. "Obesity and diabetes in mothers and their children: Can we stop the intergenerational cycle?" *Curr Diab Rep* 11 (1):20–7. doi:10.1007/s11892-010-0156-9.

Hirsch, S., H. Sanchez, C. Albala, M. P. de la Maza, G. Barrera, L. Leiva, and D. Bunout. 2009. "Colon cancer in Chile before and after the start of the flour fortification program with folic acid." *Eur J Gastroenterol Hepatol* 21 (4):436–9. doi:10.1097/MEG.0b013e328306ccdb.

Hodgetts, V., R. Morris, A. Francis, J. Gardosi, and K. Ismail. 2014. "Effectiveness of folic acid supplementation in pregnancy on reducing the risk of small-for-gestational age neonates: A population study, systematic review and meta-analysis." *BJOG* 122 (4):478–90. doi:10.1111/1471-0528.13202.

Honein, M. A., L. J. Paulozzi, T. J. Mathews, J. D. Erickson, and L. Y. Wong. 2001. "Impact of folic acid fortification of the US food supply on the occurrence of neural tube defects." *JAMA* 285 (23):2981–6.

Hou, Z. and L. H. Matherly. 2014. "Biology of the major facilitative folate transporters SLC19A1 and SLC46A1." *Curr Top Membr* 73:175–204. doi:10.1016/b978-0-12-800223-0.00004-9.

Hoyo, C., A. Murtha, J. Schildkraut, M. Forman, B. Calingaert, W. Demark-Wahnefried, J. Kurtzberg, R. Jirtle, and S. Murphy. 2011. "Folic acid supplementation before and during pregnancy in the Newborn Epigenetics STudy (NEST)." *BMC Public Health* 11 (1):46.

Huang, Y., Y. He, X. Sun, Y. Li, and C. Sun. 2014. "Maternal high folic acid supplement promotes glucose intolerance and insulin resistance in male mouse offspring fed a high-fat diet." *Int J Mol Sci* 15 (4):6298–313. doi:10.3390/ijms15046298.

Hutson, J. R., B. Stade, D. C. Lehotay, C. P. Collier, and B. M. Kapur. 2012. "Folic acid transport to the human fetus is decreased in pregnancies with chronic alcohol exposure." *PLoS One* 7 (5):e38057. doi:10.1371/journal.pone.0038057.

Jagerstad, M. and J. Jastrebova. 2013. "Occurrence, stability, and determination of formyl folates in foods." *J Agric Food Chem* 61 (41):9758–68. doi:10.1021/jf4028427.

Jansson, T. and T. L. Powell. 2007. "Role of the placenta in fetal programming: Underlying mechanisms and potential interventional approaches." *Clin Sci (Lond)* 113 (1):1–13.

Keating, E., A. Correia-Branco, J. R. Araújo, M. Meireles, R. Fernandes, L. Guardão, J. T. Guimaraes, F. Martel, and C. Calhau. 2015. "Excess perigestational folic acid exposure induces metabolic dysfunction in post-natal life." *J Endocrinol* 224 (3):245–59. doi:10.1530/JOE-14-0448.

Keating, E., P. Gonçalves, I. Campos, F. Costa, and F. Martel. 2009. "Folic acid uptake by the human syncytiotrophoblast: Interference by pharmacotherapy, drugs of abuse and pathological conditions." *Reprod Toxicol* 28 (4):511–20. doi:10.1016/j.reprotox.2009.07.001.

Keating, E., P. Gonçalves, F. Costa, I. Campos, M. J. Pinho, I. Azevedo, and F. Martel. 2009. "Comparison of the transport characteristics of bioactive substances in IUGR and normal placentas." *Pediatr Res* 66 (5):495–500. doi:10.1203/PDR.0b013e3181b9b4a3.

Keating, E., C. Lemos, I. Azevedo, and F. Martel. 2006. "Comparison of folic acid uptake characteristics by human placental choriocarcinoma cells at acidic and physiological pH." *Can J Physiol Pharmacol* 84 (2):247–55.

Keating, E., C. Lemos, P. Gonçalves, and F. Martel. 2008. "Acute and chronic effects of some dietary bioactive compounds on folic acid uptake and on the expression of folic acid transporters by the human trophoblast cell line BeWo." *J Nutr Biochem* 19 (2):91–100.

Kelly, P., J. McPartlin, M. Goggins, D. G. Weir, and J. M. Scott. 1997. "Unmetabolized folic acid in serum: Acute studies in subjects consuming fortified food and supplements." *Am J Clin Nutr* 65 (6):1790–5.

Kim, H., J. Y. Hwang, K. N. Kim, E. H. Ha, H. Park, M. Ha, K. Y. Lee, Y. C. Hong, T. Tamura, and N. Chang. 2012. "Relationship between body-mass index and serum folate concentrations in pregnant women." *Eur J Clin Nutr* 66 (1):136–8. doi:10.1038/ejcn.2011.160.

Kim, H. W., Y. J. Choi, K. N. Kim, T. Tamura, and N. Chang. 2011. "Effect of paternal folate deficiency on placental folate content and folate receptor α expression in rats." *Nutr Res Pract* 5 (2):112–6. doi:10.4162/nrp.2011.5.2.112.

Kim, J. M., K. Hong, J. H. Lee, S. Lee, and N. Chang. 2009. "Effect of folate deficiency on placental DNA methylation in hyperhomocysteinemic rats." *J Nutr Biochem* 20 (3):172–6. doi:10.1016/j.jnutbio.2008.01.010.

Kim, K.-C., S. Friso, and S.-W. Choi. 2009. "DNA methylation, an epigenetic mechanism connecting folate to healthy embryonic development and aging." *J Nutr Biochem* 20 (12):917–26. doi:10.1016/j.jnutbio.2009.06.008.

Kim, M. W., K. H. Ahn, K. J. Ryu, S. C. Hong, J. S. Lee, A. A. Nava-Ocampo, M. J. Oh, and H. J. Kim. 2014. "Preventive effects of folic acid supplementation on adverse maternal and fetal outcomes." *PLoS One* 9 (5):e97273. doi:10.1371/journal.pone.0097273.

Krishnaveni, G. V., S. R. Veena, S. C. Karat, C. S. Yajnik, and C. H. Fall. 2014. "Association between maternal folate concentrations during pregnancy and insulin resistance in Indian children." *Diabetologia* 57 (1):110–21. doi:10.1007/s00125-013-3086-7.

Landete, J. M. 2012. "Updated knowledge about polyphenols: Functions, bioavailability, metabolism, and health." *Crit Rev Food Sci Nutr* 52 (10):936–48. doi:10.1080/10408398.2010.513779.

Lappas, M., U. Hiden, G. Desoye, J. Froehlich, S. Hauguel-de Mouzon, and A. Jawerbaum. 2011. "The role of oxidative stress in the pathophysiology of gestational diabetes mellitus." *Antioxid Redox Signal* 15:3061–100. doi:10.1089/ars.2010.3765.

Lausman, A., J. Kingdom; Maternal Fetal Medicine Committee, R. Gagnon, M. Basso, H. Bos, J. Crane, G. Davies, M. F. Delisle, L. Hudon, S. Menticoglou, W. Mundle, A. Ouellet, T. Pressey, C. Pylypjuk, A. Roggensack, and F. Sanderson. 2013. "Intrauterine growth restriction: Screening, diagnosis, and management." *J Obstet Gynaecol Can* 35 (8):741–57.

Lee, H., H. C. Jang, H. K. Park, and N. H. Cho. 2007. "Early manifestation of cardiovascular disease risk factors in offspring of mothers with previous history of gestational diabetes mellitus." *Diabetes Res Clin Pract* 78:238–45. doi:10.1016/j.diabres.2007.03.023.

Lepercq, J., M. Cauzac, N. Lahlou, J. Timsit, J. Girard, J. Auwerx and S. Hauguel-de Mouzon. 1998. "Overexpression of placental leptin in diabetic pregnancy: A critical role for insulin." *Diabetes* 47:847–50. doi:10.2337/diabetes.47.5.847.

Liu, F., M. J. Soares, and K. L. Audus. 1997. "Permeability properties of monolayers of the human trophoblast cell line BeWo." *Am J Physiol* 273 (5 Pt 1):C1596–604.

Lucock, M. 2000. "Folic acid: Nutritional biochemistry, molecular biology, and role in disease processes." *Mol Genet Metab* 71 (1–2):121–38. doi:10.1006/mgme.2000.3027.

Lucock, M. and Z. Yates. 2009. "Folic acid fortification: A double-edged sword." *Curr Opin Clin Nutr Metab Care* 12 (6):555–64.

Mantovani, E., F. Filippini, R. Bortolus, and M. Franchi. 2014. "Folic acid supplementation and preterm birth: Results from observational studies." *BioMed Res Int* 2014:481914. doi:10.1155/2014/481914.

Martel, F., R. Monteiro, and C. Calhau. 2010. "Effect of polyphenols on the intestinal and placental transport of some bioactive compounds." *Nutr Res Rev* 23 (1):47–64. doi:10.1017/S0954422410000053.

Mason, J. B., A. Dickstein, P. F. Jacques, P. Haggarty, J. Selhub, G. Dallal, and I. H. Rosenberg. 2007. "A temporal association between folic acid fortification and an increase in colorectal cancer rates may be illuminating important biological principles: A hypothesis." *Cancer Epidemiol Biomarkers Prev* 16 (7):1325–9. doi:10.1158/1055-9965.EPI-07-0329.

McHugh, R. K., S. Wigderson, and S. F. Greenfield. 2014. "Epidemiology of substance use in reproductive-age women." *Obstet Gynecol Clin North Am* 41 (2):177–89. doi:10.1016/j.ogc.2014.02.001.

Metayer, C., E. Milne, J. D. Dockerty, J. Clavel, M. S. Pombo-de-Oliveira, C. Wesseling, L. G. Spector, J. Schuz, E. Petridou, S. Ezzat, B. K. Armstrong, J. Rudant, S. Koifman, P. Kaatsch, M. Moschovi, W. M. Rashed, S. Selvin, K. McCauley, R. J. Hung, A. Y. Kang, and C. Infante-Rivard. 2014. "Maternal supplementation with folic acid and other vitamins and risk of leukemia in offspring: A childhood leukemia international consortium study." *Epidemiology* 25 (6):811–22. doi:10.1097/ede.0000000000000141.

Metzger, B. E., L. P. Lowe, A. R. Dyer, E. R. Trimble, U. Chaovarindr, D. R. Coustan, D. R. Hadden, D. R. McCance, M. Hod, H. D. McIntyre, J. J. Oats, B. Persson, M. S. Rogers, and D. A. Sacks. 2008. "Hyperglycemia and adverse pregnancy outcomes." *N Engl J Med* 358:1991–2002. doi:10.1056/NEJMoa0707943.

Mills, J. L., Y. J. Lee, M. R. Conley, P. N. Kirke, J. M. McPartlin, D. G. Weir, and J. M. Scott. 1995. "Homocysteine metabolism in pregnancies complicated by neural-tube defects." *Lancet* 345 (8943):149–51. doi:10.1016/S0140-6736(95)90165-5.

Miracle, X., G. C. Di Renzo, A. Stark, A. Fanaroff, X. Carbonell-Estrany, and E. Saling. 2008. "Coordinators of World Association of Perinatal Medicine Prematurity Working Group. Guideline for the use of antenatal corticosteroids for fetal maturation." *J Perinat Med* 36 (3):191–6. doi:10.1515/JPM.2008.032.

Molloy, A. M., P. N. Kirke, L. C. Brody, J. M. Scott, and J. L. Mills. 2008. "Effects of folate and vitamin B12 deficiencies during pregnancy on fetal, infant, and child development." *Food Nutr Bull* 29 (2 Suppl):S101–11; discussion S112–5.

MRC. 1991. "Prevention of neural tube defects: Results of the Medical Research Council Vitamin Study. MRC Vitamin Study Research Group." *Lancet* 338 (8760):131–7.

Office of Dietary Supplements, National Institutes of Health. 2012. "Dietary Supplement Fact Sheet: Folate, Health Professional." Last Modified December 14, 2012. Accessed December 2, 2014. Available at http://ods.od.nih.gov/factsheets/Folate-HealthProfessional/.

Ohrvik, V. E. and C. M. Witthoft. 2011. "Human folate bioavailability." *Nutrients* 3 (4):475–90. doi:10.3390/nu3040475.

Pfeiffer, C. M., S. P. Caudill, E. W. Gunter, J. Osterloh, and E. J. Sampson. 2005. "Biochemical indicators of B vitamin status in the US population after folic acid fortification: Results from the National Health and Nutrition Examination Survey 1999–2000." *Am J Clin Nutr* 82 (2):442–50.

Plomgaard, P., A. R. Nielsen, C. P. Fischer, O. H. Mortensen, C. Broholm, M. Penkowa, R. Krogh-Madsen, C. Erikstrup, B. Lindegaard, A. M. Petersen, S. Taudorf, and B. K. Pedersen. 2007. "Associations between insulin resistance and TNF-alpha in plasma, skeletal muscle and adipose tissue in humans with and without type 2 diabetes." *Diabetologia* 50:2562–71. doi:10.1007/s00125-007-0834-6.

Ratan, S. K., K. N. Rattan, R. M. Pandey, S. Singhal, S. Kharab, M. Bala, V. Singh, and A. Jhanwar. 2008. "Evaluation of the levels of folate, vitamin B12, homocysteine and fluoride in the parents and the affected neonates with neural tube defect and their matched controls." *Pediatr Surg Int* 24 (7):803–8. doi:10.1007/s00383-008-2167-z.

Reilly, A., J. Amberg-Mueller, M. Beer, L. Busk, A.-M. Castellazzi, J. Castenmiller, M. Flynn, I. Margaritis, A. Lampen, C. Parvan, L. B. Rasmussen, H. Refsum, M. S. Szabo, D. Taruscio, A. Tedstone, G. Vansant, and A. Weissenborn. 2009. ESCO Report on Analysis of risks and benefits of fortification of food with folic acid. EFSA.

Sacks, D. A., D. R. Hadden, M. Maresh, C. Deerochanawong, A. R. Dyer, B. E. Metzger, L. P. Lowe, D. R. Coustan, M. Hod, J. J. Oats, B. Persson, E. R. Trimble, and HAPO Study Cooperative Research Group. 2012. "Frequency of gestational diabetes mellitus at collaborating centers based on IADPSG consensus panel recommended criteria: The Hyperglycemia and Adverse Pregnancy Outcome (HAPO) Study." *Diabetes Care* 35:526–8. doi:10.2337/dc11-1641.

Sauer, J., J. B. Mason, and S. W. Choi. 2009. "Too much folate: A risk factor for cancer and cardiovascular disease?" *Curr Opin Clin Nutr Metab Care* 12 (1):30–6. doi:10.1097/MCO.0b013e32831cec62.

Sengpiel, V., J. Bacelis, R. Myhre, S. Myking, A. Devold Pay, M. Haugen, A. L. Brantsaeter, H. Meltzer, R. Miodini Nilsen, P. Magnus, S. Vollset, S. Nilsson, and B. Jacobsson. 2014. "Folic acid supplementation, dietary folate intake during pregnancy and risk for spontaneous preterm delivery: A prospective observational cohort study." *BMC Pregnancy Childb* 14 (1):375. doi:10.1186/s12884-014-0375-1.

Siega-Riz, A. M., D. A. Savitz, S. H. Zeisel, J. M. Thorp, and A. Herring. 2004. "Second trimester folate status and preterm birth." *Am J Obstet Gynecol* 191 (6):1851–7. doi:10.1016/j.ajog.2004.07.076.

Sinclair, K. D., C. Allegrucci, R. Singh, D. S. Gardner, S. Sebastian, J. Bispham, A. Thurston, J. F. Huntley, W. D. Rees, C. A. Maloney, R. G. Lea, J. Craigon, T. G. McEvoy, and L. E. Young. 2007. "DNA methylation, insulin resistance, and blood pressure in offspring determined by maternal periconceptional B vitamin and methionine status." *Proc Natl Acad Sci U S A* 104 (49):19351–6. doi:10.1073/pnas.0707258104.

Smithells, R. W., S. Sheppard, and C. J. Schorah. 1976. "Vitamin deficiencies and neural tube defects." *Arch Dis Child* 51 (12):944–50.

Solanky, N., A. Requena Jimenez, S. W. D'Souza, C. P. Sibley, and J. D. Glazier. 2010. "Expression of folate transporters in human placenta and implications for homocysteine metabolism." *Placenta* 31 (2):134–43. doi:10.1016/j.placenta.2009.11.017.

Stolzenberg-Solomon, R. Z., S. C. Chang, M. F. Leitzmann, K. A. Johnson, C. Johnson, S. S. Buys, R. N. Hoover, and R. G. Ziegler. 2006. "Folate intake, alcohol use, and postmenopausal breast cancer risk in the Prostate, Lung, Colorectal, and Ovarian Cancer Screening Trial." *Am J Clin Nutr* 83 (4):895–904.

Tamura, T. and M. F. Picciano. 2006. "Folate and human reproduction." *Am J Clin Nutr* 83 (5):993–1016.

Torrens, C., L. Brawley, F. W. Anthony, C. S. Dance, R. Dunn, A. A. Jackson, L. Poston, and M. A. Hanson. 2006. "Folate supplementation during pregnancy improves offspring cardiovascular dysfunction induced by protein restriction." *Hypertension* 47 (5):982–7. doi:10.1161/01.HYP.0000215580.43711.d1.

Torricelli, M., C. Voltolini, E. Bloise, G. Biliotti, A. Giovannelli, M. De Bonis, A. Imperatore, and F. Petraglia. 2009. "Urocortin increases IL-4 and IL-10 secretion and reverses LPS-induced TNF-alpha release from human trophoblast primary cells." *Am J Reprod Immunol* 62:224–31. doi:10. 1111/j .1600-0897.2009.00729.x.

Ulrich, C. M. and J. D. Potter. 2006. "Folate supplementation: Too much of a good thing?" *Cancer Epidemiol Biomarkers Prev* 15 (2):189–93. doi:10.1158/1055-9965.epi-06-0054.

Vollset, S. E., R. Clarke, S. Lewington, M. Ebbing, J. Halsey, E. Lonn, J. Armitage, J. E. Manson, G. J. Hankey, J. D. Spence, P. Galan, K. H. Bonaa, R. Jamison, J. M. Gaziano, P. Guarino, J. A. Baron, R. F. Logan, E. L. Giovannucci, M. den Heijer, P. M. Ueland, D. Bennett, R. Collins, and R. Peto. 2013. "Effects of folic acid supplementation on overall and site-specific cancer incidence during the randomised trials: Meta-analyses of data on 50,000 individuals." *Lancet* 381 (9871):1029–36. doi:10.1016/S0140-6736(12)62001-7.

Wallingford, J. B., L. A. Niswander, G. M. Shaw, and R. H. Finnell. 2013. "The continuing challenge of understanding, preventing, and treating neural tube defects." *Science* 339 (6123):1222002. doi:10.1126/science.1222002.

Wen, S. W., J. Champagne, R. Rennicks White, D. Coyle, W. Fraser, G. Smith, D. Fergusson, and M. C. Walker. 2013. "Effect of folic acid supplementation in pregnancy on preeclampsia: The folic acid clinical trial study." *J Pregnancy* 2013:294312. doi:10.1155/2013/294312.

Wenstrom, K. D., G. L. Johanning, J. Owen, K. E. Johnston, S. Acton, S. Cliver, and T. Tamura. 2000. "Amniotic fluid homocysteine levels, 5,10-methylenetetrahydrafolate reductase genotypes, and neural tube closure sites." *Am J Med Genet* 90 (1):6–11.

Winkels, R. M., I. A. Brouwer, E. Siebelink, M. B. Katan, and P. Verhoef. 2007. "Bioavailability of food folates is 80% of that of folic acid." *Am J Clin Nutr* 85 (2):465–73.

Wolff, T., C. T. Witkop, T. Miller, and S. B. Syed. 2009. "Folic acid supplementation for the prevention of neural tube defects: An update of the evidence for the U.S. Preventive Services Task Force." *Ann Intern Med* 150 (9):632–9.

World Health Organization (WHO). 2012. Guideline: Daily iron and folic acid supplementation in pregnant women.

Wyrwoll, C. S., D. Kerrigan, M. C. Holmes, J. R. Seckl, and A. J. Drake. 2012. "Altered placental methyl donor transport in the dexamethasone programmed rat." *Placenta* 33 (3):220–3. doi:10.1016/j.placenta .2011.12.017.

Xiao, S., D. K. Hansen, E. T. Horsley, Y. S. Tang, R. A. Khan, S. P. Stabler, H. N. Jayaram, and A. C. Antony. 2005. "Maternal folate deficiency results in selective upregulation of folate receptors and heterogeneous nuclear ribonucleoprotein-E1 associated with multiple subtle aberrations in fetal tissues." *Birth Defects Res A Clin Mol Teratol* 73 (1):6–28.

Xita, N. and A. Tsatsoulis. 2010. "Fetal origins of the metabolic syndrome." *Ann N Y Acad Sci* 1205 (1):148–55. doi:10.1111/j.1749-6632.2010.05658.x.

Yajnik, C. S. and U. S. Deshmukh. 2012. "Fetal programming: Maternal nutrition and role of one-carbon metabolism." *Rev Endocr Metab Disord* 13 (2):121–7. doi:10.1007/s11154-012-9214-8.

Yajnik, C. S., S. S. Deshpande, A. A. Jackson, H. Refsum, S. Rao, D. J. Fisher, D. S. Bhat, S. S. Naik, K. J. Coyaji, C. V. Joglekar, N. Joshi, H. G. Lubree, V. U. Deshpande, S. S. Rege, and C. H. D. Fall. 2008. "Vitamin B12 and folate concentrations during pregnancy and insulin resistance in the offspring: The Pune Maternal Nutrition Study." *Diabetologia* 51 (1):29–38. doi:10.1007/s00125-007-0793-y.

Zhang, T., R. Xin, X. Gu, F. Wang, L. Pei, L. Lin, G. Chen, J. Wu, and X. Zheng. 2009. "Maternal serum vitamin B12, folate and homocysteine and the risk of neural tube defects in the offspring in a high-risk area of China." *Public Health Nutr* 12 (5):680–6. doi: 10.1017/S1368980008002735.

Zhao, R., L. H. Matherly, and I. D. Goldman. 2009. "Membrane transporters and folate homeostasis: Intestinal absorption and transport into systemic compartments and tissues." *Expert Rev Mol Med* 11:e4. doi:10.1017/S1462399409000969.

Zhao, R., N. Diop-Bove, M. Visentin, and I. D. Goldman. 2011. "Mechanisms of membrane transport of folates into cells and across epithelia." *Annu Rev Nutr* 31:177–201. doi:10.1146/annurev-nutr-072610-145133.

13 Vitamin D Effects on Pregnancy and Trophoblast Function
Limited Data yet Endless Possibilities

Bryanne Colvin, Mark S. Longtine, and D. Michael Nelson

CONTENTS

ABSTRACT

Vitamin D is a family of steroid-hormones, derived from the diet and by *de novo* synthesis from 7-hydroxy-cholesterol, that plays multiple roles in human health and disease. Vitamin D is converted to 25(OH)D (25-hydroxycycholecalciferol) in the liver and to the most biologically active form, $1,25(OH)_2D$ (calcitriol), in the kidney and other tissues, including the placenta. $1,25(OH)_2D$ binds the intracellular vitamin D receptor, eliciting both rapid nongenomic responses and slower genomic responses. The endocrine activity of circulating $1,25(OH)_2D$ generated by the kidney is responsible for the classic genomic actions of vitamin D in calcium metabolism and bone health. Recent work highlights the importance of the nonclassic actions of vitamin D, which result from conversion of 25(OH)D to $1,25(OH)_2D$ in selected tissues, including the placenta, to yield autocrine and paracrine responses. These multifaceted affects include modulation of innate and adaptive immunity. The intake of vitamin D that results in adequate, insufficient, or deficient, 25(OH)D levels during pregnancy is debated, but most agree that circulating 25(OH)D levels are a reasonable reflection of the vitamin D status of women. Vitamin D has been assigned roles in implantation, gestational diabetes mellitus, preeclampsia, preterm birth, bacterial vaginosis, neonatal skeletal health, and the placental response to pathogens. Notably, placental trophoblasts exhibit the 1-α hydroxylase that converts 25(OH)D to active $1,25(OH)_2D$ and the 24, 25-hydroxylase that inactivates $1,25(OH)_2D$. We discuss the chemistry, metabolism, and roles of vitamin D during pregnancy and in the biology of placental trophoblasts.

KEY WORDS

Trophoblast, placenta, pregnancy, vitamin D.

13.1 INTRODUCTION

German researcher Dr. Adolf Windaus received the Nobel Prize for chemistry in 1928 for his work on sterols and their relationship with vitamins (Wolf, 2004). Notably, he was the first to discover three forms of vitamin D, which he called D_1, D_2, and D_3. Vitamin D_1 was later found to be a mixture of compounds rather than a pure vitamin product, so the term D_1 is no longer used. *Vitamin D* now refers to a group of steroid-derived molecules that modulate multiple pathways in human biology. The classic action of vitamin D regulates the expression of genes to allow calcium homeostasis and skeletal health, with extreme deficiency resulting in rickets and other bone-associated problems (reviewed in DeLuca, 2004; Hollis and Wagner, 2013; Verstuyf et al., 2010). Study of vitamin D has undergone a renaissance because of recent findings of nonclassic roles for vitamin D in modulation of the immune system, cell proliferation, and disease.

Relative deficiency of vitamin D in women is linked to infertility, preeclampsia, gestational diabetes mellitus (GDM), infectious diseases, premature birth, and increased rates of Caesarean section (Aghajafari et al., 2013; Brannon and Picciano, 2011; Lapillonne, 2010; Mulligan et al., 2010; Paffoni et al., 2014; Shin et al., 2010; Wei et al., 2013; Zhou et al., 2014). Offspring of vitamin D-deficient women show suboptimal intrauterine growth, defects in skeletal and muscle maldevelopment, and elevated rates of autoimmune disease, respiratory infections, atopic disorders, and schizophrenia (Hollis and Wagner, 2013; Wagner et al., 2012; Wei et al., 2013). Notably, vitamin D has recently gained the attention of those devoted to placental research, as vitamin D in the human placenta modulates immune cell functions (Liu et al., 2009), regulates inflammation (Diaz et al., 2009; Liu et al., 2011), and alters secretion of pregnancy hormones (Avila et al., 2007, Stephanou et al., 1994), among other activities (Gysler et al., 2015; Sun et al., 2014). Our review will first briefly describe the metabolism and actions of vitamin D outside pregnancy. We will then address the controversies about the levels of vitamin D to optimize pregnancy outcomes and finish with a more detailed discussion of the metabolism and actions of vitamin D in the placenta. Vitamin D-induced responses in pregnancy, in general, and the placenta, specifically, are blossoming into an exciting area of placental trophoblast research.

13.2 THE CHEMISTRY AND ACTIONS OF VITAMIN D

Vitamin D is a general term referring to a family of hormones derived from cleavage of a ring in a steroid, thereby making them *secosteroids*. The nomenclature of vitamin D as discussed in this review is shown in Table 13.1. The pathways that generate active vitamin D are shown in Figure 13.1, and important chemical structures in vitamin D metabolism are shown in Figure 13.2. Vitamin D_2 and Vitamin D_3 derive from different sources (Table 13.1), with the major source of vitamin D_3 being from *de novo* synthesis in the skin (DeLuca, 2004; Verstuyf et al., 2010). Henceforth, we will use the term *vitamin D* to refer to vitamin D_2 or vitamin D_3 with no distinction. With this stated, we note that vitamin D_3, compared with vitamin D_2, is at least three times more potent on a per gram basis in increasing circulating levels of 25(OH)D (Armas et al., 2004; Houghton and Vieth, 2006).

Vitamin D is hydroxylated in the liver to form 25-hydroxyvitamin D (25(OH)D) by cytochrome P450 enzymes, especially CYP2R1 (Zhu et al., 2013), and 25(OH)D enters the circulation. 25(OH)D has a long half-life (weeks), in contrast to the short half-life (hours) of 1,25(OH)$_2$D (1,25 dihydroxyvitamin D). Because of its stability, 25(OH)D is the molecule measured to determine if an individual has sufficient or insufficient vitamin D levels. Most, but not all, of the circulating 25(OH)D is hydroxylated in renal proximal tubule epithelial cells to the biologically active derivative of vitamin D, 1,25(OH)$_2$D, by the CYP27B1-encoded cytochrome P450 (Figures 13.1 and 13.2). Kidney-produced 1,25(OH)$_2$D accounts for the majority of the circulating 1,25(OH)$_2$D and is key for the endocrine effects of vitamin D on bone metabolism through the classical pathway. Importantly, kidney cells are not the only ones that can produce 1,25(OH)$_2$D. Prostate, breast, colon, and lung cells; macrophages; as well as uterine decidual cells and placental trophoblasts all express CYP27B1 and

TABLE 13.1

Vitamin D and Its Derivatives and Proteins Involved in Metabolism

7-dehydrocholesterol: A sterol that is converted to previtamin D_3 by ultraviolet-B (UVB) light induced β-ring cleavage.

Previtamin D_3: Product of 7-dehydrocholesterol after UVB-mediated cleavage but before spontaneous isomerization.

Vitamin D_2 (ergocalciferol, ercalciol): The precursor to $25(OH)D_2$ produced by plants and fungi and obtained from the diet.

Vitamin D_3 (cholecalciferol, calciol): The precursor to $25(OH)D_3$ formed by isomerization of previtamin D_3. Synthesized by UVB light in the body (major source) or obtained from the diet (minor source).

25(OH)D (calcidiol, 25-hydroxyvitamin D, calcifediol, 25-hydroxycholecalciferol): Generated in the liver by hydroxylation of vitamin D by 25-hydroxylase and is the most abundant circulating vitamin D-derived molecule. Circulating 25(OH)D levels are measured to determine vitamin D adequacy or inadequacy, as 25(OH)D has a half-life of 14–21 days.

$1,25(OH)_2D$ (calcitriol, dihydroxyvitamin D, 1,25-dihydroxyvitamin D, 1,25-dihydroxycholecalciferol): Generated from 25(OH)D by 1-α-hydroxylase. The kidney is the major site of conversion of 25(OH)D to $1,25(OH)_2D$. Some immune cells, uterine decidual cells, and placental trophoblasts also produce $1,25(OH)_2D$ from 25(OH) D.

$24,25(OH)_2D$ (24,25 dihydroxycholecalciferol): Inactivated molecule from 24-hydroxylase activity on 25(OH)D that will be eliminated by excretion.

$1,24,25(OH)_3D$ (calcitetrol, 1α,24R,25 trihydroxycholecalciferol): Inactivated molecule from 24-hydroxylase activity on $1,25(OH)_2D$ that will be eliminated by excretion.

DBP (VDBP, *Gc*-globulin): Vitamin D-binding protein, a 58-kDa transport protein to which most circulating vitamin D and its derivatives are bound.

Cubilin: ~400-kDa multiligand transmembrane receptor protein that interacts with megalin to bind and internalize DBP (and bound 25(OH)D) by endocytosis.

Megalin: ~517-kDa multiligand transmembrane receptor protein that interacts with cubilin to bind and internalize DBP (and bound 25(OH)D) by endocytosis.

VDR: ~58-kDa intracellular nuclear hormone receptor protein that binds $1,25(OH)_2D$, dimerizes with retinoid-X receptor (RXR), and binds vitamin D response elements in nuclear DNA to activate or repress target gene transcription.

25 hydroxylase: The enzyme that converts vitamin D to 25(OH)D in the liver. The major activity is from the CYP2B1 cytochrome P450, with contributions by other enzymes.

1-α-hydroxylase: The cytochrome P450 enzyme encoded by CYP27B1 that converts 25(OH)D to $1,25(OH)_2D$. The majority of circulating $1,25(OH)_2D$ is generated by 25(OH)D hydroxylation in the kidney. 1-α-hydroxylase activity is also high in macrophages, dendritic cells, uterine decidual cells, and placental trophoblasts.

24-hydroxylase: The cytochrome P450 enzyme encoded by CYP24A1 that inactivates both 25(OH)D and $1,25(OH)_2D$ by hydroxylation to form $24,25(OH)_2D$ and $1,24,25(OH)_3D$. CYP24A1 shows negative feedback regulation by $1,25(OH)_2D$ via VDR-mediated transcriptional repression in responsive cell types, including placental trophoblasts.

Research pearls: $25(OH)D_3$ (MW 400.6 g/mol), 40 ng/mL = 100 nmol/Li. Vitamin D_3 (MW 384.6 g/mol), 400 IU = 10 μg.

produce $1,25(OH)_2D$ from circulating 25(OH)D (Verstuyf et al., 2010). Importantly, the $1,25(OH)_2D$ from nonrenal cells accounts for only a minor proportion of the total circulating $1,25(OH)_2$ and is unlikely to contribute significantly to the classical pathway. Instead, the $1,25(OH)_2D$ generated outside the kidney serves autocrine or paracrine functions, notably in reproductive tissues and immune cells in pregnancy.

All vitamin D metabolites are hydrophobic and travel in the circulation largely bound to carrier proteins. The major chauffeur is vitamin D-binding protein (DBP; Table 13.1), which transports over 90% of vitamin D and its metabolites. Much of the remainder is bound by albumin and lipoproteins, with <1% existing in the free (unbound) form (Bikle, 2014). In addition to transport, DBP plays a pivotal role in the entry of 25(OH)D into kidney epithelial cells in the proximal tubule, where DBP and bound 25(OH)D interact with the heteromeric megalin/cubilin endocytic receptor pair (Christensen and Birn, 2002; Negri, 2006) and are endocytosed. The intracellular 25(OH)D is then released and becomes the substrate for hydroxylation by the CYP27B1 cytochrome P450 to form active $1,25(OH)_2D$, which then enters the circulation. Megalin/cubilin-mediated import of

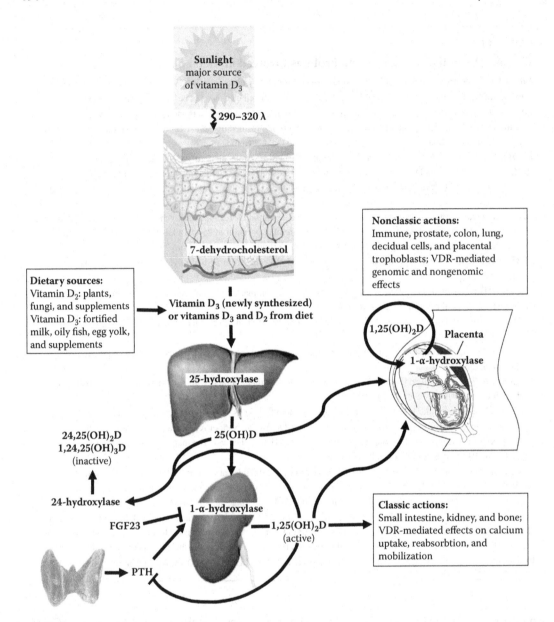

FIGURE 13.1   Pathways of vitamin D metabolism and action. See text for details.

DBP-25(OH)D is also important in mammary (Rowling et al., 2006), prostate, and colon (Ternes and Rowling, 2013) cells. Whether megalin/cubilin is important in other cell types is largely unknown.

The biological activity of 1,25(OH)$_2$D occurs via two pathways, both of which involve binding to the vitamin D receptor (VDR). VDR is a member of the super family of nuclear receptors for steroid hormones, and 1,25(OH)$_2$D-bound VDR heterodimerizes with the retinoic acid X receptor (RXR). This 1,25(OH)$_2$D/VDR/RXR trimeric complex enters the nucleus, binds coactivators and corepressors, and influences transcription of target genes by binding vitamin D response elements (VDREs) in the nuclear DNA (Carlberg and Seuter, 2009; Haussler et al., 2011; Pike and Meyer, 2010). This genomic response can involve the induction or repression of transcription and can be widespread, as ~3000 genes contain potential VDREs (Chun et al., 2014a; Wang et al., 2005). In the second pathway of action, 1,25(OH)$_2$D binding to the VDR can trigger rapid nongenomic responses,

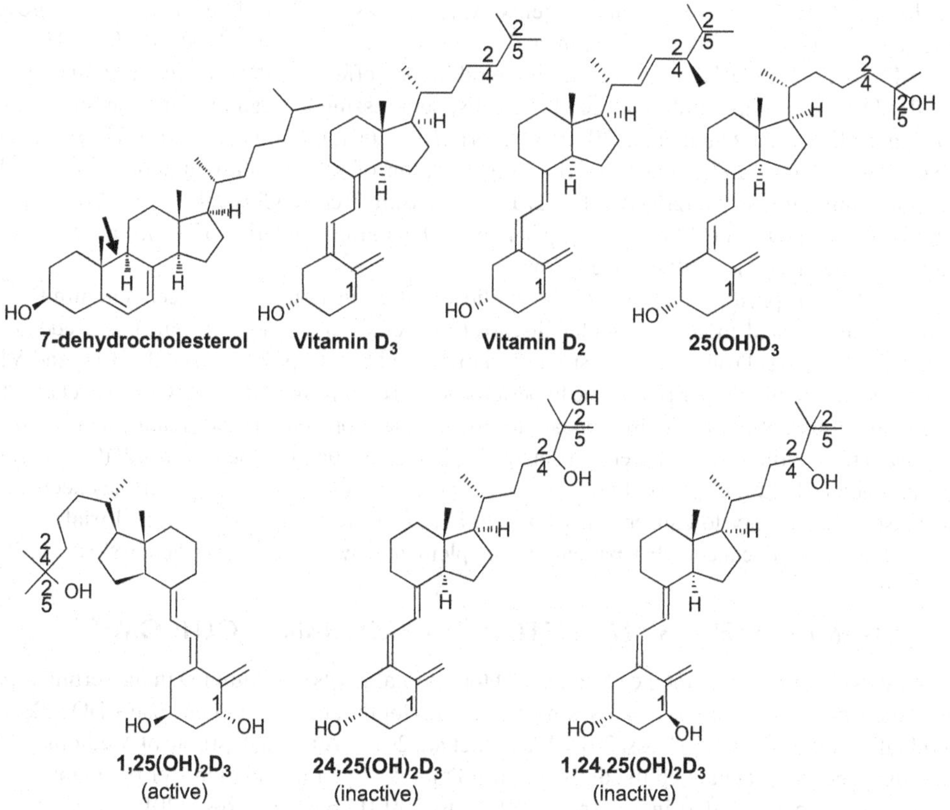

FIGURE 13.2 Structures of key molecules of vitamin D metabolism. In select molecules, the 1, 24, and 25 positions are indicated. Arrow indicates bond cleaved by UV light in 7-dehydrocholesterol, the precursor to vitamin D_3. Other than vitamin D_2 itself, the structures shown are the precursor or derivatives of vitamin D_3.

which can occur within minutes of hormone exposure (Bikle, 2014; Haussler et al., 2011). The nongenomic actions of $1,25(OH)_2D$ are mediated by the interaction of ligand-bound VDR with signal transduction pathways, including the protein kinase C and mitogen-activated protein kinases, with additional pathways, some of which are likely not yet identified. Ligand stimulation yields exocytosis, or opens chloride or calcium channels, that associates with membrane responses in pancreatic β-cells, endothelial cells, osteoblasts, and Sertoli cells (Bikle, 2014; Haussler et al., 2011). $1,25(OH)_2D$ and $25(OH)D$ are inactivated in the kidney and other responsive cell types by 24-hydroxylase (CYP24A1), a mitochondrial cytochrome P450 enzyme (Table 13.1, Figures 13.1 and 13.2). CYP24A1 transcription is itself induced by $1,25(OH)_2D$, thus providing a negative feedback mechanism to limit vitamin D activity.

Classically, $1,25(OH)_2D$ acts to maintain calcium homeostasis in three separate ways, all of which involve VDR-mediated effects on gene expression (Bikle, 2014; DeLuca, 2004). First, $1,25(OH)_2D$ increases absorption of calcium and phosphorus in the intestine. Second, in the absence of intestinal absorption of calcium, $1,25(OH)_2D$ acts in concert with parathyroid hormone to increase calcium mobilization from bone. Third, $1,25(OH)_2D$ acts in the distal renal tubule to increase reabsorption of calcium. The production of $1,25(OH)_2D$ in the kidney is stimulated by parathyroid hormone and is inhibited by fibroblast growth factor 23 (Figure 13.1) as well as by elevated calcium and phosphate concentrations (DeLuca, 2004; Quarles, 2012). Because prolonged severe deficiency of vitamin D leads to impaired calcium absorption and hypocalcemia, rickets can ensue.

Multiple effects of vitamin D over the last decade have been identified that regulate immune cells. Antigen presenting cells from the innate immune system express CYP27B1, and many cells from the innate and adaptive immune systems express VDR. Vitamin D enhances the expression of the antibacterial proteins cathelicidin and β-defensin 2 (Fabri and Modlin, 2009; Hewison, 2010). Moreover, 1,25(OH)$_2$D has an immunomodulatory effect on the adaptive immune system. 1,25(OH)$_2$D decreases maturation of dendritic cells, suppressing antigen presentation and decreasing T-cell proliferation (Chun et al., 2014a; Gregori et al., 2001; Griffin et al., 2001; Hewison, 2011; Penna et al., 2007). 1,25(OH)$_2$D supports the generation of tolerogenic regulatory T cells while suppressing inflammatory interleukin-17 (IL-17)-expressing T cells (Christakos et al., 2013; Joshi et al., 2011). Thus, one key nonclassic effect of vitamin D is in the regulation of the immune response, including in the placenta, as described below.

Vitamin D also appears to have effects on cardiovascular function and in cancer. Vitamin D levels are strongly implicated in cardiovascular disease (Nigwekar and Thadhani, 2013). Indeed, in animal models, 1,25(OH)$_2$D reverses agonist-induced myocyte hypertrophy (Chen et al., 2011) and VDR-deficient rodents display hyper-reninemic hypertension and cardiac hypertrophy (Gezmish et al., 2010; Xiang et al., 2005). Vitamin D also appears to affect cancer prevention and treatment (Deeb et al., 2007). Data from animal studies (Feldman et al., 2014) suggest that treatment with 1,25(OH)$_2$D inhibits progression of breast, colon, and prostate cancer cells, and knockout of the VDR has been shown to increase susceptibility to cancer (Christakos et al., 2013). Randomized controlled trials report a decreased incidence of cancer when patients are supplemented with vitamin D (Pludowski et al., 2013).

13.3   VITAMIN D LEVELS AND EFFECTS ON PREGNANCY OUTCOMES

Debate rages about the daily intake of vitamin D for optimal levels of vitamin D in the serum of pregnant women, but what is clear is that assessment of serum for the stable metabolite 25(OH)D reflects an individual's vitamin D status (Ross, 2011; Wagner et al., 2012). A recent Institute of Medicine (IOM) consensus panel report changed the daily vitamin D intake recommendations for pregnant women, increasing the recommended intake from 400 IU to 600 IU per day (Ross, 2011): see the report at http://www.iom.edu/Reports/2010/Dietary-Reference-Intakes-for-Calcium-and-Vitamin-D.aspx. The IOM report also defined vitamin D deficiency as 25(OH)D levels of <20 ng/mL (<50 nmol/L), insufficiency as 21–29 ng/mL (51–74 nmol/L), and sufficiency as >30 ng/mL (>75 nmol/L). Both the IOM and the Endocrine Society recommend ≤100 ng/mL (250 nmol/L) as maximal blood level in all patients (Holick et al., 2011; Ross, 2011). Although the recent IOM report increased the recommended daily intake of vitamin D for pregnant women (Ross, 2011: see the report at http://www.iom.edu/Reports/2010/Dietary-Reference-Intakes-for-Calcium-and-Vitamin-D.aspx), others have argued that a 10-fold higher amount, 4000 IU per day, may be required for pregnant women to achieve levels of 40 ng/mL, where sufficiency is "optimal" (Hollis and Wagner, 2013; Wagner et al., 2012). Reassuringly, vitamin D intoxication rarely occurs, as this requires ingestion of >10,000 IU per day (Wagner et al., 2012) and serum levels must rise to >150 ng/mL (375 nmol/L).

In normal pregnancy, circulating 1,25(OH)$_2$D levels rise twofold to fourfold in the first trimester compared with nonpregnant levels, and this upward trend continues into the second and third trimesters. The increase in 1,25(OH)$_2$D is not driven by a change in calcium homeostasis in pregnancy (Hollis and Wagner, 2013) and is unlikely to be placental in origin, as women with nonfunctioning renal CYP27B1 and normal placental function fail to increase 1,25(OH)$_2$D during pregnancy. Placental methylation of CYP24A1 prevents catabolism of 1,25(OH)$_2$D and the rise of calcitonin in pregnancy (Novakovic et al., 2009). These changes stimulate renal CYP27B1 and may contribute to the increase in bioactive vitamin D (Novakovic et al., 2009; Zhong et al., 2009). The role of prolactin is also debated. Prolactin stimulates CYP27B1 during pregnancy, and the elevated 1,25(OH)$_2$D levels during pregnancy fall postpartum, even though prolactin remains elevated postpartum during lactation (Ajibade et al., 2010). Further research is clearly needed in this field to elucidate the factors contributing to higher bioactive vitamin D in pregnant vs. nonpregnant women.

Although widespread consensus is lacking, as noted above, clinical trials have addressed the issue of what might be the optimal daily ingestion of vitamin D. Six randomized controlled trials have been conducted with pregnant women, and each study aimed to achieve a 25(OH)D level of >30 ng/mL (75 nmol/L) as a definition of vitamin D sufficiency. Four trials used a daily oral dose of 2000 or 4000 IU of vitamin D (Dawodu et al., 2013; Hollis et al., 2011; Hossain et al., 2014; Wagner et al., 2013), and two trials used weekly intramuscular vitamin D injections of either 35,000 IU or 50,000 IU (Hashemipour et al., 2013; Roth et al., 2013). All studies reported a higher level of 25(OH)D in both mothers and neonates in the supplemented group, compared with the control group, and no study reported an adverse event related to vitamin D supplementation. Notably, the two studies that utilized weekly vitamin D therapy (Hashemipour et al., 2013; Roth et al., 2013) recorded 100% success in reaching sufficiency of vitamin D levels in mothers and neonates.

Whether the serum level of vitamin D influences the incidence of preeclampsia is also hotly debated. Recent meta-analyses of observational data concluded that there was an increased risk of preeclampsia in women with lower maternal levels of vitamin D (Aghajafari et al., 2013; Hypponen et al., 2013; Wei et al., 2013). A meta-analysis of four randomized controlled trials of vitamin D supplementation during pregnancy also concluded that vitamin D was protective (Hypponen et al., 2013). However, only one of these trials was conducted recently (Hollis et al., 2011), with the others from 1937, 1946, and 1987. Notably, a 2014 trial failed to support this protective association (Hossain et al., 2014). Clearly, sufficiently powered randomized controlled trials are necessary to resolve this issue, while the mechanisms of action for any protection from preeclampsia remain to be discovered.

The second half of pregnancy is a diabetogenic state for women with suboptimal insulin reserves, and this makes the carbohydrate intolerance of obesity and type 2 diabetes mellitus worse. Observational studies are mixed on whether GDM and vitamin D sufficiency are related (Cho et al., 2013; Farrant et al., 2009; Fernandez-Alonso et al., 2012; Lacroix et al., 2014; Lau et al., 2011; McManus et al., 2014; Rodriguez et al., 2014; Schneuer et al., 2014; Whitelaw et al., 2014). Three recent meta-analyses found an inverse relationship between maternal vitamin D status and the diagnosis of GDM (Aghajafari et al., 2013; Poel et al., 2012; Wei et al., 2013). However, emerging data from randomized controlled trials suggest no difference in the risk of developing GDM in women based on vitamin D levels (Hollis et al., 2011; Wagner et al., 2013; Yap et al., 2014). Vitamin D supplementation for mothers already diagnosed with GDM may improve glycemic control and the overall metabolic profile (Asemi et al., 2014). A multicentered, multinational trial is ongoing in Europe to evaluate the efficacy of supplemental vitamin D, along with healthy eating and physical activity, for prevention of GDM in high-risk women (Jelsma et al., 2013), and further trials are encouraged (Burris and Camargo, 2014). Notably, no study has yet to identify a risk for vitamin D toxicity from supplementation. Placentas from women with GDM, compared with placentas from nondiabetic control patients, express higher CYP24A1 mRNA and protein levels, with no difference in CYP27B1 or VDR levels (Cho et al., 2013). Upregulation of VDR in response to low vitamin D levels occurs in extravillous trophoblasts and fetoplacental endothelial cells in placentas of mothers with GDM compared with controls (Knabl et al., 2015). These findings suggest that there is increased metabolism of the bioactive 1,25(OH)$_2$D in the placentas of women with GDM, compared with normoglycemic controls (Cho et al., 2013). Collectively, the studies to date indicate that metabolism of vitamin D is altered in placentas from mothers with GDM, but the specific effects of this change in bioactive vitamin D in the placenta requires more research.

Although vitamin D clearly affects the innate immune system and the antimicrobial properties of the placenta, whether these affects modulate the risk of infection is unknown. A recent randomized controlled trial of vitamin D supplementation reported no difference in the incidence of infection during pregnancy (Hollis et al., 2011). Bodnar et al. (2014), in a retrospective case-control study, examined vitamin D levels as well as placental pathology for mothers with spontaneous preterm birth. The authors reported an increased risk of preterm birth among nonwhite mothers with lower vitamin D levels. This increased risk was associated with placental pathology, implicating low vitamin D and the predisposition to inflammation as parts of the pathogenesis of preterm birth (Bodnar et al., 2014).

Three observational studies examining the association between vitamin D status and diagnosis of bacterial vaginosis in pregnant women also found an increased incidence of bacterial vaginosis in women with lower vitamin D levels (Aghajafari et al., 2013; Bodnar et al., 2009; Dunlop et al., 2011). However, a very recent vitamin D supplementation trial in pregnancy showed no difference in the incidence of bacterial vaginosis between the supplemented and standard care groups (Turner et al., 2014).

Vitamin D is critical to mineral homeostasis in both mother and fetus. This is especially notable because circulating levels of $1,25(OH)_2D$ are not subject to as much modulation by the classical regulatory factors, such as low calcium or increased parathyroid hormone (PTH). Pregnant women have normal serum and urinary calcium levels, despite markedly elevated $1,25(OH)_2D$ level (Hollis et al., 2011). Recent randomized controlled trials have shown that mothers and neonates who have improved vitamin D status also have improved calcium status (Harrington et al., 2014; Hashemipour et al., 2013). These data support the conjecture that vitamin D supplementation maintains calcium in the neonate in the first few days after birth (Specker, 2004).

Vitamin D status may impact fetal growth through calcium availability and skeletal growth (Specker, 2012) and by modulation of placental pathologies, contributing to decreased fetal growth. Two recent meta-analyses of observational data have revealed up to a twofold increased risk for small for gestational age with suboptimal maternal vitamin D status (Aghajafari et al., 2013; Wei et al., 2013). Subsequent observational studies have had mixed results, with some studies finding a positive (Gernand et al., 2014; van den Berg et al., 2013), and others a negative (Rodriguez et al., 2014; Schneuer et al., 2014; Zhou et al., 2014), association. For example, other randomized controlled trials of vitamin D supplementation during pregnancy found no difference in the incidence of small-for-gestational-age infants between supplemented and control groups (Hollis and Wagner, 2013; Hossain et al., 2014). However, a recent randomized controlled trial of women identified as insufficient or deficient for 25(OH) D, at <30 ng/mL, were supplemented with 400 IU vitamin D daily by mouth, plus or minus 50,000 IU intramuscular per week. The data showed that the mothers supplemented with the intramuscular vitamin D had infants with higher birth weight (3429 g vs. 3258 g) and longer lengths than controls did. Indeed, these measurements correlated with maternal vitamin D levels (Hashemipour et al., 2014). Thus, vitamin D may be an important modifiable factor for improving birth weight of infants of at-risk mothers.

13.4 PLACENTAL METABOLISM AND TROPHOBLAST RESPONSES TO VITAMIN D

The placenta is a site of extrarenal conversion of 25(OH)D to $1,25(OH)_2D$ (Weisman et al., 1979), mediated by the 1α-hydroxylase enzyme activity (Figures 13.1 and 13.3). CYP27B1 and CYP24A1 are expressed in syncytiotrophoblasts (Avila et al., 2004, 2007; Barrera et al., 2008; Diaz et al., 2000), and CYP27B1 is expressed in trophoblasts and decidua (Zehnder et al., 2002). CYP27B1 is inhibited by its product, $1,25(OH)_2D$, through a feedback mechanism present in both the kidney and the placenta (Prosser and Jones, 2004). Notably, CYP27B1 shows higher expression in the first and second trimesters of pregnancy, compared with levels in the third trimester (Zehnder et al., 2002). Increased placental expression of CYP27B1 is associated with increasing maternal circulating 25(OH)D levels, although mechanistic data for this association are lacking (O'Brien et al., 2014).

In cultured human placental syncytiotrophoblasts, catabolism of $1,25(OH)_2D$ by CYP24A1 is induced by a negative feedback mechanism. This effect is limited by an inhibitor of VDR, suggesting that CYP24A1 induction by $1,25(OH)_2D$ is mediated through the VDR (Avila et al., 2007). Moreover, the regulatory region of CYP24A1 is variably methylated in term placental tissue, chorionic villous samples, and first-trimester cytotrophoblasts. Methylation down-regulates basal gene activity and abolishes vitamin D induction by promoters (Novakovic et al., 2009). Interestingly, almost complete methylation of CYP24A1, VDR, and CYP27B1 is seen in JEG-3, BeWo, and JAR cells, three choriocarcinoma cell lines frequently used in trophoblast research (Novakovic et al., 2009). Therefore, while CYP24A1 may be induced by 1,25(OH)$_2$D, methylation also decreases its expression, potentially providing a partial explanation for increased 1,25(OH)$_2$D levels seen in pregnancy.

The VDR is expressed in placental trophoblasts (Barrera et al., 2008; Ma et al., 2012; Pospechova et al., 2009; Shahbazi et al., 2011), and VDR expressed is higher in early compared with late gestation (Zehnder et al., 2002). We have found that VDR mRNA is expressed in *in vitro* cultured primary human cytotrophoblasts and syncytiotrophoblasts and in villous explants from term placenta (our unpublished results). Placental VDR expression is inversely associated with neonatal 25(OH)D levels in cord blood and positively associated with 1,25(OH)$_2$D levels but is not associated with maternal 25(OH)D levels. These observations yield the speculation that there is a signal from the fetus to the placenta to increase placental VDR expression when fetal 25(OH)D levels are low (Young et al., 2014). This hypothesis awaits testing.

DBP levels increase during pregnancy (Brannon and Picciano, 2011; Wagner et al., 2012). The source for the increased DBP is conjectured to be secondary to high estrogen levels, analogous to the higher DBP in women supplemented with estrogen through oral contraceptives or for menopausal symptoms (Brannon and Picciano, 2011). Increased levels of DBP are found as early as 8 weeks' gestation (Ritchie et al., 1998), and DBP concentrations progressively rise for the remainder of the pregnancy. Despite the increase in DBP, the amount of free 1,25(OH)$_2$D rises in pregnant women above those of nonpregnant women (Hollis et al., 2011). The mechanisms by which trophoblasts uptake 25(OH)D are poorly understood (Figure 13.3). One possibility is that transport of 25(OH)D

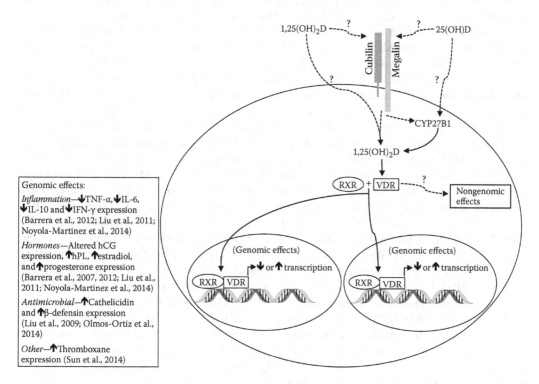

FIGURE 13.3 Vitamin D responses in placental trophoblasts. Simplified diagram of a placental syncytiotrophoblast with two nuclei shown. 25(OH)D and 1,25(OH)$_2$D may enter trophoblasts via DBP-mediated binding to the megalin/cubilin complex and endocytosis, or alternatively, "free hormone" (unbound to DBP) may enter by diffusion through the plasma membrane. 1,25(OH)$_2$D, which can be generated inside the trophoblast by the CYP27B1 hydroxylase, has genomic effects in trophoblasts, as described in the text box. Whether vitamin D has nongenomic effects in trophoblasts remains unknown.

into trophoblasts is mediated through the actions of megalin and cubilin, which are expressed in trophoblasts (Burke et al., 2013 and our unpublished results), although this remains uninvestigated. An alternative idea, the "free hormone hypothesis," suggests that the effects of vitamin D in extrarenal cells are mediated by circulating unbound 1,25(OH)$_2$D, which enters cells by diffusion (Chun et al., 2014b). Of course, both these mechanisms may exist. The expression of CYP27B1 (Ma et al., 2012) in trophoblasts suggests that 25(OH)D can be converted to active 1,25(OH)$_2$D within these cells, consistent with the demonstrated action of 25(OH)D in affecting gene expression in trophoblasts (Barrera et al., 2008; Diaz et al., 2009; Liu et al., 2009; our unpublished results).

Surprisingly, there are no direct data examining the mechanism of transport of vitamin D derivatives from the maternal to fetal circulations across the placenta. Observational data acquired years ago showed that plasma levels of 1,25(OH)$_2$D were higher in mothers than in the neonates (Kovacs and Kronenberg, 1997). Later studies with simultaneous sampling and subsequent assay of umbilical arterial and venous blood revealed higher 1,25(OH)$_2$D levels in arterial compared with venous blood, suggesting fetal participation in the synthesis of 1,25(OH)$_2$D (Wieland et al., 1980). However, using state-of-the-art approaches, the most recent studies failed to associate maternal and neonatal 1,25(OH)$_2$D concentrations at delivery (Young et al., 2014). Instead, levels of 25(OH)D in the neonate, while lower, correlate with maternal levels of the more stable 25(OH)D, suggesting that this is the metabolite that is transported across the placenta. Studies using rats support this theory (Weisman et al., 1978), indicating 25(OH)D. Such a conclusion emphasizes the importance of 25(OH)D status in the mother during pregnancy. An important yet unanswered series of questions include the following: By what mechanism does 25(OH)D enter the villous trophoblast? Does all or most 25(OH)D undergo hydroxylation in the trophoblast layer? How much 25(OH)D is transported from the trophoblast into the fetal circulation and by what means does this occur?

Successful implantation and completion of pregnancy require the maternal immune system to develop tolerance to paternal antigens derived from the placenta and fetus. This is nowhere more obvious than in the maternal decidua during implantation. Vitamin D affects the adaptive immune system (Hewison, 2011), with 1,25(OH)$_2$D promoting type 2 helper T cells, which produce more anti-inflammatory cytokines and which suppress cellular Th1 responses (Boonstra et al., 2001). Vitamin D also induces the differentiation of CD4$^+$ T cells into regulatory T cells, another immunosuppressive cell (Barrat et al., 2002). The maternal decidua has an abundance of immune cells, including CD56+ uterine natural killer (NK) cells. The NK cells are modulated by both 25(OH)D and 1,25(OH)$_2$D, suppressing inflammatory cytokine production *in vitro* (Evans et al., 2006). 1,25(OH)$_2$D inhibits the expression of inflammatory cytokines in trophoblasts challenged with tumor necrosis factor-α (TNF-α) (Diaz et al., 2009) and suppresses cyclooxygenase-2 up-regulation and consequent thromboxane production, in response to the hypoxia mimetic CoCl$_2$ (Sun et al., 2014). Mouse placentas exposed to lipopolysaccharide (LPS) exhibit increased expression of *Cyp27b1* and *VDR*, and mouse knockouts for these genes exhibit dysregulation of inflammatory reactions in response to immune challenges (Liu et al., 2011). In the presence of 25(OH)D or 1,25(OH)$_2$D, wild-type mouse placentas showed suppressed inflammatory responses to an *ex vivo* LPS challenge (Liu et al., 2011). 1,25(OH)$_2$D decreases IL-10 expression in human trophoblasts from normal and preeclamptic pregnancies and from control trophoblasts challenged with TNF-α (Barrera et al., 2012). Moreover, 1,25(OH)$_2$D stimulated the expression of β-defensins and cathelicidin, while IL-10 inhibited the expression of these antimicrobial peptides. Thus, 1,25(OH)$_2$D might restrict IL-10 permissive actions toward microbial invasion while restraining inflammation to allow pregnancy continuance (Olmos-Ortiz et al., 2014). Collectively, these studies indicate that vitamin D plays an important role in placental immunomodulation.

Vitamin D affects the synthesis of multiple hormones secreted by the placental trophoblasts (Figure 13.3). Supplementation with 1,25(OH)$_2$D alters the expression of human chorionic gonadotropin and increases the expression of estradiol, progesterone, and human placental lactogen (Barrera et al., 2007, 2008; Stephanou et al., 1994), all of which are important for the maintenance of a normal pregnancy. Whether the effect of vitamin D on trophoblast secretory activities include nongenomic affects, and exactly how the genomic affects are mediated, is an area worthy of future study.

Vitamin D influences the innate immune system by stimulating antimicrobial activity (Hewison, 2011), and vitamin D also stimulates the placenta to produce antibacterial proteins (Figure 13.3). Toll-like receptor (TLR) activation in monocytes induces the expression of the VDR and CYP27B1 (increasing 1,25(OH)$_2$D) and induces elevated production by trophoblasts of the antimicrobial proteins cathelicidin (CAMP) (Liu et al., 2009) and β-defensin (Olmos-Ortiz et al., 2014), as noted above. *In vitro* studies of the maternal decidua have shown that exposure to either 25(OH)D or 1,25(OH)$_2$D increases mRNA production for cathelicidin (Evans et al., 2006). Cord blood monocytes in vitamin D-deficient plasma (25(OH)D <30 nmol/L) show decreased TLR-induced cathelicidin expression (Walker et al., 2011), compared with culture with sufficient levels of vitamin D (>75 nmol/L). Moreover, supplementation of vitamin D-deficient plasma with 25(OH)D also increased cathelicidin expression (Walker et al., 2011). In placental trophoblasts, 1,25(OH)$_2$D induces cathelicidin in a dose-dependent fashion, although it is not enhanced by costimulation with TLR ligands, such as LPS, suggesting that induction of the innate immune system in the placenta is independent of TLR involvement (Liu et al., 2009). 25(OH)D and 1,25(OH)$_2$D significantly enhance antibacterial responses in trophoblastic cells, showing decreased numbers of bacterial colony-forming units and decreased trophoblast cell death after *Escherichia coli* infection, an important gram-negative pathogen in pregnancy (Liu et al., 2009). Recent work has also shown that when exposed to an array of proinflammatory cytokines, trophoblasts increase levels of both CYP27B1 and CYP24A1, affecting the metabolism and, therefore, availability of 1,25(OH)$_2$D (Noyola-Martinez et al., 2014). Similar to findings in the innate immune system, vitamin D-mediated antimicrobial effects on placental trophoblasts are likely an important factor in protecting the placenta from pathogens.

There are several mechanisms implicated in the etiology of preeclampsia, including those that involve abnormal inflammatory responses and endothelial cell dysfunction (Chaiworapongsa et al., 2014). There is evidence that vitamin D metabolism is altered in trophoblasts from preeclamptic pregnancies, although data are conflicting as to the nature of the alteration. Some report decreased synthesis of 1,25(OH)$_2$D and CYP27B1 mRNA levels in placentas from preeclamptic women, compared with placentas from normal pregnancies (Diaz et al., 2002; Halhali et al., 2014). Others report increased CYP27B1 protein expression in addition to increased CYP24A1 and decreased VDR protein expression compared with normal pregnancies (Ma et al., 2012). Increased CYP27B1 and decreased CYP24A1 and VDR mRNA levels in preeclamptic pregnancies have also been reported (Fischer et al., 2007). These conflicting results may be related to the nature of the preparations used when performing experiments or may be a result of the functional capability of the mRNA or protein. In addition, examination of the serum of preeclamptic women revealed elevated levels of autoantibodies to DBP, which may diminish the influence of 1,25(OH)$_2$D on trophoblasts (Behrouz et al., 2013).

Trophoblasts from placentas of preeclamptic pregnancies with 1,25(OH)$_2$D show decreased secretion and mRNA expression of the proinflammatory cytokines TNF-α and IL-6, suggesting that the protective effect of vitamin D for preeclampsia may be related to its anti-inflammatory properties (Noyola-Martinez et al., 2014). Endothelial progenitor cells that participate in vasculogenesis and endothelial repair are implicated in preeclampsia, and 1,25(OH)$_2$D improves endothelial colony forming cell functional properties that are otherwise decreased in preeclampsia (Brodowski et al., 2014; von Versen-Hoynck et al., 2014). Collectively, the above data show that the vitamin D pathway is dysregulated in placentas of preeclamptic women, but the specific relationship between this dysregulation and the evolution of the preeclamptic syndrome remains open for further studies.

13.5 TAKE-HOME POINTS

- Vitamin D is a family of secosteroids derived from sun exposure or dietary sources.
- Most circulating 25(OH) is generated by hydroxylation in the liver. Further hydroxylation in the kidney forms the majority of circulating 1,25(OH)$_2$D with resultant endocrine function.

- The VDR binds active $1,25(OH)_2D$ to effect genomic and nongenomic signaling in target tissues.
- Vitamin D has pleiotropic biological effects, including on bone and calcium metabolism, immune functions, and responses to infections.
- Vitamin D sufficiency in pregnancy is defined as a 25(OH)D level >30 ng/mL in blood, but the optimal daily intake of vitamin D to achieve this goal is not clear.
- Although controversy abounds concerning the specific roles for vitamin D in pregnancy complications such as preeclampsia, gestational diabetes, infection, and abnormal fetal and newborn outcomes, the data suggest that achieving vitamin D sufficiency is a worthy goal.
- The placenta is an active site of extra renal conversion of 25(OH)D to biologically active $1,25(OH)_2D$ through the action of 1α-hydroxylase.
- $1,25(OH)_2D$ from 25(OH)D in nonrenal cells, including trophoblasts, results in autocrine or paracrine functions.
- The VDR is expressed in human villous trophoblasts. Trophoblasts may modulate placental vitamin D responses through methylation of pathway genes and expression of pathway enzymes.
- Vitamin D modulates hormone secretion, immune function, and responses to infection in the placenta.
- Further study of vitamin D will likely unveil additional important functions for vitamin D in pregnancy, the placenta, and trophoblasts.

REFERENCES

Aghajafari, F., Nagulesapillai, T., Ronksley, P.E., Tough, S.C., O'Beirne, M., and Rabi, D.M. 2013. Association between maternal serum 25-hydroxyvitamin D level and pregnancy and neonatal outcomes: Systematic review and meta-analysis of observational studies. *BMJ*. 346:f1169.

Ajibade, D.V., Dhawan, P., Fechner, A.J., Meyer, M.B., Pike, J.W., and Christakos, S. 2010. Evidence for a role of prolactin in calcium homeostasis: Regulation of intestinal transient receptor potential vanilloid type 6, intestinal calcium absorption, and the 25-hydroxyvitamin D(3) 1α hydroxylase gene by prolactin. *Endocrinology*. 151:2974–84.

Armas, L.A., Hollis, B.W., and Heaney, R.P. 2004. Vitamin D2 is much less effective than vitamin D3 in humans. *J Clin Endocrinol Metab*. 89:5387–91.

Asemi, Z., Karamali, M., and Esmaillzadeh, A. 2014. Effects of calcium–vitamin D co-supplementation on glycaemic control, inflammation and oxidative stress in gestational diabetes: A randomised placebo-controlled trial. *Diabetologia*. 57:1798–806.

Avila, E., Diaz, L., Halhali, A., and Larrea, F. 2004. Regulation of 25-hydroxyvitamin D3 1α-hydroxylase, 1,25-dihydroxyvitamin D3 24-hydroxylase and vitamin D receptor gene expression by 8-bromo cyclic AMP in cultured human syncytiotrophoblast cells. *J Steroid Biochem Mol Biol*. 89–90:115–9.

Avila, E., Diaz, L., Barrera, D., Halhali, A., Mendez, I., Gonzalez, L., Zuegel, U., Steinmeyer, A., and Larrea, F. 2007. Regulation of vitamin D hydroxylases gene expression by 1,25-dihydroxyvitamin D3 and cyclic AMP in cultured human syncytiotrophoblasts. *J Steroid Biochem Mol Biol*. 103:90–6.

Barrat, F.J., Cua, D.J., Boonstra, A., Richards, D.F., Crain, C., Savelkoul, H.F., de Waal-Malefyt, R., Coffman, R.L., Hawrylowicz, C.M., and O'Garra, A. 2002. In vitro generation of interleukin 10-producing regulatory CD4(+) T cells is induced by immunosuppressive drugs and inhibited by T helper type 1 (Th1)- and Th2-inducing cytokines. *J Exp Med*. 195:603–16.

Barrera, D., Avila, E., Hernandez, G., Halhali, A., Biruete, B., Larrea, F., and Diaz, L. 2007. Estradiol and progesterone synthesis in human placenta is stimulated by calcitriol. *J Steroid Biochem Mol Biol*. 103:529–32.

Barrera, D., Avila, E., Hernandez, G., Mendez, I., Gonzalez, L., Halhali, A., Larrea, F., Morales, A., and Diaz, L. 2008. Calcitriol affects hCG gene transcription in cultured human syncytiotrophoblasts. *Reprod Biol Endocrinol*. 6:3.

Barrera, D., Noyola-Martinez, N., Avila, E., Halhali, A., Larrea, F., and Diaz, L. 2012. Calcitriol inhibits interleukin-10 expression in cultured human trophoblasts under normal and inflammatory conditions. *Cytokine*. 57:316–21.

Behrouz, G.F., Farzaneh, G.S., Leila, J., Jaleh, Z., and Eskandar, K.S. 2013. Presence of auto-antibody against two placental proteins, annexin A1 and vitamin D binding protein, in sera of women with pre-eclampsia. *J Reprod Immunol.* 99:10–6.

Bikle, D.D. 2014. Vitamin D metabolism, mechanism of action, and clinical applications. *Chem Biol.* 21:319–29.

Bodnar, L.M., Krohn, M.A., and Simhan, H.N. 2009. Maternal vitamin D deficiency is associated with bacterial vaginosis in the first trimester of pregnancy. *J Nutr.* 139:1157–61.

Bodnar, L.M., Klebanoff, M.A., Gernand, A.D., Platt, R.W., Parks, W.T., Catov, J.M., and Simhan, H.N. 2014. Maternal vitamin D status and spontaneous preterm birth by placental histology in the US Collaborative Perinatal Project. *Am J Epidemiol.* 179:168–76.

Boonstra, A., Barrat, F.J., Crain, C., Heath, V.L., Savelkoul, H.F., and O'Garra, A. 2001. 1α,25-dihydroxyvitamin D3 has a direct effect on naive CD4(+) T cells to enhance the development of Th2 cells. *J Immunol.* 167:4974–80.

Brannon, P.M. and Picciano, M.F. 2011. Vitamin D in pregnancy and lactation in humans. *Annu Rev Nutr.* 31:89–115.

Brodowski, L., Burlakov, J., Myerski, A.C., von Kaisenberg, C.S., Grundmann, M., Hubel, C.A., and von Versen-Hoynck, F. 2014. Vitamin D prevents endothelial progenitor cell dysfunction induced by sera from women with preeclampsia or conditioned media from hypoxic placenta. *PLoS One.* 9:e98527.

Burke, K.A., Jauniaux, E., Burton, G.J., and Cindrova-Davies, T. 2013. Expression and immunolocalisation of the endocytic receptors megalin and cubilin in the human yolk sac and placenta across gestation. *Placenta.* 34:1105–9.

Burris, H.H. and Camargo, C.A.J. 2014. Time for large randomised trials of vitamin D for women with gestational diabetes mellitus to improve perinatal health outcomes. *Diabetologia.* 57:1746–8.

Carlberg, C. and Seuter, S. 2009. A genomic perspective on vitamin D signaling. *Anticancer Res.* 29:3485–93.

Chaiworapongsa, T., Chaemsaithong, P., Yeo, L., and Romero, R. 2014. Pre-eclampsia part 1: Current understanding of its pathophysiology. *Nat Rev Nephrol.* 10:466–80.

Chen, S., Law, C.S., Grigsby, C.L., Olsen, K., Hong, T.T., Zhang, Y., Yeghiazarians, Y., and Gardner, D.G. 2011. Cardiomyocyte-specific deletion of the vitamin D receptor gene results in cardiac hypertrophy. *Circulation.* 124:1838–47.

Cho, G.J., Hong, S.C., Oh, M.J., and Kim, H.J. 2013. Vitamin D deficiency in gestational diabetes mellitus and the role of the placenta. *Am J Obstet Gynecol.* 209:560.e1–8.

Christakos, S., Hewison, M., Gardner, D.G., Wagner, C.L., Sergeev, I.N., Rutten, E., Pittas, A.G., Boland, R., Ferrucci, L., and Bikle, D.D. 2013. Vitamin D: Beyond bone. *Ann N Y Acad Sci.* 1287:45–58.

Christensen, E.I. and Birn, H. 2002. Megalin and cubilin: Multifunctional endocytic receptors. *Nat Rev Mol Cell Biol.* 3:256–66.

Chun, R.F., Liu, P.T., Modlin, R.L., Adams, J.S., and Hewison, M. 2014a. Impact of vitamin D on immune function: Lessons learned from genome-wide analysis. *Front Physiol.* 5:151.

Chun, R.F., Peercy, B.E., Orwoll, E.S., Nielson, C.M., Adams, J.S., and Hewison, M. 2014b. Vitamin D and DBP: The free hormone hypothesis revisited. *J Steroid Biochem Mol Biol.* 144 Pt A:132–7.

Dawodu, A., Saadi, H.F., Bekdache, G., Javed, Y., Altaye, M., and Hollis, B.W. 2013. Randomized controlled trial (RCT) of vitamin D supplementation in pregnancy in a population with endemic vitamin D deficiency. *J Clin Endocrinol Metab.* 98:2337–46.

Deeb, K.K., Trump, D.L., and Johnson, C.S. 2007. Vitamin D signalling pathways in cancer: Potential for anticancer therapeutics. *Nat Rev Cancer.* 7:684–700.

DeLuca, H.F. 2004. Overview of general physiologic features and functions of vitamin D. *Am J Clin Nutr.* 80:1689S–96S.

Diaz, L., Sanchez, I., Avila, E., Halhali, A., Vilchis, F., and Larrea, F. 2000. Identification of a 25-hydroxyvitamin D3 1α-hydroxylase gene transcription product in cultures of human syncytiotrophoblast cells. *J Clin Endocrinol Metab.* 85:2543–9.

Diaz, L., Arranz, C., Avila, E., Halhali, A., Vilchis, F., and Larrea, F. 2002. Expression and activity of 25-hydroxyvitamin D-1α-hydroxylase are restricted in cultures of human syncytiotrophoblast cells from preeclamptic pregnancies p. *J Clin Endocrinol Metab.* 87:3876–82.

Diaz, L., Noyola-Martinez, N., Barrera, D., Hernandez, G., Avila, E., Halhali, A., and Larrea, F. 2009. Calcitriol inhibits TNF-α-induced inflammatory cytokines in human trophoblasts. *J Reprod Immunol.* 81:17–24.

Dunlop, A.L., Taylor, R.N., Tangpricha, V., Fortunato, S., and Menon, R. 2011. Maternal vitamin D, folate, and polyunsaturated fatty acid status and bacterial vaginosis during pregnancy. *Infect Dis Obstet Gynecol.* 2011:216217.

Evans, K.N., Nguyen, L., Chan, J., Innes, B.A., Bulmer, J.N., Kilby, M.D., and Hewison, M. 2006. Effects of 25-hydroxyvitamin D3 and 1,25-dihydroxyvitamin D3 on cytokine production by human decidual cells. *Biol Reprod.* 75:816–22.

Fabri, M. and Modlin, R.L. 2009. A vitamin for autophagy. *Cell Host Microbe.* 6:201–3.

Farrant, H.J., Krishnaveni, G.V., Hill, J.C., Boucher, B.J., Fisher, D.J., Noonan, K., Osmond, C., Veena, S.R., and Fall, C.H. 2009. Vitamin D insufficiency is common in Indian mothers but is not associated with gestational diabetes or variation in newborn size. *Eur J Clin Nutr.* 63:646–52.

Feldman, D., Krishnan, A.V., Swami, S., Giovannucci, E., and Feldman, B.J. 2014. The role of vitamin D in reducing cancer risk and progression. *Nat Rev Cancer.* 14:342–57.

Fernandez-Alonso, A.M., Dionis-Sanchez, E.C., Chedraui, P., Gonzalez-Salmeron, M.D., and Perez-Lopez, F.R. 2012. First-trimester maternal serum 25-hydroxyvitamin D(3) status and pregnancy outcome. *Int J Gynaecol Obstet.* 116:6–9.

Fischer, D., Schroer, A., Ludders, D., Cordes, T., Bucker, B., Reichrath, J., and Friedrich, M. 2007. Metabolism of vitamin D3 in the placental tissue of normal and preeclampsia complicated pregnancies and premature births. *Clin Exp Obstet Gynecol.* 34:80–4.

Gernand, A.D., Simhan, H.N., Caritis, S., and Bodnar, L.M. 2014. Maternal vitamin D status and small-for-gestational-age offspring in women at high risk for preeclampsia. *Obstet Gynecol.* 123:40–8.

Gezmish, O., Tare, M., Parkington, H.C., Morley, R., Porrello, E.R., Bubb, K.J., and Black, M.J. 2010. Maternal vitamin D deficiency leads to cardiac hypertrophy in rat offspring. *Reprod Sci.* 17:168–76.

Gregori, S., Casorati, M., Amuchastegui, S., Smiroldo, S., Davalli, A.M., and Adorini, L. 2001. Regulatory T cells induced by 1α,25-dihydroxyvitamin D3 and mycophenolate mofetil treatment mediate transplantation tolerance. *J Immunol.* 167:1945–53.

Griffin, M.D., Lutz, W., Phan, V.A., Bachman, L.A., McKean, D.J., and Kumar, R. 2001. Dendritic cell modulation by 1α,25 dihydroxyvitamin D3 and its analogs: A vitamin D receptor-dependent pathway that promotes a persistent state of immaturity in vitro and in vivo. *Proc Natl Acad Sci U S A.* 98:6800–5.

Gysler, S.M., Mulla, M.J., Stuhlman, M., Sfakianaki, A.K., Paidas, M.J., Stanwood, N.L., Gariepy, A., Brosens, J.J., Chamley, L.W., and Abrahams, V.M. 2015. Vitamin D reverses aPL-induced inflammation and LMWH-induced sFlt-1 release by human trophoblast. *Am J Reprod Immunol.* 73:242–50.

Halhali, A., Diaz, L., Barrera, D., Avila, E., and Larrea, F. 2014. Placental calcitriol synthesis and IGF-I levels in normal and preeclamptic pregnancies. *J Steroid Biochem Mol Biol.* 144 Pt A:44–9.

Harrington, J., Perumal, N., Al Mahmud, A., Baqui, A., and Roth, D.E. 2014. Vitamin D and fetal–neonatal calcium homeostasis: Findings from a randomized controlled trial of high-dose antenatal vitamin D supplementation. *Pediatr Res.* 76:302–9.

Hashemipour, S., Lalooha, F., Zahir Mirdamadi, S., Ziaee, A., and Dabaghi Ghaleh, T. 2013. Effect of vitamin D administration in vitamin D-deficient pregnant women on maternal and neonatal serum calcium and vitamin D concentrations: A randomised clinical trial. *Br J Nutr.* 110:1611–6.

Hashemipour, S., Ziaee, A., Javadi, A., Movahed, F., Elmizadeh, K., Javadi, E.H., and Lalooha, F. 2014. Effect of treatment of vitamin D deficiency and insufficiency during pregnancy on fetal growth indices and maternal weight gain: A randomized clinical trial. *Eur J Obstet Gynecol Reprod Biol.* 172:15–9.

Haussler, M.R., Jurutka, P.W., Mizwicki, M., and Norman, A.W. 2011. Vitamin D receptor (VDR)-mediated actions of 1α,25(OH)(2)vitamin D(3): Genomic and non-genomic mechanisms. *Best Pract Res Clin Endocrinol Metab.* 25:543–59.

Hewison, M. 2010. Vitamin D and the immune system: New perspectives on an old theme. *Endocrinol Metab Clin North Am.* 39:365–79.

Hewison, M. 2011. Vitamin D and innate and adaptive immunity. *Vitam Horm.* 86:23–62.

Holick, M.F., Binkley, N.C., Bischoff-Ferrari, H.A., Gordon, C.M., Hanley, D.A., Heaney, R.P., Murad, M.H., and Weaver, C.M. 2011. Evaluation, treatment, and prevention of vitamin D deficiency: An Endocrine Society clinical practice guideline. *J Clin Endocrinol Metab.* 96:1911–30.

Hollis, B.W. and Wagner, C.L. 2013. Vitamin D and pregnancy: Skeletal effects, nonskeletal effects, and birth outcomes. *Calcif Tissue Int.* 92:128–39.

Hollis, B.W., Johnson, D., Hulsey, T.C., Ebeling, M., and Wagner, C.L. 2011. Vitamin D supplementation during pregnancy: Double-blind, andomized clinical trial of safety and effectiveness. *J Bone Miner Res.* 26:2341–57.

Hossain, N., Kanani, F.H., Ramzan, S., Kausar, R., Ayaz, S., Khanani, R., and Pal, L. 2014. Obstetric and neonatal outcomes of maternal vitamin D supplementation: Results of an open-label, randomized controlled trial of antenatal vitamin D supplementation in Pakistani women. *J Clin Endocrinol Metab.* 99:2448–55.

Houghton, L.A. and Vieth, R. 2006. The case against ergocalciferol (vitamin D2) as a vitamin supplement. *Am J Clin Nutr.* 84:694–7.

Hypponen, E., Cavadino, A., Williams, D., Fraser, A., Vereczkey, A., Fraser, W.D., Banhidy, F., Lawlor, D., and Czeizel, A.E. 2013. Vitamin D and pre-eclampsia: Original data, systematic review and meta-analysis. *Ann Nutr Metab.* 63:331–40.

Jelsma, J.G., van Poppel, M.N., Galjaard, S., Desoye, G., Corcoy, R., Devlieger, R., van Assche, A., Timmerman, D., Jans, G., Harreiter, J. et al. 2013. DALI: Vitamin D and lifestyle intervention for gestational diabetes mellitus (GDM) prevention: An European multicentre, randomised trial—Study protocol. *BMC Pregnancy Childbirth.* 13:142.

Joshi, S., Pantalena, L.C., Liu, X.K., Gaffen, S.L., Liu, H., Rohowsky-Kochan, C., Ichiyama, K., Yoshimura, A., Steinman, L., Christakos, S. et al. 2011. 1,25-dihydroxyvitamin D(3) ameliorates Th17 autoimmunity via transcriptional modulation of interleukin-17A. *Mol Cell Biol.* 31:3653–69.

Knabl, J., Huttenbrenner, R., Hutter, S., Gunthner-Biller, M., Riedel, C., Hiden, U., Kainer, F., Desoye, G., and Jeschke, U. 2015. Gestational diabetes mellitus upregulates vitamin D receptor in extravillous trophoblasts and fetoplacental endothelial cells. *Reprod Sci.* 22:358–66.

Kovacs, C.S. and Kronenberg, H.M. 1997. Maternal–fetal calcium and bone metabolism during pregnancy, puerperium, and lactation. *Endocr Rev.* 18:832–72.

Lacroix, M., Battista, M.C., Doyon, M., Houde, G., Menard, J., Ardilouze, J.L., Hivert, M.F., and Perron, P. 2014. Lower vitamin D levels at first trimester are associated with higher risk of developing gestational diabetes mellitus. *Acta Diabetol.* 51:609–16.

Lapillonne, A. 2010. Vitamin D deficiency during pregnancy may impair maternal and fetal outcomes. *Med Hypotheses.* 74:71–5.

Lau, S.L., Gunton, J.E., Athayde, N.P., Byth, K., and Cheung, N.W. 2011. Serum 25-hydroxyvitamin D and glycated haemoglobin levels in women with gestational diabetes mellitus. *Med J Aust.* 194:334–7.

Liu, N., Kaplan, A.T., Low, J., Nguyen, L., Liu, G.Y., Equils, O., and Hewison, M. 2009. Vitamin D induces innate antibacterial responses in human trophoblasts via an intracrine pathway. *Biol Reprod.* 80:398–406.

Liu, N.Q., Kaplan, A.T., Lagishetty, V., Ouyang, Y.B., Ouyang, Y., Simmons, C.F., Equils, O., and Hewison, M. 2011. Vitamin D and the regulation of placental inflammation. *J Immunol.* 186:5968–74.

Ma, R., Gu, Y., Zhao, S., Sun, J., Groome, L.J., and Wang, Y. 2012. Expressions of vitamin D metabolic components VDBP, CYP2R1, CYP27B1, CYP24A1, and VDR in placentas from normal and preeclamptic pregnancies. *Am J Physiol Endocrinol Metab.* 303:E928–35.

McManus, R., Summers, K., de Vrijer, B., Cohen, N., Thompson, A., and Giroux, I. 2014. Maternal, umbilical arterial and umbilical venous 25-hydroxyvitamin D and adipocytokine concentrations in pregnancies with and without gestational diabetes. *Clin Endocrinol (Oxf).* 80:635–41.

Mulligan, M.L., Felton, S.K., Riek, A.E., and Bernal-Mizrachi, C. 2010. Implications of vitamin D deficiency in pregnancy and lactation. *Am J Obstet Gynecol.* 202:429.e1–9.

Negri, A.L. 2006. Proximal tubule endocytic apparatus as the specific renal uptake mechanism for vitamin D-binding protein/25-(OH)D3 complex. *Nephrology (Carlton).* 11:510–5.

Nigwekar, S.U. and Thadhani, R. 2013. Vitamin D receptor activation: Cardiovascular and renal implications. *Kidney Int Suppl (2011).* 3(5):427–30.

Novakovic, B., Sibson, M., Ng, H.K., Manuelpillai, U., Rakyan, V., Down, T., Beck, S., Fournier, T., Evain-Brion, D., Dimitriadis, E. et al. 2009. Placenta-specific methylation of the vitamin D 24-hydroxylase gene: Implications for feedback autoregulation of active vitamin D levels at the fetomaternal interface. *J Biol Chem.* 284:14838–48.

Noyola-Martinez, N., Diaz, L., Zaga-Clavellina, V., Avila, E., Halhali, A., Larrea, F., and Barrera, D. 2014. Regulation of CYP27B1 and CYP24A1 gene expression by recombinant pro-inflammatory cytokines in cultured human trophoblasts. *J Steroid Biochem Mol Biol.* 144 Pt A:106–9.

O'Brien, K.O., Li, S., Cao, C., Kent, T., Young, B.V., Queenan, R.A., Pressman, E.K., and Cooper, E.M. 2014. Placental CYP27B1 and CYP24A1 expression in human placental tissue and their association with maternal and neonatal calcitropic hormones. *J Clin Endocrinol Metab.* 99:1348–56.

Olmos-Ortiz, A., Noyola-Martinez, N., Barrera, D., Zaga-Clavellina, V., Avila, E., Halhali, A., Biruete, B., Larrea, F., and Diaz, L. 2014. IL-10 inhibits while calcitriol reestablishes placental antimicrobial peptides gene expression. *J Steroid Biochem Mol Biol.* doi:10.1016/j.jsbmb.2014.7.012.

Paffoni, A., Ferrari, S., Vigano, P., Pagliardini, L., Papaleo, E., Candiani, M., Tirelli, A., Fedele, L., and Somigliana, E. 2014. Vitamin D deficiency and infertility: Insights from in vitro fertilization cycles. *J Clin Endocrinol Metab.* 99:E2372–6.

Penna, G., Amuchastegui, S., Giarratana, N., Daniel, K.C., Vulcano, M., Sozzani, S., and Adorini, L. 2007. 1,25-Dihydroxyvitamin D3 selectively modulates tolerogenic properties in myeloid but not plasmacytoid dendritic cells. *J Immunol.* 178:145–53.

Pike, J.W. and Meyer, M.B. 2010. The vitamin D receptor: New paradigms for the regulation of gene expression by 1,25-dihydroxyvitamin D(3). *Endocrinol Metab Clin North Am.* 39:255–69.

Pludowski, P., Holick, M.F., Pilz, S., Wagner, C.L., Hollis, B.W., Grant, W.B., Shoenfeld, Y., Lerchbaum, E., Llewellyn, D.J., Kienreich, K. et al. 2013. Vitamin D effects on musculoskeletal health, immunity, autoimmunity, cardiovascular disease, cancer, fertility, pregnancy, dementia and mortality—A review of recent evidence. *Autoimmun Rev.* 12:976–89.

Poel, Y.H., Hummel, P., Lips, P., Stam, F., van der Ploeg, T., and Simsek, S. 2012. Vitamin D and gestational diabetes: A systematic review and meta-analysis. *Eur J Intern Med.* 23:465–9.

Pospechova, K., Rozehnal, V., Stejskalova, L., Vrzal, R., Pospisilova, N., Jamborova, G., May, K., Siegmund, W., Dvorak, Z., Nachtigal, P. et al. 2009. Expression and activity of vitamin D receptor in the human placenta and in choriocarcinoma BeWo and JEG-3 cell lines. *Mol Cell Endocrinol.* 299:178–87.

Prosser, D.E. and Jones, G. 2004. Enzymes involved in the activation and inactivation of vitamin D. *Trends Biochem Sci.* 29:664–73.

Quarles, L.D. 2012. Skeletal secretion of FGF-23 regulates phosphate and vitamin D metabolism. *Nat Rev Endocrinol.* 8:276–86.

Ritchie, L.D., Fung, E.B., Halloran, B.P., Turnlund, J.R., Van Loan, M.D., Cann, C.E., and King, J.C. 1998. A longitudinal study of calcium homeostasis during human pregnancy and lactation and after resumption of menses. *Am J Clin Nutr.* 67:693–701.

Rodriguez, A., Garcia-Esteban, R., Basterretxea, M., Lertxundi, A., Rodriguez-Bernal, C., Iniguez, C., Rodriguez-Dehli, C., Tardon, A., Espada, M., Sunyer, J. et al. 2014. Associations of maternal circulating 25-hydroxyvitamin D3 concentration with pregnancy and birth outcomes. *BJOG.* doi:10.1111/1471–0528.13074.

Ross, A.C., Taylor, C.R., Yaktine, A.L., and Del Valle, H.B. 2011. Dietary Reference Intakes for Calcium and Vitamin D. *JCEM* 96:53–8.

Roth, D.E., Al Mahmud, A., Raqib, R., Akhtar, E., Perumal, N., Pezzack, B., and Baqui, A.H. 2013. Randomized placebo-controlled trial of high-dose prenatal third-trimester vitamin D3 supplementation in Bangladesh: the AViDD trial. *Nutr J.* 12:47.

Rowling, M.J., Kemmis, C.M., Taffany, D.A., and Welsh, J. 2006. Megalin-mediated endocytosis of vitamin D binding protein correlates with 25-hydroxycholecalciferol actions in human mammary cells. *J Nutr.* 136:2754–9.

Schneuer, F.J., Roberts, C.L., Guilbert, C., Simpson, J.M., Algert, C.S., Khambalia, A.Z., Tasevski, V., Ashton, A.W., Morris, J.M., and Nassar, N. 2014. Effects of maternal serum 25-hydroxyvitamin D concentrations in the first trimester on subsequent pregnancy outcomes in an Australian population. *Am J Clin Nutr.* 99:287–95.

Shahbazi, M., Jeddi-Tehrani, M., Zareie, M., Salek-Moghaddam, A., Akhondi, M.M., Bahmanpoor, M., Sadeghi, M.R., and Zarnani, A.H. 2011. Expression profiling of vitamin D receptor in placenta, decidua and ovary of pregnant mice. *Placenta.* 32:657–64.

Shin, J.S., Choi, M.Y., Longtine, M.S., and Nelson, D.M. 2010. Vitamin D effects on pregnancy and the placenta. *Placenta.* 31:1027–34.

Specker, B. 2004. Vitamin D requirements during pregnancy. *Am J Clin Nutr.* 80:1740S–7S.

Specker, B.L. 2012. Does vitamin D during pregnancy impact offspring growth and bone? *Proc Nutr Soc.* 71:38–45.

Stephanou, A., Ross, R., and Handwerger, S. 1994. Regulation of human placental lactogen expression by 1,25-dihydroxyvitamin D3. *Endocrinology.* 135:2651–6.

Sun, J., Zhong, W., Gu, Y., Groome, L.J., and Wang, Y. 2014. 1,25(OH)2D3 suppresses COX-2 up-regulation and thromboxane production in placental trophoblast cells in response to hypoxic stimulation. *Placenta.* 35:143–5.

Ternes, S.B. and Rowling, M.J. 2013. Vitamin D transport proteins megalin and disabled-2 are expressed in prostate and colon epithelial cells and are induced and activated by all-trans-retinoic acid. *Nutr Cancer.* 65:900–7.

Turner, A.N., Carr Reese, P., Fields, K.S., Anderson, J., Ervin, M., Davis, J.A., Fichorova, R.N., Roberts, M.W., Klebanoff, M.A., and Jackson, R.D. 2014. A blinded, randomized controlled trial of high-dose vitamin D supplementation to reduce recurrence of bacterial vaginosis. *Am J Obstet Gynecol.* 211:479.e1–13.

van den Berg, G., van Eijsden, M., Vrijkotte, T.G., and Gemke, R.J. 2013. Suboptimal maternal vitamin D status and low education level as determinants of small-for-gestational-age birth weight. *Eur J Nutr.* 52:273–9.

Verstuyf, A., Carmeliet, G., Bouillon, R., and Mathieu, C. 2010. Vitamin D: A pleiotropic hormone. *Kidney Int.* 78:140–5.

von Versen-Hoynck, F., Brodowski, L., Dechend, R., Myerski, A.C., and Hubel, C.A. 2014. Vitamin D antagonizes negative effects of preeclampsia on fetal endothelial colony forming cell number and function. *PLoS One.* 9:e98990.

Wagner, C.L., Taylor, S.N., Johnson, D.D., and Hollis, B.W. 2012. The role of vitamin D in pregnancy and lactation: Emerging concepts. *Womens Health (Lond Engl).* 8:323–40.

Wagner, C.L., McNeil, R., Hamilton, S.A., Winkler, J., Rodriguez Cook, C., Warner, G., Bivens, B., Davis, D.J., Smith, P.G., Murphy, M. et al. 2013. A randomized trial of vitamin D supplementation in 2 community health center networks in South Carolina. *Am J Obstet Gynecol.* 208:137.e1–13.

Walker, V.P., Zhang, X., Rastegar, I., Liu, P.T., Hollis, B.W., Adams, J.S., and Modlin, R.L. 2011. Cord blood vitamin D status impacts innate immune responses. *J Clin Endocrinol Metab.* 96:1835–43.

Wang, T.T., Tavera-Mendoza, L.E., Laperriere, D., Libby, E., MacLeod, N.B., Nagai, Y., Bourdeau, V., Konstorum, A., Lallemant, B., Zhang, R. et al. 2005. Large-scale in silico and microarray-based identification of direct 1,25-dihydroxyvitamin D3 target genes. *Mol Endocrinol.* 19:2685–95.

Wei, S.Q., Qi, H.P., Luo, Z.C., and Fraser, W.D. 2013. Maternal vitamin D status and adverse pregnancy outcomes: A systematic review and meta-analysis. *J Matern Fetal Neonatal Med.* 26:889–99.

Weisman, Y., Vargas, A., Duckett, G., Reiter, E., and Root, A.W. 1978. Synthesis of 1,25-dihydroxyvitamin D in the nephrectomized pregnant rat. *Endocrinology.* 103:1992–6.

Weisman, Y., Harell, A., Edelstein, S., David, M., Spirer, Z., and Golander, A. 1979. 1α,25-Dihydroxyvitamin D3 and 24,25-dihydroxyvitamin D3 in vitro synthesis by human decidua and placenta. *Nature.* 281:317–9.

Whitelaw, D.C., Scally, A.J., Tuffnell, D.J., Davies, T.J., Fraser, W.D., Bhopal, R.S., Wright, J., and Lawlor, D.A. 2014. Associations of circulating calcium and 25-hydroxyvitamin D with glucose metabolism in pregnancy: A cross-sectional study in European and South Asian women. *J Clin Endocrinol Metab.* 99:938–46.

Wieland, P., Fischer, J.A., Trechsel, U., Roth, H.R., Vetter, K., Schneider, H., and Huch, A. 1980. Perinatal parathyroid hormone, vitamin D metabolites, and calcitonin in man. *Am J Physiol.* 239:E385–90.

Wolf, G. 2004. The discovery of vitamin D: The contribution of Adolf Windaus. *J Nutr.* 134:1299–302.

Xiang, W., Kong, J., Chen, S., Cao, L.P., Qiao, G., Zheng, W., Liu, W., Li, X., Gardner, D.G., and Li, Y.C. 2005. Cardiac hypertrophy in vitamin D receptor knockout mice: Role of the systemic and cardiac renin–angiotensin systems. *Am J Physiol Endocrinol Metab.* 288:E125–32.

Yap, C., Cheung, N.W., Gunton, J.E., Athayde, N., Munns, C.F., Duke, A., and McLean, M. 2014. Vitamin D supplementation and the effects on glucose metabolism during pregnancy: A randomized controlled trial. *Diabetes Care.* 37:1837–44.

Young, B.E., Cooper, E.M., McIntyre, A.W., Kent, T., Witter, F., Harris, Z.L., and O'Brien, K.O. 2014. Placental vitamin D receptor (VDR) expression is related to neonatal vitamin D status, placental calcium transfer, and fetal bone length in pregnant adolescents. *FASEB J.* 28:2029–37.

Zehnder, D., Evans, K.N., Kilby, M.D., Bulmer, J.N., Innes, B.A., Stewart, P.M., and Hewison, M. 2002. The ontogeny of 25-hydroxyvitamin D(3) 1α-hydroxylase expression in human placenta and decidua. *Am J Pathol.* 161:105–14.

Zhong, Y., Armbrecht, H.J., and Christakos, S. 2009. Calcitonin, a regulator of the 25-hydroxyvitamin D3 1α-hydroxylase gene. *J Biol Chem.* 284:11059–69.

Zhou, J., Su, L., Liu, M., Liu, Y., Cao, X., Wang, Z., and Xiao, H. 2014. Associations between 25-hydroxyvitamin D levels and pregnancy outcomes: A prospective observational study in southern China. *Eur J Clin Nutr.* 68:925–30.

Zhu, J.G., Ochalek, J.T., Kaufmann, M., Jones, G., and Deluca, H.F. 2013. CYP2R1 is a major, but not exclusive, contributor to 25-hydroxyvitamin D production in vivo. *Proc Natl Acad Sci U S A.* 110:15650–5.

14 Choline and Placental Trophoblast Development

Sze Ting (Cecilia) Kwan, Julia H. King, and Marie A. Caudill

CONTENTS

ABSTRACT

Choline is an essential micronutrient whose metabolic derivatives play important roles in many biological processes that are crucial to placental development and functioning. Dietary choline recommendations of 450 mg/day were established for pregnant women in 1998; however, recent data indicate that choline intakes exceeding current recommendations may improve placental development by modulating its epigenome, acetylcholine signaling, and vasculature. Abnormal placental development is a key contributor to the pathology of many pregnancy complications. By optimizing various aspects of placental development, increasing maternal choline intake during pregnancy may be a safe and effective strategy to reduce the risk of these undesirable pregnancy outcomes. As the placenta has an influential role in determining fetal development, maternal choline supplementation may also impact fetal long-term health. Given that most US women do not consume choline at recommended intake levels, public health efforts are needed to promote awareness of choline among pregnant women and to provide strategies for enhancing choline intake during this reproductive state.

KEY WORDS

Choline, placenta, methylation, epigenome, acetylcholine signaling, protein kinase C, preeclampsia, fetal programming.

14.1 INTRODUCTION

Choline, a bioactive nutrient commonly grouped with the B vitamins, was first recognized as an essential nutrient in 1991 when men consuming a choline-deficient diet developed liver dysfunction (Zeisel et al. 1991). This finding led to the establishment of dietary choline recommendations by the Institute of Medicine (IOM) in 1998 (IOM 1998). Choline functions as the precursor molecule for several key metabolites that have essential roles in one-carbon metabolism, neurotransmission, cell signaling pathways, as well as lipid and phospholipid metabolism (see Figure 14.1). These choline-dependent biological processes are critical to normal placental development and a successful pregnancy.

14.1.1 Importance of Choline Metabolites in Biological Processes

14.1.1.1 Betaine: A Methyl Donor for One-Carbon Metabolism

Betaine is the oxidized derivative of choline (see Figure 14.2), which functions in the remethylation of homocysteine, a non-protein-coding amino acid that is elevated in several disorders of pregnancy (e.g., preeclampsia) (Kalhan and Marczewski 2012), to methionine, an essential amino acid. Methionine is ultimately converted to S-adenosylmethionine (SAM), the universal methyl donor for cellular methylation reactions, including methylation of DNA (Jiang, Yan, and Caudill 2013). In this way, methyl groups originating from choline can have wide-ranging effects on epigenetic regulation

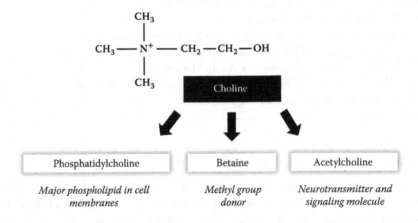

FIGURE 14.1 The metabolic fates and functions of choline and its metabolites.

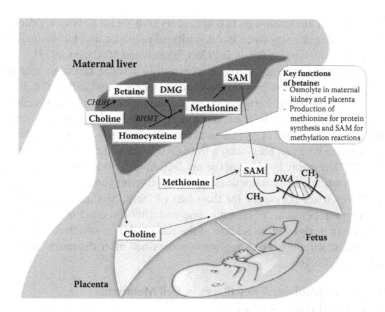

FIGURE 14.2 In the liver, choline is oxidized to betaine by choline dehydrogenase (*CHDH*), which donates a methyl group for the conversion of homocysteine to methionine via the enzyme betaine homocysteine methyltransferase (*BHMT*), producing dimethylglycine (DMG). Methionine and *S*-adenosylmethionine (SAM) can be transported into the placenta, where they are used for methylation reactions.

and gene expression. Betaine is also a source of one-carbons for folate-mediated nucleotide synthesis. Conversion of homocysteine to methionine yields dimethylglycine, a molecule with two labile one-carbon moieties that can be used for purine and pyrimidine biosynthesis.

Betaine has an additional function as an osmolyte, a molecule that aids in the regulation of cell volume (Lever and Slow 2010) and the prevention of osmotic stress, which induces apoptosis and DNA damage (Arroyo et al. 2012). Placental trophoblasts require effective osmoregulation because of their high rates of division with accompanying cell volume shifts. During early embryonic development and implantation, betaine and other osmolytes protect embryos from elevated osmolarity (Dawson and Baltz 1997). Betaine is a major organic osmolyte in the rat placenta (Miller, Hanson, and Yancey 2000); however, the importance of betaine as an osmolyte in human placenta has yet to be ascertained.

14.1.1.2 Acetylcholine: A Signaling Molecule in Neuronal and Nonneuronal Tissues

Choline is also used to synthesize acetylcholine, a neurotransmitter of the central and peripheral nervous systems. Acetylcholine also functions in many nonneuronal tissues (Kawashima and Fujii 2008; Wessler et al. 2003), including the human placenta, which contains roughly seven times more acetylcholine than that found in the nervous system (Sastry 1997). Since placenta is not innervated and is not an excitable tissue, this unexpected finding led to research seeking to characterize the function of placental acetylcholine.

Acetylcholine is found in the syncytiotrophoblast in a bound form (Sastry et al. 1976), and unlike neuronal acetylcholine, it is not stored in vesicles (Wessler et al. 2003). Placental acetylcholine concentration varies according to gestational age. The highest concentrations are observed during the second trimester of pregnancy at gestational weeks 21 to 24 (Sastry et al. 1976), whereas a dramatic decrease in placental acetylcholine occurs at the onset of labor (Brennecke et al. 1988). Choline acetyltransferase activity, the enzyme that synthesizes acetylcholine from choline and acetyl coenzyme A, shows a similar expression pattern, peaking at gestational weeks 16 to 20 and attenuating at parturition (Sastry et al. 1976). Notably, the placenta's ability to produce acetylcholine is highly related to the integrity of the syncytiotrophoblast. When the syncytiotrophoblast develops abnormally, as in the case of preeclampsia, acetylcholine synthesis is impaired (Satyanarayana 1986).

The high acetylcholine concentration and choline acetyltransferase activity appears to be a unique characteristic of human placentas since the majority of domestic and lab animals have very low amounts of this choline metabolite (Welsch 1976b; Welsch and McCarthy 1977).

Nonneuronal acetylcholine plays a role in controlling cellular functions that are critical for growth and development, such as proliferation, differentiation, and cell–cell contact (Wessler et al. 2003). Placental acetylcholine is suggested to play an important role in placental development through its effects on blood flow regulation, transport of amino acids, and hormone release (King et al. 1991, Sastry 1997) (see Figure 14.3). Placental acetylcholine may also be involved in the process of parturition. Acetylcholine has been shown to stimulate the myometrium directly (Brennecke et al. 1988; Sastry 1997), possibly by altering the production of prostaglandins (Sastry 1997). During pregnancy, prostaglandins cause contractions in the myometrium and trigger cervical ripening and dilation, both of which are necessary for the onset of labor. Studies comparing the amount of acetylcholine content in placentas obtained before and after the onset of labor suggest that there may be an increase in acetylcholine release at the time of labor, which could explain the lower acetylcholine concentration observed in placentas obtained after the onset of labor (Brennecke et al. 1988; King et al. 1991).

14.1.1.3 Phosphatidylcholine: A Key Player in Cell Membrane Integrity and Lipid Metabolism

Phosphatidylcholine (PC), another molecule generated from choline, is a major component of cell membranes and plays a critical role in maintaining their structural integrity. The demand for PC is high during pregnancy because of accelerations in cellular division and rapid expansion of fetal tissue. PC synthesis occurs mainly in the liver, and it can be produced by two pathways (see Figure 14.4). The majority of PC is produced from choline through the cytidine diphosphate (CDP)–choline pathway (Zeisel and Blusztajn 1994). An alternative pathway for PC synthesis is via the phosphatidylethanolamine N-methyltransferase (PEMT) pathway, which involves sequential methylation of phosphatidylethanolamine (a noncholine metabolite) to PC using SAM as the methyl

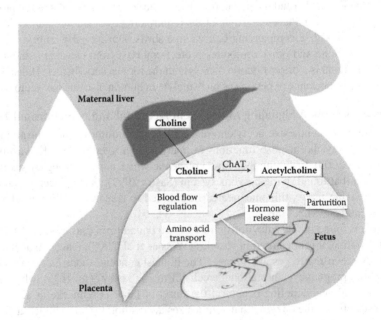

FIGURE 14.3 After choline is transported into the placenta, it is converted into acetylcholine by choline acetyltransferase (ChAT). Placental acetylcholine is suggested to serve four important functions: it regulates placental blood flow, it modulates placental amino acid transport, it affects placental hormonal release, and it is involved in parturition.

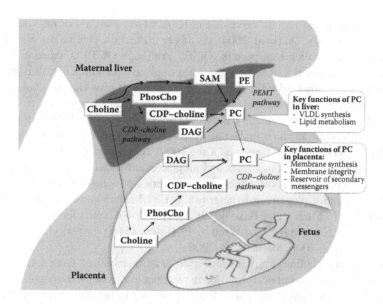

FIGURE 14.4 Phosphatidylcholine (PC) performs several important functions during pregnancy: it forms the cell membrane and maintains its integrity, it is a reservoir of important secondary signaling molecules, and it is involved in lipid metabolism. PC is produced in two different pathways: cytidine diphosphosphate (CDP)–choline pathway, which uses choline as a substrate, and the endogenous phosphatidylethanolamine *N*-methyltransferase (PEMT) pathway. DAG, diacylglycerol; SAM, *S*-adenosylmethionine; VLDL, very-low-density lipoprotein.

donor (Zeisel and Blusztajn 1994). The PEMT pathway, which enables endogenous biosynthesis of choline and is upregulated during pregnancy (Resseguie et al. 2007), produces a molecule that is enriched in docosahexaenoic acid (DHA) (DeLong et al. 1999), a long-chain unsaturated fatty acid required for proper brain development. Human studies employing stable isotope methodology have shown that PEMT–PC, rather than CDP–PC (enriched in medium chain saturated fatty acids), is selectively transferred by the placenta to the developing fetus (Yan et al. 2013).

PC metabolism can also influence the abundance of several signaling molecules and processes involved in lipid transport. Perturbations in PC metabolism have been shown to increase accumulation of diacylglycerol (DAG), with undesirable effects on the protein kinase C (PKC) signaling pathway and placental development (Jiang et al. 2014; Yen, Mar, and Zeisel 1999; Zeisel and Blusztajn 1994). Perturbations in PC metabolism can also impair hepatic lipid export because PC is required for the synthesis of very-low-density lipoproteins. Notably, production of triglycerides in the maternal liver increases dramatically during gestation, and efficient removal is critical for the prevention of fatty liver in the mothers (Caudill 2010).

14.1.2 CHOLINE UPTAKE BY PLACENTA

A maternal source of choline is critical to fetal development secondary to low PEMT activity in placenta (Welsch 1978) and fetal liver (Garner et al. 1993). Hence, the only way for the fetus to obtain choline is through placental uptake from the maternal circulation with subsequent secretion into fetal circulation.

Choline transport into the placenta occurs against a concentration gradient, is weakly sodium dependent, and is strongly inhibited by hemicholinium 3, a drug that blocks the reuptake of choline by the choline transporters (Eaton and Sooranna 1998; Grassl 1994; van der Aa et al. 1994; Welsch 1976a). High-affinity choline transporters (CHT1), which are abundant in the brain, do not appear to play a predominant role in placental choline uptake because these transporters function only in the presence of sodium and are not expressed in human term placenta or rat syncytiotrophoblast (Lee, Choi, and Kang 2009; Oda et al. 2004). As an organic cation, choline can also be transported by polyspecific organic cation transporters (OCTs). Although OCT3 is abundantly expressed in the human placenta (Lee et al. 2013), its importance in placental choline uptake is unclear because OCT3 transports many other substrates even in the presence of high choline (Kekuda et al. 1998). The recently identified intermediate-affinity choline transporter-like proteins (CTLs), which are expressed in both neuronal and nonneuronal tissues, are emerging as candidates for placental uptake of choline. CTL1, the main member in the family, is sensitive to inhibition by hemicholinium 3 and is weakly sodium dependent (Lee, Choi, and Kang 2009). In addition, *CTL1* has two splice variants, one of which is highly expressed in human and rat placenta (Michel et al. 2006) and is involved in transporting choline in rat syncytiotrophoblasts (Lee, Choi, and Kang 2009). Interestingly, extracellular choline concentration plays a role in determining CTL1 expression such that choline deficiency down-regulates CTL1 (Michel and Bakovic 2012). This down-regulation of CTL1, and reduced placental uptake of choline, may be mediated by PKC-dependent phosphorylation and inactivation of CTL1 (Fullerton et al. 2006; Michel et al. 2006).

Within the placenta, choline is rapidly converted to its metabolites, most notably acetylcholine (Welsch 1976a). The synthesis of acetylcholine in placenta may require the coupling of the choline transporter activity with choline acetyltransferase as shown in human cholinergic neuroblastoma cells (Yamada et al. 2011). After production, acetylcholine can remain in the placenta or can be released into fetal circulation by OCT1 and OCT3 (Wessler et al. 2001). Choline in the placenta can also be used to make PC. Although small amounts of betaine are found in placenta, this choline metabolite is likely derived from maternal circulation. Notably, betaine is not used as a methyl donor in placenta because betaine homocysteine methyltransferase (BHMT) is not expressed in this tissue. Human studies employing isotopically labeled choline support placental entry of choline-derived methyl groups as methionine and SAM.

14.1.3 DIETARY RECOMMENDATIONS FOR CHOLINE

The current adequate intake (AI) for women is 425 mg choline/day with upward adjustments to 450 and 550 mg choline/day for pregnant and lactating women, respectively (IOM 1998). However, recent data suggest that pregnant women require choline intakes that exceed current recommendations (Jiang et al. 2012; Yan et al. 2012, 2013). In a 12-week feeding study providing 480 mg choline/day, third-trimester pregnant women (versus control women) exhibited 40%–60% lower plasma concentrations of choline-derived methyl donors and altered partitioning of choline in favor of PC synthesis through the CDP–choline pathway rather than betaine synthesis via the oxidative pathway. Notably, consumption of 930 mg choline/day (~twice the AI) improved circulating levels of choline-derived methyl donors among pregnant women, normalized the partitioning of choline between the CDP–choline and oxidative pathways, and did not increase the urinary loss of choline, indicating that this dose did not exceed the metabolic requirement for choline during the third trimester of pregnancy (Yan et al. 2012, 2013). Unfortunately, the majority of women are not consuming choline at recommended intake levels (Cho et al. 2006; Chester et al. 2011; Jensen et al. 2007; Shaw et al. 2004). As shown in Figure 14.5, meeting this requirement may be especially difficult for vegetarian and vegan women, as the richest sources of choline are animal products.

14.1.3.1 Genetic Variation and Choline Requirements

In addition to reproductive status, numerous genetic variants (i.e., single-nucleotide polymorphisms [SNPs]) have been reported to alter choline metabolism and requirements (da Costa, Kozyreva et al. 2006; da Costa et al. 2014; Kohlmeier et al. 2005). These SNPs tend to vary in their distribution among ethnic groups, leading to further heterogeneity of the choline requirement within a population (da Costa et al. 2014).

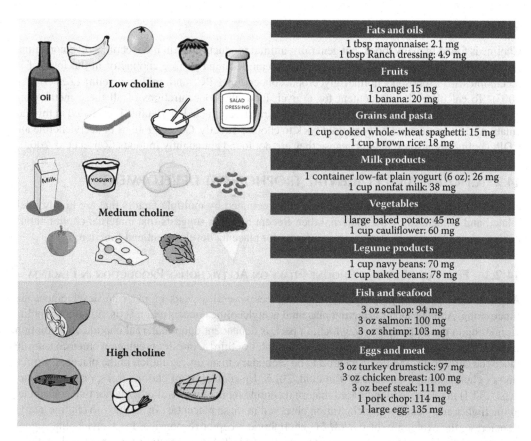

| Fats and oils |
| 1 tbsp mayonnaise: 2.1 mg |
| 1 tbsp Ranch dressing: 4.9 mg |

| Fruits |
| 1 orange: 15 mg |
| 1 banana: 20 mg |

| Grains and pasta |
| 1 cup cooked whole-wheat spaghetti: 15 mg |
| 1 cup brown rice: 18 mg |

| Milk products |
| 1 container low-fat plain yogurt (6 oz): 26 mg |
| 1 cup nonfat milk: 38 mg |

| Vegetables |
| 1 large baked potato: 45 mg |
| 1 cup cauliflower: 60 mg |

| Legume products |
| 1 cup navy beans: 70 mg |
| 1 cup baked beans: 78 mg |

| Fish and seafood |
| 3 oz scallop: 94 mg |
| 3 oz salmon: 100 mg |
| 3 oz shrimp: 103 mg |

| Eggs and meat |
| 3 oz turkey drumstick: 97 mg |
| 3 oz chicken breast: 100 mg |
| 3 oz beef steak: 111 mg |
| 1 pork chop: 114 mg |
| 1 large egg: 135 mg |

Low choline

Medium choline

High choline

FIGURE 14.5 Choline is found in many foods. Animal products such as eggs, meats, and seafood are rich sources of choline (i.e., provide at least 90 mg choline/serving). Moderate amounts of choline (i.e., provides at least 25 mg choline/serving) are found in legume products, select vegetables, and milk products. Fruits, grain products, fats, and oils contain low amounts of choline. (The values for choline content may vary slightly depending on the method of preparation. Information on choline content was obtained from USDA National Nutrient Database for Standard Reference, Release 27.)

Premenopausal women are less susceptible to developing choline deficiency symptoms than postmenopausal women and men because of upregulation of PEMT by estrogen and enhanced de novo biosynthesis of choline (da Costa, Kozyreva et al. 2006). However, this effect can be countered by SNPs in the *PEMT* gene, including a promoter region SNP (−744 G>C, rs12325817), which reduces binding of estrogen to its response element, thus attenuating upregulation of PEMT. Additional SNPs in the choline-metabolizing enzymes choline kinase (*CHK*), *BHMT*, choline dehydrogenase (*CHDH*), and the choline transporter *CTL1* have been characterized and may also influence choline requirements (da Costa, Kozyreva et al. 2006, da Costa et al. 2014).

Several folate metabolizing enzymes have been shown to influence choline requirements (Kohlmeier et al. 2005; Yan et al. 2011). Individuals with at least one copy of the 1958 G>A SNP in the *MTHFD1* gene (5,10-methylene tetrahydrofolate dehydrogenase; rs2236225) were found to have a 7 times higher risk of developing organ dysfunction on a choline-deficient diet (Kohlmeier et al. 2005). This effect was particularly pronounced in premenopausal women, since 88% of women with the variant developed organ dysfunction. This SNP may restrict supply of methyl groups for endogenous PC synthesis via the PEMT pathway. Notably, the effect was not seen in folate-supplemented individuals, suggesting that folic acid (or choline) supplementation during pregnancy may be especially crucial for women carrying genetic variants that limit endogenous choline synthesis (Kohlmeier et al. 2005).

14.1.4 COMMON FOOD SOURCES

Choline is found in many foods, but generally, animal products contain more choline than nonanimal products do (see Figure 14.5). Choline in foods can be found as free choline or in the form of its metabolites (e.g., phosphocholine, glycerophosphocholine, PC, and sphingomyelin) (Zeisel et al. 2003). To calculate choline content for a given food, the concentrations of all these metabolites, except betaine, acetylcholine, and CDP–choline directly, are included. Betaine is excluded in this calculation because it cannot be converted back to choline directly. Concentrations of acetylcholine and CDP–choline are also excluded because they are not found abundantly in foods (Zeisel et al. 2003).

14.2 CHOLINE AND PLACENTAL TROPHOBLAST DEVELOPMENT

Normal placenta development and function are regulated by multiple factors that are highly interrelated and influenced by the maternal diet. Recent research suggests that maternal choline intake during pregnancy may be especially important for placenta development and function.

14.2.1 EFFECT OF MATERNAL CHOLINE INTAKE ON ACETYLCHOLINE PRODUCTION IN PLACENTA

As mentioned previously, acetylcholine influences several aspects of placenta development and functioning. A major factor affecting placental acetylcholine concentration is the amount of choline circulating in the maternal body, which, in part, is dependent upon maternal choline consumption. Indeed, more acetylcholine accumulated in placentas of third-trimester pregnant women consuming twice the current AI, and this appeared to be secondary to an up-regulation in the placental expression of choline acetyltransferase (Yan et al. 2012). Up-regulation of choline transporter expression (e.g., CTL1) in response to increased maternal choline intake may be another factor that contributed to the higher acetylcholine concentration observed in these placentas. In addition to choline acetyltransferase, the expression of *CHRM4* (a cholinergic receptor responsible for acetylcholine signaling) was also elevated in these placentas (Jiang et al. 2013), suggesting that increased maternal choline intake may enhance signaling through the acetylcholine pathway, with possible downstream effects on biological processes occurring in the placenta.

14.2.2 EFFECT OF MATERNAL CHOLINE INTAKE ON THE EPIGENOME DURING DEVELOPMENT

The term *epigenetics* refers to changes in gene function that arise from chemical modifications of DNA rather than alterations in the DNA nucleotide sequence. The most frequently studied epigenetic modifications are DNA and histone methylation, both of which are crucial factors in the regulation of placental and fetal development (Nelissen et al. 2011). DNA methylation involves the addition of methyl groups to cytosine bases, typically at sites where the cytosine is immediately followed by a guanine (Cytosine-phosphate-Guanine dinucleotide [CpG] site), and is carried out by enzymes of the DNA methyltransferase (DNMT) family. Gene promoters often contain CpG islands, regions of CpG clusters that are important in regulating gene expression. Typically, DNA methylation is associated with transcriptional silencing via inhibition of transcription factor binding and recruitment of methyl–CpG-binding domain proteins that modify histones (Klose and Bird 2006). Because of this, an unmethylated promoter CpG island will lead to active transcription of the gene. However, there are exceptions to this rule, including some imprinted genes where methylation can act as a transcription activator (Holmes and Soloway 2006). Histone proteins, together with the DNA wrapped around them, form nucleosomes that are responsible for organizing and condensing chromatin in the nucleus (Holmes and Soloway 2006). Histones may be modified by the addition of methyl groups on various amino acid residues of their tails, which can have an activating or silencing effect on the gene depending on location (Strahl and Allis 2000). These modifications, catalyzed by euchromatin histone methyltransferases (EHMTs), form a code that controls gene expression by regulating the configuration of chromatin and its interaction with transcription factors (Bannister and Kouzarides 2011).

As a methyl group donor, choline has been studied for its role in modulating the epigenome during early development, which may have lifelong effects on offspring health. Maternal choline supplementation during rodent pregnancy alters DNA and histone methylation in a variety of fetal tissues such as liver and brain (Davison et al. 2009; Kovacheva et al. 2007). Similar findings have been observed in human pregnancy. Third-trimester pregnant women consuming twice the AI of choline (930 vs. 480 mg/day) showed 22% higher global DNA methylation and 20% higher global H3K9me2 (a silencing mark on histone 3) in the placenta (Jiang et al. 2012). In addition, the placental gene expression of *DNMT1* was 33% higher (nonstatistically significant trend) and the expression of *EHMT2* was increased by 36%. These results collectively indicate that increased maternal choline intake during pregnancy can modulate the placental epigenome, which may induce widespread effects on gene expression, placental function, and offspring health.

A large number of genes in the placenta are imprinted, being expressed from only one parental allele and silenced on the other (Nelissen et al. 2011). These genes encode for proteins that influence nutrient uptake and delivery, thus regulating placental growth as well as prenatal and postnatal fetal development (Fowden et al. 2006). Abnormal expression of these genes contributes to the pathology of pregnancy disorders such as preeclampsia and intrauterine growth restriction (Lim and Ferguson-Smith 2010). One of the well-studied imprinted genes is insulin-like growth factor 2 (*IGF2*), which is expressed paternally and up-regulated by DNA methylation of specific differentially methylated regions. IGF2 is a major determinant of fetal and placental growth and has been shown to be highly responsive to perinatal maternal choline intake in rodent models (Napoli, Blusztajn, and Mellott 2008). Interestingly, the effects of choline on *Igf2* expression may be tissue-specific and time-sensitive. Prenatal choline supplementation induced higher expression of *Igf2* and *Igf2r* in several brain regions in rat offspring (Napoli, Blusztajn, and Mellott 2008). Conversely, in fetal rat liver, *Igf2* was down-regulated in late gestation by maternal choline supplementation as a consequence of higher methylation and lower expression of the methyltransferase *Dnmt1* (Kovacheva et al. 2007). Choline ingestion during pregnancy has also been shown to regulate histone methylation and histone-modifying enzymes at gestational day 17 in the rat fetus (Davison et al. 2009). Maternal choline supplementation increased levels of transcription-repressing marks H3K9me2 and H3K27me3 in fetal liver, while decreasing levels of the activating mark H3K4me2. Supplementing the maternal diet with choline also increased the expression of the histone methylated enzyme *Suv39H1* in the fetal cortex. These results add to the growing body of evidence on the modulatory effects of maternal diet on epigenetic changes and gene expression in the fetal compartments.

Few studies have investigated choline's effects on the placental imprinting profile. Using a microarray discovery approach, one study found that consuming twice the current choline AI during the third trimester of pregnancy decreased placental expression of *HOXD10* (Jiang et al. 2013), which is imprinted in human placenta (Lambertini et al. 2012) and adversely impacts placental vascular development (Chen et al. 2009). How the expression of other placental imprinted genes respond to a higher maternal choline intake remains to be discovered.

14.2.3 Effect of Choline Supply on Placental Vascular Development

The development of the placenta requires extensive angiogenesis and vasculogenesis. Maternal spiral arteries must be invaded and remodeled by cytotrophoblasts to allow for increased perfusion to the fetus (Whitley and Cartwright 2009), a process that requires adequate expression of proangiogenic genes. The vascular endothelial growth factor (VEGF) family consists of two important proangiogenic genes, VEGF and placental growth factor (PlGF), and two receptors that transduce their functions, VEGFR1 (FLT1) and VEGFR2 (KDR) (Andraweera, Dekker, and Roberts 2012). An additional splice variant of VEGFR1, known as soluble fms-like tyrosine kinase (sFLT1), is an antiangiogenic factor that sequesters VEGF and PlGF in maternal and placental circulation, thereby preventing its binding to the membrane-bound endothelial receptor VEGFR1 (mFLT1) (Maynard et al. 2003; Tsatsaris et al. 2003). Because functions of VEGF during placentation include stimulating angiogenesis, reducing apoptosis, inducing vasodilation, and potentially regulating trophoblast invasion and remodeling of the spiral arteries (Andraweera, Dekker, and Roberts 2012), alterations in the normal balance between proangiogenic and antiangiogenic factors contribute to placental disorders such as preeclampsia (Boij et al. 2012). An additional antiangiogenic factor implicated in the development of preeclampsia is the soluble form of endoglin (ENG). ENG is an accessory receptor in the transforming growth factor β (TGFβ) signaling family, which facilitates the binding of the proangiogenic factor TGFβ1 to its receptors TGFBR1 and TGFBR2 to promote endothelial cell proliferation and migration (Lebrin and Mummery 2008; ten Dijke and Arthur 2007). However, the soluble form (sENG), which is generated by matrix metalloproteinase-14 (MMP14) cleaving of ENG, antagonizes the binding process (Kaitu'u-Lino et al. 2012) and impairs angiogenesis.

Maternal choline intake during pregnancy has been shown to affect angiogenesis in fetal mouse hippocampus (Mehedint, Craciunescu, and Zeisel 2010). Choline deficiency reduced endothelial cell proliferation and blood vessel number in the hippocampus at embryonic day 17, whereas the expression of proangiogenic factors *Vegfc* and *Angpt2* (angiopoietin-2) was significantly increased. These gene expression changes may have resulted in enhanced cell differentiation, which lowered the number of dividing cells, thereby limiting proliferation. The increased gene expression corresponded with a decrease in site-specific methylation at CpG islands in the *Vegfc* and *Angpt2* genes. In another study using chorioallantoic membrane of the chick embryo as an *in vivo* model for the study of angiogenesis (Ribatti 2008), choline chloride stimulated angiogenesis with an efficacy similar to VEGF (Wang et al. 2013).

The ability of choline to regulate angiogenesis in human placenta has recently been investigated. Among third-trimester pregnant women, higher maternal choline intake (930 versus 480 mg/day) reduced placental transcription of *sFLT1* by 30% (Jiang et al. 2013). Using a whole-genome microarray, the authors also detected differential expression of 166 placental genes as a result of maternal choline supplementation. The gene ontology categories of Circulatory System Development and Blood Circulation were strongly represented. Down-regulated genes included *ADORA3* (adenosine A3 receptor), *RBP4* (retinol binding protein 4, plasma), *OXTR* (oxytocin receptor), and *ERRFI1* (ERBB receptor feedback inhibitor 1), while *GHRL* (ghrelin/obestatin prepropeptide), *NPY5R* (neuropeptide Y receptor Y5), and *ELN* (elastin) were upregulated (Jiang et al. 2013). The significance of these differentially expressed genes remains to be elucidated but likely plays a role in choline's influence on placental vascularization.

Similarly, in a human cell culture model of placental trophoblasts, choline deficiency increased not only the production of the angiogenic factor sFLT1 but also the secretion of VEGFA. This increase in VEGF may be a compensatory response by the placenta to offset disturbances in vascular function arising from choline deficiency. sENG was below detectable concentrations; however, the ENG-cleaving proteinase MMP14, typically linked with elevated sENG levels, was increased by choline deficiency (Jiang et al. 2014). In addition, tube length and number of branch points (indicative of angiogenesis) were reduced in human umbilical vein endothelial cells cultured in the media from the low choline placental cell line (Jiang et al. 2014). Overall, these results demonstrate a regulatory role of choline on angiogenic processes in the developing placenta, with extra choline improving vascular function and possibly lowering the risk of preeclampsia.

14.2.4 EFFECT OF CHOLINE SUPPLY ON PLACENTAL INFLAMMATION

As the immune interface between the maternal and the fetal compartments, the placenta plays a crucial role in regulating the production of proinflammatory cytokines such as tumor necrosis factor-α (TNF-α), interferon-γ (IFN-γ), and interleukin-1β (IL-1β), as well as the production of anti-inflammatory cytokines such as IL-10 (Saito and Sakai 2003). Normal pregnancy is characterized as a mild inflammatory state, which gradually strengthens as the pregnancy continues (Redman and Sargent 2004). However, an intensified inflammatory state caused by an abnormal elevation of the proinflammatory cytokines, especially during early gestation, has adverse consequences on placental development. Elevations in placental TNF-α increase the amount of vasoconstrictors and contribute to placental endothelial cell dysfunction (Marusic et al. 2013). The TNF-α pathway may also mediate abnormal placental vascular development because TNF-α reduces acetylcholine-induced vascular relaxation in other tissues (Conrad and Benyo 1997). Notably, placental production of the antiangiogenic factor sFLT1 can initiate an inflammatory response (Redman and Sargent 2004), which further exemplifies the close connection between inflammation and angiogenesis. Abnormal increases in proinflammatory cytokines can also harm the fetus, resulting in fetal death (e.g., IFN-γ) and preterm labor (e.g., IL-6) (Challis et al. 2009; Lin et al. 1993). Given these undesirable effects, it is important to regulate the production of the proinflammatory cytokines to ensure a successful pregnancy.

Increased choline supply has been shown to mitigate inflammation under different pathological conditions. Extra choline administered to a mouse model of airway disease or individuals with asthma reduced the production of IL-5 and TNF-α as well as suppressed the activity of nuclear factor κB (NFκB) (Mehta et al. 2009, 2010). In addition, alveolar macrophages isolated from rats consuming a diet rich in choline produced less TNF-α when exposed to lipopolysaccharide *in vitro* (Rivera et al. 1998). In the placenta, not only does choline modulate the angiogenic process, but it also influences the production of inflammatory cytokines. Specifically, *IL-6* and *IL-1β* were upregulated when placental trophoblast cells were cultured in medium containing a low choline concentration. The mRNA levels of genes encoding two subunits of NFκB were also upregulated. This caused the activation of NFκB (Jiang et al. 2014), which contributed to the proinflammatory state. Overall, these data demonstrate the modulatory role of choline on inflammation and highlight the importance of an adequate maternal choline intake during pregnancy.

14.2.5 EFFECT OF CHOLINE SUPPLY ON PLACENTAL APOPTOSIS

Apoptosis, a process of programmed cell death, plays an essential role in normal placental development throughout pregnancy. As described previously, to form the vascular structure, invasion of the cytotrophoblast cells into the maternal decidua and remodeling of the maternal spiral arteries are needed. Both of these processes are mediated, in part, by inducing the cells lining the lumen to undergo apoptosis (Straszewski-Chavez, Abrahams, and Mor 2005). Moreover, the placenta also undergoes constant renewal to ensure the removal of aged trophoblast cells so that placental functioning will not be affected (Straszewski-Chavez, Abrahams, and Mor 2005). However, dysregulation of the apoptotic stimuli, such as high level of the proinflammatory cytokine TNF-α, can lead to excessive trophoblast apoptosis (Bowen et al. 2002; Christiaens et al. 2008), generating a large amount of placental apoptotic fragments. Once released into the maternal circulation, these fragments can trigger an intensified inflammatory response, decreased proliferation of the endothelial cells, and reduced vascular relaxation (Heazell et al. 2008). These perturbations contribute to abnormal placental development and adverse pregnancy outcomes, indicating that the process of apoptosis must be tightly regulated. Multiple apoptotic pathways are identified in the placenta, with caspase-3 being the major component of these pathways because of its central role in the execution phase of apoptosis (Straszewski-Chavez, Abrahams, and Mor 2005).

Choline's ability to modulate apoptosis has been shown in different tissues. When PC12 cells, a cell line derived from the rat adrenal medulla, were cultured in choline-free medium, more apoptotic cells were observed (Yen, Mar, and Zeisel 1999). Choline deficiency also triggered cultured hepatocytes and myocytes to undergo apoptosis (da Costa, Niculescu et al. 2006). This effect was also observed *in vivo*. Peripheral lymphocytes of individuals who developed liver or muscle dysfunction caused by a very low choline intake had more activated caspase-3 and a higher number of TUNEL-positive lymphocytes, an indicator of DNA damage (da Costa, Niculescu et al. 2006). Similar effects of choline are seen in placenta trophoblast cells. *In vitro* experiments using placenta trophoblast cells found that the number of cells detached from the culture dish (an indicator of apoptosis) was inversely proportional to the amount of choline in the culture medium. Low choline in the culture medium also increased mRNA and protein abundance as well as the activation of caspase-3 and p53 (another widely studied protein involved in placental apoptosis) (Heazell and Crocker 2008; Jiang et al. 2014). Collectively, these findings demonstrate that choline insufficiency detrimentally increases placental trophoblast apoptosis and highlight the importance of an adequate choline supply during pregnancy.

14.2.6 EFFECT OF CHOLINE SUPPLY ON OXIDATIVE STRESS IN PLACENTA

The imbalance between cellular production of reactive oxygen species (ROS) and the cell's ability to generate sufficient antioxidants to detoxify these species causes oxidative stress. By affecting cellular integrity and genomic stability, as well as enzymatic activities, the presence of an excessive amount of ROS results in cellular damage (Borzychowski, Sargent, and Redman 2006) and thus impairs normal placental development. Indeed, incomplete trophoblast invasion into the maternal decidua during early gestation, coupled with disturbances in remodeling of the maternal spiral arteries, leads to placental hypoxia, an initiating factor in ROS production. ROS are themselves proinflammatory, and their presence triggers an inflammatory response (Borzychowski, Sargent, and Redman 2006), leading to trophoblast apoptosis and endothelial cell dysfunction.

In addition to angiogenesis, inflammation, and apoptosis, choline also has an influential role in ROS production, as supported by data generated from both *in vitro* and *in vivo* studies using a variety of tissues. For example, choline deficiency in both human and mouse caused an increase in oxidative stress, a higher production and leakage of ROS, as well as an elevated level of DNA damage, all of which were corrected by the administration of choline (da Costa, Niculescu et al. 2006; Mehta et al. 2009, 2010; Yoshida et al. 2006). Consistent with these data, when placenta trophoblast cells were cultured in medium with a low choline concentration, intracellular ROS concentration increased. Membrane fluidity was also increased (an indicator of reduced membrane integrity), and more DNA damage was observed in these cells (Jiang et al. 2014). Together, these findings suggest that adverse placental development due to choline inadequacy is mediated partly by the induction of oxidative stress.

14.2.7 POTENTIAL MECHANISMS THROUGH WHICH CHOLINE SUPPLY AFFECTS BIOLOGICAL PROCESSES IN THE PLACENTA

14.2.7.1 Methylation

As discussed previously, a higher maternal choline intake influences both global and site-specific DNA methylation in the placenta (see Figure 14.2). Increased maternal choline intake during pregnancy can augment placental SAM supply as well as placental expression of the epigenetic enzymes DNMT1 and EHMT2 (Jiang et al. 2012). Because of the crucial role of methylation in controlling trophoblast development, choline has the potential to modulate a wide range of metabolic and physiologic processes.

14.2.7.2 Acetylcholine Signaling

Large amounts of acetylcholine are produced in the placenta from maternally derived choline. In addition to signaling through the cholinergic receptor CHRM4, placental acetylcholine acts through activation of alpha-7 nicotinic receptor, which is one of the nicotinic receptors expressed in human placental cells (Dowling et al. 2007). In third-trimester pregnant women, placental acetylcholine concentrations and *CHRM4* expression were inversely correlated with mRNA expression and maternal circulating levels of sFLT1 (Jiang et al. 2013). Interestingly, smoking during pregnancy reduces risk of PE, possibly through the actions of nicotine on nicotinic receptors and activation of the acetylcholine signaling pathway. Indeed, nicotine is associated with lower sFLT1 and improved angiogenesis (Kahn et al. 2011), enhanced vasodilation through release of NO and endothelium-derived relaxing factor (Rama Sastry, Hemontolor, and Olenick 1999), and lower release of inflammatory cytokines (Dowling et al. 2007). Taken together, these data suggest that maternal choline supplementation may beneficially influence angiogenic and inflammatory processes through activation of acetylcholine signaling pathways.

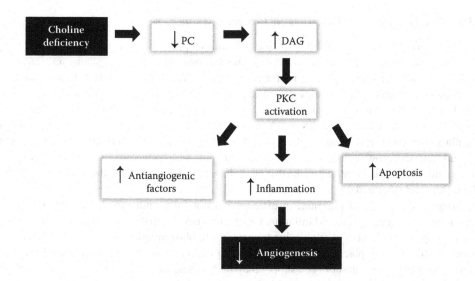

FIGURE 14.6 Choline deficiency adversely impacts placental development by increasing accumulation of diacylglycerol (DAG) in the placenta. DAG accumulation activates the protein kinase C (PKC) signaling pathway, leading to increased production of antiangiogenic factors, proinflammatory cytokines, and apoptotic fragments. All these factors contribute to poor placental vascular development.

14.2.7.3 PKC Signaling

Effects of choline on placental development may also be mediated via the PKC signaling pathway (see Figure 14.6). PKCs, notably PKCδ and PKCε, can be activated by polyunsaturated species of DAG (Rosse et al. 2010). In the situation of choline deficiency, these species accumulate because choline is not available for PC generation. Accumulation of these DAG species up-regulates the transcription of PKCδ and PKCε as well as their translocation to the cellular membrane (indicative of activation). Consequences of PKC activation in trophoblast cells include a higher expression of antiangiogenic factors and proinflammatory cytokines as well as more apoptotic cells (Jiang et al. 2014). These alterations can severely impair the development of placental vasculature, subsequently increasing the risk for pregnancy complications such as preeclampsia.

14.3 POTENTIAL CLINICAL IMPLICATIONS

Given the beneficial impact of increased choline supply on biological processes involved in placental development, supplementing the maternal diet with extra choline during pregnancy may be a nutritional strategy to reduce the risk of pregnancy disorders (see Figure 14.7). In addition, by improving placental development and functioning, increased maternal choline intake during pregnancy may have an influential role in determining the lifelong health of the child.

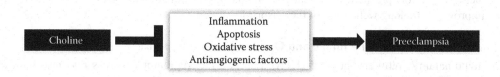

FIGURE 14.7 Choline has been shown to attenuate numerous biological processes implicated in the development of preeclampsia, including inflammation, apoptosis, oxidative stress, and antiangiogenic factors.

14.3.1 PREECLAMPSIA AND INTRAUTERINE GROWTH RESTRICTION

Placental insufficiency, or an inability of the placenta to provide adequate nutrients and oxygen to the fetus, can lead to numerous adverse complications, including preeclampsia, intrauterine growth restriction, miscarriage, and preterm delivery (Chaddha et al. 2004). Preeclampsia is a life-threatening disease of pregnancy that results in maternal hypertension and proteinuria (Duley 2003). It affects 3%–6% of pregnancies in the United States and has risen in prevalence over the previous two decades (Ananth, Keyes, and Wapner 2013). The only cure for preeclampsia is delivery of the placenta; however, this early delivery can have detrimental health effects for the fetus (Duley 2003). Intrauterine growth restriction may also contribute to lifelong adverse health consequences for the child, including increased risk of type 2 diabetes and cardiovascular disease in later life (Salam, Das, and Bhutta 2014).

Although the etiology of placental insufficiency is not fully understood, an imbalance of pro-angiogenic and antiangiogenic and inflammatory factors may contribute (Azizieh, Raghupathy, and Makhseed 2005; Chaddha et al. 2004). Inadequate trophoblast invasion of maternal decidua is also a characteristic of many placental pathologies. When this process is incomplete, blood flow to the placenta is compromised, and oxygen supply may be sporadic, leading to placental hypoxic injury. Oxidative stress, excessive apoptosis, and inflammation result, compromising trophoblast function and preventing efficient transfer of nutrients (Cheng and Wang 2009). Antiangiogenic factors in the maternal circulation, including sFLT1 and sENG, are elevated in preeclampsia and can be used as biomarkers or predictors of risk when measured in early gestation (Boij et al. 2012; Venkatesha et al. 2006). Increases in maternal circulating sFLT1 and sENG may contribute to preeclampsia pathogenesis by impairing endothelial cell function. sFLT1 reduces the expression of specific MMPs, which may lead to the accumulation of collagen that impedes maternal decidua invasion by trophoblasts (Li et al. 2014).

Nutritional interventions using bioactive nutrients, as a highly safe and acceptable treatment option during pregnancy, represent a promising area of study to improve placental function and, ultimately, maternal and fetal health (Xu et al. 2009). The unique bioactive properties of choline in modulating angiogenesis, inflammation, apoptosis, and oxidative stress (see Figure 14.7) suggest that choline supplementation during pregnancy may improve placental functioning and fetal outcomes especially among women at high risk of preeclampsia. Notably, preeclamptic placentas produce less acetylcholine (Sastry 1997), suggesting impairments in acetylcholine signaling, which could be rectified with a higher maternal choline intake during these reproductive states.

14.3.2 IMPROVED FETAL DEVELOPMENT

As an interface between the maternal and fetal compartments, the placenta is increasingly recognized to play an essential role in fetal programming, which asserts that an adverse *in utero* environment (e.g., poor maternal nutrition) increases the risk of developing metabolic diseases in the adult offspring. As a compensatory response to a suboptimal prenatal environment, the fetal genome undergoes epigenetic modifications that facilitate fetal survival but may be incompatible with the postnatal environment, ultimately increasing metabolic disease risk in later life (Godfrey 2002). By beneficially modulating placental vascular development (improving placental function) and acting as a methyl donor for epigenetic modifications, choline has the potential to affect fetal programming and improve the lifelong well-being of the offspring.

14.3.2.1 Maternal Choline Intake and Offspring Stress Response

The hypothalamic–pituitary–adrenal (HPA) axis is a key regulator of stress response both *in utero* and in later life. Disturbances in placental HPA axis activity during gestation are associated with greater risk of several metabolic diseases (e.g., hypertension, type 2 diabetes, and cardiovascular diseases) in the adult offspring (Braun et al. 2013; Huh et al. 2008). Abnormal activity of placental HPA axis can also affect infant neurobehavioral development, as indicated by attention scores, stress abstinence scores, and quality of movement scores (Lesseur, Paquette, and Marsit 2014). Additionally, disturbances in the HPA axis have been noted in preeclampsia and pregnancy complicated with intrauterine growth restriction, including higher placental corticotropin-releasing hormone (CRH) expression and elevated cord blood cortisol (Goland et al. 1993; Wadhwa et al. 2004).

Many genes of the HPA axis are regulated by DNA and histone methylation, identifying them as potential targets for modulation by maternal choline intake. A higher choline intake (930 versus 480 mg/day) across the third trimester of human pregnancy increased placental methylation of CpG sites in the *CRH* promoter, which was associated with approximately 40% lower placental *CRH* gene expression and 33% lower cord blood cortisol concentrations (Jiang et al. 2012). These findings suggest that HPA axis reactivity among infants can be attenuated by maternal choline supplementation, with possible long-term consequences of reduced risk for stress-related diseases in later life.

14.3.2.2 Maternal Choline Intake and Offspring Cognitive Development

Many animal studies indicate that increasing maternal choline consumption during pregnancy has long-lasting beneficial effects on offspring memory and attention. Choline supplementation of pregnant rodents alters the structural integrity and morphology of the fetal hippocampus, which may contribute to improved cognitive functioning as well as the prevention of age-related cognitive decline (Blusztajn and Mellott 2013).

In the brain, choline metabolites are required for proper development and function. First, PC is necessary to synthesize the membranes of newly generated neuronal cells and can be a source of DHA (Yan et al. 2013). Second, DAG and ceramide are important signaling molecules that regulate neuron apoptosis (Yen, Mar, and Zeisel 1999). Third, methyl groups derived from choline are used to modify the methylation status of histones and genes that are critical to (1) proliferation and differentiation of neuronal cells, (2) angiogenic processes in the hippocampus, as well as (3) memory and learning (Davison et al. 2009; Mehedint, Craciunescu, and Zeisel 2010; Niculescu, Craciunescu, and Zeisel 2006). These choline-derived methyl groups can also be used to change the methylation status of the *Igf2* gene (Kovacheva et al. 2007), which may increase the hippocampal release of acetylcholine, a mediator of neurogenesis, cholinergic neurotransmission, and several high-order cognitive processes (Napoli, Blusztajn, and Mellott 2008).

Choline's beneficial effects in improving placental development may also contribute to the offspring's enhanced cognitive development. Altered placental angiogenesis may cause a hypoxic *in utero* environment, resulting in brain injury and poor cognitive functioning (Hsiao and Patterson 2012). A higher maternal choline intake has been shown to improve placental angiogenesis, which may enhance oxygen supply to the developing brain, thereby improving offspring brain development. Proinflammatory cytokines produced by the placenta can be released into the fetal circulation and subsequently delivered to the fetal brain, since the blood–brain barrier is not yet fully established (Coe and Lubach 2014). Since choline deficiency increases the trophoblast production of proinflammatory cytokines, a higher maternal choline intake may improve offspring brain development by attenuating placental production of proinflammatory cytokines and minimizing their harmful effects on the fetal brain.

The placental epigenetic profile may also play an important role in programming the offspring's brain development and influencing their postnatal behaviors. Many imprinted genes that are found in the placenta are also expressed in the brain, and their expression in the placenta may indicate future cognitive performance. For example, the expression of *HOXD10* and other imprinted genes in the placenta were found to associate with the infant's quality of movement (Lesseur, Paquette, and Marsit 2014). Given that choline is capable of altering the placental expression of *HOXD10*, it is also possible that a higher maternal choline intake can beneficially modify the expression of other placental imprinted genes to improve offspring cognition.

14.3.2.3 Maternal Choline Intake and Developmental Disorders

Choline supplementation during pregnancy and lactation in rodents mitigates the neurocognitive dysfunction associated with Down syndrome, including better performance on tests evaluating attention, spatial cognition, and emotional regulation (Moon et al. 2010; Velazquez et al. 2013). The adverse effects of a trisomic genome are not limited to the fetal brain but are also observed in the placenta. One such effect is the abnormal vasculature in the labyrinth compartment (Bersu, Mossman, and Kornguth 1989), which may be normalized by maternal choline supplementation.

Prenatal alcohol exposure has harmful effects on placental development, such as impaired remodeling of maternal spiral arteries and abnormal morphological development in different placental trophoblast compartments (Gundogan et al. 2008). The amount of DNA damage and expression of caspase-3 in placental trophoblast cells are elevated when trophoblast cells are exposed to a culture medium high in alcohol concentration, which subsequently results in the activation of apoptotic pathway in these cells (Clave et al. 2014). All these can negatively impact placental blood flow and placental ability to transport nutrients and oxygen to the fetus, causing the range of abnormalities seen in individuals with fetal alcohol syndrome. In rats, maternal choline supplementation reduces some of the adverse developmental consequences associated with prenatal alcohol exposure, including reduced birth weight and brain weight as well as altered reflex development (Thomas, Abou, and Dominguez 2009). Although the mechanisms underlying these improvements remain to be fully determined, choline's role in improving placental development may contribute to these beneficial effects.

14.3.2.4 Maternal Choline Intake and Other Defects or Diseases

Consuming a diet high in choline during pregnancy has additional benefits. For example, a higher maternal choline intake during the periconceptional period was associated with a lower risk of neural tube defects (NTDs) (Shaw et al. 2004). This lowering of NTD risk could arise from choline's central role in one-carbon metabolism and regulation of apoptosis, both of which are important to neural tube development (Shaw et al. 2004). As another example, compared with female rats born to dams in the choline-deficient group, those born to dams in the choline-supplemented group had mammary tumors that progressed slower and showed a desirable gene expression profile (Kovacheva et al. 2009). These protective effects may arise from epigenetic modifications (Davison et al. 2009) and possibly improved vascularization, which would be expected to enhance placental delivery of choline and other methyl-donor nutrients to the developing fetus.

14.4 CONCLUDING REMARKS AND FUTURE PERSPECTIVES

Placenta development and function are influenced by the regulation of epigenetics, angiogenesis, inflammation, apoptosis, and oxidative stress. Because increased choline supply appears to modify these processes in a desirable manner, maternal choline supplementation may be a nutritional strategy to improve placental development and pregnancy outcomes. Nevertheless, more human studies are needed to determine the bioefficacy of choline in the prevention and treatment of placental-related disorders and in the promotion of the long-term health of the offspring.

REFERENCES

Ananth, C. V., K. M. Keyes, and R. J. Wapner. 2013. "Pre-eclampsia rates in the United States, 1980–2010: Age-period-cohort analysis." *BMJ* no. 347:f6564.

Andraweera, P. H., G. A. Dekker, and C. T. Roberts. 2012. "The vascular endothelial growth factor family in adverse pregnancy outcomes." *Hum Reprod Update* no. 18 (4):436–57.

Arroyo, J. A., P. Garcia-Jones, A. Graham, C. C. Teng, F. C. Battaglia, and H. L. Galan. 2012. "Placental TonEBP/NFAT5 osmolyte regulation in an ovine model of intrauterine growth restriction." *Biol Reprod* no. 86 (3):94.

Azizieh, F., R. Raghupathy, and M. Makhseed. 2005. "Maternal cytokine production patterns in women with pre-eclampsia." *Am J Reprod Immunol* no. 54 (1):30–7.

Bannister, A. J. and T. Kouzarides. 2011. "Regulation of chromatin by histone modifications." *Cell Res* no. 21 (3):381–95.

Bersu, E. T., H. W. Mossman, and S. E. Kornguth. 1989. "Altered placental morphology associated with murine trisomy 16 and murine trisomy 19." *Teratology* no. 40 (5):513–23.

Blusztajn, J. K. and T. J. Mellott. 2013. "Neuroprotective actions of perinatal choline nutrition." *Clin Chem Lab Med* no. 51 (3):591–9.

Boij, R., J. Svensson, K. Nilsson-Ekdahl, K. Sandholm, T. L. Lindahl, E. Palonek, M. Garle, G. Berg, J. Ernerudh, M. Jenmalm, and L. Matthiesen. 2012. "Biomarkers of coagulation, inflammation, and angiogenesis are independently associated with preeclampsia." *Am J Reprod Immunol* no. 68 (3):258–70.

Borzychowski, A. M., I. L. Sargent, and C. W. Redman. 2006. "Inflammation and pre-eclampsia." *Semin Fetal Neonatal Med* no. 11 (5):309–16.

Bowen, J. M., L. Chamley, J. A. Keelan, and M. D. Mitchell. 2002. "Cytokines of the placenta and extra-placental membranes: Roles and regulation during human pregnancy and parturition." *Placenta* no. 23 (4):257–73.

Braun, T., J. R. Challis, J. P. Newnham, and D. M. Sloboda. 2013. "Early-life glucocorticoid exposure: The hypothalamic–pituitary–adrenal axis, placental function, and long-term disease risk." *Endocr Rev* no. 34 (6):885–916.

Brennecke, S. P., S. Chen, R. G. King, and A. L. Boura. 1988. "Human placental acetylcholine content and release at parturition." *Clin Exp Pharmacol Physiol* no. 15 (9):715–25.

Caudill, M. A. 2010. "Pre- and postnatal health: Evidence of increased choline needs." *J Am Diet Assoc* no. 110 (8):1198–206.

Chaddha, V., S. Viero, B. Huppertz, and J. Kingdom. 2004. "Developmental biology of the placenta and the origins of placental insufficiency." *Semin Fetal Neonatal Med* no. 9 (5):357–69.

Challis, J. R., C. J. Lockwood, L. Myatt, J. E. Norman, J. F. Strauss 3rd, and F. Petraglia. 2009. "Inflammation and pregnancy." *Reprod Sci* no. 16 (2):206–15.

Chen, A., I. Cuevas, P. A. Kenny, H. Miyake, K. Mace, C. Ghajar, A. Boudreau, M. J. Bissell, and N. Boudreau. 2009. "Endothelial cell migration and vascular endothelial growth factor expression are the result of loss of breast tissue polarity." *Cancer Res* no. 69 (16):6721–9.

Cheng, M. H. and P. H. Wang. 2009. "Placentation abnormalities in the pathophysiology of preeclampsia." *Expert Rev Mol Diagn* no. 9 (1):37–49.

Chester, D., J. Goldman, J. Ahuja, and A. Moshfegh. 2011. Dietary intakes of choline. What we eat in America, NHANES 2007–2008. Agricultural Research Service, U.S. Department of Agriculture.

Cho, E., S. H. Zeisel, P. Jacques, J. Selhub, L. Dougherty, G. A. Colditz, and W. C. Willett. 2006. "Dietary choline and betaine assessed by food-frequency questionnaire in relation to plasma total homocysteine concentration in the Framingham Offspring Study." *Am J Clin Nutr* no. 83 (4):905–11.

Christiaens, I., D. B. Zaragoza, L. Guilbert, S. A. Robertson, B. F. Mitchell, and D. M. Olson. 2008. "Inflammatory processes in preterm and term parturition." *J Reprod Immunol* no. 79 (1):50–7.

Clave, S., X. Joya, J. Salat-Batlle, O. Garcia-Algar, and O. Vall. 2014. "Ethanol cytotoxic effect on trophoblast cells." *Toxicol Lett* no. 225 (2):216–21.

Coe, C. L. and G. R. Lubach. 2014. "Vital and vulnerable functions of the primate placenta critical for infant health and brain development." *Front Neuroendocrinol* no. 35 (4):439–46.

Conrad, K. P. and D. F. Benyo. 1997. "Placental cytokines and the pathogenesis of preeclampsia." *Am J Reprod Immunol* no. 37 (3):240–9.

da Costa, K. A., O. G. Kozyreva, J. Song, J. A. Galanko, L. M. Fischer, and S. H. Zeisel. 2006. "Common genetic polymorphisms affect the human requirement for the nutrient choline." *FASEB J* no. 20 (9):1336–44.

da Costa, K. A., M. D. Niculescu, C. N. Craciunescu, L. M. Fischer, and S. H. Zeisel. 2006. "Choline deficiency increases lymphocyte apoptosis and DNA damage in humans." *Am J Clin Nutr* no. 84 (1):88–94.

da Costa, K. A., K. D. Corbin, M. D. Niculescu, J. A. Galanko, and S. H. Zeisel. 2014. "Identification of new genetic polymorphisms that alter the dietary requirement for choline and vary in their distribution across ethnic and racial groups." *FASEB J* no. 28 (7):2970–8.

Davison, J. M., T. J. Mellott, V. P. Kovacheva, and J. K. Blusztajn. 2009. "Gestational choline supply regulates methylation of histone H3, expression of histone methyltransferases G9a (Kmt1c) and Suv39h1 (Kmt1a), and DNA methylation of their genes in rat fetal liver and brain." *J Biol Chem* no. 284 (4):1982–9.

Dawson, K. M. and J. M. Baltz. 1997. "Organic osmolytes and embryos: Substrates of the Gly and beta transport systems protect mouse zygotes against the effects of raised osmolarity." *Biol Reprod* no. 56 (6):1550–8.

DeLong, C. J., Y. J. Shen, M. J. Thomas, and Z. Cui. 1999. "Molecular distinction of phosphatidylcholine synthesis between the CDP–choline pathway and phosphatidylethanolamine methylation pathway." *J Biol Chem* no. 274 (42):29683–8.

Dowling, O., B. Rochelson, K. Way, Y. Al-Abed, and C. N. Metz. 2007. "Nicotine inhibits cytokine production by placenta cells via NFkappaB: Potential role in pregnancy-induced hypertension." *Mol Med* no. 13 (11–12):576–83.

Duley, L. 2003. "Pre-eclampsia and the hypertensive disorders of pregnancy." *Br Med Bull* no. 67:161–76.

Eaton, B. M. and S. R. Sooranna. 1998. "Regulation of the choline transport system in superfused microcarrier cultures of BeWo cells." *Placenta* no. 19 (8):663–9.

Fowden, A. L., C. Sibley, W. Reik, and M. Constancia. 2006. "Imprinted genes, placental development and fetal growth." *Horm Res* no. 65 Suppl 3:50–8.

Fullerton, M. D., L. Wagner, Z. Yuan, and M. Bakovic. 2006. "Impaired trafficking of choline transporter-like protein-1 at plasma membrane and inhibition of choline transport in THP-1 monocyte-derived macrophages." *Am J Physiol Cell Physiol* no. 290 (4):C1230–8.

Garner, S. C., S. C. Chou, M. H. Mar, R. A. Coleman, and S. H. Zeisel. 1993. "Characterization of choline metabolism and secretion by human placental trophoblasts in culture." *Biochim Biophys Acta* no. 1168 (3):358–64.

Godfrey, K. M. 2002. "The role of the placenta in fetal programming—A review." *Placenta* no. 23 Suppl A:S20–7.

Goland, R. S., S. Jozak, W. B. Warren, I. M. Conwell, R. I. Stark, and P. J. Tropper. 1993. "Elevated levels of umbilical cord plasma corticotropin-releasing hormone in growth-retarded fetuses." *J Clin Endocrinol Metab* no. 77 (5):1174–9.

Grassl, S. M. 1994. "Choline transport in human placental brush-border membrane vesicles." *Biochim Biophys Acta* no. 1194 (1):203–13.

Gundogan, F., G. Elwood, L. Longato, M. Tong, A. Feijoo, R. I. Carlson, J. R. Wands, and S. M. de la Monte. 2008. "Impaired placentation in fetal alcohol syndrome." *Placenta* no. 29 (2):148–57.

Heazell, A. E. and I. P. Crocker. 2008. "Live and let die—Regulation of villous trophoblast apoptosis in normal and abnormal pregnancies." *Placenta* no. 29 (9):772–83.

Heazell, A. E., H. R. Buttle, P. N. Baker, and I. P. Crocker. 2008. "Altered expression of regulators of caspase activity within trophoblast of normal pregnancies and pregnancies complicated by preeclampsia." *Reprod Sci* no. 15 (10):1034–43.

Holmes, R. and P. D. Soloway. 2006. "Regulation of imprinted DNA methylation." *Cytogenet Genome Res* no. 113 (1–4):122–9.

Hsiao, E. Y. and P. H. Patterson. 2012. "Placental regulation of maternal–fetal interactions and brain development." *Dev Neurobiol* no. 72 (10):1317–26.

Huh, S. Y., R. Andrew, J. W. Rich-Edwards, K. P. Kleinman, J. R. Seckl, and M. W. Gillman. 2008. "Association between umbilical cord glucocorticoids and blood pressure at age 3 years." *BMC Med* no. 6:25.

Institute of Medicine, Food and Nutrition Board. 1998. *Dietary Reference Intakes for Thiamin, Riboflavin, Niacin, Vitamin B6, Folate, Vitamin B12, Pantothenic Acid, Biotin and Choline.* Washington, DC: National Academies Press.

Jensen, H. H., S. P. Batres-Marquez, A. Carriquiry, and K. L. Schalinske. 2007. "Choline in the diets of the US population: NHANES, 2003–2004." *FASEB J* no. 21:1b219.

Jiang, X., J. Yan, A. A. West, C. A. Perry, O. V. Malysheva, S. Devapatla, E. Pressman, F. Vermeylen, and M. A. Caudill. 2012. "Maternal choline intake alters the epigenetic state of fetal cortisol-regulating genes in humans." *FASEB J* no. 26 (8):3563–74.

Jiang, X., H. Y. Bar, J. Yan, S. Jones, P. M. Brannon, A. A. West, C. A. Perry, A. Ganti, E. Pressman, S. Devapatla, F. Vermeylen, M. T. Wells, and M. A. Caudill. 2013. "A higher maternal choline intake among third-trimester pregnant women lowers placental and circulating concentrations of the antiangiogenic factor fms-like tyrosine kinase-1 (sFLT1)." *FASEB J* no. 27 (3):1245–53.

Jiang, X., J. Yan, and M. A. Caudill. 2013. "Choline," 5th ed. In *Handbook of Vitamins.* Taylor & Francis LLC.

Jiang, X., S. Jones, B. Y. Andrew, A. Ganti, O. V. Malysheva, N. Giallourou, P. M. Brannon, M. S. Roberson, and M. A. Caudill. 2014. "Choline inadequacy impairs trophoblast function and vascularization in cultured human placental trophoblasts." *J Cell Physiol* no. 229 (8):1016–27.

Kahn, S. R., N. D. Almeida, H. McNamara, G. Koren, J. Genest Jr., M. Dahhou, R. W. Platt, and M. S. Kramer. 2011. "Smoking in preeclamptic women is associated with higher birthweight for gestational age and lower soluble fms-like tyrosine kinase-1 levels: A nested case control study." *BMC Pregnancy Childbirth* no. 11:91.

Kaitu'u-Lino, T. J., K. R. Palmer, C. L. Whitehead, E. Williams, M. Lappas, and S. Tong. 2012. "MMP-14 is expressed in preeclamptic placentas and mediates release of soluble endoglin." *Am J Pathol* no. 180 (3):888–94.

Kalhan, S. C. and S. E. Marczewski. 2012. "Methionine, homocysteine, one carbon metabolism and fetal growth." *Rev Endocr Metab Disord* no. 13 (2):109–19.

Kawashima, K. and T. Fujii. 2008. "Basic and clinical aspects of non-neuronal acetylcholine: Overview of non-neuronal cholinergic systems and their biological significance." *J Pharmacol Sci* no. 106 (2):167–73.

Kekuda, R., P. D. Prasad, X. Wu, H. Wang, Y. J. Fei, F. H. Leibach, and V. Ganapathy. 1998. "Cloning and functional characterization of a potential-sensitive, polyspecific organic cation transporter (OCT3) most abundantly expressed in placenta." *J Biol Chem* no. 273 (26):15971–9.

King, R. G., N. M. Gude, B. R. Krishna, S. Chen, S. P. Brennecke, A. L. Boura, and T. J. Rook. 1991. "Human placental acetylcholine." *Reprod Fertil Dev* no. 3 (4):405–11.

Klose, R. J. and A. P. Bird. 2006. "Genomic DNA methylation: The mark and its mediators." *Trends Biochem Sci* no. 31 (2):89–97.

Kohlmeier, M., K. A. da Costa, L. M. Fischer, and S. H. Zeisel. 2005. "Genetic variation of folate-mediated one-carbon transfer pathway predicts susceptibility to choline deficiency in humans." *Proc Natl Acad Sci U S A* no. 102 (44):16025–30.

Kovacheva, V. P., T. J. Mellott, J. M. Davison, N. Wagner, I. Lopez-Coviella, A. C. Schnitzler, and J. K. Blusztajn. 2007. "Gestational choline deficiency causes global and Igf2 gene DNA hypermethylation by up-regulation of Dnmt1 expression." *J Biol Chem* no. 282 (43):31777–88.

Kovacheva, V. P., J. M. Davison, T. J. Mellott, A. E. Rogers, S. Yang, M. J. O'Brien, and J. K. Blusztajn. 2009. "Raising gestational choline intake alters gene expression in DMBA-evoked mammary tumors and prolongs survival." *FASEB J* no. 23 (4):1054–63.

Lambertini, L., M. Lee, C. J. Marsit, and J. Chen. 2012. "Genomic imprinting in human placenta." In *Recent Advances in Research on the Human Placenta*, edited by Jing Zheng. 438 pp., InTech. doi: 10.5772/1211.

Lebrin, F. and C. L. Mummery. 2008. "Endoglin-mediated vascular remodeling: Mechanisms underlying hereditary hemorrhagic telangiectasia." *Trends Cardiovasc Med* no. 18 (1):25–32.

Lee, N. Y., H. M. Choi, and Y. S. Kang. 2009. "Choline transport via choline transporter-like protein 1 in conditionally immortalized rat syncytiotrophoblast cell lines TR-TBT." *Placenta* no. 30 (4):368–74.

Lee, N., M. F. Hebert, B. Prasad, T. R. Easterling, E. J. Kelly, J. D. Unadkat, and J. Wang. 2013. "Effect of gestational age on mRNA and protein expression of polyspecific organic cation transporters during pregnancy." *Drug Metab Dispos* no. 41 (12):2225–32.

Lesseur, C., A. G. Paquette, and C. J. Marsit. 2014. "Epigenetic regulation of infant neurobehavioral outcomes." *Med Epigenet* no. 2 (2):71–9.

Lever, M. and S. Slow. 2010. "The clinical significance of betaine, an osmolyte with a key role in methyl group metabolism." *Clin Biochem* no. 43 (9):732–44.

Li, W., K. M. Mata, M. Q. Mazzuca, and R. A. Khalil. 2014. "Altered matrix metalloproteinase-2 and -9 expression/activity links placental ischemia and anti-angiogenic sFlt-1 to uteroplacental and vascular remodeling and collagen deposition in hypertensive pregnancy." *Biochem Pharmacol* no. 89 (3):370–85.

Lim, A. L. and A. C. Ferguson-Smith. 2010. "Genomic imprinting effects in a compromised *in utero* environment: Implications for a healthy pregnancy." *Semin Cell Dev Biol* no. 21 (2):201–8.

Lin, H., T. R. Mosmann, L. Guilbert, S. Tuntipopipat, and T. G. Wegmann. 1993. "Synthesis of T helper 2-type cytokines at the maternal–fetal interface." *J Immunol* no. 151 (9):4562–73.

Marusic, J., I. K. Prusac, S. Z. Tomas, J. R. Karara, and D. Roje. 2013. "Expression of inflammatory cytokines in placentas from pregnancies complicated with preeclampsia and HELLP syndrome." *J Matern Fetal Neonatal Med* no. 26 (7):680–5.

Maynard, S. E., J. Y. Min, J. Merchan, K. H. Lim, J. Li, S. Mondal, T. A. Libermann, J. P. Morgan, F. W. Sellke, I. E. Stillman, F. H. Epstein, V. P. Sukhatme, and S. A. Karumanchi. 2003. "Excess placental soluble fms-like tyrosine kinase 1 (sFlt1) may contribute to endothelial dysfunction, hypertension, and proteinuria in preeclampsia." *J Clin Invest* no. 111 (5):649–58.

Mehedint, M. G., C. N. Craciunescu, and S. H. Zeisel. 2010. "Maternal dietary choline deficiency alters angiogenesis in fetal mouse hippocampus." *Proc Natl Acad Sci U S A* no. 107 (29):12834–9.

Mehta, A. K., N. Arora, S. N. Gaur, and B. P. Singh. 2009. "Choline supplementation reduces oxidative stress in mouse model of allergic airway disease." *Eur J Clin Invest* no. 39 (10):934–41.

Mehta, A. K., B. P. Singh, N. Arora, and S. N. Gaur. 2010. "Choline attenuates immune inflammation and suppresses oxidative stress in patients with asthma." *Immunobiology* no. 215 (7):527–34.

Michel, V. and M. Bakovic. 2012. "The ubiquitous choline transporter SLC44A1." *Cent Nerv Syst Agents Med Chem* no. 12 (2):70–81.

Michel, V., Z. Yuan, S. Ramsubir, and M. Bakovic. 2006. "Choline transport for phospholipid synthesis." *Exp Biol Med (Maywood)* no. 231 (5):490–504.

Miller, T. J., R. D. Hanson, and P. H. Yancey. 2000. "Developmental changes in organic osmolytes in prenatal and postnatal rat tissues." *Comp Biochem Physiol A Mol Integr Physiol* no. 125 (1):45–56.

Moon, J., M. Chen, S. U. Gandhy, M. Strawderman, D. A. Levitsky, K. N. Maclean, and B. J. Strupp. 2010. "Perinatal choline supplementation improves cognitive functioning and emotion regulation in the Ts65Dn mouse model of Down syndrome." *Behav Neurosci* no. 124 (3):346–61.

Napoli, I., J. K. Blusztajn, and T. J. Mellott. 2008. "Prenatal choline supplementation in rats increases the expression of IGF2 and its receptor IGF2R and enhances IGF2-induced acetylcholine release in hippocampus and frontal cortex." *Brain Res* no. 1237:124–35.

Nelissen, E. C., A. P. van Montfoort, J. C. Dumoulin, and J. L. Evers. 2011. "Epigenetics and the placenta." *Hum Reprod Update* no. 17 (3):397–417.

Niculescu, M. D., C. N. Craciunescu, and S. H. Zeisel. 2006. "Dietary choline deficiency alters global and gene-specific DNA methylation in the developing hippocampus of mouse fetal brains." *FASEB J* no. 20 (1):43–9.

Oda, Y., Y. Muroishi, H. Misawa, and S. Suzuki. 2004. "Comparative study of gene expression of cholinergic system-related molecules in the human spinal cord and term placenta." *Neuroscience* no. 128 (1):39–49.

Rama Sastry, B. V., M. E. Hemontolor, and M. Olenick. 1999. "Prostaglandin E2 in human placenta: Its vascular effects and activation of prostaglandin E2 formation by nicotine and cotinine." *Pharmacology* no. 58 (2):70–86.

Redman, C. W. and I. L. Sargent. 2004. "Preeclampsia and the systemic inflammatory response." *Semin Nephrol* no. 24 (6):565–70.

Resseguie, M., J. Song, M. D. Niculescu, K. A. da Costa, T. A. Randall, and S. H. Zeisel. 2007. "Phosphatidylethanolamine N-methyltransferase (PEMT) gene expression is induced by estrogen in human and mouse primary hepatocytes." *FASEB J* no. 21 (10):2622–32.

Ribatti, D. 2008. "Chick embryo chorioallantoic membrane as a useful tool to study angiogenesis." *Int Rev Cell Mol Biol* no. 270:181–224.

Rivera, C. A., M. D. Wheeler, N. Enomoto, and R. G. Thurman. 1998. "A choline-rich diet improves survival in a rat model of endotoxin shock." *Am J Physiol* no. 275 (4 Pt 1):G862–7.

Rosse, C., M. Linch, S. Kermorgant, A. J. Cameron, K. Boeckeler, and P. J. Parker. 2010. "PKC and the control of localized signal dynamics." *Nat Rev Mol Cell Biol* no. 11 (2):103–12.

Saito, S. and M. Sakai. 2003. "Th1/Th2 balance in preeclampsia." *J Reprod Immunol* no. 59 (2):161–73.

Salam, R. A., J. K. Das, and Z. A. Bhutta. 2014. "Impact of intrauterine growth restriction on long-term health." *Curr Opin Clin Nutr Metab Care* no. 17 (3):249–54.

Sastry, B. V. 1997. "Human placental cholinergic system." *Biochem Pharmacol* no. 53 (11):1577–86.

Sastry, B. V., J. Olubadewo, R. D. Harbison, and D. E. Schmidt. 1976. "Human placental cholinergic system. Occurrence, distribution and variation with gestational age of acetylcholine in human placenta." *Biochem Pharmacol* no. 25 (4):425–31.

Satyanarayana, M. 1986. "A correlative review of acetylcholine synthesis in relation to histopathology of the human syncytiotrophoblast." *Acta Obstet Gynecol Scand* no. 65 (6):567–72.

Shaw, G. M., S. L. Carmichael, W. Yang, S. Selvin, and D. M. Schaffer. 2004. "Periconceptional dietary intake of choline and betaine and neural tube defects in offspring." *Am J Epidemiol* no. 160 (2):102–9.

Strahl, B. D. and C. D. Allis. 2000. "The language of covalent histone modifications." *Nature* no. 403 (6765):41–5.

Straszewski-Chavez, S. L., V. M. Abrahams, and G. Mor. 2005. "The role of apoptosis in the regulation of trophoblast survival and differentiation during pregnancy." *Endocr Rev* no. 26 (7):877–97.

ten Dijke, P. and H. M. Arthur. 2007. "Extracellular control of TGFbeta signalling in vascular development and disease." *Nat Rev Mol Cell Biol* no. 8 (11):857–69.

Thomas, J. D., E. J. Abou, and H. D. Dominguez. 2009. "Prenatal choline supplementation mitigates the adverse effects of prenatal alcohol exposure on development in rats." *Neurotoxicol Teratol* no. 31 (5):303–11.

Tsatsaris, V., F. Goffin, C. Munaut, J. F. Brichant, M. R. Pignon, A. Noel, J. P. Schaaps, D. Cabrol, F. Frankenne, and J. M. Foidart. 2003. "Overexpression of the soluble vascular endothelial growth factor receptor in preeclamptic patients: Pathophysiological consequences." *J Clin Endocrinol Metab* no. 88 (11):5555–63.

van der Aa, E. M., A. C. Wouterse, J. H. Peereboom-Stegeman, and F. G. Russel. 1994. "Uptake of choline into syncytial microvillus membrane vesicles of human term placenta." *Biochem Pharmacol* no. 47 (3):453–6.

Velazquez, R., J. A. Ash, B. E. Powers, C. M. Kelley, M. Strawderman, Z. I. Luscher, S. D. Ginsberg, E. J. Mufson, and B. J. Strupp. 2013. "Maternal choline supplementation improves spatial learning and adult hippocampal neurogenesis in the Ts65Dn mouse model of Down syndrome." *Neurobiol Dis* no. 58:92–101.

Venkatesha, S., M. Toporsian, C. Lam, J. Hanai, T. Mammoto, Y. M. Kim, Y. Bdolah, K. H. Lim, H. T. Yuan, T. A. Libermann, I. E. Stillman, D. Roberts, P. A. D'Amore, F. H. Epstein, F. W. Sellke, R. Romero, V. P. Sukhatme, M. Letarte, and S. A. Karumanchi. 2006. "Soluble endoglin contributes to the pathogenesis of preeclampsia." *Nat Med* no. 12 (6):642–9.

Wadhwa, P. D., T. J. Garite, M. Porto, L. Glynn, A. Chicz-DeMet, C. Dunkel-Schetter, and C. A. Sandman. 2004. "Placental corticotropin-releasing hormone (CRH), spontaneous preterm birth, and fetal growth restriction: A prospective investigation." *Am J Obstet Gynecol* no. 191 (4):1063–9.

Wang, H., X. Z. Zeng, W. Y. Cui, and L. Duan. 2013. "[Choline promotes angiogenesis in chick embryo chorioallantoic membrane]." *Zhongguo Ying Yong Sheng Li Xue Za Zhi* no. 29 (3):229–31.

Welsch, F. 1976a. "Studies on accumulation and metabolic fate of (N-Me3h)choline in human term placenta fragments." *Biochem Pharmacol* no. 25 (9):1021–30.

Welsch, F. 1976b. "Uptake of acetylcholine by human placenta fragments and slices from guinea pig and rat placenta." *Biochem Pharmacol* no. 25 (1):81–9.

Welsch, F. 1978. "Choline metabolism in human term placenta—Studies on de novo synthesis and the effects of some drugs on the metabolic fate of [N-methyl 3H]choline." *Biochem Pharmacol* no. 27 (8):1251–7.

Welsch, F. and S. K. McCarthy. 1977. "Choline acetyltransferase and carnitine acetyltransferase in the placenta of the mouse." *Comp Biochem Physiol C* no. 56 (2):163–9.

Wessler, I., E. Roth, C. Deutsch, P. Brockerhoff, F. Bittinger, C. J. Kirkpatrick, and H. Kilbinger. 2001. "Release of non-neuronal acetylcholine from the isolated human placenta is mediated by organic cation transporters." *Br J Pharmacol* no. 134 (5):951–6.

Wessler, I., H. Kilbinger, F. Bittinger, R. Unger, and C. J. Kirkpatrick. 2003. "The non-neuronal cholinergic system in humans: Expression, function and pathophysiology." *Life Sci* no. 72 (18–19):2055–61.

Whitley, G. S. and J. E. Cartwright. 2009. "Trophoblast-mediated spiral artery remodelling: A role for apoptosis." *J Anat* no. 215 (1):21–6.

Xu, H., B. Shatenstein, Z. C. Luo, S. Wei, and W. Fraser. 2009. "Role of nutrition in the risk of preeclampsia." *Nutr Rev* no. 67 (11):639–57.

Yamada, T., M. Inazu, H. Tajima, and T. Matsumiya. 2011. "Functional expression of choline transporter-like protein 1 (CTL1) in human neuroblastoma cells and its link to acetylcholine synthesis." *Neurochem Int* no. 58 (3):354–65.

Yan, J., W. Wang, J. F. Gregory 3rd, O. Malysheva, J. T. Brenna, S. P. Stabler, R. H. Allen, and M. A. Caudill. 2011. "MTHFR C677T genotype influences the isotopic enrichment of one-carbon metabolites in folate-compromised men consuming d9-choline." *Am J Clin Nutr* no. 93 (2):348–55.

Yan, J., X. Jiang, A. A. West, C. A. Perry, O. V. Malysheva, S. Devapatla, E. Pressman, F. Vermeylen, S. P. Stabler, R. H. Allen, and M. A. Caudill. 2012. "Maternal choline intake modulates maternal and fetal biomarkers of choline metabolism in humans." *Am J Clin Nutr* no. 95 (5):1060–71.

Yan, J., X. Jiang, A. A. West, C. A. Perry, O. V. Malysheva, J. T. Brenna, S. P. Stabler, R. H. Allen, J. F. Gregory 3rd, and M. A. Caudill. 2013. "Pregnancy alters choline dynamics: Results of a randomized trial using stable isotope methodology in pregnant and nonpregnant women." *Am J Clin Nutr* no. 98 (6):1459–67.

Yen, C. L., M. H. Mar, and S. H. Zeisel. 1999. "Choline deficiency-induced apoptosis in PC12 cells is associated with diminished membrane phosphatidylcholine and sphingomyelin, accumulation of ceramide and diacylglycerol, and activation of a caspase." *FASEB J* no. 13 (1):135–42.

Yoshida, Y., N. Itoh, M. Hayakawa, Y. Habuchi, R. Inoue, Z. H. Chen, J. Cao, O. Cynshi, and E. Niki. 2006. "Lipid peroxidation in mice fed a choline–deficient diet as evaluated by total hydroxyoctadecadienoic acid." *Nutrition* no. 22 (3):303–11.

Zeisel, S. H. and J. K. Blusztajn. 1994. "Choline and human nutrition." *Annu Rev Nutr* no. 14:269–96.

Zeisel, S. H., K. A. Da Costa, P. D. Franklin, E. A. Alexander, J. T. Lamont, N. F. Sheard, and A. Beiser. 1991. "Choline, an essential nutrient for humans." *FASEB J* no. 5 (7):2093–8.

Zeisel, S. H., M. H. Mar, J. C. Howe, and J. M. Holden. 2003. "Concentrations of choline-containing compounds and betaine in common foods." *J Nutr* no. 133 (5):1302–7.

15 Role of Calcium in Fetal Development

Evemie Dubé and Julie Lafond

CONTENTS

ABSTRACT

Calcium is a critical element for the fetus during pregnancy as it has been highlighted in various pathologies associated with fetal growth problems, such as preeclampsia, gestational mellitus diabetes, and intrauterine growth retardation. Most of the calcium is provided by the maternal metabolism that needs to adapt to the exponential fetal needs in calcium and goes through the placenta. The transplacental transport of calcium from the mother to the fetus is a complex process that is tightly regulated and involves numerous proteins. This chapter will focus mainly on the description of these various key players involved in the transport of calcium in the human placenta.

KEY WORDS

Calcium, pregnancy, placenta, VDCC, SOC, CaSR, S100 proteins, PMCA, pregnancy-associated pathologies.

15.1 INTRODUCTION

Calcium constitutes a crucial element for proper fetal development and growth and mostly originates from the maternal circulation. Thus, fetal demands lead to adaptations of maternal homeostasis to provide the required calcium, especially in the last trimester of pregnancy. These adaptations also induce changes in the numerous key players involved in placental calcium homeostasis. In addition, several factors are known to influence the pool of calcium in the blood and bones. Therefore, it is important to clearly understand the role and transport of calcium during pregnancy as well as the impact of any impairment of calcium homeostasis during pregnancy that could have major consequences on the future health of the offspring. Thus, this chapter will discuss the proteins associated with calcium and homeostasis in the placenta during normal and pathological pregnancies.

15.2 FETOMATERNAL CALCIUM HOMEOSTASIS DURING PREGNANCY

15.2.1 ROLE OF CALCIUM IN FETAL DEVELOPMENT

Fetal needs in calcium increase progressively throughout pregnancy, especially in the last trimester, to allow the fetus to accumulate up to 30 mg of calcium. The fetal calcium accretion rate is about 50 mg/day at 20 weeks and increases to approximately 350 mg/day at 35 weeks of pregnancy (Prentice and Bates 1994). This calcium, which is present in higher levels in the fetal circulation than in the maternal circulation, is essential for fetal skeletal mineralization and multiple cellular processes such as gene regulation, cell differentiation, and apoptosis (Kovacs 2014).

15.2.2 MATERNAL CALCIUM HOMEOSTASIS DURING PREGNANCY

Multiple changes occur in the maternal calcium homeostasis during pregnancy to ensure proper calcium transfer to the fetus. Indeed, studies have noted that the total maternal plasma concentration of calcium is lower in pregnant women compared with nonpregnant women (Wisser et al. 2005). Adaptations of the maternal calcium metabolism during pregnancy include increased intestinal absorption, decreased renal excretion, and increased resorption from the skeleton (Olausson et al. 2012). Even in the presence of maternal calcium deficiency, active transport of calcium to the fetus and fetal hypercalcemia are maintained (Vargas Zapata et al. 2004). It has been demonstrated that calcium absorption efficiency increases by twofold during the second half of pregnancy in association with increased expression of intestinal calcium ATPase plasma membrane calcium ATPase 1 (PMCA1) and calcium binding protein CaBP9K (Cross et al. 1995; Zhu et al. 1998). In addition, the circulating levels of the active form of vitamin D known as calcitriol rise progressively during pregnancy (Cross et al. 1995). These increased levels of calcitriol are probably due to enhanced renal synthesis of calcitriol (resulting from increased stimulation of renal 1-α-hydroxylase activity, the enzyme that converts vitamin D to calcitriol) in addition to the synthesis of calcitriol by the placenta and the fetus (Evans et al. 2004). Surprisingly, the levels of parathyroid hormone (PTH), which is the key hormone that stimulates renal calcitriol synthesis, are unchanged during pregnancy (Cross et al. 1995). The increased levels of calcitriol during pregnancy are likely due to high circulating levels of parathyroid hormone-related protein (PTHrP) originating from fetal, placental, and mammary tissues. Indeed, PTHrP is known to activate the PTH/PTHrP receptor and exhibit PTH-like effects (Kovacs 2014).

15.3 TRANSPLACENTAL TRANSPORT OF CALCIUM

To satisfy fetal needs, calcium is actively transported across the human placenta from the maternal to the fetal circulation at a rate of 140 mg/kg/day. This active transport begins by week 12 of gestation and peaks at week 36 (Salle et al. 1987). Human syncytiotrophoblast, which forms a barrier between the mother and fetus, are responsible for most of this transport that requires several channels, transporters and exchangers located on both of its microvillous (MVMs) and basal plasma (BPMs) membranes (Figure 15.1). These proteins are going to be described in the following sections.

15.3.1 Voltage-Dependent Calcium Channels

Calcium channels are divided into two main families, voltage-dependent calcium channels (VDCCs) and non-voltage-gated channels. VDCCs are transmembrane channels divided into two groups, low-voltage activated (LVA) and high-voltage activated (HVA) channels, based on their activation threshold. The HVA channels include the L-type, N-type, P-type, R-type, and Q-type, while the LVA channels include the T-type. Two types of VDCCs have been shown to be expressed by human trophoblast cells: L-type and T-type VDCCs (Liu, Hill, and Khan 2005; Meuris et al. 1994; Robidoux et al. 2000). T-type channels are composed of α_1 subunits ($Ca_v3.1$, $Ca_v3.2$, and $Ca_v3.3$), but little is known about their role in the human placenta. On the other hand, L-type channels are composed of five subunits: α_1, α_2, β, γ, and δ. The α_1 is the pore forming subunit, the β subunit regulates the translocation of the α_1 subunit to the plasma membrane, and the others are considered as accessory subunits (Neely and Hidalgo 2014). In the human placenta, mRNAs of both α_{1C} and α_{1D} subunits of the L-type VDCC are expressed by cytotrophoblast and syncytiotrophoblast cells (Bernucci et al. 2006). Moreover the activation of L-type channels in placental explants has been shown to stimulate the release of human chorionic gonadotrophin and placental lactogen (Meuris

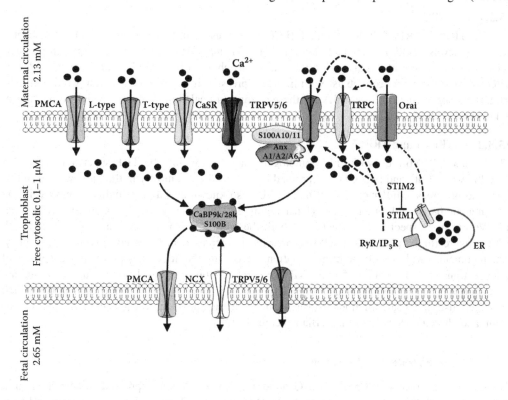

FIGURE 15.1 Schematic representation of calcium transport in human syncytiotrophoblast. Anx, annexin; Ca^{2+}, calcium; CaBP, calcium-binding protein; CaSR, calcium sensing receptor; ER, endoplasmic reticulum; IP_3R, inositol-1,4,5-triphosphate receptor; NCX, Na^+/Ca^{2+}-exchanger; PMCA, plasma membrane Ca^{2+} ATPase; RyR, ryanodine receptor; STIM, stromal interaction molecule; TRPC, transient receptor potential cation channels family; TRPV, transient receptor potential vanilloid family.

et al. 1994), suggesting that L-type VDCCs are involved in placental hormonal regulation in addition to calcium homeostasis.

15.3.2 STORE-OPERATED CALCIUM CHANNELS

Store-operated calcium channels (SOCs) are non-voltage-gated channels that are activated by the release of calcium from the endoplasmic reticulum (ER). They comprise the transient receptor potential (TRP) (transient receptor potential canonical [TRPC], transient receptor potential vanilloid [TRPV], transient receptor potential metastatin [TRPM], transient receptor potential channel [TRPA], transient receptor potential polycystic [TRPP], TRPML, and transient receptor potential ion channels with no mechanoreceptor potential [TRPN]). In the following sections, we will focus on the SOCs expressed in the placenta and their partners Orai (Orai1–3) and stromal interaction molecule (STIM1–2).

15.3.2.1 STIMs and Orais

STIM1 is ubiquitously expressed in human tissues, including the placenta and the myometrium. Its splice variant STIM1L is also found in the placenta (Horinouchi et al. 2012). Unfortunately, little information exists on these proteins, their interactions, and their function in the placenta. In other cell types, STIM1 is expressed at the cell surface and ER, whereas STIM2 is found only in the intracellular space. SOCs can be activated in a STIM1-independent manner, following the activation of the IP$_3$ receptor (IP$_3$R) or ryanodine receptors (RyRs) (Choi et al. 2014). Interestingly, IP$_3$R1, IP$_3$R2, RyR1, RyR2, and RyR3 are down-regulated in preeclamptic placentas (Hache et al. 2011).

15.3.2.2 TRPC

TRPC1, TRPC3, TRPC4, TRCP5, and TRPC6 are expressed in first-trimester and term placentas at varying levels. TRPC7 is not at all detected. TRPC3 and TRPC4 are localized to cytotrophoblast cells in first-trimester placentas and to the syncytiotrophoblast in term placentas, while TRPC6 is detected in the syncytiotrophoblast with higher expression in term placentas compared with first trimesters, suggesting different roles for these channels in calcium homeostasis during pregnancy (Clarson et al. 2003).

15.3.2.3 TRPV5 and TRPV6

TRPV5 and TRPV6 are two highly homologous members within the TRP superfamily. TRPV5 (also known as Cat2 and ECAC1) is expressed in various tissues, mostly in the kidney, small intestine, and pancreas (Muller et al. 2000). TRPV6 (also known as Cat1) is highly expressed in the placenta compared with other organs (Hirnet et al. 2003). In the syncytiotrophoblast, TRPV5 and TRPV6 are more specifically detected on both the basal and apical membranes (Bernucci et al. 2006). Interestingly, placental TRPV6 expression is increased in the second half of pregnancy, which coincides with fetal bone mineralization, suggesting that it is a key player in transplacental calcium transfer. Indeed, TRPV5 and TRPV6 could be involved in basal calcium uptake of human syncytiotrophoblast (Moreau et al. 2002). This was confirmed by TRPV6 knockout mice, which presented disordered calcium homeostasis, reduced fertility, deficient transplacental transfer of calcium, and altered bone homeostasis (Bianco et al. 2007).

15.3.3 CALCIUM-SENSING RECEPTOR

Calcium-sensing receptor (CaSR) is a G-protein coupled receptor expressed in several tissues, including in both the villous (mainly on the MVM) and extravillous regions of first-term and term placentas (Bradbury et al. 2002), thus suggesting a role for CaSR in the regulation of transplacental calcium transport and placental development. In the adult, the role of CaSR is to maintain the normal serum calcium level, mostly by regulating the PTH synthesis and secretion from the parathyroid glands. Animal models confirmed that CaSR had a similar role during fetal development.

Indeed, the heterozygous and homozygous disruption of CaSR results in fetal hyperparathyroidism, fetal hypercalcemia, and reduced placental calcium transfer (Ho et al. 1995). In pregnancies associated with gestational diabetes mellitus (GDM), CaSR is less expressed compared with control placentas (Papadopoulou et al. 2014).

15.3.4 CALCIUM-BINDING PROTEINS

Calcium-binding proteins (CaBPs) of the troponin-C superfamily are cytosolic proteins with epidermal factor (EF) hand motifs that have a high affinity for calcium. This large family of more than 200 members is present in many calcium-transporting tissues such as the bone, kidney, and placenta. In the placenta, a number of CaBPs have been identified, such as HCaBP, CaBP57k, CaBP9k, CaBP28k, oncomodulin, and a few S100 proteins (Lafond and Simoneau 2006). We will focus on the most important ones in the following sections.

15.3.4.1 CaBP57k

CaBP57k is high-molecular weight CaBP exclusively expressed by trophoblasts in both human and rodent placentas (Tuan, Lamb, and Jesinkey 1988). Following diffferentiation of Rcho-1 cells (a rat choriocarcinoma cell line) into trophoblastic giant cells, the expression of this CaBP is upregulated as well as the calcium uptake, suggesting that this protein is involved in placental calcium uptake and trophoblast differentiation. Not surprisingly, the expression of this protein also increases during pregnancy. Moreover, both the expression of this CaBP and the calcium uptake in Rcho-1 cells and placental organ cultures can be stimulated by PTHrP 67-84, but not by calcitriol, estrogen, PTH, or PTHrP 1–34 (Hershberger and Tuan 1998).

15.3.4.2 S100 Proteins

The S100 protein family consists of 24 members expressed exclusively in vertebrates that exhibit a cell-specific expression pattern. These proteins act either as intracellular regulators or as extracellular signaling proteins. S100 proteins have been involved in multiple cellular processes such as the regulation of proliferation, differentiation, apoptosis, calcium homeostasis, and inflammation (Donato et al. 2013).

a. S100A1

S100A1 (also known as S100) has been detected in the placenta and umbilical cord, more specifically in the syncytiotrophoblast, in myofibroblats, smooth muscle cells of the vascular walls, and in macrophages (Wijnberger et al. 2002). The presence of this protein in amniotic fluid and fetal cerebrospinal fluid is usually indicative of neonatal brain damage (Gazzolo et al. 1999). Studies in double knockout mice for both S100A1 and S100B revealed that these proteins are not essential for normal endochondral ossification during skeletal development, suggesting the existence of a compensatory mechanism (Mori et al. 2014). However, the role of S100A1 in the placenta is unknown.

b. S100A6

S100A6 mRNA expression was detected in mice in the uterus, decidua, and placenta (Waterhouse et al. 1992). Interestingly, S100A6 can be released by trophoblast cells and stimulate the secretion of mouse placental lactogen type II (Thordarson, Southard, and Talamantes 1991). Targets of S100A6 include lumican and PRELP in Wharton's jelly as well as insulin-like growth factor-binding protein 1 (IGFBP-1), but only in preeclamptic Wharton's jelly, suggesting that S100A6 plays a role in the development of preeclampsia (Jurewicz et al. 2014).

c. S100A9

S100A9 (also known as myeloid-related protein [MRP]-14, macrophage migration inhibitory factor [MIF], or calgranulin-B) is expressed by trophoblasts of the chorionic villi (Arcuri et al. 1999). Circulating levels of S100A9 are increased in women with GDM and preeclampsia (Todros et al. 2005; Yilmaz et al. 2012). Although its function in the placenta is not clear, it has been suggested that the action of this protein on macrophages could play a role in the implantation and early development of the embryo during the first trimester of pregnancy.

d. S100A10

S100A10 (also known as p11) is present with annexin A2 and A6 on the surface of the syncytiotrophoblast MVMs, and its expressions increases progressively during pregnancy (Kaczan-Bourgois et al. 1996; Riquelme et al. 2004). Moreover, this complex binds to TRPV6 and TRPV5 in various epithelia and plays a crucial role in the routing of TRPV5 and TRPV6 to the plasma membrane (van de Graaf et al. 2003). Interestingly, circulating levels of S100A10 are upregulated in early-onset preeclampsia (Chaiworapongsa et al. 2013).

e. S100B

S100B is localized in the cytoplasm of villous and intermediate trophoblasts, and its expression increases progressively during pregnancy. In addition, this protein is present in amnion and decidual cells of fetal membranes at all gestational ages (Cai et al. 2012; Marinoni et al. 2002). S100B is also detectable in the umbilical cord blood and urine of preterm and term fetuses, with increased levels in intrauterine growth-retarded fetuses, without any changes in its placental expression (Gazzolo et al. 2000, 2002). Moreover, up-regulation of S100B has been observed after oxidative stress in endothelial cells from villous and amniotic tissues (Tskitishvili et al. 2010) as well as in preeclamptic placentas (Cai et al. 2012).

f. CaBP9k

CaBP9k, initially identified in the intestine, has been detected in various tissues and has been shown to be involved in active calcium transport (Bouhtiauy et al. 1994b). In the placenta, CaBP9k is expressed by trophoblasts and fetal chorionic epithelium, with the highest expression in the second half of pregnancy, except in the baboon (Belkacemi, Simoneau, and Lafond 2002; Belkacemi et al. 2004; Jeung et al. 1995; Krisinger et al. 1992, 1995; Nikitenko et al. 1998). CaBP9K is also present in the endometrium and myometrium, suggesting that it may be involved in the regulation of implantation and uterine smooth muscle function during pregnancy (Miller et al. 1994; Tatsumi et al. 1999). However, the role of this protein in the placenta is still not clear. Studies have shown that the expression of this protein can be regulated by calcium, vitamin D, estrogens, PTHrP, and hypoxia, but its regulation is tissue specific (Brehier and Thomasset 1990; Kovacs et al. 2002; L'Horset et al. 1990; Romagnolo et al. 1996; Yang et al. 2013). In the placenta, its expression is vitamin D independent (Shamley et al. 1996). CaBP9k, CaBP28k, and CaBP-k/28k double knockout mouse models revealed possible compensatory mechanisms involving TRPV6. Indeed, TRPV6 was upregulated, which means that the enhanced expression of this channel in CaBP9k and CaBP28k knockout mice may compensate for calbindin deficiency in the placenta. Na^+/Ca^{2+}-exchanger 1 (NCX1) expression was also higher in the fetal placenta in CaBP-9k knockout mice (Koo et al. 2012; Lee et al. 2007).

15.3.4.3 CaBP28k

CaBP28k, initially identified in the intestine, is expressed in many tissues, including the endometrium, and by trophoblasts in the placenta (Belkacemi et al. 2003; Yang et al. 2011). Moreover, CaBP28k is upregulated in the presence of vitamin D in the choriocarcinoma cell line JEG-3 (Belkacemi et al. 2005). In other tissues, CaBP28k is regulated by vitamin D (Inpanbutr et al. 1996), corticosteroids, (Iacopino and Christakos 1990; Tohmon et al. 1988), nerve growth factor (Iacopino et al. 1992), and estrogen (Yang et al. 2011), but not by calcitonin (Hsu et al. 2010). Even if the role of this protein is unclear in the placenta, CaBP28k has been shown to act as a calcium buffer by interacting with TRPV5 in renal epithelial cells (Bouhtiauy et al. 1994a; Lambers et al. 2006). However, knockout animals revealed that deletion of CaBP28k alone does not affect body calcium homeostasis; it is rather the deletion of both CaBP9k and CaBP28k that has a significant effect on calcium processing under calcium-deficient conditions (Ko et al. 2009). This could be due to a compensatory mechanism involving TRPV6 (Koo et al. 2012). Interestingly, a significant decrease in protein levels of TRPV5, TRPV6, CaBP9k, and CaBP28k was observed in preeclamptic placentas; thus, TRPV6 is not able to compensate for CaBP deficiency in preeclamptic placentas (Hache et al. 2011).

15.3.5 PLASMA MEMBRANE CALCIUM ATPASE

PMCA is a high-affinity and low-capacity calcium pump responsible of the removal of excessive intracellular calcium. Studies have demonstrated the existence of four isoforms (PMCA1, PMCA2, PMCA3, and PMCA4) that share a high degree of sequence homology. More than 20 splice variants also exist. Although PMCA1 and PMCA4 are widely expressed, PMCA2 is mostly expressed by cerebellar Purkinje cells, uterus, liver, kidney, and lactating mammary gland, while PMCA3 is present in the brain and in the skeletal muscle (reviewed in Di Leva et al. 2008). Most PMCA knockout animals are viable, except for PMCA1 knockouts that suffer from embryonic lethality, suggesting an important role for this protein in fetal development (Kozel et al. 1998; Okunade et al. 2004; Penheiter et al. 2001). Several studies have demonstrated the involvement of PMCA in calcium extrusion from placental cells (Lafond, Leclerc, and Brunette 1991; Moreau et al. 2003; Moreau, Simoneau, and Lafond 2003; Strid et al. 2003). In addition, in the human placenta, a higher expression and activity of PMCA1 and PMCA4 were observed on the MVM of the syncytiotrophoblast compared with the BPM (Marin et al. 2008; Strid and Powell 2000). Interestingly, the expression and activity of these pumps increase during the last trimester of pregnancy on the BPM of syncytiotrophoblast (Glazier et al. 1992; Strid and Powell 2000), suggesting an important role for these proteins in cell calcium extrusion from the placenta toward the fetal circulation in the last trimester of pregnancy. Moreover, a study has suggested that placental mRNA expression of PMCA3 at term could be predictive of neonatal whole-body bone mineral content (Martin et al. 2007). Additionally, a significant decrease in protein levels of PMCA1/4 was noted in preeclamptic placentas (Hache et al. 2011).

15.3.6 NA⁺/CA²⁺-EXCHANGER

NCXs, which are plasma membrane transporters, are important components of intracellular calcium homeostasis and electrical conduction. Three mammalian isoforms have been discovered, NCX1, NCX2, and NCX3, that are expressed in different tissues (reviewed in Lytton 2007). Both NCX1 and NCX3 are expressed in the human placenta, more specifically by the syncytiotrophoblast (Kamath and Smith 1994; Moreau et al. 2003). In the human placenta, NCXs are possibly involved in transplacental transfer of calcium and in regulating intracellular levels. But only a minimal role of NCX in the transplacental transfer of calcium was observed *in vitro* in human term placental lobules, primary trophoblast cultures as well as in BeWo cells (Lafond, Leclerc, and Brunette 1991; Moreau et al. 2003; Moreau, Simoneau, and Lafond 2003; Williams et al. 1991). Knockout of NCX1 in mice resulted in embryonic lethality, most likely because of a lack of vascular morphogenesis within the placental yolk sac (Cho et al. 2003; Koushik et al. 2001; Wakimoto et al. 2000). Thus, NCX1 in the placenta could instead be involved in the establishment of placental vascularization. On the other hand, the role of NCX3 may be different since NCX3 knockout mice were viable and fertile (Sokolow et al. 2004).

15.4 IMPACT OF PREGNANCY COMPLICATIONS ON CALCIUM HOMEOSTASIS

Several placental pathologies, such as preeclampsia, GDM, and intrauterine growth retardation, are associated with alterations in maternal and placental calcium homeostasis as described in the above sections (Dodd, O'Brien, and Grivell 2014). Low calcium levels in the cord blood of GDM and in intrauterine growth retardated infants with asphyxia have been measured, as well as decreased total body bone mineral content at birth in small-for-gestational-age infants (Chen et al. 1995; Papadopoulou et al. 2014; Tsang et al. 1975). Preeclampsia in particular is associated with low urinary calcium excretion, low circulating levels of calcitriol, PTH-related peptide and calcitonin gene-related peptide, and altered placental calcium transport (Hache et al. 2011; Halhali et al. 2000). Epidemiological data even suggest an inverse correlation between dietary calcium uptake and incidence of gestational hypertensive disorders. But the efficiency of calcium supplementation in the prevention of hypertensive disorders and programmed adult bone deficits associated with perinatal growth restriction is still controversial (Hofmeyr, Duley, and Atallah 2007). Calcium and vitamin D cosupplementation is also currently studied in case of GDM (Asemi, Karamali, and Esmaillzadeh 2014).

15.5 CONCLUSIONS

Our understanding of the mechanisms involved in calcium homeostasis has greatly improved over the last decades. However, even if the placental transfer of maternal calcium to the fetus represents a vital mechanism for fetal development, little meaningful information is currently available regarding the functional mechanisms involved in this process in normal and pathological pregnancies. Therefore, it is important to continue research on these mechanisms since poor maternal and newborn health and nutrition are significant contributors to the development of adult diseases. Calcium supplementation could have the potential to reduce adverse gestational outcomes, in particular by decreasing the risk of developing hypertensive disorders during pregnancy. Thus, it is important to understand the effects of calcium supplementation on maternal and infant outcomes in conjunction with other nutrients such as vitamin D.

REFERENCES

Arcuri, F., M. T. del Vecchio, M. M. de Santi, A. V. Lalinga, V. Pallini, L. Bini, S. Bartolommei, S. Parigi, and M. Cintorino. 1999. "Macrophage migration inhibitory factor in the human prostate: Identification and immunocytochemical localization." *The Prostate* no. 39 (3):159–65.

Asemi, Z., M. Karamali, and A. Esmaillzadeh. 2014. "Effects of calcium–vitamin D co-supplementation on glycaemic control, inflammation and oxidative stress in gestational diabetes: A randomised placebo-controlled trial." *Diabetologia* no. 57 (9):1798–806. doi:10.1007/s00125-014-3293-x.

Belkacemi, L., L. Simoneau, and J. Lafond. 2002. "Calcium-binding proteins: Distribution and implication in mammalian placenta." *Endocrine* no. 19 (1):57–64. doi:10.1385/ENDO:19:1:57.

Belkacemi, L., G. Gariepy, C. Mounier, L. Simoneau, and J. Lafond. 2003. "Expression of calbindin-D28k (CaBP28k) in trophoblasts from human term placenta." *Biology of Reproduction* no. 68 (6):1943–50. doi:10.1095/biolreprod.102.009373.

Belkacemi, L., G. Gariepy, C. Mounier, L. Simoneau, and J. Lafond. 2004. "Calbindin-D9k (CaBP9k) localization and levels of expression in trophoblast cells from human term placenta." *Cell and Tissue Research* no. 315 (1):107–17. doi:10.1007/s00441-003-0811-4.

Belkacemi, L., U. Zuegel, A. Steinmeyer, J. P. Dion, and J. Lafond. 2005. "Calbindin-D28k (CaBP28k) identification and regulation by 1,25-dihydroxyvitamin D3 in human choriocarcinoma cell line JEG-3." *Molecular and Cellular Endocrinology* no. 236 (1–2):31–41. doi:10.1016/j.mce.2005.03.002.

Bernucci, L., M. Henriquez, P. Diaz, and G. Riquelme. 2006. "Diverse calcium channel types are present in the human placental syncytiotrophoblast basal membrane." *Placenta* no. 27 (11–12):1082–95. doi:10.1016/j.placenta.2005.12.007.

Bianco, S. D., J. B. Peng, H. Takanaga, Y. Suzuki, A. Crescenzi, C. H. Kos, L. Zhuang, M. R. Freeman, C. H. Gouveia, J. Wu, H. Luo, T. Mauro, E. M. Brown, and M. A. Hediger. 2007. "Marked disturbance of calcium homeostasis in mice with targeted disruption of the Trpv6 calcium channel gene." *Journal of Bone and Mineral Research: The Official Journal of the American Society for Bone and Mineral Research* no. 22 (2):274–85. doi:10.1359/jbmr.061110.

Bouhtiauy, I., D. Lajeunesse, S. Christakos, and M. G. Brunette. 1994a. "Two vitamin D3-dependent calcium binding proteins increase calcium reabsorption by different mechanisms. I. Effect of CaBP 28K." *Kidney International* no. 45 (2):461–8.

Bouhtiauy, I., D. Lajeunesse, S. Christakos, and M. G. Brunette. 1994b. "Two vitamin D3-dependent calcium binding proteins increase calcium reabsorption by different mechanisms. II. Effect of CaBP 9K." *Kidney International* no. 45 (2):469–74.

Bradbury, R. A., J. Cropley, O. Kifor, F. J. Lovicu, R. U. de Iongh, E. Kable, E. M. Brown, E. W. Seely, B. B. Peat, and A. D. Conigrave. 2002. "Localization of the extracellular Ca(2+)-sensing receptor in the human placenta." *Placenta* no. 23 (2–3):192–200. doi:10.1053/plac.2001.0765.

Brehier, A. and M. Thomasset. 1990. "Stimulation of calbindin-D9K (CaBP9K) gene expression by calcium and 1,25-dihydroxycholecalciferol in fetal rat duodenal organ culture." *Endocrinology* no. 127 (2):580–7. doi:10.1210/endo-127-2-580.

Cai, R. M., Z. P. Weng, Y. Y. Wang, Y. T. Li, and X. H. Ji. 2012. "[Relationship of S100B protein expression and the pathogenesis of early-onset and late-onset preeclampsia]." *Zhonghua fu chan ke za zhi* no. 47 (7):510–3.

Chaiworapongsa, T., R. Romero, A. Whitten, A. L. Tarca, G. Bhatti, S. Draghici, P. Chaemsaithong, J. Miranda, and S. S. Hassan. 2013. "Differences and similarities in the transcriptional profile of peripheral whole blood in early and late-onset preeclampsia: Insights into the molecular basis of the phenotype of pre-eclampsiaa." *Journal of Perinatal Medicine* no. 41 (5):485–504. doi:10.1515/jpm-2013-0082.

Chen, J. Y., U. P. Ling, W. L. Chiang, C. B. Liu, and S. P. Chanlai. 1995. "Total body bone mineral content in small-for-gestational-age, appropriate-for-gestational-age, large-for-gestational-age term infants, and appropriate-for-gestational-age preterm infants." *Zhonghua yi xue za zhi = Chinese Medical Journal; Free China ed* no. 56 (2):109–14.

Cho, C. H., S. Y. Lee, H. S. Shin, K. D. Philipson, and C. O. Lee. 2003. "Partial rescue of the Na^+–Ca^{2+} exchanger (NCX1) knock-out mouse by transgenic expression of NCX1." *Experimental & Molecular Medicine* no. 35 (2):125–35. doi:10.1038/emm.2003.18.

Choi, S., J. Maleth, A. Jha, K. P. Lee, M. S. Kim, I. So, M. Ahuja, and S. Muallem. 2014. "The TRPCs–STIM1–Orai interaction." *Handbook of Experimental Pharmacology* no. 223:1035–54. doi:10.1007/978-3-319-05161-1_13.

Clarson, L. H., V. H. Roberts, B. Hamark, A. C. Elliott, and T. Powell. 2003. "Store-operated Ca^{2+} entry in first trimester and term human placenta." *The Journal of Physiology* no. 550 (Pt 2):515–28. doi:10.1113/jphysiol.2003.044149.

Cross, N. A., L. S. Hillman, S. H. Allen, G. F. Krause, and N. E. Vieira. 1995. "Calcium homeostasis and bone metabolism during pregnancy, lactation, and postweaning: A longitudinal study." *The American Journal of Clinical Nutrition* no. 61 (3):514–23.

Di Leva, F., T. Domi, L. Fedrizzi, D. Lim, and E. Carafoli. 2008. "The plasma membrane Ca^{2+} ATPase of animal cells: Structure, function and regulation." *Archives of Biochemistry and Biophysics* no. 476 (1):65–74. doi:10.1016/j.abb.2008.02.026.

Dodd, J. M., C. O'Brien, and R. M. Grivell. 2014. "Preventing pre-eclampsia—Are dietary factors the key?" *BMC Medicine* no. 12:176. doi:10.1186/s12916-014-0176-4.

Donato, R., B. R. Cannon, G. Sorci, F. Riuzzi, K. Hsu, D. J. Weber, and C. L. Geczy. 2013. "Functions of S100 proteins." *Current Molecular Medicine* no. 13 (1):24–57.

Evans, K. N., J. N. Bulmer, M. D. Kilby, and M. Hewison. 2004. "Vitamin D and placental–decidual function." *Journal of the Society for Gynecologic Investigation* no. 11 (5):263–71. doi:10.1016/j.jsgi.2004.02.002.

Gazzolo, D., P. Vinesi, M. Bartocci, M. C. Geloso, W. Bonacci, G. Serra, K. G. Haglid, and F. Michetti. 1999. "Elevated S100 blood level as an early indicator of intraventricular hemorrhage in preterm infants. Correlation with cerebral Doppler velocimetry." *Journal of the Neurological Sciences* no. 170 (1):32–5.

Gazzolo, D., P. Vinesi, E. Marinoni, R. Di Iorio, M. Marras, M. Lituania, P. Bruschettini, and F. Michetti. 2000. "S100B protein concentrations in cord blood: Correlations with gestational age in term and preterm deliveries." *Clinical Chemistry* no. 46 (7):998–1000.

Gazzolo, D., E. Marinoni, R. di Iorio, M. Lituania, P. L. Bruschettini, and F. Michetti. 2002. "Circulating S100beta protein is increased in intrauterine growth-retarded fetuses." *Pediatric Research* no. 51 (2):215–9. doi:10.1203/00006450-200202000-00015.

Glazier, J. D., D. E. Atkinson, K. L. Thornburg, P. T. Sharpe, D. Edwards, R. D. Boyd, and C. P. Sibley. 1992. "Gestational changes in Ca^{2+} transport across rat placenta and mRNA for calbindin9K and Ca(2+)-ATPase." *The American Journal of Physiology* no. 263 (4 Pt 2):R930–5.

Hache, S., L. Takser, F. LeBellego, H. Weiler, L. Leduc, J. C. Forest, Y. Giguere, A. Masse, B. Barbeau, and J. Lafond. 2011. "Alteration of calcium homeostasis in primary preeclamptic syncytiotrophoblasts: Effect on calcium exchange in placenta." *Journal of Cellular and Molecular Medicine* no. 15 (3):654–67. doi:10.1111/j.1582-4934.2010.01039.x.

Halhali, A., A. R. Tovar, N. Torres, H. Bourges, M. Garabedian, and F. Larrea. 2000. "Preeclampsia is associated with low circulating levels of insulin-like growth factor I and 1,25-dihydroxyvitamin D in maternal and umbilical cord compartments." *The Journal of Clinical Endocrinology and Metabolism* no. 85 (5):1828–33. doi:10.1210/jcem.85.5.6528.

Hershberger, M. E. and R. S. Tuan. 1998. "Placental 57-kDa Ca(2+)-binding protein: Regulation of expression and function in trophoblast calcium transport." *Developmental Biology* no. 199 (1):80–92. doi:10.1006/dbio .1998.8926.

Hirnet, D., J. Olausson, C. Fecher-Trost, M. Bodding, W. Nastainczyk, U. Wissenbach, V. Flockerzi, and M. Freichel. 2003. "The TRPV6 gene, cDNA, and protein." *Cell Calcium* no. 33 (5–6):509–18.

Ho, C., D. A. Conner, M. R. Pollak, D. J. Ladd, O. Kifor, H. B. Warren, E. M. Brown, J. G. Seidman, and C. E. Seidman. 1995. "A mouse model of human familial hypocalciuric hypercalcemia and neonatal severe hyperparathyroidism." *Nature Genetics* no. 11 (4):389–94. doi:10.1038/ng1295–389.

Hofmeyr, G. J., L. Duley, and A. Atallah. 2007. "Dietary calcium supplementation for prevention of preeclampsia and related problems: A systematic review and commentary." *BJOG: An International Journal of Obstetrics and Gynaecology* no. 114 (8):933–43. doi:10.1111/j.1471-0528.2007.01389.x.

Horinouchi, T., T. Higashi, T. Higa, K. Terada, Y. Mai, H. Aoyagi, C. Hatate, P. Nepal, M. Horiguchi, T. Harada, and S. Miwa. 2012. "Different binding property of STIM1 and its novel splice variant STIM1L to Orai1, TRPC3, and TRPC6 channels." *Biochemical and Biophysical Research Communications* no. 428 (2):252–8. doi:10.1016/j.bbrc.2012.10.034.

Hsu, Y. J., H. Dimke, J. G. Hoenderop, and R. J. Bindels. 2010. "Calcitonin-stimulated renal Ca^{2+} reabsorption occurs independently of TRPV5." *Nephrology, Dialysis, Transplantation: Official Publication of the European Dialysis and Transplant Association—European Renal Association* no. 25 (5):1428–35. doi:10.1093/ndt/gfp645.

Iacopino, A. M. and S. Christakos. 1990. "Corticosterone regulates calbindin–D28k mRNA and protein levels in rat hippocampus." *The Journal of Biological Chemistry* no. 265 (18):10177–80.

Iacopino, A. M., S. Christakos, P. Modi, and C. A. Altar. 1992. "Nerve growth factor increases calcium binding protein (calbindin–D28K) in rat olfactory bulb." *Brain Research* no. 578 (1–2):305–10.

Inpanbutr, N., J. D. Reiswig, W. L. Bacon, R. D. Slemons, and A. M. Iacopino. 1996. "Effect of vitamin D on testicular CaBP28K expression and serum testosterone in chickens." *Biology of Reproduction* no. 54 (1):242–8.

Jeung, E. B., N. C. Fan, P. C. Leung, J. C. Herr, A. Freemerman, and J. Krisinger. 1995. "The baboon expresses the calbindin–D9k gene in intestine but not in uterus and placenta: Implication for conservation of the gene in primates." *Molecular Reproduction and Development* no. 40 (4):400–7. doi:10.1002/mrd.1080400403.

Jurewicz, E., I. Kasacka, E. Bankowski, and A. Filipek. 2014. "S100A6 and its extracellular targets in Wharton's jelly of healthy and preeclamptic patients." *Placenta* no. 35 (6):386–91. doi:10.1016/j .placenta.2014.03.017.

Kaczan-Bourgois, D., J. P. Salles, F. Hullin, J. Fauvel, A. Moisand, I. Duga-Neulat, A. Berrebi, G. Campistron, and H. Chap. 1996. "Increased content of annexin II (p36) and p11 in human placenta brush-border membrane vesicles during syncytiotrophoblast maturation and differentiation." *Placenta* no. 17 (8):669–76.

Kamath, S. G. and C. H. Smith. 1994. "Na^+/Ca^{2+} exchange, Ca2+ binding, and electrogenic Ca^{2+} transport in plasma membranes of human placental syncytiotrophoblast." *Pediatric Research* no. 36 (4):461–7. doi:10.1203/00006450-199410000-00008.

Ko, S. H., K. C. Choi, G. T. Oh, and E. B. Jeung. 2009. "Effect of dietary calcium and 1,25-(OH)2D3 on the expression of calcium transport genes in calbindin-D9k and -D28k double knockout mice." *Biochemical and Biophysical Research Communications* no. 379 (2):227–32. doi:10.1016/j.bbrc.2008.12.029.

Koo, T. H., H. Yang, B. S. An, K. C. Choi, S. H. Hyun, and E. B. Jeung. 2012. "Calcium transport genes are differently regulated in maternal and fetal placenta in the knockout mice of calbindin-D(9k) and -D(28k)." *Molecular Reproduction and Development* no. 79 (5):346–55. doi:10.1002/mrd.22033.

Koushik, S. V., J. Wang, R. Rogers, D. Moskophidis, N. A. Lambert, T. L. Creazzo, and S. J. Conway. 2001. "Targeted inactivation of the sodium-calcium exchanger (Ncx1) results in the lack of a heartbeat and abnormal myofibrillar organization." *FASEB Journal: Official Publication of the Federation of American Societies for Experimental Biology* no. 15 (7):1209–11.

Kovacs, C. S. 2014. "Bone development and mineral homeostasis in the fetus and neonate: Roles of the calciotropic and phosphotropic hormones." *Physiological Reviews* no. 94 (4):1143–218. doi:10.1152 /physrev.00014.2014.

Kovacs, C. S., L. L. Chafe, M. L. Woodland, K. R. McDonald, N. J. Fudge, and P. J. Wookey. 2002. "Calcitropic gene expression suggests a role for the intraplacental yolk sac in maternal–fetal calcium exchange." *American Journal of Physiology. Endocrinology and Metabolism* no. 282 (3):E721–32. doi:10.1152/ajpendo.00369.2001.

Kozel, P. J., R. A. Friedman, L. C. Erway, E. N. Yamoah, L. H. Liu, T. Riddle, J. J. Duffy, T. Doetschman, M. L. Miller, E. L. Cardell, and G. E. Shull. 1998. "Balance and hearing deficits in mice with a null mutation in the gene encoding plasma membrane Ca^{2+}-ATPase isoform 2." *The Journal of Biological Chemistry* no. 273 (30):18693–6.

Krisinger, J., J. L. Dann, E. B. Jeung, and P. C. Leung. 1992. "Calbindin-D9k gene expression during pregnancy and lactation in the rat." *Molecular and Cellular Endocrinology* no. 88 (1–3):119–28.

Krisinger, J., E. B. Jeung, R. C. Simmen, and P. C. Leung. 1995. "Porcine calbindin-D9k gene: Expression in endometrium, myometrium, and placenta in the absence of a functional estrogen response element in intron A." *Biology of Reproduction* no. 52 (1):115–23.

L'Horset, F., C. Perret, A. Brehier, and M. Thomasset. 1990. "17 beta-estradiol stimulates the calbindin-D9k (CaBP9k) gene expression at the transcriptional and posttranscriptional levels in the rat uterus." *Endocrinology* no. 127 (6):2891–7. doi:10.1210/endo-127-6-2891.

Lafond, J. and L. Simoneau. 2006. "Calcium homeostasis in human placenta: Role of calcium-handling proteins." *International Review of Cytology* no. 250:109–74. doi:10.1016/S0074-7696(06)50004-X.

Lafond, J., M. Leclerc, and M. G. Brunette. 1991. "Characterization of calcium transport by basal plasma membranes from human placental syncytiotrophoblast." *Journal of Cellular Physiology* no. 148 (1):17–23. doi:10.1002/jcp.1041480103.

Lambers, T. T., F. Mahieu, E. Oancea, L. Hoofd, F. de Lange, A. R. Mensenkamp, T. Voets, B. Nilius, D. E. Clapham, J. G. Hoenderop, and R. J. Bindels. 2006. "Calbindin-D28K dynamically controls TRPV5-mediated Ca^{2+} transport." *The EMBO Journal* no. 25 (13):2978–88. doi:10.1038/sj.emboj.7601186.

Lee, G. S., K. Y. Lee, K. C. Choi, Y. H. Ryu, S. G. Paik, G. T. Oh, and E. B. Jeung. 2007. "Phenotype of a calbindin-D9k gene knockout is compensated for by the induction of other calcium transporter genes in a mouse model." *Journal of Bone and Mineral Research: The Official Journal of the American Society for Bone and Mineral Research* no. 22 (12):1968–78. doi:10.1359/jbmr.070801.

Liu, B., S. J. Hill, and R. N. Khan. 2005. "Oxytocin inhibits T-type calcium current of human decidual stromal cells." *The Journal of Clinical Endocrinology and Metabolism* no. 90 (7):4191–7. doi:10.1210/jc.2005-0480.

Lytton, J. 2007. "Na^+/Ca^{2+} exchangers: Three mammalian gene families control Ca^{2+} transport." *The Biochemical Journal* no. 406 (3):365–82. doi:10.1042/BJ20070619.

Marin, R., G. Riquelme, P. Godoy, P. Diaz, C. Abad, R. Caires, T. Proverbio, S. Pinero, and F. Proverbio. 2008. "Functional and structural demonstration of the presence of Ca-ATPase (PMCA) in both microvillous and basal plasma membranes from syncytiotrophoblast of human term placenta." *Placenta* no. 29 (8):671–9. doi:10.1016/j.placenta.2008.06.003.

Marinoni, E., R. Di Iorio, D. Gazzolo, C. Lucchini, F. Michetti, V. Corvino, and E. V. Cosmi. 2002. "Ontogenetic localization and distribution of S-100beta protein in human placental tissues." *Obstetrics and Gynecology* no. 99 (6):1093–9.

Martin, R., N. C. Harvey, S. R. Crozier, J. R. Poole, M. K. Javaid, E. M. Dennison, H. M. Inskip, M. Hanson, K. M. Godfrey, C. Cooper, and R. Lewis. 2007. "Placental calcium transporter (PMCA3) gene expression predicts intrauterine bone mineral accrual." *Bone* no. 40 (5):1203–8. doi:10.1016/j.bone.2006.12.060.

Meuris, S., B. Polliotti, C. Robyn, and P. Lebrun. 1994. "Ca^{2+} entry through L-type voltage-sensitive Ca^{2+} channels stimulates the release of human chorionic gonadotrophin and placental lactogen by placental explants." *Biochimica et Biophysica Acta* no. 1220 (2):101–6.

Miller, E. K., R. A. Word, C. A. Goodall, and A. M. Iacopino. 1994. "Calbindin-D9K gene expression in human myometrium during pregnancy and labor." *The Journal of Clinical Endocrinology and Metabolism* no. 79 (2):609–15. doi:10.1210/jcem.79.2.8045984.

Moreau, R., G. Daoud, R. Bernatchez, L. Simoneau, A. Masse, and J. Lafond. 2002. "Calcium uptake and calcium transporter expression by trophoblast cells from human term placenta." *Biochimica et Biophysica Acta* no. 1564 (2):325–32.

Moreau, R., G. Daoud, A. Masse, L. Simoneau, and J. Lafond. 2003. "Expression and role of calcium-ATPase pump and sodium–calcium exchanger in differentiated trophoblasts from human term placenta." *Molecular Reproduction and Development* no. 65 (3):283–8. doi:10.1002/mrd.10303.

Moreau, R., L. Simoneau, and J. Lafond. 2003. "Calcium fluxes in human trophoblast (BeWo) cells: Calcium channels, calcium–ATPase, and sodium–calcium exchanger expression." *Molecular Reproduction and Development* no. 64 (2):189–98. doi:10.1002/mrd.10247.

Mori, Y., D. Mori, U. I. Chung, S. Tanaka, J. Heierhorst, T. Buchou, J. Baudier, H. Kawaguchi, and T. Saito. 2014. "S100A1 and S100B are dispensable for endochondral ossification during skeletal development." *Biomedical Research* no. 35 (4):243–50.

Muller, D., J. G. Hoenderop, I. C. Meij, L. P. van den Heuvel, N. V. Knoers, A. I. den Hollander, P. Eggert, V. Garcia-Nieto, F. Claverie-Martin, and R. J. Bindels. 2000. "Molecular cloning, tissue distribution, and chromosomal mapping of the human epithelial Ca2+ channel (ECAC1)." *Genomics* no. 67 (1):48–53.

Neely, A. and P. Hidalgo. 2014. "Structure-function of proteins interacting with the alpha1 pore-forming subunit of high-voltage-activated calcium channels." *Frontiers in Physiology* no. 5:209. doi:10.3389/fphys.2014.00209.

Nikitenko, L., G. Morgan, S. I. Kolesnikov, and F. B. Wooding. 1998. "Immunocytochemical and In situ hybridization studies of the distribution of calbindin D9k in the bovine placenta throughout pregnancy." *The Journal of Histochemistry and Cytochemistry: Official Journal of the Histochemistry Society* no. 46 (5):679–88.

Okunade, G. W., M. L. Miller, G. J. Pyne, R. L. Sutliff, K. T. O'Connor, J. C. Neumann, A. Andringa, D. A. Miller, V. Prasad, T. Doetschman, R. J. Paul, and G. E. Shull. 2004. "Targeted ablation of plasma membrane Ca^{2+}-ATPase (PMCA) 1 and 4 indicates a major housekeeping function for PMCA1 and a critical role in hyperactivated sperm motility and male fertility for PMCA4." *The Journal of Biological Chemistry* no. 279 (32):33742–50. doi:10.1074/jbc.M404628200.

Olausson, H., G. R. Goldberg, M. A. Laskey, I. Schoenmakers, L. M. Jarjou, and A. Prentice. 2012. "Calcium economy in human pregnancy and lactation." *Nutrition Research Reviews* no. 25 (1):40–67. doi:10.1017/S0954422411000187.

Papadopoulou, A., E. Gole, A. Moutafi, C. Sfikas, W. Oehrl, M. Samiotaki, A. Papadimitriou, V. Papaevagelou, and P. Nicolaidou. 2014. "Calcium sensing receptor in pregnancies complicated by gestational diabetes mellitus." *Placenta* no. 35 (8):632–8. doi:10.1016/j.placenta.2014.05.001.

Penheiter, A. R., A. G. Filoteo, C. L. Croy, and J. T. Penniston. 2001. "Characterization of the deafwaddler mutant of the rat plasma membrane calcium–ATPase 2." *Hearing Research* no. 162 (1–2):19–28.

Prentice, A. and C. J. Bates. 1994. "Adequacy of dietary mineral supply for human bone growth and mineralisation." *European Journal of Clinical Nutrition* no. 48 Suppl 1:S161–76; discussion S177.

Riquelme, G., P. Llanos, E. Tischner, J. Neil, and B. Campos. 2004. "Annexin 6 modulates the maxi-chloride channel of the apical membrane of syncytiotrophoblast isolated from human placenta." *The Journal of Biological Chemistry* no. 279 (48):50601–8. doi:10.1074/jbc.M407859200.

Robidoux, J., L. Simoneau, A. Masse, and J. Lafond. 2000. "Activation of L-type calcium channels induces corticotropin-releasing factor secretion from human placental trophoblasts." *The Journal of Clinical Endocrinology and Metabolism* no. 85 (9):3356–64. doi:10.1210/jcem.85.9.6774.

Romagnolo, B., F. Cluzeaud, M. Lambert, S. Colnot, A. Porteu, T. Molina, M. Tomasset, A. Vandewalle, A. Kahn, and C. Perret. 1996. "Tissue-specific and hormonal regulation of calbindin-D9K fusion genes in transgenic mice." *The Journal of Biological Chemistry* no. 271 (28):16820–6.

Salle, B. L., J. Senterre, F. H. Glorieux, E. E. Delvin, and G. Putet. 1987. "Vitamin D metabolism in preterm infants." *Biology of the Neonate* no. 52 Suppl 1:119–30.

Shamley, D. R., G. Veale, J. M. Pettifor, and R. Buffenstein. 1996. "Trophoblastic giant cells of the mouse placenta contain calbindin-D9k but not the vitamin D receptor." *The Journal of Endocrinology* no. 150 (1):25–32.

Sokolow, S., M. Manto, P. Gailly, J. Molgo, C. Vandebrouck, J. M. Vanderwinden, A. Herchuelz, and S. Schurmans. 2004. "Impaired neuromuscular transmission and skeletal muscle fiber necrosis in mice lacking Na/Ca exchanger 3." *The Journal of Clinical Investigation* no. 113 (2):265–73. doi:10.1172/JCI18688.

Strid, H. and T. L. Powell. 2000. "ATP-dependent Ca^{2+} transport is up-regulated during third trimester in human syncytiotrophoblast basal membranes." *Pediatric Research* no. 48 (1):58–63. doi:10.1203/00006450-200007000-00012.

Strid, H., E. Bucht, T. Jansson, M. Wennergren, and T. L. Powell. 2003. "ATP dependent Ca^{2+} transport across basal membrane of human syncytiotrophoblast in pregnancies complicated by intrauterine growth restriction or diabetes." *Placenta* no. 24 (5):445–52.

Tatsumi, K., T. Higuchi, H. Fujiwara, T. Nakayama, K. Itoh, T. Mori, S. Fujii, and J. Fujita. 1999. "Expression of calcium binding protein D-9k messenger RNA in the mouse uterine endometrium during implantation." *Molecular Human Reproduction* no. 5 (2):153–61.

Thordarson, G., J. N. Southard, and F. Talamantes. 1991. "Purification and characterization of mouse decidual calcyclin: A novel stimulator of mouse placental lactogen-II secretion." *Endocrinology* no. 129 (3):1257–65. doi:10.1210/endo-129-3-1257.

Todros, T., S. Bontempo, E. Piccoli, F. Ietta, R. Romagnoli, M. Biolcati, M. Castellucci, and L. Paulesu. 2005. "Increased levels of macrophage migration inhibitory factor (MIF) in preeclampsia." *European Journal of Obstetrics, Gynecology, and Reproductive Biology* no. 123 (2):162–6. doi:10.1016/j.ejogrb.2005.03.014.

Tohmon, M., M. Fukase, M. Kishihara, S. Kadowaki, and T. Fujita. 1988. "Effect of glucocorticoid admin-istration on intestinal, renal, and cerebellar calbindin-D28K in chicks." *Journal of Bone and Mineral Research: The Official Journal of the American Society for Bone and Mineral Research* no. 3 (3):325–31. doi:10.1002/jbmr.5650030312.

Tsang, R. C., M. Gigger, W. Oh, and D. R. Brown. 1975. "Studies in calcium metabolism in infants with intra-uterine growth retardation." *The Journal of Pediatrics* no. 86 (6):936–41.

Tskitishvili, E., N. Sharentuya, K. Temma-Asano, K. Mimura, Y. Kinugasa-Taniguchi, T. Kanagawa, H. Fukuda, T. Kimura, T. Tomimatsu, and K. Shimoya. 2010. "Oxidative stress-induced S100B protein from placenta and amnion affects soluble Endoglin release from endothelial cells." *Molecular Human Reproduction* no. 16 (3):188–99. doi:10.1093/molehr/gap104.

Tuan, R. S., B. T. Lamb, and C. B. Jesinkey. 1988. "Mouse placental 57-kDa calcium-binding protein: II. Localization of mRNA in mouse and human placentae by in situ cDNA hybridization." *Differentiation; Research in Biological Diversity* no. 37 (3):198–204.

van de Graaf, S. F., J. G. Hoenderop, D. Gkika, D. Lamers, J. Prenen, U. Rescher, V. Gerke, O. Staub, B. Nilius, and R. J. Bindels. 2003. "Functional expression of the epithelial Ca(2+) channels (TRPV5 and TRPV6) requires association of the S100A10–annexin 2 complex." *The EMBO Journal* no. 22 (7):1478–87. doi:10.1093/emboj/cdg162.

Vargas Zapata, C. L., C. M. Donangelo, L. R. Woodhouse, S. A. Abrams, E. M. Spencer, and J. C. King. 2004. "Calcium homeostasis during pregnancy and lactation in Brazilian women with low calcium intakes: A longitudinal study." *The American Journal of Clinical Nutrition* no. 80 (2):417–22.

Wakimoto, K., K. Kobayashi, O. M. Kuro, A. Yao, T. Iwamoto, N. Yanaka, S. Kita, A. Nishida, S. Azuma, Y. Toyoda, K. Omori, H. Imahie, T. Oka, S. Kudoh, O. Kohmoto, Y. Yazaki, M. Shigekawa, Y. Imai, Y. Nabeshima, and I. Komuro. 2000. "Targeted disruption of Na+/Ca2+ exchanger gene leads to cardio-myocyte apoptosis and defects in heartbeat." *The Journal of Biological Chemistry* no. 275 (47):36991–8. doi:10.1074/jbc.M004035200.

Waterhouse, P., R. S. Parhar, X. Guo, P. K. Lala, and D. T. Denhardt. 1992. "Regulated temporal and spatial expression of the calcium-binding proteins calcyclin and OPN (osteopontin) in mouse tissues during pregnancy." *Molecular Reproduction and Development* no. 32 (4):315–23. doi:10.1002/mrd.1080320403.

Wijnberger, L. D., P. G. Nikkels, A. J. van Dongen, C. W. Noorlander, E. J. Mulder, L. H. Schrama, and G. H. Visser. 2002. "Expression in the placenta of neuronal markers for perinatal brain damage." *Pediatric Research* no. 51 (4):492–6. doi:10.1203/00006450-200204000-00015.

Williams, J. M., D. R. Abramovich, C. G. Dacke, T. M. Mayhew, and K. R. Page. 1991. "Inhibitor action on placental calcium transport." *Calcified Tissue International* no. 48 (1):7–12.

Wisser, J., I. Florio, M. Neff, V. Konig, R. Huch, A. Huch, and U. von Mandach. 2005. "Changes in bone den-sity and metabolism in pregnancy." *Acta Obstetricia et Gynecologica Scandinavica* no. 84 (4):349–54. doi:10.1111/j.0001-6349.2005.00766.x.

Yang, H., T. H. Kim, H. H. Lee, K. C. Choi, Y. P. Hong, P. C. Leung, and E. B. Jeung. 2011. "Expression of calbindin-D28k and its regulation by estrogen in the human endometrium during the menstrual cycle." *Reproductive Biology and Endocrinology: RB&E* no. 9:28. doi:10.1186/1477-7827-9-28.

Yang, H., B. S. An, K. C. Choi, and E. B. Jeung. 2013. "Change of genes in calcium transport channels caused by hypoxic stress in the placenta, duodenum, and kidney of pregnant rats." *Biology of Reproduction* no. 88 (2):30. doi:10.1095/biolreprod.112.103705.

Yilmaz, O., M. Kucuk, L. Kebapcilar, T. Altindag, A. Yuksel, H. O. Yuvanc, T. Dal, and Y. Savran. 2012. "Macrophage migration-inhibitory factor is elevated in pregnant women with gestational diabetes mel-litus." *Gynecological Endocrinology: The Official Journal of the International Society of Gynecological Endocrinology* no. 28 (1):76–9. doi:10.3109/09513590.2011.588757.

Zhu, Y., J. P. Goff, T. A. Reinhardt, and R. L. Horst. 1998. "Pregnancy and lactation increase vitamin D-dependent intestinal membrane calcium adenosine triphosphatase and calcium binding protein mes-senger ribonucleic acid expression." *Endocrinology* no. 139 (8):3520–4. doi:10.1210/endo.139.8.6141.

Section IV

Regulation of Trophoblast Angiogenesis and Invasion

16 Maternal Obesity and Placental Vascular Function

Louiza Belkacemi, Michael G. Ross, and Mina Desai

CONTENTS

ABSTRACT

In the United States, more than one half of pregnant women are overweight or obese, putting them at a greater risk of pregnancy complications, including gestational diabetes mellitus, hypertension, and preeclampsia. Similarly, babies of pregnant women who are overweight or obese are at increased risk of prematurity, congenital anomalies, and programmed obesity and metabolic abnormalities in adulthood. Fetal growth is largely dictated by the availability of nutrients in maternal circulation and the ability of these nutrients to be transported into fetal circulation via the placenta. The placenta is the organ through which gases, nutrients, and wastes are exchanged between the maternal–fetal circulations. Key components of healthy placental function include proper development of its vascular network and accessibility and activity of its nutrient-specific transporters. Maternal obesity is characterized by poor placental vascularization usually accompanied by alterations in the expression of nutrient transporters at the placental barrier, both of which contribute to altered fetal growth and long-term metabolic abnormalities.

This chapter discusses the vital role of placenta for optimal fetal growth and long-term health outcome and the adverse effect of maternal obesity on placental vascular development and placental nutrient transport. The focus is primarily on human placenta with some animal mechanistic studies.

KEY WORDS

Maternal obesity, pregnancy, placental vasculature, nutrient transporters.

16.1 INTRODUCTION

The prevalence of obesity and its associated metabolic abnormalities have increased dramatically worldwide over the past few decades, with continued upward trend (Bray and Bellanger 2006, Korner and Aronne 2003). In the United States, approximately 65% of adults are overweight or obese, and more alarming, about one third of all pregnant women in the United States are obese (King 2006). Obesity, which is caused by an imbalance between energy consumption and expenditure (Shoelson, Herrero, and Naaz 2007), is now acknowledged to have its origins, in part, *in utero*. This emphasizes the importance of optimal maternal environment for most advantageous fetal outcome and long-term offspring health.

In obese pregnant women, dietary energy intake, including total fat intake, is elevated before and during pregnancy (Catalano 2003). Although the usual outcome is fetal overgrowth in pregnancies of obese women (Cnattingius et al. 1998, Jansson et al. 2008, Sebire et al. 2001), intrauterine growth restriction has also been observed (Perlow et al. 1992). Irrespective of their growth, intriguingly, both large and small offspring have increased risk of developing adult obesity and metabolic syndrome (Higgins et al. 2011). More importantly, these second-generation obese females are at risk of themselves giving birth to macrosomic newborns, perpetuating the vicious cycle of an obese phenotype (Catalano 2003, Cnattingius et al. 1998, Jansson et al. 2008). While the biological mechanism of maternal obesity and its impact on fetal development is complex, undoubtedly, placental dysfunction plays an important role (Higgins et al. 2013).

The placenta, a transient organ during pregnancy, is situated at the maternal–fetal interface, where it facilitates nutrient uptake, waste elimination, and gas exchange via the mother's blood supply to support fetal growth. The highly vascular characteristic of human placenta is essential for effective maternal–fetal exchange. Hence, vasculogenesis and subsequent angiogenesis are of pivotal importance in placental development, and it is imperative that they are appropriately regulated. Failure to do so leads to poor obstetric outcome. The placental vasculogenesis and angiogenesis are regulated by an array of factors. Maternal obesity has been implicated as a perpetuating factor that adversely impacts placental vasculature development and the subsequent exchange between the maternal and fetal circulations (Reynolds and Redmer 1995). For example, maternal obesity has been shown to impact vascular development, alter cell proliferation and angiogenic factors, and promote inflammation and cytokine expression in placenta. This chapter discusses the impact of maternal obesity during pregnancy on placental vasculature and the ensuing effects on placental nutrient transport to the fetus.

16.2 HUMAN PLACENTA

16.2.1 DEVELOPMENT

During the first half of human gestation, the trophoblast undergoes critical proliferation and differentiation to form villi, whereas in the second half of gestation, extensive angiogenesis and vascularization occur, as described below.

The development of placenta is initiated upon implantation of the blastocyst into the maternal endometrium. From the point of view of its origin, the placenta has two components, the fetal placenta (chorion), which develops from trophoblast cells (outer layer of blastocyst), and the maternal placenta (decidua basalis), which develops from the maternal uterine tissue. The placenta connects to the fetus by an umbilical cord, which encloses two umbilical arteries and one umbilical vein.

Vessels branch out over the surface of the placenta and further divide to form villous tree structures. On the maternal side, these villous tree structures are grouped into lobules called cotyledons (10–40 cotyledons). Each maternal cotyledon has several anchoring villi, extending into the
maternal decidua basalis, to which they are anchored by syncytial cells and fibrin. On the fetal side,
each cotyledon is formed by one to three villous trees made of chorionic villi (Figure 16.1). These
functional structures are lined by two trophoblast layers, the underlying cytotrophoblast layer and
the overlying syncytiotrophoblast layer (Talbert and Sebire 2004). The syncytiotrophoblast is a multinucleated continuous cell layer that forms as a result of differentiation and fusion of the underlying
cytotrophoblast cells, a process that continues throughout placental development. The syncytiotrophoblast is in direct contact with maternal blood, where it directs exchange of oxygen, nutrient, and
removal of waste products occurs.

16.2.2 PLACENTAL CIRCULATION

The placenta receives blood supplies from both the maternal and the fetal systems making up the
two separate circulatory systems for blood circulation (Figure 16.1). The veins conduct oxygenated blood toward the fetus, whereas the arteries carry deoxygenated blood toward the placenta.
Uteroplacental circulation involves maternal blood flow into the intervillous space through decidual
spiral arteries. Exchange of oxygen and nutrients occurs as the maternal blood flows around the
terminal villi in the intervillous space. The in-flowing maternal arterial blood drives deoxygenated
blood into the endometrial and then uterine veins back to the maternal circulation. The fetal–
placental circulation permits the umbilical arteries to transport deoxygenated and nutrient-depleted
fetal blood from the fetus to the villous core fetal vessels. After the exchange of oxygen and nutrients, the umbilical vein transfers fresh oxygenated and nutrient-rich blood circulating back to the
fetal systemic circulation.

16.2.3 VASCULAR FORMATION

The human placental vascular system develops through two distinct processes: vasculogenesis,
which begins at day 21 postconception (p.c.), and angiogenesis, which continues from day 32 p.c.
until delivery (Arroyo and Winn 2008).

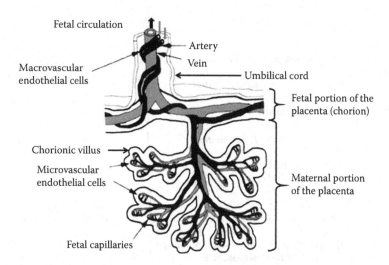

FIGURE 16.1 Diagram showing a portion of placental vasculature. (Adapted from Murthi, P. et al., *Placenta*,
29, 624–630, 2008. With permission.)

Vasculogenesis refers to a new blood vessel formation from pluripotent mesenchymal stem cells. The earliest primitive capillary formation results from *in situ* differentiation of the hemangiogenic stem into angioblast cells (the progenitors of endothelial cells) and hemangioblastic cells (the progenitors of hematopoietic cells) (Hanahan 1997, Ribatti et al. 2002) (Figure 16.2). The fetal vascularization of the human placenta results from local *de novo* formation of capillaries from mesenchymal precursor cells in the placental villi, rather than protrusion of embryonic vessels into the placenta (Demir, Seval, and Huppertz 2007).

Angiogenesis is a process involving the growth of new blood vessels from preexisting vessels (Birbrair et al. 2013) (Figure 16.2) through the remodeling of differentiated endothelial cells (Sipos et al. 2010). The angiogenic processes occur during three periods: (1) formation of capillary networks from day 32 to 25 weeks p.c. by dominance of branching angiogenesis; (2) regression of peripheral capillary webs and formation of central stem vessels between 15 and 32 weeks p.c., and finally (3) formation of terminal capillary loops by prevalence of nonbranching angiogenesis.

16.2.4 VASCULAR REGULATION

Various growth factors have been implicated in the molecular regulation and stimulation of placental vasculogenesis and angiogenesis. Among these, the most prominent are the vascular endothelial growth factor A (VEGFA) and fibroblast growth factor 2, which, when activated, induce the transition from vasculogenesis to angiogenesis. Additional regulatory include placental growth factor (PGF), angiopoietins (ANGPTs) and the insulin/insulin-like growth factor as well as hormones erythropoietin, leptin, and adiponectin, all known to specifically promote placental angiogenesis. Effects are mediated by specific cell surface receptors on the endothelium (Anthony, Limesand, and Jeckel 2001, Borowicz et al. 2007). A subgroup of these factors (VEGFA, PGF, ANGPT) is regulated acutely by the local oxygen concentration via hypoxia inducible factor (HIF-1α) transcription factor. Specifically, HIF-1α responds to hypoxia and interacts with the angiogenic factors (VEGFA and ANGPT) to promote gene transcription (Shih and Claffey 1999, Simon, Tournaire, and Pouyssegur 2008). Further, these angiogenic factors interact with the local vasodilator endothelium-derived nitric oxide (NO) to coordinate placental angiogenesis and blood flow (Krause, Hanson, and Casanello 2011, Smith et al. 1992, Ziche and Morbidelli 2000).

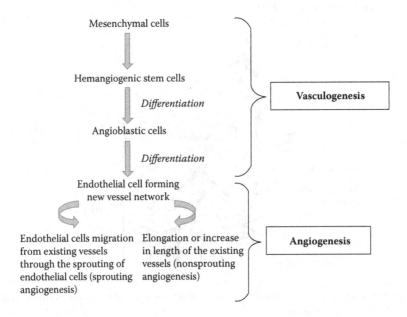

FIGURE 16.2 Vasculogenesis and angiogenesis of human placenta.

16.3 MATERNAL OBESITY AND PLACENTAL VASCULAR MODIFICATIONS

16.3.1 PLACENTA

Approximately one third of all pregnant women in the United States are obese (Desai, Beall, and Ross 2013). Maternal obesity at conception alters gestational metabolic milieu and affects placental, embryonic, and fetal growth and development. Maternal body mass index (BMI) has been shown to affect both placental properties and weight (Challier et al. 2008, Salafia et al. 2008). Higher early-pregnancy BMI and higher maternal weight gain are associated with increased placental weight as well as placental dysfunction (Becker et al. 2008, Taylor, al Busaidy, and Mellor 1991). Moreover, placental weight is independently associated with fetal growth (Friis et al. 2013, Tikellis et al. 2012).

Under physiological conditions, it is reasonable to assume that placental weight is correlated to exchange area and therefore with total transport capacity (Fowden et al. 2006, Robinson, Seamark, and Owens 1994), which is also dependent upon the density of transport proteins. The placenta is furthermore believed to act as a nutrient sensor, up- or down-regulating transport proteins according to the maternal environment (Jansson and Powell 2006). It is conceivable that some of the metabolic abnormalities associated with increasing BMI, as well as the low-grade placenta inflammatory response (Challier et al. 2008), play a role in regulating placental function.

16.3.2 PLACENTAL VASCULATURE

Overnutrition is a major compromising factor of placental vasculogenesis and angiogenesis resulting in histomorphometric abnormalities. Placental structural changes occur throughout normal gestation and in response to maternal nutritional manipulations (Sibley et al. 2005). Abnormalities in placental vascular development, as evident by reduced fetal capillary branching, malformation of the villous tree and/or alterations in the expression of angiogenic factors in the feto–maternal unit, are associated with adverse maternal outcome and fetal growth.

In humans, there are limited studies on obese pregnancies that shed some insight into the complexities of placental vascular growth. For example, maternal obesity results in higher than normal muscularity in the placental vessel walls (Roberts et al. 2011). Other studies have shown that maternal obesity is associated with reduced both placental villous proliferation and apoptosis, which may impact vascular function and increase susceptibility to adverse pregnancy outcomes (Higgins et al. 2013). In contrast to humans, high-fat-fed animals exhibit placental vascular immaturity, as indicated by the increased blood vessel density observed in the high-fat-fed mice was inversely proportional to the staining of smooth muscle actin, an indicator of blood vessel maturity (Cimpean, Raica, and Suciu 2007), suggesting impaired blood vessel maturity in the obese animals. Specifically, a significantly higher proportion of the offspring of high-fat diet dams were small for gestational age (Hayes et al. 2012). This was associated with increased endothelial cluster of differentiation 31 (CD31) protein staining in the placental labyrinth zone (zone of maternal–fetal exchange), suggesting the presence of greater numbers of blood vessels. Consistent with this, another study on high-fat diet during mice pregnancy showed that labyrinth thickness and cell proliferation were decreased at mid and late gestation in obese compared with normal-weight pregnancies (Kim et al. 2014). Similarly, dysregulation of placental cotyledon vascularization was observed in obese ewe (Akyol, Langley-Evans, and McMullen 2009).

Collectively, these results underscore that a typical feature of maternal obesity/high-fat diet includes placental vascular dysfunction. As discussed below, the underlying mechanism may be attributed to alteration in trophoblast invasion, endothelial cells and inflammation as well as hypoxia and oxidative stress (OS).

16.3.3 PLACENTAL TROPHOBLAST INVASION AND VASCULAR DYSREGULATION

Successful pregnancy is reliant on a subpopulation of placental trophoblast cells, the extravillous trophoblasts, to invade the uterine wall (interstitial invasion) and its blood vessels (endovascular invasion). In the spiral arteries, the extravillous trophoblasts interdigitate between the endothelial cells, substituting the endothelial lining and most of the musculoelastic tissue in the vessel walls (Ashton et al. 2005). This results in a high-flow, low-resistance circulation that increases maternal blood flow to the placental villi at the maternal–fetal interface. Conversely, in pregnancy, complications associated with obesity-altered trophoblast invasion and aberrant spiral artery remodeling are often observed (Berger et al. 1983). Dysfunctional spiral arteries cause decreased uteroplacental blood flow to the placenta (Frias et al. 2011). The placental deficiency can lead to placental hypoxia and placental secretion of inflammatory cytokines (Laresgoiti-Servitje and Gomez-Lopez 2012), both of which, as discussed in the next sections, will further negatively impact placental development.

16.3.4 ENDOTHELIAL CELLS/INFLAMMATION AND PLACENTAL VASCULAR DYSFUNCTION

Endothelial cells cover the entire placental vasculature, where they provide a nonthrombogenic surface to help prevent inappropriate blood clotting. Moreover, endothelial cells play a critical role in blood flow, as they are in close juxtaposition to the trophoblast. Endothelial cells produce NO, which diffuses from the endothelium to the underlying layer of vascular smooth muscle cells leading to cyclic guanosine monophosphate (GMP)-dependent vasodilatation (Moncada and Higgs 2006). In placenta vessels, all of which lack innervation (Fox and Khong 1990), the synthesis and release of vasoconstrictors and vasodilators from the endothelium regulate vascular tone (Myatt 2010).

In obese women, placental endothelial dysfunction is evident by a reduced ability of placental endothelium tissue to stimulate NO-mediated vasodilatation (Deanfield et al. 2005), in part, a consequence of increased inflammatory cytokines. The present view is that an aberrant maternal metabolic environment may generate stimuli within the placental cells, yielding increased production of inflammatory cytokines. Obese patients' placentas exhibit a higher inflammatory profile with a specific increase in the expression of interleukin-1 (IL-1), IL-8, and chemo attractant protein 1 (Roberts et al. 2011). Consistent with this, Challier et al. (2008) demonstrated an elevated expression of the pro-inflammatory cytokines IL-1, tumor necrosis factor-α (TNF-α), and IL-6 in placental macrophages of obese women compared with nonobese women. A similar placental phenotype has been reported in a baboon model of obesity (Farley et al. 2009). Based on these findings, it is possible that reduced endothelium capacity to stimulate NO-mediated vasodilatation in placentas of obese women may stem from increased inflammatory cytokines. In accordance with this, several investigators showed that when the endothelium is exposed to placental cytokines such as IL-6 and TNF-α (Kern et al. 2001, Tilg and Moschen 2006, Vozarova et al. 2001), endothelial NO synthase expression and activity are altered, which may lead to a decline in NO bioavailability (Kim et al. 2008, Nascimento et al. 2011, Suwaidi et al. 2000). Although some controversy exists as to the involvement of the NO pathway on vascular disorders induced by obesity, there is evidence that impairment of NO synthesis is a central defect triggering many of the vascular abnormalities characteristic of obesity (Deng et al. 2010, Martins et al. 2010).

Taken together, these findings indicate that placental endothelial cell NO plays a critical role in the well-being of placental vasculature, and this effect may be antagonized by obesity-associated proinflammatory cytokines.

16.3.5 HYPOXIA/OS AND VASCULAR DYSREGULATION

During early pregnancy, the placenta develops in a comparatively hypoxic environment (Jaffe, Jauniaux, and Hustin 1997) because of plugs of the inner layer of the cytotrophoblasts blocking maternal spiral arteries that supply the placental site (Burton, Jauniaux, and Watson 1999), as well as the absence of maternal erythrocytes in the intervillous space. However, by 11 weeks' gestation, the plugs are displaced, blood flow begins, and oxygenation rises with the development of placental vasculature (Burton, Jauniaux, and Watson 1999). As mentioned previously, in the first and early second trimesters of pregnancy, remodeling of the muscular wall of uterine arteries by invading extravillous trophoblasts is essential to guarantee sufficient maternal blood flow to the placenta. Should this process fail, a relative placental hypoxic environment recurs.

Placental hypoxia is coupled with increased OS (Hayes et al. 2012), which is defined as an imbalance between increased cellular reactive oxygen species (ROS) production and cellular antioxidant defenses. Some of the most commonly known ROS species are superoxide, hydroxide, and hydrogen peroxide (Fridovich 1995). High ROS levels may cause damage to several biological biomolecules (e.g., lipids, proteins, DNA), leading to loss of function and, ultimately, apoptosis (Raha and Robinson 2001). In human term placentas from obese women, redox balance was altered, as revealed by elevated lipid peroxidation and activity of antioxidant enzymes including superoxide dismutases and glutathione peroxidase (Malti et al. 2014). Myatt et al. (2000) suggested that OS can trigger vascular dysfunction in the placenta, leading to compromised fetal growth. They further suggested nitrative stress as a route to vascular dysfunction in the placentas of obese women (Myatt 2010, Myatt et al. 2000). Animal models of obesity have shown that OS and overproduction of ROS influence arterial branching of the placental exchange region from high-fat-fed mothers. For example, in C57BL/6 mice, a high-fat diet induced placental OS that caused vascular dysfunction (Jones et al. 2009). A trend of decreased placental weight in high-fat-fed mice caused by OS-induced trophoblast loss and endothelial necrosis was also observed (Liang, DeCourcy, and Prater 2010). Similar findings of altered vascular development have been reported in placentas of Sprague-Dawley rats fed a high-fat diet (Hayes et al. 2012).

HIF-1α is a transcription factor that regulates the cellular response to low oxygen tension and is central to the maintenance of oxygen homeostasis (Semenza 2011, Tal 2012). HIF-1α was highly expressed in the low-oxygen environment of the human placenta in early gestation, falling at around 9 weeks of gestation in conjunction with increased placental oxygen levels (Caniggia et al. 2000). Through transcriptional activation, HIF-1α regulates many different cellular processes in response to hypoxia, including angiogenesis. Maternal obesity is associated with decreased HIF-1α protein, suggesting a potential link between increased inflammation/OS and decreased angiogenic factors (Saben et al. 2014).

Collectively, these findings suggest that hypoxia is a key player in normal placental vascular development and a major compromising factor in suboptimal nutritional conditions. Vascular dysfunction results in placental insufficiency, which may impair exchange between the maternal and fetal circulations (Reynolds and Redmer 1995).

16.4 MATERNAL OBESITY AND PLACENTAL VASCULAR FUNCTION

16.4.1 PLACENTAL BARRIER CELL TYPES AND NUTRIENT TRANSPORT

To sustain appropriate fetal development, the mother must provide nutrients to be transferred across the placental barrier via mechanisms including passive diffusion, facilitated diffusion, and active transport. In human placenta, there are only two cell layers positioned between the maternal and fetal circulation: the syncytiotrophoblast and the fetal capillary endothelium. The endothelium is a continuous layer of blood vessels closely resembling other continuous nonbrain capillaries (Leach and Firth 1992). This type of endothelium allows for relatively unrestricted passage of nutrients, including glucose, amino acids, and fatty acids (FAs), through pores within the interendothelial cleft (Michel and Curry 1999) and is therefore unlikely to represent a significant barrier to transport of nutrients. Conversely, the transport across the polarized plasma membranes of the syncytiotrophoblast probably represents the limiting step in transplacental transfer. As a determinant of the placenta's capacity for nutrient transport, the syncytiotrophoblast is contingent on the number, density, and distribution of nutrient transporters (Jansson, Cetin et al. 2006, Jansson, Pettersson et al. 2006, Johansson et al. 2003). Notably in mice, a trilaminar layer of trophoblast cells separates the fetal capillary from the maternal sinusoids: a bilayer of syncytiotrophoblast surrounds the fetal blood vessel endothelium and a layer of mononuclear cells lines the maternal blood sinuses (Adamson et al. 2002). Subsequently, nutrient must diffuse or be transferred across four layers to get from one blood compartment to the next.

As a result of an intimate relationship between the syncytiotrophoblast and the fetal vessels, suboptimal conditions that alter vessel development (as described in previous sections) or syncytiotrophoblast transporters (reviewed in the next section) are likely to impair the transport function of the placenta. The changes in the rate of nutrient delivery to the fetus may thus result in aberrant growth and development.

16.4.2 GLUCOSE TRANSPORTERS

Glucose is the primary energy substrate required for growth of the fetus and the placenta. In humans, fetal production of glucose is negligible; therefore, the fetus is almost entirely reliant on maternal glucose passing through the placenta (Kalhan and Parimi 2000). Placental glucose transport occurs by facilitated diffusion along a concentration gradient through specific glucose transporter proteins (GLUTs, or SLC2As) (Baumann, Deborde, and Illsley 2002). There are at least 12 members of the GLUT family, among which GLUT1 is the only isoform abundantly expressed in early and at term gestation in humans (Illsley 2000), whereas both GLUT1 and GLUT3 are expressed in rodents (Ashcroft, Coster, and Smith 1977). GLUT1 is primarily responsible for placental glucose uptake from the maternal blood supply (Desoye and Shafrir 1994).

There has been limited research on the effect of maternal obesity on placental GLUTs. In obese, normoglycemic human pregnancies, there was no difference in placental GLUT1 transcript or GLUT1 protein expression and only a significantly lower GLUT4 transcript, although not protein expression, as compared with placentas from normal-weight patients (Colomiere et al. 2009). In mice fed a high-fat diet (32% fat, 52% carbohydrate, 16% protein) before mating and during gestation, fetal growth increased by 43%, in association with a significantly elevated rate of glucose clearance and expression of trophoblast plasma membranes GLUT1 protein (5-fold) (Jones et al. 2009), although placental growth was not affected. Mice fed a high-sugar, high-fat diet (30% fat, 17% protein, 53% carbohydrate) only during pregnancy resulted in enhanced fetal weights and both increased placental glucose transport and expression of GLUT3 (Sferruzzi-Perri et al. 2013). As placental weights were reduced, these results suggest that GLUT3 may represent a mechanism linking maternal high-fat diet during pregnancy to fetal overgrowth. Taken together, these data suggest that placental GLUT isoform alterations are dependent on the type of obesogenic diet and on the period of intake during pregnancy.

16.4.3 AMINO ACID TRANSPORTERS

Amino acids play a central role in the development of fetal tissue. The plasma concentrations of amino acids in fetal blood are, in general, higher than in maternal blood (Cetin et al. 1992). Thus, amino acids are transferred to the fetus by active transport (Broer 2002). The placenta expresses over 15 different amino acid transporters, and each is responsible for the uptake of several different amino acids (Jansson 2001). These transporters are classified by the types of amino acids transferred and whether there is a cotransport of sodium (Na^+) (Christensen et al. 1994). The two most studied amino acid transport systems in the placenta are System A, which consists of Na^+-coupled small neutral amino acid transporters (SNATs), and System L, which includes large Na^+-independent neutral amino acid transporters (LATs) (Jansson 2001). System A protein isoforms include SNAT1, SNAT2, and SNAT4 (Mackenzie and Erickson 2004). System L proteins consist of subtypes LAT1, LAT2, LAT3, and LAT4 (Haase et al. 2007).

In pregnancies complicated by fetal growth restriction, decreased placental System A activity has been well illustrated (Glazier et al. 1997). However, there are only few reports on the effects of maternal obesity on placental SNAT activity. In obese pregnant women, placental amino acid transport has been associated with decreased activity and expression of placental SNAT4, as compared with lean women, whereas the expression of SNAT1 and SNAT2 proteins, which were thought to be the major contributors to System A transport (Desforges et al. 2009, 2010), was unchanged (Farley et al. 2010, Waller et al. 2007). Perhaps, the comparable expression of placental SNAT1 between normal and obese women may have contributed to the similarities in offspring birth weight observed between the two groups (Farley et al. 2010). Alternatively, a protective mechanism may exist involving placental System A, as maternal obesity was associated with lower placental SNAT activity despite appropriate maternal weight gain and fetal growth (Farley et al. 2010). In a recent study, placental microvillous plasma membrane System A, but not System L, activity was positively correlated to offspring birth weight (Jansson et al. 2013). Specifically, the expression of SNAT2 was positively correlated with birth weight and maternal BMI, but neither SNAT1 nor SNAT4 was associated with birth weight or BMI (Jansson et al. 2013). A limitation of this study is that maternal serum amino acid concentrations were not evaluated. Nevertheless, these findings may support the authors' belief that decreased SNAT activity represents placental dysfunction, not adaptive regulation (Farley et al. 2010). Despite the contradictory results, there is some evidence to suggest a possible link between maternal obesity, up-regulation of specific placental amino acid transporter isoforms, and increased fetal growth (Jansson et al. 2013). Unlike in humans, in rats, high-fat diet increased SNTA4 in the placentas (Lin et al. 2012) and was positively correlated with birth weight. In mouse model, *ad libitum* access to a high-fat, high-sucrose "cafeteria diet" (58% fat, 25.5% sucrose, 16.4% protein) increased the expression of SNAT2 in male placentas and SNAT4 in female placentas (King et al. 2013). Collectively, these observations in humans and mice support a gender-selective role for placental amino acids in diet and obesity-associated gestations.

16.4.4 FA Transporters

FAs are pivotal for the development of tissues and organs, including brain development and fat accretion. FAs are precursors for essential bioactive compounds. During the third trimester of human pregnancy, fat rapidly accumulates in fetal adipose tissue and brain (Haggarty 2010). FAs are taken up by the placenta and transported to the fetus. These FAs originate from two main sources in maternal circulation: nonesterified FAs (NEFAs) and esterified FAs in triglycerides (TGs) carried by lipoproteins. Maternal TGs have been suggested as a primary source of FAs because of their significant rise in late gestation compared with NEFAs (Haggarty 2010). TGs cannot cross the syncytiotrophoblasts, although they may be broken down into free fatty acids (FFAs) by placental TG lipases (King 2006) before uptake into the placenta through FA transport proteins (Duttaroy 2009). FA transport proteins include FA transport proteins (FATPs), FA translocase (FAT/CD36), plasma membrane FA-binding protein (FABPpm), and FA-binding proteins (FABP). FATPs are part of the membrane proteins that contribute to the uptake of long-chain FAs (Kazantzis and Stahl 2012). There are six members of the FATP family, five of which have been identified in placental trophoblasts (FATP1–FATP4 and FATP6) (Schaiff et al. 2005).

There are only a few studies examining the effect of maternal obesity on the expression or activity of FA transport proteins in human pregnancies. Scifres et al. (2011) demonstrated that placentas from obese-diabetic women displayed elevated FABP4 and FABP5 mRNA and FABP4 protein expression, with no modification in FABP3 or FABPpm, compared with obese, nondiabetic or normal-weight women. Moreover, the investigators found that in primary human trophoblast cultures, FAs markedly increased the expression of FABP4 (20- to 40-fold) and cellular TG content (4-fold), and this effect was mitigated by small interfering RNA-mediated knockdown of FABP4. The lower TG content after FABP4 inhibition suggested that FABP4 was essential for trophoblast lipid accumulation (Scifres et al. 2011). Maternal obesity was also associated with significantly higher *FAT/CD36* mRNA and protein levels but lower expression of FATP4, FABP1, and FABP3 proteins than the normal-weight women (Dube et al. 2012).

Recently, it has been suggested that placental FA transfer may be fetal sex specific (Brass, Hanson, and O'Tierney-Ginn 2013, Kimura et al. 1991). Brass, Hanson, and O'Tierney-Ginn (2013) showed that placental oleic acid uptake was 43% lower in male offspring and 73% higher in female offspring of obese women, compared with those of lean women, suggesting that uptake in both male and female fetuses is susceptible to maternal BMI, but males may inadequately acquire oleic acid, when subjected to maternal obesity (Brass, Hanson, and O'Tierney-Ginn 2013). The role of FA transporters has also been studied in animal models, with results indicating that obesity-altered placental FA transport occurs through alterations in transporter levels but not TG hydrolysis. Zhu et al. (2010) found elevated fetal blood levels of cholesterol and TG and increased FATP1 and FATP4 protein levels, but no difference in lipoprotein lipase expression in midgestation cotyledons in obese sheep. The increase in nuclear receptor peroxisome proliferator-activated receptor gamma, a regulator of FA storage (Motojima et al. 1998), may represent a mechanism mediating enhanced FATP expression in cotyledonary.

Collectively, these findings establish that fetal growth in obese pregnancies is dependent not only on the level of maternal energy intake but also on the placental nutrient transfer to the fetus. Further work is warranted to examine nutrient transport effects of maternal BMI and diet, as well as sex-specific differences.

16.5 CONCLUSION

Maternal nutrition during pregnancy is a critical determining parameter of optimal fetal development, pregnancy outcome, and, eventually, adult health. Normal placental function aids the maternal–fetal transfer of nutrients that are critical for the development of a healthy fetus (Knipp, Audus, and Soares 1999). Maternal obesity affects fetal growth, in part, by impairing placental development and function, resulting in infants born with a greater birth weight than those of nonobese women (Simmonds 1979). Placental changes depend upon the nutritional setting and include altered vascular development subsequent to decreased invasion, endothelial dysfunction, diminished vasculogenesis and angiogenic growth factor expression, increased OS, and altered placental glucose, amino acid, and FA transporters. In most circumstances, the flexibility of the placenta permits this crucial organ to compensate for different nutritional status of the mother. However, when the placental response is insufficient to maintain normal fetal growth, overgrowth ensues in most cases, and suboptimal outcomes may appear not only in the newborn but with potential long-term effects on the offspring. Further studies are urgently needed to unveil the mechanism of vascular dysfunction in the obesogenic environment, either due to maternal obesity or the maternal high-fat diet, to reduce pregnancy related negative outcomes.

REFERENCES

Adamson, S. L., Y. Lu, K. J. Whiteley, D. Holmyard, M. Hemberger, C. Pfarrer, and J. C. Cross. 2002. "Interactions between trophoblast cells and the maternal and fetal circulation in the mouse placenta." *Developmental Biology* 250 (2):358–73.

Akyol, A., S. C. Langley-Evans, and S. McMullen. 2009. "Obesity induced by cafeteria feeding and pregnancy outcome in the rat." *The British Journal of Nutrition* 102 (11):1601–10. doi:10.1017/S0007114509990961.

Anthony, R. V., S. W. Limesand, and K. M. Jeckel. 2001. "Transcriptional regulation in the placenta during normal and compromised fetal growth." *Biochemical Society Transactions* 29 (Pt 2):42–8.

Arroyo, J. A. and V. D. Winn. 2008. "Vasculogenesis and angiogenesis in the IUGR placenta." *Seminars in Perinatology* 32 (3):172–7. doi:10.1053/j.semperi.2008.02.006.

Ashcroft, R. G., H. G. Coster, and J. R. Smith. 1977. "Local anaesthetic benzyl alcohol increases membrane thickness." *Nature* 269 (5631):819–20.

Ashton, S. V., G. S. Whitley, P. R. Dash, M. Wareing, I. P. Crocker, P. N. Baker, and J. E. Cartwright. 2005. "Uterine spiral artery remodeling involves endothelial apoptosis induced by extravillous trophoblasts through Fas/FasL interactions." *Arteriosclerosis, Thrombosis, and Vascular Biology* 25 (1):102–8. doi:10.1161/01.ATV.0000148547.70187.89.

Baumann, M. U., S. Deborde, and N. P. Illsley. 2002. "Placental glucose transfer and fetal growth." *Endocrine* 19 (1):13–22. doi:10.1385/ENDO:19:1:13.

Becker, T., M. J. Vermeulen, P. R. Wyatt, C. Meier, and J. G. Ray. 2008. "Maternal obesity and the risk of placental vascular disease." *Journal of Obstetrics and Gynaecology Canada: JOGC = Journal d'obstetrique et gynecologie du Canada: JOGC* 30 (12):1132–6.

Berger, M., V. Jorgens, I. Muhlhauser, and H. Zimmermann. 1983. "[The value of education of diabetics in the therapy of type 1 diabetes]." *Deutsche medizinische Wochenschrift* 108 (11):424–30. doi: 10.1055/s-2008-1069573.

Birbrair, A., T. Zhang, Z. M. Wang, M. L. Messi, A. Mintz, and O. Delbono. 2013. "Type-1 pericytes participate in fibrous tissue deposition in aged skeletal muscle." *American Journal of Physiology. Cell Physiology* 305 (11):C1098–113. doi:10.1152/ajpcell.00171.2013.

Borowicz, P. P., D. R. Arnold, M. L. Johnson, A. T. Grazul-Bilska, D. A. Redmer, and L. P. Reynolds. 2007. "Placental growth throughout the last two thirds of pregnancy in sheep: Vascular development and angiogenic factor expression." *Biology of Reproduction* 76 (2):259–67. doi:10.1095/biolreprod .106.054684.

Brass, E., E. Hanson, and P. F. O'Tierney-Ginn. 2013. "Placental oleic acid uptake is lower in male offspring of obese women." *Placenta* 34 (6):503–9. doi:10.1016/j.placenta.2013.03.009.

Bray, G. A. and T. Bellanger. 2006. "Epidemiology, trends, and morbidities of obesity and the metabolic syndrome." *Endocrine* 29 (1):109–17. doi:10.1385/ENDO:29:1:109.

Broer, S. 2002. "Adaptation of plasma membrane amino acid transport mechanisms to physiological demands." *Pflugers Archiv: European Journal of Physiology* 444 (4):457–66. doi:10.1007/s00424-002-0840-y.

Burton, G. J., E. Jauniaux, and A. L. Watson. 1999. "Maternal arterial connections to the placental intervillous space during the first trimester of human pregnancy: The Boyd collection revisited." *American Journal of Obstetrics and Gynecology* 181 (3):718–24.

Caniggia, I., H. Mostachfi, J. Winter, M. Gassmann, S. J. Lye, M. Kuliszewski, and M. Post. 2000. "Hypoxia-inducible factor-1 mediates the biological effects of oxygen on human trophoblast differentiation through TGFbeta(3)." *The Journal of Clinical Investigation* 105 (5):577–87. doi:10.1172/JCI8316.

Catalano, P. M. 2003. "Obesity and pregnancy—The propagation of a viscous cycle?" *The Journal of Clinical Endocrinology and Metabolism* 88 (8):3505–6. doi:10.1210/jc.2003-031046.

Cetin, I., A. M. Marconi, C. Corbetta, A. Lanfranchi, A. M. Baggiani, F. C. Battaglia, and G. Pardi. 1992. "Fetal amino acids in normal pregnancies and in pregnancies complicated by intrauterine growth retardation." *Early Human Development* 29 (1–3):183–6.

Challier, J. C., S. Basu, T. Bintein, J. Minium, K. Hotmire, P. M. Catalano, and S. Hauguel-de Mouzon. 2008. "Obesity in pregnancy stimulates macrophage accumulation and inflammation in the placenta." *Placenta* 29 (3):274–81. doi:10.1016/j.placenta.2007.12.010.

Christensen, H. N., L. M. Albritton, D. K. Kakuda, and C. L. MacLeod. 1994. "Gene-product designations for amino acid transporters." *The Journal of Experimental Biology* 196:51–7.

Cimpean, A. M., M. Raica, and C. Suciu. 2007. "CD105/smooth muscle actin double immunostaining discriminate between immature and mature tumor blood vessels." *Romanian Journal of Morphology and Embryology = Revue roumaine de morphologie et embryologie* 48 (1):41–5.

Cnattingius, S., R. Bergstrom, L. Lipworth, and M. S. Kramer. 1998. "Prepregnancy weight and the risk of adverse pregnancy outcomes." *The New England Journal of Medicine* 338 (3):147–52. doi:10.1056 /NEJM199801153380302.

Colomiere, M., M. Permezel, C. Riley, G. Desoye, and M. Lappas. 2009. "Defective insulin signaling in placenta from pregnancies complicated by gestational diabetes mellitus." *European Journal of Endocrinology /European Federation of Endocrine Societies* 160 (4):567–78. doi:10.1530/EJE-09-0031.

Deanfield, J., A. Donald, C. Ferri, C. Giannattasio, J. Halcox, S. Halligan, A. Lerman, G. Mancia, J. J. Oliver, A. C. Pessina, D. Rizzoni, G. P. Rossi, A. Salvetti, E. L. Schiffrin, S. Taddei, and D. J. Webb. 2005. "Endothelial function and dysfunction. Part I: Methodological issues for assessment in the different vascular beds: A statement by the Working Group on Endothelin and Endothelial Factors of the European Society of Hypertension." *Journal of Hypertension* 23 (1):7–17.

Demir, R., Y. Seval, and B. Huppertz. 2007. "Vasculogenesis and angiogenesis in the early human placenta." *Acta Histochemica* 109 (4):257–65. doi:10.1016/j.acthis.2007.02.008.

Deng, G., Y. Long, Y. R. Yu, and M. R. Li. 2010. "Adiponectin directly improves endothelial dysfunction in obese rats through the AMPK–eNOS pathway." *International Journal of Obesity* 34 (1):165–71. doi:10.1038/ijo.2009.205.

Desai, M., M. Beall, and M. G. Ross. 2013. "Developmental origins of obesity: Programmed adipogenesis." *Current Diabetes Reports* 13 (1):27–33. doi:10.1007/s11892-012-0344-x.

Desforges, M., K. J. Mynett, R. L. Jones, S. L. Greenwood, M. Westwood, C. P. Sibley, and J. D. Glazier. 2009. "The SNAT4 isoform of the system A amino acid transporter is functional in human placental microvillous plasma membrane." *The Journal of Physiology* 587 (Pt 1):61–72. doi:10.1113/jphysiol .2008.161331.

Desforges, M., S. L. Greenwood, J. D. Glazier, M. Westwood, and C. P. Sibley. 2010. "The contribution of SNAT1 to system A amino acid transporter activity in human placental trophoblast." *Biochemical and Biophysical Research Communications* 398 (1):130–4. doi:10.1016/j.bbrc.2010.06.051.

Desoye, G. and E. Shafrir. 1994. "Placental metabolism and its regulation in health and diabetes." *Molecular Aspects of Medicine* 15 (6):505–682.

Dube, E., A. Gravel, C. Martin, G. Desparois, I. Moussa, M. Ethier-Chiasson, J. C. Forest, Y. Giguere, A. Masse, and J. Lafond. 2012. "Modulation of fatty acid transport and metabolism by maternal obesity in the human full-term placenta." *Biology of Reproduction* 87 (1):14, 1–11. doi:10.1095/biolreprod.111.098095.

Duttaroy, A. K. 2009. "Transport of fatty acids across the human placenta: A review." *Progress in Lipid Research* 48 (1):52–61. doi:10.1016/j.plipres.2008.11.001.

Farley, D., M. E. Tejero, A. G. Comuzzie, P. B. Higgins, L. Cox, S. L. Werner, S. L. Jenkins, C. Li, J. Choi, E. J. Dick Jr., G. B. Hubbard, P. Frost, D. J. Dudley, B. Ballesteros, G. Wu, P. W. Nathanielsz, and N. E. Schlabritz-Loutsevitch. 2009. "Fetoplacental adaptations to maternal obesity in the baboon." *Placenta* 30 (9):752–60. doi:10.1016/j.placenta.2009.06.007.

Farley, D. M., J. Choi, D. J. Dudley, C. Li, S. L. Jenkins, L. Myatt, and P. W. Nathanielsz. 2010. "Placental amino acid transport and placental leptin resistance in pregnancies complicated by maternal obesity." *Placenta* 31 (8):718–24. doi:10.1016/j.placenta.2010.06.006.

Fowden, A. L., J. W. Ward, F. P. Wooding, A. J. Forhead, and M. Constancia. 2006. "Programming placental nutrient transport capacity." *The Journal of Physiology* 572 (Pt 1):5–15. doi:10.1113/jphysiol.2005.104141.

Fox, S. B. and T. Y. Khong. 1990. "Lack of innervation of human umbilical cord. An immunohistological and histochemical study." *Placenta* 11 (1):59–62.

Frias, A. E., T. K. Morgan, A. E. Evans, J. Rasanen, K. Y. Oh, K. L. Thornburg, and K. L. Grove. 2011. "Maternal high-fat diet disturbs uteroplacental hemodynamics and increases the frequency of stillbirth in a nonhuman primate model of excess nutrition." *Endocrinology* 152 (6):2456–64. doi:10.1210/en.2010-1332.

Fridovich, I. 1995. "Superoxide radical and superoxide dismutases." *Annual Review of Biochemistry* 64:97–112. doi:10.1146/annurev.bi.64.070195.000525.

Friis, C. M., E. Qvigstad, M. C. Paasche Roland, K. Godang, N. Voldner, J. Bollerslev, and T. Henriksen. 2013. "Newborn body fat: Associations with maternal metabolic state and placental size." *PLoS One* 8 (2):e57467. doi:10.1371/journal.pone.0057467.

Glazier, J. D., I. Cetin, G. Perugino, S. Ronzoni, A. M. Grey, D. Mahendran, A. M. Marconi, G. Pardi, and C. P. Sibley. 1997. "Association between the activity of the system A amino acid transporter in the microvillous plasma membrane of the human placenta and severity of fetal compromise in intrauterine growth restriction." *Pediatric Research* 42 (4):514–9. doi:10.1203/00006450-199710000-00016.

Haase, C., R. Bergmann, F. Fuechtner, A. Hoepping, and J. Pietzsch. 2007. "L-type amino acid transporters LAT1 and LAT4 in cancer: Uptake of 3-O-methyl-6-18F-fluoro-L-dopa in human adenocarcinoma and squamous cell carcinoma in vitro and in vivo." *Journal of Nuclear Medicine: Official Publication, Society of Nuclear Medicine* 48 (12):2063–71. doi:10.2967/jnumed.107.043620.

Haggarty, P. 2010. "Fatty acid supply to the human fetus." *Annual Review of Nutrition* 30:237–55. doi:10.1146 /annurev.nutr.012809.104742.

Hanahan, D. 1997. "Signaling vascular morphogenesis and maintenance." *Science* 277 (5322):48–50.

Hayes, E. K., A. Lechowicz, J. J. Petrik, Y. Storozhuk, S. Paez-Parent, Q. Dai, I. A. Samjoo, M. Mansell, A. Gruslin, A. C. Holloway, and S. Raha. 2012. "Adverse fetal and neonatal outcomes associated with a life-long high fat diet: Role of altered development of the placental vasculature." *PLoS One* 7 (3):e33370. doi:10.1371/journal.pone.0033370.

Higgins, L., S. L. Greenwood, M. Wareing, C. P. Sibley, and T. A. Mills. 2011. "Obesity and the placenta: A consideration of nutrient exchange mechanisms in relation to aberrant fetal growth." *Placenta* 32 (1):1–7. doi:10.1016/j.placenta.2010.09.019.

Higgins, L., T. A. Mills, S. L. Greenwood, E. J. Cowley, C. P. Sibley, and R. L. Jones. 2013. "Maternal obesity and its effect on placental cell turnover." *The Journal of Maternal–Fetal & Neonatal Medicine: The Official Journal of the European Association of Perinatal Medicine, the Federation of Asia and Oceania Perinatal Societies, the International Society of Perinatal Obstetricians* 26 (8):783–8. doi:10.3109/147 67058.2012.760539.

Illsley, N. P. 2000. "Glucose transporters in the human placenta." *Placenta* 21 (1):14–22. doi:10.1053 /plac.1999.0448.

Jaffe, R., E. Jauniaux, and J. Hustin. 1997. "Maternal circulation in the first-trimester human placenta—Myth or reality?" *American Journal of Obstetrics and Gynecology* 176 (3):695–705.

Jansson, T. 2001. "Amino acid transporters in the human placenta." *Pediatric Research* 49 (2):141–7. doi:10.1203/00006450-200102000-00003.

Jansson, T., and T. L. Powell. 2006. "IFPA 2005 Award in Placentology Lecture. Human placental transport in altered fetal growth: Does the placenta function as a nutrient sensor?—A review." *Placenta* 27 Suppl A:S91–7. doi:10.1016/j.placenta.2005.11.010.

Jansson, N., J. Pettersson, A. Haafiz, A. Ericsson, I. Palmberg, M. Tranberg, V. Ganapathy, T. L. Powell, and T. Jansson. 2006. "Down-regulation of placental transport of amino acids precedes the development of intrauterine growth restriction in rats fed a low protein diet." *The Journal of Physiology* 576 (Pt 3):935–46. doi:10.1113/jphysiol.2006.116509.

Jansson, T., I. Cetin, T. L. Powell, G. Desoye, T. Radaelli, A. Ericsson, and C. P. Sibley. 2006. "Placental transport and metabolism in fetal overgrowth—A workshop report." *Placenta* 27 Suppl A:S109–13. doi:10.1016/j.placenta.2006.01.017.

Jansson, N., A. Nilsfelt, M. Gellerstedt, M. Wennergren, L. Rossander-Hulthen, T. L. Powell, and T. Jansson. 2008. "Maternal hormones linking maternal body mass index and dietary intake to birth weight." *The American Journal of Clinical Nutrition* 87 (6):1743–9.

Jansson, N., F. J. Rosario, F. Gaccioli, S. Lager, H. N. Jones, S. Roos, T. Jansson, and T. L. Powell. 2013. "Activation of placental mTOR signaling and amino acid transporters in obese women giving birth to large babies." *The Journal of Clinical Endocrinology and Metabolism* 98 (1):105–13. doi:10.1210/jc.2012-2667.

Johansson, M., L. Karlsson, M. Wennergren, T. Jansson, and T. L. Powell. 2003. "Activity and protein expression of Na+/K+ ATPase are reduced in microvillous syncytiotrophoblast plasma membranes isolated from pregnancies complicated by intrauterine growth restriction." *The Journal of Clinical Endocrinology and Metabolism* 88 (6):2831–7. doi:10.1210/jc.2002-021926.

Jones, H. N., L. A. Woollett, N. Barbour, P. D. Prasad, T. L. Powell, and T. Jansson. 2009. "High-fat diet before and during pregnancy causes marked up-regulation of placental nutrient transport and fetal overgrowth in C57/BL6 mice." *FASEB Journal: Official Publication of the Federation of American Societies for Experimental Biology* 23 (1):271–8. doi:10.1096/fj.08-116889.

Kalhan, S. and P. Parimi. 2000. "Gluconeogenesis in the fetus and neonate." *Seminars in Perinatology* 24 (2):94–106.

Kazantzis, M. and A. Stahl. 2012. "Fatty acid transport proteins, implications in physiology and disease." *Biochimica et Biophysica Acta* 1821 (5):852–7. doi:10.1016/j.bbalip.2011.09.010.

Kern, P. A., S. Ranganathan, C. Li, L. Wood, and G. Ranganathan. 2001. "Adipose tissue tumor necrosis factor and interleukin-6 expression in human obesity and insulin resistance." *American Journal of Physiology. Endocrinology and Metabolism* 280 (5):E745–51.

Kim, F., M. Pham, E. Maloney, N. O. Rizzo, G. J. Morton, B. E. Wisse, E. A. Kirk, A. Chait, and M. W. Schwartz. 2008. "Vascular inflammation, insulin resistance, and reduced nitric oxide production precede the onset of peripheral insulin resistance." *Arteriosclerosis, Thrombosis, and Vascular Biology* 28 (11):1982–8. doi:10.1161/ATVBAHA.108.169722.

Kim, D. W., S. L. Young, D. R. Grattan, and C. L. Jasoni. 2014. "Obesity during pregnancy disrupts placental morphology, cell proliferation, and inflammation in a sex-specific manner across gestation in the mouse." *Biology of Reproduction* 90 (6):130. doi:10.1095/biolreprod.113.117259.

Kimura, M., K. Kowari, M. Inokuti, I. K. Bronic, D. Srdoc, and B. Obelic. 1991. "Theoretical study of W values in hydrocarbon gases." *Radiation Research* 125 (3):237–42.

King, J. C. 2006. "Maternal obesity, metabolism, and pregnancy outcomes." *Annual Review of Nutrition* 26:271–91. doi:10.1146/annurev.nutr.24.012003.132249.

King, V., N. Hibbert, J. R. Seckl, J. E. Norman, and A. J. Drake. 2013. "The effects of an obesogenic diet during pregnancy on fetal growth and placental gene expression are gestation dependent." *Placenta* 34 (11):1087–90. doi:10.1016/j.placenta.2013.09.006.

Knipp, G. T., K. L. Audus, and M. J. Soares. 1999. "Nutrient transport across the placenta." *Advanced Drug Delivery Reviews* 38 (1):41–58.

Korner, J. and L. J. Aronne. 2003. "The emerging science of body weight regulation and its impact on obesity treatment." *The Journal of Clinical Investigation* 111 (5):565–70. doi:10.1172/JCI17953.

Krause, B. J., M. A. Hanson, and P. Casanello. 2011. "Role of nitric oxide in placental vascular development and function." *Placenta* 32 (11):797–805. doi:10.1016/j.placenta.2011.06.025.

Laresgoiti-Servitje, E. and N. Gomez-Lopez. 2012. "The pathophysiology of preeclampsia involves altered levels of angiogenic factors promoted by hypoxia and autoantibody-mediated mechanisms." *Biology of Reproduction* 87 (2):36. doi:10.1095/biolreprod.112.099861.

Leach, L. and J. A. Firth. 1992. "Fine structure of the paracellular junctions of terminal villous capillaries in the perfused human placenta." *Cell and Tissue Research* 268 (3):447–52.

Liang, C., K. DeCourcy, and M. R. Prater. 2010. "High-saturated-fat diet induces gestational diabetes and placental vasculopathy in C57BL/6 mice." *Metabolism: Clinical and Experimental* 59 (7):943–50. doi:10.1016/j.metabol.2009.10.015.

Lin, Y., Y. Zhuo, Z. F. Fang, L. Q. Che, and D. Wu. 2012. "Effect of maternal dietary energy types on placenta nutrient transporter gene expressions and intrauterine fetal growth in rats." *Nutrition* 28 (10):1037–43. doi:10.1016/j.nut.2012.01.002.

Mackenzie, B. and J. D. Erickson. 2004. "Sodium-coupled neutral amino acid (System N/A) transporters of the SLC38 gene family." *Pflugers Archiv: European Journal of Physiology* 447 (5):784–95. doi:10.1007/s00424-003-1117-9.

Malti, N., H. Merzouk, S. A. Merzouk, B. Loukidi, N. Karaouzene, A. Malti, and M. Narce. 2014. "Oxidative stress and maternal obesity: Fetoplacental unit interaction." *Placenta* 35 (6):411–6. doi:10.1016/j.placenta.2014.03.010.

Martins, M. A., M. Catta-Preta, C. A. Mandarim-de-Lacerda, M. B. Aguila, T. C. Brunini, and A. C. Mendes-Ribeiro. 2010. "High fat diets modulate nitric oxide biosynthesis and antioxidant defence in red blood cells from C57BL/6 mice." *Archives of Biochemistry and Biophysics* 499 (1–2):56–61. doi:10.1016/j.abb.2010.04.025.

Michel, C. C. and F. E. Curry. 1999. "Microvascular permeability." *Physiological Reviews* 79 (3):703–61.

Moncada, S. and E. A. Higgs. 2006. "The discovery of nitric oxide and its role in vascular biology." *British Journal of Pharmacology* 147 Suppl 1:S193–201. doi:10.1038/sj.bjp.0706458.

Motojima, K., P. Passilly, J. M. Peters, F. J. Gonzalez, and N. Latruffe. 1998. "Expression of putative fatty acid transporter genes are regulated by peroxisome proliferator-activated receptor alpha and gamma activators in a tissue- and inducer-specific manner." *The Journal of Biological Chemistry* 273 (27):16710–4.

Murthi, P., U. Hiden, G. Rajaraman, H. Liu, A. J. Borg, F. Coombes, G. Desoye, S. P. Brennecke, and B. Kalionis. 2008. "Novel homeobox genes are differentially expressed in placental microvascular endothelial cells compared with macrovascular cells." *Placenta* 29 (7):624–30. doi:10.1016/j.placenta.2008.04.006.

Myatt, L. 2010. "Review: Reactive oxygen and nitrogen species and functional adaptation of the placenta." *Placenta* 31 Suppl:S66–9. doi:10.1016/j.placenta.2009.12.021.

Myatt, L., W. Kossenjans, R. Sahay, A. Eis, and D. Brockman. 2000. "Oxidative stress causes vascular dysfunction in the placenta." *The Journal of Maternal–Fetal Medicine* 9 (1):79–82. doi:10.1002/(SICI)1520-6661(200001/02)9:1<79::AID-MFM16>3.0.CO;2-O.

Nascimento, T. B., F. Baptista Rde, P. C. Pereira, D. H. Campos, A. S. Leopoldo, A. P. Leopoldo, S. A. Oliveira Junior, C. R. Padovani, A. C. Cicogna, and S. Cordellini. 2011. "Vascular alterations in high-fat diet-obese rats: Role of endothelial L-arginine/NO pathway." *Arquivos brasileiros de cardiologia* 97 (1):40–5.

Perlow, J. H., M. A. Morgan, D. Montgomery, C. V. Towers, and M. Porto. 1992. "Perinatal outcome in pregnancy complicated by massive obesity." *American Journal of Obstetrics and Gynecology* 167 (4 Pt 1):958–62.

Raha, S. and B. H. Robinson. 2001. "Mitochondria, oxygen free radicals, and apoptosis." *American Journal of Medical Genetics* 106 (1):62–70. doi:10.1002/ajmg.1398.

Reynolds, L. P. and D. A. Redmer. 1995. "Utero-placental vascular development and placental function." *Journal of Animal Science* 73 (6):1839–51.

Ribatti, D., A. Vacca, B. Nico, R. Ria, and F. Dammacco. 2002. "Cross-talk between hematopoiesis and angio-genesis signaling pathways." *Current Molecular Medicine* 2 (6):537–43.

Roberts, K. A., S. C. Riley, R. M. Reynolds, S. Barr, M. Evans, A. Statham, K. Hor, H. N. Jabbour, J. E. Norman, and F. C. Denison. 2011. "Placental structure and inflammation in pregnancies associated with obesity." *Placenta* 32 (3):247–54. doi:10.1016/j.placenta.2010.12.023.

Robinson, J. S., R. F. Seamark, and J. A. Owens. 1994. "Placental function." *The Australian & New Zealand Journal of Obstetrics & Gynaecology* 34 (3):240–6.

Saben, J., F. Lindsey, Y. Zhong, K. Thakali, T. M. Badger, A. Andres, H. Gomez-Acevedo, and K. Shankar. 2014. "Maternal obesity is associated with a lipotoxic placental environment." *Placenta* 35 (3):171–7. doi:10.1016/j.placenta.2014.01.003.

Salafia, C. M., J. Zhang, A. K. Charles, M. Bresnahan, P. Shrout, W. Sun, and E. M. Maas. 2008. "Placental characteristics and birthweight." *Paediatric and Perinatal Epidemiology* 22 (3):229–39. doi:10.1111/j.1365-3016.2008.00935.x.

Schaiff, W. T., I. Bildirici, M. Cheong, P. L. Chern, D. M. Nelson, and Y. Sadovsky. 2005. "Peroxisome proliferator-activated receptor-gamma and retinoid X receptor signaling regulate fatty acid uptake by primary human placental trophoblasts." *The Journal of Clinical Endocrinology and Metabolism* 90 (7):4267–75. doi:10.1210/jc.2004-2265.

Scifres, C. M., B. Chen, D. M. Nelson, and Y. Sadovsky. 2011. "Fatty acid binding protein 4 regulates intracellular lipid accumulation in human trophoblasts." *The Journal of Clinical Endocrinology and Metabolism* 96 (7):E1083–91. doi:10.1210/jc.2010-2084.

Sebire, N. J., M. Jolly, J. P. Harris, J. Wadsworth, M. Joffe, R. W. Beard, L. Regan, and S. Robinson. 2001. "Maternal obesity and pregnancy outcome: A study of 287,213 pregnancies in London." *International Journal of Obesity and Related Metabolic Disorders: Journal of the International Association for the Study of Obesity* 25 (8):1175–82. doi:10.1038/sj.ijo.0801670.

Semenza, G. L. 2011. "Oxygen sensing, homeostasis, and disease." *The New England Journal of Medicine* 365 (6):537–47. doi:10.1056/NEJMra1011165.

Sferruzzi-Perri, A. N., O. R. Vaughan, M. Haro, W. N. Cooper, B. Musial, M. Charalambous, D. Pestana, S. Ayyar, A. C. Ferguson-Smith, G. J. Burton, M. Constancia, and A. L. Fowden. 2013. "An obesogenic diet during mouse pregnancy modifies maternal nutrient partitioning and the fetal growth trajectory." *FASEB Journal: Official Publication of the Federation of American Societies for Experimental Biology* 27 (10):3928–37. doi:10.1096/fj.13-234823.

Shih, S. C. and K. P. Claffey. 1999. "Regulation of human vascular endothelial growth factor mRNA stability in hypoxia by heterogeneous nuclear ribonucleoprotein L." *The Journal of Biological Chemistry* 274 (3):1359–65.

Shoelson, S. E., L. Herrero, and A. Naaz. 2007. "Obesity, inflammation, and insulin resistance." *Gastroenterology* 132 (6):2169–80. doi:10.1053/j.gastro.2007.03.059.

Sibley, C. P., M. A. Turner, I. Cetin, P. Ayuk, C. A. Boyd, S. W. D'Souza, J. D. Glazier, S. L. Greenwood, T. Jansson, and T. Powell. 2005. "Placental phenotypes of intrauterine growth." *Pediatric Research* 58 (5):827–32. doi:10.1203/01.PDR.0000181381.82856.23.

Simmonds, H. A. 1979. "2,8-Dihydroxyadeninuria—Or when is a uric acid stone not a uric acid stone?" *Clinical Nephrology* 12 (5):195–7.

Simon, M. P., R. Tournaire, and J. Pouyssegur. 2008. "The angiopoietin-2 gene of endothelial cells is up-regulated in hypoxia by a HIF binding site located in its first intron and by the central factors GATA-2 and Ets-1." *Journal of Cellular Physiology* 217 (3):809–18. doi:10.1002/jcp.21558.

Sipos, P. I., I. P. Crocker, C. A. Hubel, and P. N. Baker. 2010. "Endothelial progenitor cells: their potential in the placental vasculature and related complications." *Placenta* 31 (1):1–10. doi:10.1016/j.placenta.2009.10.006.

Smith, D. K., S. B. Leonard, J. M. Greene, S. Skelley, and K. A. Parker. 1992. "Physician's and dietitian's role in obese care." *The Journal of the Florida Medical Association* 79 (6):385–7.

Suwaidi, J. A., S. Hamasaki, S. T. Higano, R. A. Nishimura, D. R. Holmes Jr., and A. Lerman. 2000. "Long-term follow-up of patients with mild coronary artery disease and endothelial dysfunction." *Circulation* 101 (9):948–54.

Tal, R. 2012. "The role of hypoxia and hypoxia-inducible factor-1alpha in preeclampsia pathogenesis." *Biology of Reproduction* 87 (6):134. doi:10.1095/biolreprod.112.102723.

Talbert, D. and N. J. Sebire. 2004. "The dynamic placenta: I. Hypothetical model of a placental mechanism matching local fetal blood flow to local intervillus oxygen delivery." *Medical Hypotheses* 62 (4):511–9. doi:10.1016/j.mehy.2003.10.025.

Taylor, W. P., S. M. al Busaidy, and P. S. Mellor. 1991. "Bluetongue in the Sultanate of Oman, a preliminary epidemiological study." *Epidemiology and Infection* 107 (1):87–97.

Tikellis, G., A. L. Ponsonby, J. C. Wells, A. Pezic, J. Cochrane, and T. Dwyer. 2012. "Maternal and infant factors associated with neonatal adiposity: Results from the Tasmanian Infant Health Survey (TIHS)." *International Journal of Obesity* 36 (4):496–504. doi:10.1038/ijo.2011.261.

Tilg, H. and A. R. Moschen. 2006. "Adipocytokines: Mediators linking adipose tissue, inflammation and immunity." *Nature Reviews. Immunology* 6 (10):772–83. doi:10.1038/nri1937.

Vozarova, B., C. Weyer, K. Hanson, P. A. Tataranni, C. Bogardus, and R. E. Pratley. 2001. "Circulating interleukin-6 in relation to adiposity, insulin action, and insulin secretion." *Obesity Research* 9 (7):414–7. doi:10.1038/oby.2001.54.

Waller, D. K., G. M. Shaw, S. A. Rasmussen, C. A. Hobbs, M. A. Canfield, A. M. Siega-Riz, M. S. Gallaway, and A. Correa. 2007. "Prepregnancy obesity as a risk factor for structural birth defects." *Archives of Pediatrics & Adolescent Medicine* 161 (8):745–50. doi:10.1001/archpedi.161.8.745.

Zhu, M. J., Y. Ma, N. M. Long, M. Du, and S. P. Ford. 2010. "Maternal obesity markedly increases placental fatty acid transporter expression and fetal blood triglycerides at midgestation in the ewe." *American Journal of Physiology. Regulatory, Integrative and Comparative Physiology* 299 (5):R1224–31. doi:10.1152/ajpregu.00309.2010.

Ziche, M. and L. Morbidelli. 2000. "Nitric oxide and angiogenesis." *Journal of Neuro-Oncology* 50 (1–2):139–48.

17 Placental Dysfunction and Future Maternal Cardiovascular Disease

Anne Cathrine Staff and Christopher W.G. Redman

CONTENTS

ABSTRACT

Preeclampsia is a placentally mediated pregnancy complication. It is potentially lethal for mother and offspring. Women who develop preeclampsia have an increased long-term risk of cardiovascular disease (CVD) and premature death.

This review summarizes the current pathophysiological understanding of the major placental dysfunction disorders, namely, preeclampsia and fetal growth restriction. We review the relation between placental dysfunction and future maternal health burden, focusing on CVD. Pregnancy is regarded as a metabolic and vascular "stress test for life," and women who "fail" the test, for example by developing preeclampsia, are at increased risk of long-term cardiovascular disorders, including coronary heart disease and stroke. The risk is highest in pregnancies with both maternal and fetal manifestations of abnormal placentation, which is associated with preterm delivery.

Possible mechanisms of the associations are discussed. Women developing placental dysfunction may have risk factors in common with older persons developing CVD. Additionally, pregnancy in itself, and especially placental dysfunction, could also represent an added risk factor for CVD. We present our hypothesis that the presence of uteroplacental acute atherosis, which is strongly associated with preeclampsia and resembles early atherosclerosis, could identify a specific subset of women at increased risk of future atherosclerotic CVD. Possible strategies for follow-up after placentally mediated complications of pregnancy to prevent manifest CVD are discussed.

KEY WORDS

Preeclampsia, cardiovascular disease, atherosclerosis, atherosis, hypertension, pregnancy, spiral artery.

17.1 INTRODUCTION: THE BURDEN OF CARDIOVASCULAR DISEASE AND ITS ASSOCIATION TO PREGNANCY AND PLACENTAL DYSFUNCTION

Cardiovascular disease (CVD), including coronary heart disease, stroke, and other atherosclerotic conditions, is the leading cause of death for men and women in developed countries and most emerging economies (Mosca et al. 2011). CVD is a noncommunicable epidemic, with high costs for the patient and family and for the society. In the United States, CVD is registered as the cause of death in 52% of women (Ahmed et al. 2014). There are significant epidemiological gender differences: coronary artery disease kills more women than men (Lawton 2011). Women develop CVD 10–15 years later than men do but may present with more atypical CVD symptoms. Women less often have angina before myocardial infarction, and younger women are more likely to die of their first heart attack than men are. Thus, preventing CVD may be especially crucial for women (Mosca et al. 2011). Classic risk factors for CVD are gender nonspecific and include insulin resistance/diabetes mellitus, obesity, lack of exercise, tobacco smoking, hypertension, and hyperlipidemia. In 2011, the American Heart Association added preeclampsia (PE), gestational diabetes, and delivery of a growth-restricted child as gender-specific and pregnancy-related risk factors for CVD (Mosca et al. 2011). Women who have suffered from such pregnancy complications are, however, nowadays not routinely followed up after pregnancy, despite recommendations (Mosca et al. 2011).

Pregnancy has been described as a "screening test" for later CVD (Roberts and Catov 2012). It has been proposed that pregnancy could be viewed as a metabolic and vascular "stress test for life" (Williams 2003). According to this concept, a pregnant woman who does not develop gestational syndromes during her pregnancy is in a privileged position with a reduced risk of developing several diseases later in life as compared with a pregnant woman with a gestational syndrome (Sattar and Greer 2002). Women who "fail" the test (developing PE and/or gestational diabetes and/or fetal growth restriction [FGR] and/or preterm delivery) are at increased risk of long-term cardiovascular complications (Magee and von Dadelszen 2007; Newstead, von Dadelszen, and Magee 2007; Roberts and Gammill 2005; Williams 2003).

Many of the major obstetric complications, such as FGR and PE, include placenta pathology, hereafter broadly named "placental dysfunction." Some text books use the term *placental dysfunction* as synonymous with *placenta insufficiency* and define this as the situation when the placenta cannot deliver sufficient nutrients and oxygen to the growing baby. The term *placental dysfunction* is however lacking a uniform definition, and we use the term in this chapter to describe any placenta where the placentation process is impaired and/or the placenta is functioning differently from what is viewed as normal or healthy at that relevant stage of gestation, owing to some form of placental stress (Redman and Sargent 2009). Placental dysfunction may clinically be diagnosed as FGR, altered fetoplacental or uteroplacental blood flow patterns, as well as by placental structural and functional changes. There are, however, no universally accepted criteria that describe what is abnormal, either for single or combined placental parameters.

The preclinical stages of CVD, including foam cell development, fatty streaks, and atherosclerosis, begin early in life and are influenced by modifiable risk factors (Weintraub et al. 2011). Consequently, pregnancy complications involving placenta dysfunction, such as PE and FGR, represent underused opportunities to improve women's cardiovascular health (Rich-Edwards et al. 2014) and, thereby, to reduce society cost in the long run.

17.2 PLACENTAL DYSFUNCTION PATHOPHYSIOLOGY: PE AND FGR

PE has traditionally been defined as a syndrome of pregnancy-induced hypertension (PIH; blood pressure ≥140/90 mm Hg) and proteinuria, developing after gestational week 20 in a previously normotensive woman. Recently, the definition has been expanded to include PIH without proteinuria when associated with the onset of other known features of the syndrome, such as thrombocytopenia, impaired liver function, renal insufficiency, pulmonary edema, or cerebral or visual disturbances (Report of the American College of Obstetricians and Gynecologists' Task Force on Hypertension in Pregnancy 2013). PE affects 3%–5% of pregnancies in industrialized countries and is possibly more frequent in developing countries. PE is a leading cause of maternal death and perinatal morbidity and mortality, causing more than 50,000 maternal deaths annually worldwide (Ghulmiyyah and Sibai 2012). At present, it is "cured" by delivery, which may be premature, with added morbidity and mortality for the newborn. The exact etiology of PE is unknown, but the placenta is central to its pathogenesis, as reviewed by us (Redman and Sargent 2005).

Early- and late-onset PE, pragmatically often defined as a delivery before or after gestational week 37 (or 34), seems to be distinct subtypes differing in many attributes (Staff et al. 2013). Early-onset PE is more often associated with poor remodeling of the uteroplacental arterial blood supply, which occurs during the first half of pregnancy. The normal process of structural adaptation of the spiral arteries is termed *placentation*, while the deficiency that occurs in PE is often described as poor or restricted placentation. The remodeling of the spiral arteries is in early-onset PE, often restricted to the decidual part of the uterine wall, whereas much of the smooth muscle cells remain unremodeled in the deeper myometrial part of the uterine wall. Immunological factors with fetal–maternal interactions are assumed to be important contributors to failed remodeling, contributing to the clinical development of PE, which presents later, usually before 34 weeks. This sequence is described in the two-stage model of PE (Redman 1991). Poor placentation causes dysfunctional placental perfusion and release of placental stress signals to the maternal circulation, which induce excessive maternal vascular inflammation with endothelial dysfunction and the maternal features of PE, including hypertension and proteinuria (Redman and Sargent 2005).

Poor placentation with abnormal spiral artery remodeling is, however, not specific to PE, as it may be present in normotensive pregnancies complicated by FGR (Sheppard and Bonnar 1976) or with partial features such as PIH (without development of proteinuria). Inadequate remodeling of the spiral arteries is proposed to increase the velocity of the blood flow to the placental intervillous space, inducing hydrostatic villous damage and reduced time for extraction of nutrients from the intervillous blood to the fetal circulation (Burton et al. 2009a). Placental villous oxidative stress and endoplasmic reticulum stress may ensue, the latter resulting in the "unfolded protein response" (UPR). UPR turns off protein synthesis and is proposed to account for the small placentas and the association with FGR (Burton et al. 2009b).

Poor placentation may cause FGR, but FGR is not a consistent feature of PE, being confined largely to the early-onset disease and affecting 30% of all preeclamptic pregnancies (Walker 2000). At and beyond term PE, neonates are not growth restricted and even may be large for dates (Xiong et al. 2002). In late-onset PE, where remodeling of the uteroplacental spiral arteries usually appears to have been normal, we have suggested that placental perfusion becomes inadequate because intervillous perfusion is increasingly impaired by compression by the placenta growing in the confined space of the uterine cavity (Redman, Sargent, and Staff 2014).

FGR is usually defined as the failure of the fetus to achieve its genetic growth potential. There are no universally accepted criteria to diagnose FGR in utero or postpartum (Mayer and Joseph 2013), not surprisingly because the full growth potential of any specific fetus cannot be accurately known. Placental dysfunction is not the only cause of FGR, but it is a major one (Mayer and Joseph 2013). Simplified measures of fetal size are often used in epidemiological studies as proxy estimates of FGR unless there is access to definitions based on the use of longitudinal ultrasound assessments of fetal growth and umbilical or uterine arterial blood flow ultrasound Doppler waveforms. Using small for gestational age (SGA), either defined as below 3, 5, or 10 birth weight percentiles, as a proxy for FGR implies that many genetically small fetuses (with normal placenta function) are incorrectly included in this FGR category. The crucial point is that not all SGA fetuses are growth restricted, they are just constitutionally small, nor are all growth-restricted fetuses SGA (Mayer and Joseph 2013).

We have recently reviewed (Redman, Sargent, and Staff 2014) how PE concepts were changed by the discovery of how "proangiogenic" and "antiangiogenic" factors of placental origin (Levine et al. 2006; Maynard et al. 2003, 2005), secondary to placental dysfunction and stress, could contribute to the PE syndrome. These placenta-derived proteins include soluble vascular endothelial growth receptor-1, also known as soluble fms-like tyrosine kinase-1 (sFlt-1), soluble endoglin (sEng), and placental growth factor (PlGF). They have been widely investigated over the last decade as "diagnostic" and prediction biomarkers for PE and other placentally mediated disorders (Chappell et al. 2013; Staff et al. 2013). In PE, typically of early onset, there is often a circulating excess of sFlt-1 and sEng and a deficiency of PlGF compared with normotensive pregnancies. This is proposed to deprive the endothelium of the support of vascular endothelial growth factor (VEGF), which specifically causes glomerular endotheliosis, a virtually pathognomonic lesion of PE. The precision and predictive value of these angiogenic markers are, however, much less precise for late-onset than for early-onset PE (Sunderji et al. 2010; Vatten et al. 2007a). We have proposed that the angiogenic biomarkers of PE are better considered as markers not of PE but of the placental cell (syncytiotrophoblast) stress response (Redman, Sargent, and Staff 2014). The implication is that it is too simplistic to consider them to be specific biomarkers of PE; instead, they are circulating indicators of the state of health of the syncytiotrophoblast, which may be disturbed also in situations other than PE.

It is not understood why some pregnancies with placental dysfunction develop PE, others merely FGR without maternal disease, and others a combination of both (Staff et al. 2013). It is likely that both PE and FGR are unspecific syndromic entities, with overlapping, but not identical, pathophysiological steps. Epidemiologically, pregnancies developing PE seem to have more clinical maternal risk factors, such as obesity, compared with pregnancies with only FGR. Ness and Roberts (1996) argue that both PE and FGR share a complex placenta pathophysiology, but that women with medical disorders that cause chronic endothelial dysfunction will be specifically more at risk for developing the PE syndrome. The use of pregnancy biomarkers does not seem to aid in the distinction between these syndromes, as FGR, similarly to PE, is diagnosed (Benton et al. 2012; Herraiz et al. 2014; Molvarec et al. 2013; Triunfo et al. 2014) and partially predicted (Ghosh et al. 2013; Schoofs et al. 2014) by dysregulated angiogenic factors (elevated sFLt-1 and low PlGF in the maternal circulation).

17.3 PLACENTAL DYSFUNCTION AFFECTS MANY ASPECTS OF MATERNAL AND FETAL LONG-TERM HEALTH

The long-term risks of CVD for women who have had pregnancies complicated by PE and/or FGR are reviewed below. There are, however, also several other long-term effects on the health of both mother and offspring. This includes an increased risk of maternal hypothyroidism (Levine et al. 2009) and premature deliveries (van der Zanden et al. 2013). It is suggested that this association is mediated by the effect of high maternal circulating concentrations of sFlt-1, causing permanent damage to maternal fenestrated endothelium (Levine et al. 2009). As reviewed above, circulating sFlt-1 is elevated in pregnancy and is especially high in most preterm preeclamptic pregnancies (Maynard et al. 2003).

Women with chronic renal disease are at increased risk for developing PE; but PE is in itself also a risk factor for future renal disease. The typical lesion after PE is focal segmental glomerulosclerosis with development of chronic hypertension (Williams 2011). The relative risk of end-stage renal disease is 4.7 after PE in first pregnancy, and the risk augments with repeated PE and offspring low birth weight, as shown in a Norwegian population-based study (Vikse et al. 2008). It is not yet clear how much of this final outcome is directly caused by PE.

Both pregestational diabetes and gestational diabetes mellitus are associated with a two to four times increased risk of developing PE in pregnancy (Barden et al. 2004; Garner et al. 1990; Roach et al. 2000). Also, women with PE have augmented risk for developing type II diabetes after pregnancy (Carr et al. 2009; Libby et al. 2007; Magnussen et al. 2009; Pouta et al. 2004). The association is believed to be mediated through the sharing of many pathophysiological features, including endothelial dysfunction, insulin resistance, oxidative stress, and inflammation (Kaaja 1998; Patrono and FitzGerald 1997; Schram et al. 2003).

In contrast to the increased risk of several chronic diseases after PE, women who have had PE or PIH have a significantly reduced future breast cancer risk compared with women with uncomplicated pregnancies (Troisi et al. 2007; Vatten et al. 2007b).

PE and FGR also affect fetal long-term health, including increased risk of CVD, obesity, diabetes, and hypertension for the offspring (Oglaend et al. 2009; Ozanne, Fernandez-Twinn, and Hales 2004; Tenhola et al. 2003; Vatten et al. 2003), but this important topic is beyond the scope of this chapter.

17.4   LONG-TERM MATERNAL CVD AFTER PLACENTAL DYSFUNCTION: PE AND FGR

A group of common pregnancy complications, including FGR and preterm delivery (often combined as low birth weight), PIH, PE, and gestational diabetes, are associated with increased risk for CVD later in life for the mother (Rich-Edwards et al. 2014). PE and delivery of a growth-restricted baby are independent risk factors for developing CVD, and their risks synergize when both are present (Ness and Sibai 2006). The association strengthens with more severe PE, including early-onset, clinically severe PE, recurrent disease, and neonatal morbidity (Harskamp and Zeeman 2007; Ness and Hubel 2005; Wikstrom et al. 2005). The association strengthens in pregnancies with both maternal and fetal evidence of a placental syndrome, such as PE, PIH, placental abruption, or infarction in combination with FGR (Ray et al. 2005).

As stated above, reduced intrauterine growth is associated with augmented maternal risk for CVD in adult life (Barker 2002, 2006), even when present in a normotensive pregnancy (Davey et al. 1997; Smith, Harding, and Rosato 2000; Smith, Pell, and Walsh 2001). This association is sustained with preterm deliveries without PE development (Catov et al. 2010; Irgens et al. 2001; Smith, Pell, and Walsh 2001). A recent meta-analysis concluded that four of five studies showed that women with a history of preterm birth had twice the risk of CVD death compared with women who had term births, even after excluding pregnancy hypertension (Robbins et al. 2014). Spontaneous preterm labor is a syndrome caused by multiple pathologic processes (Romero, Dey, and Fisher 2014), including PE. Interestingly, women with early-onset PE in their first pregnancy have higher risk of preterm birth in a subsequent "normal pregnancy" (Lain, Krohn, and Roberts 2005), suggesting a potential relationship between PE and spontaneous preterm birth.

The associations between pregnancy and future CVD may be even more complex because mothers of large newborns (<4000–4500 g) may also have increased CVD risk. However, not all studies are consistent and the association may depend on the population prevalence of gestational diabetes mellitus and pregestational diabetes, of which both are known to cause large for gestation babies and an increased long-term CVD risk. Placental weight and birth weight are highly correlated; therefore, it is not surprising that the increased maternal risk of future CVD associated with low birth weight is similar after deliveries with low placental weight (Eskild, Romundstad, and Vatten 2009; Risnes et al. 2009).

The relative risk of future CVD after a pregnancy complicated by PE has been reported varying from 1.3 to 3.3, with a higher risk range of 2.7–8.1 in more severe PE (Newstead, von Dadelszen, and Magee 2007). Also, the association with future CVD strengthens if PE is repeated (Lykke et al. 2009; Wikstrom et al. 2005). When the severity of PE is graded, there appears to be a "dose–response" relationship with future CVD. Women with PIH (without proteinuria) have a moderately elevated CVD risk, similar to the risk of late-onset PE (Bellamy et al. 2007; Ray et al. 2005).

Several large population-based studies have shown that women who have had PE are at increased risk for later CVD, as well as increased risk of premature death later in life, compared with women with healthy pregnancies. A study of 600,000 Norwegian births to primiparous women revealed increased risks of dying of CVD (eightfold) or of stroke (fivefold) after PE and premature delivery (Irgens et al. 2001), but an increase after term PE (1.65-fold). A study by Smith et al. of 130,000 Scottish women demonstrated a twofold risk of CVD after a history of PE as well as a sevenfold risk of CVD if PE was associated with a delivery of a baby below 2.5 kg (Smith, Pell, and Walsh 2001), after adjusting for maternal age, socioeconomic status, and essential hypertension. A systematic review and meta-analysis by Bellamy et al. (2007) of 200,000 PE cases showed twofold risk for hypertension, ischemic heart disease, and cerebrovascular stroke 10 years or more postpartum of PE. A large study by Lykke et al. (2009) from Denmark showed a threefold to sixfold risk for hypertension, correlated to PE severity, with increasing risk if PE is recurrent.

17.5 WHY ARE PLACENTAL DYSFUNCTION AND CVD ASSOCIATED?

One of the most important components of CVD is atherosclerosis. There are two possible explanations to link PE and later CVD, which are not necessarily mutually exclusive. They also encompass the issue of FGR as an independent but closely related risk factor. The first is that PE and atherosclerosis share risk factors for systemic inflammation and endothelial dysfunction, including obesity, dyslipidemia, diabetes mellitus, other insulin resistance, hypertension, endothelial dysfunction, and family history (reviewed in Staff, Dechend, and Pijnenborg 2010). An important paradox is, however, smoking, which is associated with an augmented risk of atherosclerosis and CVD, as well as FGR, but with a reduced risk of PE. The alternative explanation is that pregnancy, in general, and placental dysfunction, in particular, cause permanent cardiovascular changes de novo.

As PE, FGR, and atherosclerotic CVD are syndromes with likely multifactorial pathophysiologies, the interaction between them is also likely to be heterogeneous and may differ between subgroups of placenta dysfunction syndromes. Hence, a dysfunctional placenta may play different roles for the future CVD risk in different patient groups.

17.5.1 SHARED RISK FACTORS FOR PLACENTAL DYSFUNCTION AND CVD

It is well known that conditions that cause systemic vascular (endothelial) inflammation predispose to PE. These include chronic hypertension (Bateman et al. 2012; Zetterstrom et al. 2005) and insulin resistance (Catalano 2010; Valdes et al. 2014) with or without obesity (Bodnar et al. 2007; Mbah et al. 2010) and dyslipidemia (Magnussen et al. 2007), which are also classic risk factors for CVD. Combinations of all these factors are encapsulated in the concept of the metabolic syndrome, which brings a very high risk of PE. Factors that increase the risk of the underlying medical problem that leads on to PE can be expected to lead to an association between PE and later CVD.

Both PE (Redman, Sacks, and Sargent 1999) and atherosclerosis (Ross 1999a,b) are inflammatory diseases and are characterized by augmented circulating concentrations of proinflammatory cytokines, such as interleukin-6 and tumor necrosis factor-α. Acute phase reactants such as C-reactive protein (CRP) (Belo et al. 2003; Braekke et al. 2005; Freeman et al. 2004; Teran et al. 2001; Ustun, Engin-Ustun, and Kamaci 2005) and markers of leukocyte activation are also augmented (Belo et al. 2003; Greer et al. 1989) in both conditions. Elevated CRP levels have been associated with higher risk of CVD (Blake and Ridker 2001; Danesh et al. 1998). There is an increasing understanding that CRP not only is a marker of inflammation but also may have a pathogenic role in atherosclerosis and CVD (Arici and Walls 2001; Blake and Ridker 2001; Pepys and Berger 2001; Yu and Rifai 2000). The association of elevated CRP with CVD risk has, however, been suggested to be mediated mainly through obesity, as metabolic factors are strongly associated with CRP, especially body mass index (Laugsand et al. 2012).

The genetic risk factors for PE and FGR are complex and multifactorial, as are the genetic risk factors for CVD. Nevertheless, it is likely that the conditions share susceptibility genes. In line with this, our findings from our own pregnancy biobank show that women with a polymorphism of the *RGS2* (regulator of G protein signaling) gene (C1114G, *RGS2* 1114G allele) are at augmented risk for PE (Kvehaugen et al. 2013) as well as for future hypertension (Kvehaugen et al. 2014). RGS2 is a member of a large family of regulators of G protein signaling and is involved in the control of blood pressure. Another study has presented novel empirical evidence of possible shared genetic mechanisms underlying both PE and other CVD-related risk factors (Johnson et al. 2013).

17.5.2 Placental Dysfunction as New Risk Factor for CVD

The second theory that links PE and atherosclerotic CVD risk after pregnancy is that pregnancy, especially if complicated by PE, may induce permanent arterial changes, mediating risk for future CVD. In general, many adaptive responses of normal pregnancy, such as insulin resistance, with maternal dyslipidemia, are exaggerated in PE. In PE, there is a dysregulation of lipid metabolism, leading to changes in maternal plasma lipids as compared with normal pregnancy (Hubel et al. 1996; Lorentzen et al. 1995). Hypertriglyceridemia is a prominent component of the changes. But even normal pregnancies are characterized by a degree of maternal dyslipidemia, including hypertriglyceridemia, as compared with nonpregnant fertile women.

It has been suggested that normal pregnancy imposes a transient atherogenic burden in terms of changes in circulating lipids (Martin et al. 1999). The more intense dyslipidemia of PE, compared with normotensive pregnancies, could add even more to such atherogenicity. We suggest that the changes in at least some preeclamptic women could activate lipid-dependent arterial wall inflammation that fails to resolve after delivery, with induction of potential life-long effects.

There is some epidemiological evidence that also normal pregnancies, even without hypertension, could increase the risk of maternal CVD (Lawlor et al. 2003; Ness et al. 1993), whereas this does not seem to be the case for the male partners, after correcting for obesity and metabolic risks (Lawlor et al. 2003). Accordingly, paternal CVD risk factors were not elevated after PE in a Norwegian population-based registry study (Myklestad et al. 2011), in contrast to the situation of the mother. These gender differences between parents of the same pregnancies suggest that the pregnancy metabolic burden is itself a risk factor for multiparous women, increasing the risk of CVD, rather than shared socioeconomic factors per se. As many pregnancies are hyperlipidemic compared with nonpregnancy, a pregnancy per se could be viewed as atherogenic (Martin et al. 1999). PE and gestational diabetes may add to this burden owing to more intense hyperlipidemia.

We speculate that it is possible that a stressed placenta, such as seen in PE and in pregnancies with placentally growth-restricted babies, which includes shedding of proinflammatory (e.g., angiogenic) factors into the maternal circulation, could have potential permanent effects on the maternal vasculature, either directly or indirectly.

As reviewed above, excess maternal circulating sFlt-1 and low PlGF characterize PE, especially of early-onset, secondary to an oxidatively stressed placenta (as reviewed in Staff et al. 2013). Although sFlt-1 falls rapidly after delivery, we (Kvehaugen et al. 2011) and others (Wolf et al. 2004) have shown a persistent modest dysregulation many months and years after a preeclamptic pregnancy. Whether such antiangiogenic balance was also present prepregnancy and/or could mediate later CVD is not known.

Another speculative long-lasting effect after placental dysfunction and dysregulated circulating inflammatory mediators could be an effect on endothelial progenitor cells (EPCs), which are reported to be reduced in PE (Lin et al. 2009). EPCs reflect endothelial health and are reduced in patients with essential hypertension, and their senescence is accelerated. PlGF and VEGF act in concert in adult angiogenesis (Autiero et al. 2003) and increase EPC recruitment, mobilization, as well as survival (Li et al. 2006). Whether a reduction in EPC in pregnancy (and PE) could affect long-term maternal endothelial function and whether such an effect in pregnancy is mediated through an angiogenic imbalance with low circulating maternal VEGF and PlGF are not known.

Based on the findings of a Norwegian population-based study (Helseundersøkelsen i Nord-Trøndelag: The Nord-Trøndelag Health Study [HUNT]) (Romundstad et al. 2010), it was suggested that the contribution of prepregnancy risk factors to long-term cardiovascular risk may be larger than the contribution from a hypertensive pregnancy. We would argue that a paternal effect on placental function and, thereby, fetal and placental weight and risk of PE may, however, be difficult to discern from epidemiological studies. A previous study has, for example, concluded that the risk of PE is augmented in certain combinations of fetal (specifically paternally derived) Human Leukocyte Antigen-C (HLA-C) (expressed on fetal invading trophoblast) and maternal Killer-cell immunoglobulin-like receptors (KIR) receptor (expressed on uterine natural killer cell) genotypes, especially when an HLA-C2 allele was inherited from the father (Hiby et al. 2004). The same group has recently demonstrated that paternal HLA-C genotype regulates fetal birth weight (Hiby et al. 2014), possibly through the effectiveness of uteroplacental artery remodeling processes during placentation.

A mouse model of PE is consistent with the idea that PE may be an independent risk factor for CVD. Experimental PE (induced by overexpression of sFlt-1) showed proteomic changes associated with CVD. This could suggest that long-term adverse outcomes that are associated with PE may be a consequence rather than a mere unmasking of an underlying predisposition (Bytautiene et al. 2013).

Cardiac tissue maladaptation in normal pregnancy, in general, and in preeclamptic pregnancies, in particular, may also be relevant to long-term cardiovascular risk. The hemodynamic work of Melchiorre et al. (2011) supports that early-onset PE may have long-lasting effects on maternal myocardial function.

17.6 A NOVEL HYPOTHESIS LINKING PLACENTAL DYSFUNCTION, UTEROPLACENTAL ACUTE ATHEROSIS, AND MATERNAL CVD

Acute atherosis is a uteroplacental arterial wall lesion that resembles early stages of atherosclerosis and affects many preeclamptic pregnancies (Harsem et al. 2007). The hallmark of uteroplacental acute atherosis is a subendothelial arterial wall lesion with CD68-positive lipid-filled foam cells (Hanssens et al. 1998). As reviewed above, spiral artery remodeling is often defective in PE, particularly in the myometrial segments (Pijnenborg, Vercruysse, and Hanssens 2006), but it also occurs in some cases of FGR, PIH (without proteinuria), and even rarely in normal pregnancy (Staff, Dechend, and Pijnenborg 2010). We have shown that 14% of uncomplicated pregnancies, with presumed normal artery remodeling, may be affected by acute atherosis (Harsem et al. 2007). Acute atherosis narrows spiral artery lumina, exacerbating dysfunctional uteroplacental flow, predisposing to thrombosis and placental infarction (Staff, Dechend, and Pijnenborg 2010) and, thereby, placental dysfunction. We have previously proposed that acute atherosis may represent an accelerated process that resembles the early stages of atherosclerosis, developing during the few months of pregnancy owing to excessive pregnancy-induced vascular inflammation of normal pregnancy but more particularly of PE (Staff and Redman 2014; Staff et al. 2014). We have suggested that the presence of acute atherosis in the uteroplacental spiral arteries, identified after delivery, may identify a subset of women that are more susceptible to CVD later in life (Staff, Dechend, and Pijnenborg 2010; Staff, Dechend, and Redman 2013; Staff and Redman 2014; Staff et al. 2014). If our work confirms this, women affected by acute atherosis could receive appropriate follow-up postpartum with the option of preventive medication and management if these can be proved to be beneficial in future well-designed randomized controlled trials.

17.7 WHY AND HOW TO FOLLOW-UP WITH WOMEN AFTER PLACENTA-RELATED PREGNANCY COMPLICATIONS

In 2011, The American Heart Association added pregnancy complications such as PE, gestational diabetes, and delivery of a growth-restricted child to the list of risk factors for developing CVD (Mosca et al. 2011). It has been recommended that these women, failing the "stress test" of pregnancy, should be followed up with after pregnancy for CVD risk (Mosca et al. 2011). Such routine follow-up is, however, not the standard of care globally today, including in the United States and Europe. We suggest that information on pregnancy outcome and placenta function could be used to identify women at risk for severe CVD, up to decades before clinical disease, enabling follow-up and targeted intervention.

A major challenge in the long-term follow-up of women with previous pregnancies involving placental dysfunction is that there is little evidence-based knowledge regarding efficient strategies for intensified follow-up or intervention. The advice for clinical follow-up of women with previous PE or FGR with regard to increased risks in the next pregnancy is more standardized and includes intake of low-dose aspirin to reduce risk of recurrent PE in high-risk pregnancies (Report of the American College of Obstetricians and Gynecologists' Task Force on Hypertension in Pregnancy 2013; Visintin et al. 2010). Whether avoiding repeated PE or FGR also reduces the risk for future CVD is unknown.

A challenge is that there is currently no population-based follow-up studies that have assessed the costs–benefits of cardiovascular evaluation and follow-up of women with previous placental dysfunction pregnancies. Also, whether the use of pregnancy or postpartum biomarkers, either placenta derived or cardiovascular derived, such as sFlt1-1 (Kvehaugen et al. 2011) or Mid-regional Pro-atrial Natriuretic Peptide (MRproANP) (Sugulle et al. 2012), would aid in stratifying women at risk for CVD for more targeted follow-up and intervention is not known.

The revised guidelines from the American College of Obstetrics and Gynecologists (Report of the American College of Obstetricians and Gynecologists' Task Force on Hypertension in Pregnancy 2013) suggest that women with previous PE delivered preterm (before gestational week 37) or repeated PE should be followed for augmented CVD risk, with yearly assessment of blood pressure, lipid and fasting blood glucose levels, and body mass index. This recommendation is characterized as "qualified," although the quality of evidence for the recommendation is graded as "low" ("despite clear evidence for the association"). The task force does not suggest any differences between the premenopausal and postmenopausal follow-up in these women, although the CVD risk is much larger in the latter group, whereas the first group may possibly profit more from potential long-term interventions and prophylaxis. Also, "the task force cautiously recommends lifestyle modification," which includes maintaining healthy weight, increasing physical activity, and not smoking (Report of the American College of Obstetricians and Gynecologists' Task Force on Hypertension in Pregnancy 2013). There is no reason why such recommendations should not be offered to any woman or man in general; the challenge is, of course, that the general population not always follows the best intended health recommendations. If we had more specific markers for a woman at risk for increased future CVD, we could offer improved individualized follow-up of women at risk after delivery. In addition to intensified prophylactic advice, including weight control and physical exercise, we could do more than closely follow up women at risk. As early stages of atherosclerosis is reversible, we could also offer early intervention randomized controlled trials (for example, with statins and metformin) to women at excessive risk for future CVD, aiming at identifying improved prophylactic options. The hope is that intensified follow-up and prevention will reduce the risk for and severity of cardiovascular morbidity in these women. Thus, the use of pregnancy information and placental function could have effects many decades after pregnancy.

17.8 CONCLUSIONS

Despite the clearly documented increased risk of CVD after a pregnancy complicated by PE or FGR, we lack today a mechanistic understanding of the association and also an appropriate targeting of the women at highest risk. We propose that the placental dysfunction in preeclamptic and growth-restricted pregnancies could add to the future CVD burden by disseminating factors that may directly or indirectly affect long-term vascular health. Despite no available evidence-based studies, it seems rational to advice women after PE to keep a healthy weigh (BMI <25 kg/m^2) and to perform physical exercise, with the aim to reduce CVD risk factors, in addition to smoke cessation advice. Further research is needed to ascertain whether women with previous PE or FGR benefit from prevention strategies, such as oral statins, similarly to other population groups at CVD risk.

We recommend all health personnel, in general, and those involved in preventive medicine, in particular, to ask their patients about pregnancy complications (Roberts and Catov 2012) and to increase the follow-up of patients at CVD risk. This information can prove vital to the future health of the woman and may reduce the large costs that CVD mediates for the woman, her family, and for the society in general. We argue that pregnancy information can be used to create healthier and more productive societies.

REFERENCES

Ahmed R, Dunford J, Mehran R, Robson S, and Kunadian V. 2014. Pre-eclampsia and future cardiovascular risk among women: A review. *J. Am. Coll. Cardiol.* 63 (18): 1815–1822.

Arici M and Walls J. 2001. End-stage renal disease, atherosclerosis, and cardiovascular mortality: Is C-reactive protein the missing link? *Kidney Int.* 59 (2): 407–414.

Autiero M, Waltenberger J, Communi D, Kranz A, Moons L, Lambrechts D, Kroll J, Plaisance S, De Mol M, Bono F, Kliche S, Fellbrich G, Ballmer-Hofer K, Maglione D, Mayr-Beyrle U, Dewerchin M, Dombrowski S, Stanimirovic D, Van Hummelen P, Dehio C, Hicklin DJ, Persico G, Herbert JM, Communi D, Shibuya M, Collen D, Conway EM, and Carmeliet P. 2003. Role of PlGF in the intra- and intermolecular cross talk between the VEGF receptors Flt1 and Flk1. *Nat. Med.* 9 (7): 936–943.

Barden A, Singh R, Walters BN, Ritchie J, Roberman B, and Beilin LJ. 2004. Factors predisposing to preeclampsia in women with gestational diabetes. *J. Hypertens.* 22 (12): 2371–2378.

Barker DJ. 2002. Fetal programming of coronary heart disease. *Trends Endocrinol. Metab.* 13 (9): 364–368.

Barker DJ. 2006. Adult consequences of fetal growth restriction. *Clin. Obstet. Gynecol.* 49 (2): 270–283.

Bateman BT, Bansil P, Hernandez-Diaz S, Mhyre JM, Callaghan WM, and Kuklina EV. 2012. Prevalence, trends, and outcomes of chronic hypertension: A nationwide sample of delivery admissions. *Am. J. Obstet. Gynecol.* 206 (2): 134–138.

Bellamy L, Casas JP, Hingorani AD, and Williams DJ. 2007. Pre-eclampsia and risk of cardiovascular disease and cancer in later life: Systematic review and meta-analysis. *BMJ* 335 (7627): 974.

Belo L, Santos-Silva A, Caslake M, Cooney J, Pereira-Leite L, Quintanilha A, and Rebelo I. 2003. Neutrophil activation and C-reactive protein concentration in preeclampsia. *Hypertens. Pregnancy* 22 (2): 129–141.

Benton SJ, Hu Y, Xie F, Kupfer K, Lee SW, Magee LA, and von Dadelszen P. 2012. Can placental growth factor in maternal circulation identify fetuses with placental intrauterine growth restriction? *Am. J. Obstet. Gynecol.* 206 (2): 163–167.

Blake GJ and Ridker PM. 2001. Novel clinical markers of vascular wall inflammation. *Circ. Res.* 89 (9): 763–771.

Bodnar LM, Catov JM, Klebanoff MA, Ness RB, and Roberts JM. 2007. Prepregnancy body mass index and the occurrence of severe hypertensive disorders of pregnancy. *Epidemiology* 18 (2): 234–239.

Braekke K, Holthe MR, Harsem NK, Fagerhol MK, and Staff AC. 2005. Calprotectin, a marker of inflammation, is elevated in the maternal but not in the fetal circulation in preeclampsia. *Am. J. Obstet. Gynecol.* 193 (1): 227–233.

Burton GJ, Woods AW, Jauniaux E, and Kingdom JC. 2009a. Rheological and physiological consequences of conversion of the maternal spiral arteries for uteroplacental blood flow during human pregnancy. *Placenta* 30 (6): 473–482.

Burton GJ, Yung HW, Cindrova-Davies T, and Charnock-Jones DS. 2009b. Placental endoplasmic reticulum stress and oxidative stress in the pathophysiology of unexplained intrauterine growth restriction and early onset preeclampsia. *Placenta* 30 Suppl A: S43–S48.

Bytautiene E, Bulayeva N, Bhat G, Li L, Rosenblatt KP, and Saade GR. 2013. Long-term alterations in maternal plasma proteome after sFlt1-induced preeclampsia in mice. *Am. J. Obstet. Gynecol.* 208 (5): 388.

Carr DB, Newton KM, Utzschneider KM, Tong J, Gerchman F, Kahn SE, Easterling TR, and Heckbert SR. 2009. Preeclampsia and risk of developing subsequent diabetes. *Hypertens. Pregnancy* 28 (4): 435–447.

Catalano PM. 2010. Obesity, insulin resistance, and pregnancy outcome. *Reproduction* 140 (3): 365–371.

Catov JM, Wu CS, Olsen J, Sutton-Tyrrell K, Li J, and Nohr EA. 2010. Early or recurrent preterm birth and maternal cardiovascular disease risk. *Ann. Epidemiol.* 20 (8): 604–609.

Chappell LC, Duckworth S, Seed PT, Griffin M, Myers J, Mackillop L, Simpson N, Waugh J, Anumba D, Kenny LC, Redman CW, and Shennan AH. 2013. Diagnostic accuracy of placental growth factor in women with suspected preeclampsia: A prospective multicenter study. *Circulation* 128 (19): 2121–2131.

Danesh J, Collins R, Appleby P, and Peto R. 1998. Association of fibrinogen, C-reactive protein, albumin, or leukocyte count with coronary heart disease: Meta-analyses of prospective studies. *JAMA* 279 (18): 1477–1482.

Davey SG, Hart C, Ferrell C, Upton M, Hole D, Hawthorne V, and Watt G. 1997. Birth weight of offspring and mortality in the Renfrew and Paisley study: Prospective observational study. *BMJ* 315 (7117): 1189–1193.

Eskild A, Romundstad PR, and Vatten LJ. 2009. Placental weight and birthweight: Does the association differ between pregnancies with and without preeclampsia? *Am. J. Obstet. Gynecol.* 201 (6): 595.

Freeman DJ, McManus F, Brown EA, Cherry L, Norrie J, Ramsay JE, Clark P, Walker ID, Sattar N, and Greer IA. 2004. Short- and long-term changes in plasma inflammatory markers associated with preeclampsia. *Hypertension* 44 (5): 708–714.

Garner PR, D'Alton ME, Dudley DK, Huard P, and Hardie M. 1990. Preeclampsia in diabetic pregnancies. *Am. J. Obstet. Gynecol.* 163 (2): 505–508.

Ghosh SK, Raheja S, Tuli A, Raghunandan C, and Agarwal S. 2013. Can maternal serum placental growth factor estimation in early second trimester predict the occurrence of early onset preeclampsia and/or early onset intrauterine growth restriction? A prospective cohort study. *J. Obstet. Gynaecol. Res.* 39 (5): 881–890.

Ghulmiyyah L and Sibai B. 2012. Maternal mortality from preeclampsia/eclampsia. *Semin. Perinatol.* 36 (1): 56–59.

Greer IA, Haddad NG, Dawes J, Johnstone FD, and Calder AA. 1989. Neutrophil activation in pregnancy-induced hypertension. *Br. J. Obstet. Gynaecol.* 96 (8): 978–982.

Hanssens M, Pijnenborg R, Keirse MJ, Vercruysse L, Verbist L, and Van Assche FA. 1998. Renin-like immunoreactivity in uterus and placenta from normotensive and hypertensive pregnancies. *Eur. J. Obstet. Gynecol. Reprod. Biol.* 81 (2): 177–184.

Harsem NK, Roald B, Braekke K, and Staff AC. 2007. Acute atherosis in decidual tissue: Not associated with systemic oxidative stress in preeclampsia. *Placenta* 28 (8–9): 958–964.

Harskamp RE and Zeeman GG. 2007. Preeclampsia: At risk for remote cardiovascular disease. *Am. J. Med. Sci.* 334 (4): 291–295.

Herraiz I, Droge LA, Gomez-Montes E, Henrich W, Galindo A, and Verlohren S. 2014. Characterization of the soluble fms-like tyrosine kinase-1 to placental growth factor ratio in pregnancies complicated by fetal growth restriction. *Obstet. Gynecol.* 124 (2 Pt 1): 265–273.

Hiby SE, Walker JJ, O'Shaughnessy KM, Redman CW, Carrington M, Trowsdale J, and Moffett A. 2004. Combinations of maternal KIR and fetal HLA-C genes influence the risk of preeclampsia and reproductive success. *J. Exp. Med.* 200 (8): 957–965.

Hiby SE, Apps R, Chazara O, Farrell LE, Magnus P, Trogstad L, Gjessing HK, Carrington M, and Moffett A. 2014. Maternal KIR in combination with paternal HLA-C2 regulate human birth weight. *J. Immunol.* 192 (11): 5069–5073.

Hubel CA, McLaughlin MK, Evans RW, Hauth BA, Sims CJ, and Roberts JM. 1996. Fasting serum triglycerides, free fatty acids, and malondialdehyde are increased in preeclampsia, are positively correlated, and decrease within 48 hours post partum. *Am. J. Obstet. Gynecol.* 174 (3): 975–982.

Irgens HU, Reisaeter L, Irgens LM, and Lie RT. 2001. Long term mortality of mothers and fathers after preeclampsia: Population based cohort study. *BMJ* 323 (7323): 1213–1217.

Johnson MP, Brennecke SP, East CE, Dyer TD, Roten LT, Proffitt JM, Melton PE, Fenstad MH, Aalto-Viljakainen T, Makikallio K, Heinonen S, Kajantie E, Kere J, Laivuori H, Austgulen R, Blangero J, and Moses EK. 2013. Genetic dissection of the pre-eclampsia susceptibility locus on chromosome 2q22 reveals shared novel risk factors for cardiovascular disease. *Mol. Hum. Reprod.* 19 (7): 423–437.

Kaaja R. 1998. Insulin resistance syndrome in preeclampsia. *Sem. Reprod. Endocrinol.* 16 (1): 41–46.

Kvehaugen AS, Dechend R, Ramstad HB, Troisi R, Fugelseth D, and Staff AC. 2011. Endothelial function and circulating biomarkers are disturbed in women and children after preeclampsia. *Hypertension* 58 (1): 63–69.

Kvehaugen AS, Melien O, Holmen O, Dechend R, Laivuori H, Oian P, Andersgaard A, and Staff A. 2013. Single nucleotide polymorphisms in G protein signaling pathway genes in preeclampsia. *Hypertension.* 61 (3): 655–661.

Kvehaugen AS, Melien O, Holmen OL, Laivuori H, Dechend R, and Staff AC. 2014. Hypertension after preeclampsia and relation to the C1114G polymorphism (rs4606) in RGS2: Data from the Norwegian HUNT2 study. *BMC. Med. Genet.* 15: 28.

Lain KY, Krohn MA, and Roberts JM. 2005. Second pregnancy outcomes following preeclampsia in a first pregnancy. *Hypertens. Pregnancy* 24 (2): 159–169.

Laugsand LE, Asvold BO, Vatten LJ, Romundstad PR, Wiseth R, Hveem K, and Janszky I. 2012. Metabolic factors and high-sensitivity C-reactive protein: The HUNT study. *Eur. J. Prev. Cardiol.* 19 (5): 1101–1110.

Lawlor DA, Emberson JR, Ebrahim S, Whincup PH, Wannamethee SG, Walker M, and Smith GD. 2003. Is the association between parity and coronary heart disease due to biological effects of pregnancy or adverse lifestyle risk factors associated with child-rearing? Findings from the British Women's Heart and Health Study and the British Regional Heart Study. *Circulation* 107 (9): 1260–1264.

Lawton JS. 2011. Sex and gender differences in coronary artery disease. *Semin. Thorac. Cardiovasc. Surg.* 23 (2): 126–130.

Levine RJ, Lam C, Qian C, Yu KF, Maynard SE, Sachs BP, Sibai BM, Epstein FH, Romero R, Thadhani R, and Karumanchi SA. 2006. Soluble endoglin and other circulating antiangiogenic factors in preeclampsia. *N. Engl. J. Med.* 355 (10): 992–1005.

Levine RJ, Vatten LJ, Horowitz GL, Qian C, Romundstad PR, Yu KF, Hollenberg AN, Hellevik AI, Asvold BO, and Karumanchi SA. 2009. Pre-eclampsia, soluble fms-like tyrosine kinase 1, and the risk of reduced thyroid function: Nested case-control and population based study. *BMJ* 339: b4336.

Li B, Sharpe EE, Maupin AB, Teleron AA, Pyle AL, Carmeliet P, and Young PP. 2006. VEGF and PlGF promote adult vasculogenesis by enhancing EPC recruitment and vessel formation at the site of tumor neovascularization. *FASEB J.* 20 (9): 1495–1497.

Libby G, Murphy DJ, McEwan NF, Greene SA, Forsyth JS, Chien PW, and Morris AD. 2007. Pre-eclampsia and the later development of type 2 diabetes in mothers and their children: An intergenerational study from the Walker cohort. *Diabetologia* 50 (3): 523–530.

Lin C, Rajakumar A, Plymire DA, Verma V, Markovic N, and Hubel CA. 2009. Maternal Endothelial progenitor colony-forming units with macrophage characteristics are reduced in preeclampsia. *Am. J. Hypertens.* 22 (9): 1014–1019.

Lorentzen B, Drevon CA, Endresen MJ, and Henriksen T. 1995. Fatty acid pattern of esterified and free fatty acids in sera of women with normal and pre-eclamptic pregnancy. *Br. J. Obstet. Gynaecol.* 102 (7): 530–537.

Lykke JA, Langhoff-Roos J, Sibai BM, Funai EF, Triche EW, and Paidas MJ. 2009. Hypertensive pregnancy disorders and subsequent cardiovascular morbidity and type 2 diabetes mellitus in the mother. *Hypertension* 53 (6): 944–951.

Magee LA and von Dadelszen P. 2007. Pre-eclampsia and increased cardiovascular risk. *BMJ* 335 (7627): 945–946.

Magnussen EB, Vatten LJ, Lund-Nilsen TI, Salvesen KA, Davey SG, and Romundstad PR. 2007. Prepregnancy cardiovascular risk factors as predictors of pre-eclampsia: Population based cohort study. *BMJ* 335 (7627): 978.

Magnussen EB, Vatten LJ, Smith GD, and Romundstad PR. 2009. Hypertensive disorders in pregnancy and subsequently measured cardiovascular risk factors. *Obstet. Gynecol.* 114 (5): 961–970.

Martin U, Davies C, Hayavi S, Hartland A, and Dunne F. 1999. Is normal pregnancy atherogenic? *Clin. Sci. (Lond.)* 96 (4): 421–425.

Mayer C and Joseph KS. 2013. Fetal growth: A review of terms, concepts and issues relevant to obstetrics. *Ultrasound Obstet. Gynecol.* 41 (2): 136–145.

Maynard SE, Min JY, Merchan J, Lim KH, Li J, Mondal S, Libermann TA, Morgan JP, Sellke FW, Stillman IE, Epstein FH, Sukhatme VP, and Karumanchi SA. 2003. Excess placental soluble fms-like tyrosine kinase 1 (sFlt1) may contribute to endothelial dysfunction, hypertension, and proteinuria in preeclampsia. *J. Clin. Invest.* 111 (5): 649–658.

Maynard SE, Venkatesha S, Thadhani R, and Karumanchi SA. 2005. Soluble Fms-like tyrosine kinase 1 and endothelial dysfunction in the pathogenesis of preeclampsia. *Pediatr. Res.* 57 (5 Pt 2): 1R–7R.

Mbah AK, Kornosky JL, Kristensen S, August EM, Alio AP, Marty PJ, Belogolovkin V, Bruder K, and Salihu HM. 2010. Super-obesity and risk for early and late pre-eclampsia. *BJOG* 117 (8): 997–1004.

Melchiorre K, Sutherland GR, Liberati M, and Thilaganathan B. 2011. Preeclampsia is associated with persistent postpartum cardiovascular impairment. *Hypertension* 58 (4): 709–715.

Molvarec A, Gullai N, Stenczer B, Fugedi G, Nagy B, and Rigo J, Jr. 2013. Comparison of placental growth factor and fetal flow Doppler ultrasonography to identify fetal adverse outcomes in women with hypertensive disorders of pregnancy: An observational study. *BMC Pregnancy Childbirth* 13: 161.

Mosca L, Benjamin EJ, Berra K, Bezanson JL, Dolor RJ, Lloyd-Jones DM, Newby LK, Pina IL, Roger VL, Shaw LJ, Zhao D, Beckie TM, Bushnell C, D'Armiento J, Kris-Etherton PM, Fang J, Ganiats TG, Gomes AS, Gracia CR, Haan CK, Jackson EA, Judelson DR, Kelepouris E, Lavie CJ, Moore A, Nussmeier NA, Ofili E, Oparil S, Ouyang P, Pinn VW, Sherif K, Smith SC, Jr., Sopko G, Chandra-Strobos N, Urbina EM, Vaccarino V, and Wenger NK. 2011. Effectiveness-based guidelines for the prevention of cardiovascular disease in women—2011 update: A guideline from the American Heart Association. *Circulation* 123 (11): 1243–1262.

Myklestad K, Vatten LJ, Salvesen KA, Davey SG, and Romundstad PR. 2011. Hypertensive disorders in pregnancy and paternal cardiovascular risk: A population-based study. *Ann. Epidemiol.* 21 (6): 407–412.

Ness RB and Roberts JM. 1996. Heterogeneous causes constituting the single syndrome of preeclampsia: A hypothesis and its implications. *Am. J. Obstet. Gynecol.* 175 (5): 1365–1370.

Ness RB and Hubel CA. 2005. Risk for coronary artery disease and morbid preeclampsia: A commentary. *Ann. Epidemiol.* 15 (9): 726–733.

Ness RB and Sibai BM. 2006. Shared and disparate components of the pathophysiologies of fetal growth restriction and preeclampsia. *Am. J. Obstet. Gynecol.* 195 (1): 40–49.

Ness RB, Harris T, Cobb J, Flegal KM, Kelsey JL, Balanger A, Stunkard AJ, and D'Agostino RB. 1993. Number of pregnancies and the subsequent risk of cardiovascular disease. *N. Engl. J. Med.* 328 (21): 1528–1533.

Newstead J, von Dadelszen P, and Magee LA. 2007. Preeclampsia and future cardiovascular risk. *Expert Rev. Cardiovasc. Ther.* 5 (2): 283–294.

Oglaend B, Forman MR, Romundstad PR, Nilsen ST, and Vatten LJ. 2009. Blood pressure in early adolescence in the offspring of preeclamptic and normotensive pregnancies. *J. Hypertens.* 27 (10): 2051–2054.

Ozanne SE, Fernandez-Twinn D, and Hales CN. 2004. Fetal growth and adult diseases. *Semin. Perinatol.* 28 (1): 81–87.

Patrono C and FitzGerald GA. 1997. Isoprostanes: Potential markers of oxidant stress in atherothrombotic disease. *Arterioscler. Thromb. Vasc. Biol.* 17 (11): 2309–2315.

Pepys MB and Berger A. 2001. The renaissance of C reactive protein. *BMJ* 322 (7277): 4–5.

Pijnenborg R, Vercruysse L, and Hanssens M. 2006. The uterine spiral arteries in human pregnancy: Facts and controversies. *Placenta* 27 (9–10): 939–958.

Pouta A, Hartikainen AL, Sovio U, Gissler M, Laitinen J, McCarthy MI, Ruokonen A, Elliott P, and Jarvelin MR. 2004. Manifestations of metabolic syndrome after hypertensive pregnancy. *Hypertension* 43 (4): 825–831.

Ray JG, Vermeulen MJ, Schull MJ, and Redelmeier DA. 2005. Cardiovascular health after maternal placental syndromes (CHAMPS): Population-based retrospective cohort study. *Lancet* 366 (9499): 1797–1803.

Redman CW. 1991. Current topic: Pre-eclampsia and the placenta. *Placenta* 12 (4): 301–308.

Redman CW and Sargent IL. 2005. Latest advances in understanding preeclampsia. *Science* 308 (5728): 1592–1594.

Redman CW and Sargent IL. 2009. Placental stress and pre-eclampsia: A revised view. *Placenta* 30 Suppl A: S38–S42.

Redman CW, Sacks GP, and Sargent IL. 1999. Preeclampsia: An excessive maternal inflammatory response to pregnancy. *Am. J. Obstet. Gynecol.* 180 (2 Pt 1): 499–506.

Redman CW, Sargent IL, and Staff AC. 2014. IFPA Senior Award Lecture: Making sense of pre-eclampsia—Two placental causes of preeclampsia? *Placenta* 35 Suppl: S20–S25.

Report of the American College of Obstetricians and Gynecologists' Task Force on Hypertension in Pregnancy. 2013. Hypertension in pregnancy. *Obstet. Gynecol.* 122 (5): 1122–1131.

Rich-Edwards JW, Fraser A, Lawlor DA, and Catov JM. 2014. Pregnancy characteristics and women's future cardiovascular health: An underused opportunity to improve women's health? *Epidemiol. Rev.* 36 (1): 57–70.

Risnes KR, Romundstad PR, Nilsen TI, Eskild A, and Vatten LJ. 2009. Placental weight relative to birth weight and long-term cardiovascular mortality: Findings from a cohort of 31,307 men and women. *Am. J. Epidemiol.* 170 (5): 622–631.

Roach VJ, Hin LY, Tam WH, Ng KB, and Rogers MS. 2000. The incidence of pregnancy-induced hypertension among patients with carbohydrate intolerance. *Hypertens. Pregnancy* 19 (2): 183–189.

Robbins CL, Hutchings Y, Dietz PM, Kuklina EV, and Callaghan WM. 2014. History of preterm birth and subsequent cardiovascular disease: A systematic review. *Am. J. Obstet. Gynecol.* 210 (4): 285–297.

Roberts JM and Gammill H. 2005. Pre-eclampsia and cardiovascular disease in later life. *Lancet* 366 (9490): 961–962.

Roberts JM and Catov JM. 2012. Pregnancy is a screening test for later life cardiovascular disease: Now what? Research recommendations. *Womens Health Issues* 22 (2): e123–e128.

Romero R, Dey SK, and Fisher SJ. 2014. Preterm labor: One syndrome, many causes. *Science* 345 (6198): 760–765.

Romundstad PR, Magnussen EB, Smith GD, and Vatten LJ. 2010. Hypertension in pregnancy and later cardiovascular risk: Common antecedents? *Circulation* 122 (6): 579–584.

Ross R. 1999a. Atherosclerosis is an inflammatory disease. *Am. Heart J.* 138 (5 Pt 2): S419–S420.

Ross R. 1999b. Atherosclerosis—An inflammatory disease. *N. Engl. J. Med.* 340 (2): 115–126.

Sattar N and Greer IA. 2002. Pregnancy complications and maternal cardiovascular risk: Opportunities for intervention and screening? *BMJ* 325 (7356): 157–160.

Schoofs K, Grittner U, Engels T, Pape J, Denk B, Henrich W, and Verlohren S. 2014. The importance of repeated measurements of the sFlt-1/PlGF ratio for the prediction of preeclampsia and intrauterine growth restriction. *J. Perinat. Med.* 42 (1): 61–68.

Schram MT, Chaturvedi N, Schalkwijk C, Giorgino F, Ebeling P, Fuller JH, and Stehouwer CD. 2003. Vascular risk factors and markers of endothelial function as determinants of inflammatory markers in type 1 diabetes: The EURODIAB Prospective Complications Study. *Diabetes Care* 26 (7): 2165–2173.

Sheppard BL and Bonnar J. 1976. The ultrastructure of the arterial supply of the human placenta in pregnancy complicated by fetal growth retardation. *Br. J. Obstet. Gynaecol.* 83 (12): 948–959.

Smith GD, Harding S, and Rosato M. 2000. Relation between infants' birth weight and mothers' mortality: Prospective observational study. *BMJ* 320 (7238): 839–840.

Smith GC, Pell JP, and Walsh D. 2001. Pregnancy complications and maternal risk of ischaemic heart disease: A retrospective cohort study of 129,290 births. *Lancet* 357 (9273): 2002–2006.

Staff AC and Redman CW. 2014. IFPA Award in Placentology Lecture: Preeclampsia, the decidual battleground and future maternal cardiovascular disease. *Placenta* 35 Suppl: S26–S31.

Staff AC, Dechend R, and Pijnenborg R. 2010. Learning from the placenta: Acute atherosis and vascular remodeling in preeclampsia—Novel aspects for atherosclerosis and future cardiovascular health. *Hypertension* 56 (6): 1026–1034.

Staff AC, Benton SJ, von DP, Roberts JM, Taylor RN, Powers RW, Charnock-Jones DS, and Redman CW. 2013. Redefining preeclampsia using placenta-derived biomarkers. *Hypertension* 61 (5): 932–942.

Staff AC, Dechend R, and Redman CW. 2013. Review: Preeclampsia, acute atherosis of the spiral arteries and future cardiovascular disease: Two new hypotheses. *Placenta* 34 Suppl: S73–S78.

Staff AC, Johnsen GM, Dechend R, and Redman CW. 2014. Preeclampsia and uteroplacental acute atherosis: Immune and inflammatory factors. *J. Reprod. Immunol.* 101–102: 120–126.

Sugulle M, Herse F, Hering L, Mockel M, Dechend R, and Staff AC. 2012. Cardiovascular biomarker midregional proatrial natriuretic peptide during and after preeclamptic pregnancies. *Hypertension* 59 (2): 395–401.

Sunderji S, Gaziano E, Wothe D, Rogers LC, Sibai B, Karumanchi SA, and Hodges-Savola C. 2010. Automated assays for sVEGF R1 and PlGF as an aid in the diagnosis of preterm preeclampsia: A prospective clinical study. *Am. J. Obstet. Gynecol.* 202 (1): 40–47.

Tenhola S, Rahiala E, Martikainen A, Halonen P, and Voutilainen R. 2003. Blood pressure, serum lipids, fasting insulin, and adrenal hormones in 12-year-old children born with maternal preeclampsia. *J. Clin. Endocrinol. Metab.* 88 (3): 1217–1222.

Teran E, Escudero C, Moya W, Flores M, Vallance P, and Lopez-Jaramillo P. 2001. Elevated C-reactive protein and pro-inflammatory cytokines in Andean women with pre-eclampsia. *Int. J. Gynaecol. Obstet.* 75 (3): 243–249.

Triunfo S, Lobmaier S, Parra-Saavedra M, Crovetto F, Peguero A, Nadal A, Gratacos E, and Figueras F. 2014. Angiogenic factors at diagnosis of late-onset small-for-gestational age and histological placental underperfusion. *Placenta* 35 (6): 398–403.

Troisi R, Innes KE, Roberts JM, and Hoover RN. 2007. Preeclampsia and maternal breast cancer risk by offspring gender: Do elevated androgen concentrations play a role? *Br. J. Cancer* 97 (5): 688–690.

Ustun Y, Engin-Ustun Y, and Kamaci M. 2005. Association of fibrinogen and C-reactive protein with severity of preeclampsia. *Eur. J. Obstet. Gynecol. Reprod. Biol.* 121 (2): 154–158.

Valdes E, Sepulveda-Martinez A, Manukian B, and Parra-Cordero M. 2014. Assessment of pregestational insulin resistance as a risk factor of preeclampsia. *Gynecol. Obstet. Invest.* 77 (2): 111–116.

van der Zanden M, Hop-de Groot RJ, Sweep FC, Ross HA, den Heijer M, and Spaanderman ME. 2013. Subclinical hypothyroidism after vascular complicated pregnancy. *Hypertens. Pregnancy* 32 (1): 1–10.

Vatten LJ, Romundstad PR, Holmen TL, Hsieh CC, Trichopoulos D, and Stuver SO. 2003. Intrauterine exposure to preeclampsia and adolescent blood pressure, body size, and age at menarche in female offspring. *Obstet. Gynecol.* 101 (3): 529–533.

Vatten LJ, Eskild A, Nilsen TI, Jeansson S, Jenum PA, and Staff AC. 2007a. Changes in circulating level of angiogenic factors from the first to second trimester as predictors of preeclampsia. *Am. J. Obstet. Gynecol.* 196 (3): 239–236.

Vatten LJ, Forman MR, Nilsen TI, Barrett JC, and Romundstad PR. 2007b. The negative association between preeclampsia and breast cancer risk may depend on the offspring's gender. *Br. J. Cancer* 96 (9): 1436–1438.

Vikse BE, Irgens LM, Leivestad T, Skjaerven R, and Iversen BM. 2008. Preeclampsia and the risk of end-stage renal disease. *N. Engl. J. Med.* 359 (8): 800–809.

Visintin C, Mugglestone MA, Almerie MQ, Nherera LM, James D, and Walkinshaw S. 2010. Management of hypertensive disorders during pregnancy: Summary of NICE guidance. *BMJ* 341: c2207.

Walker JJ. 2000. Pre-eclampsia. *Lancet* 356 (9237): 1260–1265.

Weintraub WS, Daniels SR, Burke LE, Franklin BA, Goff DC, Jr., Hayman LL, Lloyd-Jones D, Pandey DK, Sanchez EJ, Schram AP, and Whitsel LP. 2011. Value of primordial and primary prevention for cardiovascular disease: A policy statement from the American Heart Association. *Circulation* 124 (8): 967–990.

Wikstrom AK, Haglund B, Olovsson M, and Lindeberg SN. 2005. The risk of maternal ischaemic heart disease after gestational hypertensive disease. *BJOG* 112 (11): 1486–1491.

Williams D. 2003. Pregnancy: A stress test for life. *Curr. Opin. Obstet. Gynecol.* 15 (6): 465–471.

Williams D. 2011. Long-term complications of preeclampsia. *Semin. Nephrol.* 31 (1): 111–122.

Wolf M, Hubel CA, Lam C, Sampson M, Ecker JL, Ness RB, Rajakumar A, Daftary A, Shakir AS, Seely EW, Roberts JM, Sukhatme VP, Karumanchi SA, and Thadhani R. 2004. Preeclampsia and future cardiovascular disease: Potential role of altered angiogenesis and insulin resistance. *J. Clin. Endocrinol. Metab.* 89 (12): 6239–6243.

Xiong X, Demianczuk NN, Saunders LD, Wang FL, and Fraser WD. 2002. Impact of preeclampsia and gestational hypertension on birth weight by gestational age. *Am. J. Epidemiol.* 155 (3): 203–209.

Yu H and Rifai N. 2000. High-sensitivity C-reactive protein and atherosclerosis: From theory to therapy. *Clin. Biochem.* 33 (8): 601–610.

Zetterstrom K, Lindeberg SN, Haglund B, and Hanson U. 2005. Maternal complications in women with chronic hypertension: A population-based cohort study. *Acta Obstet. Gynecol. Scand.* 84 (5): 419–424.

18 Trophoblast–Uterine Natural Killer Cell Interactions and Their Effect on Cytokines and Angiogenic Growth Factors

Gendie E. Lash and Judith N. Bulmer

CONTENTS

ABSTRACT

Regulation of trophoblast cell invasion of the maternal uterine tissues and subsequent remodeling of the uterine spiral arteries requires the coordinated activity of several different cell types. Recent research has indicated a clear role for the uterine natural killer cells, a distinct leucocyte subpopulation found within the endometrium and decidua, in regulating these processes and the activity of extravillous trophoblast cells, while in turn being educated and modified by this trophoblast cell population. This chapter examines some of these complex interactions, with focus on alterations in secretion profiles of cytokines and angiogenic growth factors.

KEY WORDS

Decidua, uterine leucocytes, extravillous trophoblast cells, spiral artery remodeling, cytokines, angiogenic growth factors.

18.1 INTRODUCTION

Invasion of the maternal uterus and remodeling of the uterine spiral arteries, decidua, and inner third of the myometrium by placental extravillous trophoblast (EVT) cells are two of the key steps in the establishment of a successful human pregnancy. Inadequate EVT invasion and spiral artery remodeling are associated with several complications of pregnancy, including preeclampsia (Pijnenborg et al., 1991), fetal growth restriction (Khong et al., 1986), late miscarriage (Ball et al., 2006), premature rupture of membranes (Kim et al., 2002), and preterm birth (Kim et al., 2003). As EVTs invade the maternal uterine tissues, they interact with a number of different cell types, including decidual stromal cells, vascular smooth muscle and endothelial cells of the spiral arteries, and decidual leucocytes. In early pregnancy, leucocytes account for approximately 30% of decidual stromal cells, with the most predominant leucocyte being the uterine natural killer (uNK) cells. Other populations of decidual leucocytes include macrophages, T lymphocytes, and dendritic cells. This chapter focuses on the interactions between EVT and uNK cells and the potential consequences of those interactions in terms of regulation of EVT invasion, cytokine secretion, and angiogenic growth factor secretion. Before discussing EVT–uNK cell interactions, it is necessary to introduce the salient points of each of these individual cell types.

18.2 TROPHOBLAST

The human placenta is an intricate organ that is made up from a variety of different specialist cell types and vascular networks, which allows it to achieve its main functional role of promoting fetal growth and viability. The major cell type of the placenta is the trophoblast, which has three main subtypes; villous cytotrophoblast (CTB), syncytiotrophoblast, and EVT, also termed *intermediate trophoblast* (Gude et al., 2004; Fitzgerald et al., 2008). EVT and CTB can be distinguished by differential expression of various phenotypic markers, including cell adhesion molecules, integrins, growth factors, and human leucocyte antigen (HLA) molecules (Norwitz et al., 2001). The villous CTB cells fuse to form the multinucleated syncytiotrophoblast cell layer that covers floating chorionic villi in the intervillous space. Villous syncytiotrophoblasts are in contact with maternal leucocytes in the intervillous space and do not express Class I or Class II major histocompatibility (MHC) antigens. In contrast, the CTB cells of the anchoring villi differentiate from a proliferative phenotype into an invasive phenotype (EVT), anchoring the placenta to the underlying decidua (Irving et al., 1995). The EVTs invade through the decidua and into the inner third of the myometrium via two distinct pathways, interstitial and endovascular.

Interstitial EVT cells invade through the decidua and inner myometrium. Mononuclear interstitial EVTs are found throughout the decidua and inner myometrium and are thought to fuse at these sites to form multinuclear interstitial EVT, although the underlying mechanism is not known. Endovascular EVT cells move up the lumen of the spiral arteries in a retrograde fashion, again ceasing in the inner third of the myometrium. During the process of spiral artery remodeling or transformation, vascular smooth muscle cells (VSMCs) are lost from the spiral artery wall and are replaced by intramural EVT cells embedded in fibrinoid material within the spiral artery wall (Pijnenborg et al., 2006). It is commonly reported that endovascular EVTs completely replace the spiral artery endothelium and undergo vascular mimicry changes. However, as imaging techniques have improved, it is now clear that the spiral artery endothelial cells undergo morphological changes, with initial swelling and rounding up, and are lost in the presence of endovascular EVT plugs only when they are in contact with the vessel wall. As the plugs dissipate and the vessel becomes fully remodeled, endothelial cells regenerate and reline the vessels (Pijnenborg et al., 2006). The regenerated endothelium has a more classic appearance, being thin, long, and flat, and covers the underlying intramural EVT (Ellis et al., 2011).

18.2.1 TROPHOBLAST INVASION

Cellular invasion is a complex process that is tightly regulated in EVT, unlike in metastatic spread of malignant neoplastic cells (Lala et al., 2002). In simple terms, there are three features of cellular invasion: attachment to the extracellular matrix (ECM), proteolytic breakdown of the ECM, and then movement into that cleared space before reattachment. EVT cells are a naturally highly invasive cell type, although their ability to invade in *in vitro* models decreases with increasing gestational age, with EVT cells from 8 to 10 weeks' gestational age being twice as invasive as those from 12 to 14 weeks, 16 to 20 weeks, or term (Genbacev et al., 1996; Lash et al., 2006a). EVT cell invasiveness is associated with their phenotype, which is distinct from villous CTB. For example, EVT cells express a unique repertoire of cell surface integrins, distinct from those expressed by villous CTB. In particular, EVTs are characterized by the expression of $\alpha 1\beta 1$ and $\alpha 5\beta 1$ integrins, while CTBs express $\alpha 6\beta 4$ integrin (Damsky et al., 1992). This switch in integrin expression appears to be essential for the invasive phenotype of EVT cells (Damsky et al., 1994). Disruptions in the tightly controlled process of EVT invasion, especially into uterine spiral arteries, can lead to placental deficiencies, which affect maternal vascular homeostasis, resulting in pregnancy complications such as early miscarriage (Khong et al., 1987; Hustin et al., 1990), late miscarriage (Ball et al., 2006), preeclampsia (Pijnenborg et al., 1991), fetal growth restriction (Khong et al., 1986), premature rupture of membranes (Kim et al., 2002), preterm birth (Kim et al., 2003), and placenta accreta (Khong and Robertson, 1987; Hannon et al., 2012). Despite the importance of trophoblast invasion for successful healthy pregnancy, very little is understood about the factors that control this process *in vivo*, although decidual factors are likely to play an important role (Fitzgerald et al., 2008; Knöfler and Pollheimer, 2012).

18.3 uNK CELLS

uNK cells are the most abundant of all decidual leucocytes, accounting for up to approximately 70% of decidual stromal leucocytes in the first trimester of human pregnancy. uNK cells are CD56^{bright} but are CD16$^-$, differing from peripheral blood natural killer (NK) cells, which are CD56^{dim}CD16$^+$. Although a small population of CD56^{bright}CD16$^-$ NK cells are detectable in peripheral blood, these are usually agranular, in contrast to uNK cells, which are CD56^{bright}CD16$^-$CD57$^-$ and are highly granulated.

The origin of uNK cells in the endometrium and decidua remains the subject of debate; there is evidence supporting both trafficking of differentiated uNK cells from the peripheral circulation and, alternatively, *in situ* differentiation and proliferation of precursor cells locally in the endometrium. Several recent reviews cover this subject in detail (Manaster and Mandelboim, 2008; Yagel, 2009; Bulmer et al., 2010).

18.3.1 DISTRIBUTION OF uNK CELLS IN PREGNANT UTERINE DECIDUA

CD56$^+$ uNK cells are present in proliferative and early secretory phase endometrium, albeit in small numbers (King et al., 1989; Bulmer et al., 1991), with numbers increasing in the late secretory phase of the menstrual cycle and increasing further into early pregnancy. In normal human placental bed during the first half of pregnancy, CD56$^+$ uNK cell numbers do not alter between first-trimester (8–12 weeks' gestation) and early second-trimester (13–20 weeks' gestation) decidua (Williams et al., 2009), although the number of cells immunostaining for perforin and granzyme B and showing phloxinophilic granules in phloxine/tartrazine stained samples are reduced across this same period (Bulmer et al., 2010). A decline in CD56$^+$ cell numbers is observed at term, although substantial numbers of CD56$^+$ uNK cells remain in both decidua basalis and decidua parietalis (Williams et al., 2009). The loss of cytoplasmic granules may reflect functional differences between uNK cells in early and late pregnancy, and electron microscopy studies have suggested that degranulation occurs in pregnancy (Spornitz, 1992).

In early pregnancy, decidua uNK cells are found associated with invading interstitial EVT cells. Several studies have compared the distribution and number of uNK cells between decidua basalis and decidua parietalis in pregnancy, with varying results (reviewed in Bulmer and Lash, 2005; Bulmer et al., 2010); some groups have noted no difference between the two decidual areas, whereas others have reported increased numbers of uNK cells in decidua basalis in association with EVT. Most recently, Helige et al. (2014) reported increased density of uNK cells in close proximity (within 20 μm) of invading EVT, with uNK cell density decreasing in areas distant from invading EVT.

18.3.2 FUNCTIONAL INVESTIGATIONS

The precise *in vivo* functions of uNK cells are still not clear, but *in vitro* studies are providing clues to their functions in early human pregnancy.

18.3.2.1 Cytotoxicity

uNK cells isolated from early pregnancy decidua (Ritson and Bulmer, 1989) exhibit cytotoxic activity against the NK cell target K562, although this cytotoxic activity is consistently lower than that of peripheral blood NK cells (Kopcow et al., 2005). uNK cells are noncytolytic to EVT cells, due in part to EVT expression of HLA-G and uNK cell expression of inhibitory receptors (Chumbly et al., 1994; Rouas-Freiss et al., 1997; Chen et al., 2010). In addition, uNK cell secreted vascular endothelial growth factor (VEGF)-C up-regulates EVT expression of anti-transporter protein antibody (TAP-1), which plays a role in peptide loading for MHC class I assembly and antigen presentation in EVT cells, protecting them from cytolytic attack by uNK cells (Kalkunte et al., 2009).

18.3.2.2 Cytokine, Growth Factor, and Protease Secretion

uNK cells are a rich source of many cytokines and growth factors, including tumor necrosis factor (TNF)-α, interleukin (IL)-10, granulocyte macrophage colony stimulating factor (GM-CSF), IL-1β, transforming growth factor (TGF)-β1, macrophage colony stimulating factor (M-CSF), leukemia inhibitor factor (LIF), and interferon (IFN)-γ (Saito et al., 1993; Jokhi et al., 1994; Lash et al., 2010a). It has been shown that uNK cell secretion of IL-1β, GM-CSF (Lash et al., 2010a), IL-6 (Champion et al., 2012), IL-8 (De Oliveira et al., 2010), and IFN-γ (Lash et al., 2006b) increases with gestational age from 8–10 to 12–14 weeks' gestational age. It has also been demonstrated that uNK cells are a major decidual source of angiogenic growth factors, including angiopoietin (Ang)-1, Ang-2, VEGF-C, placental growth factor (PlGF), and TGF-β1 (Li et al., 2001; Lash et al., 2006c). In contrast with cytokine production, uNK cell secretion of Ang-2 and VEGF-C was reduced at 12–14 weeks' gestation compared with 8–10 weeks' gestation (Lash et al., 2006c). Differences in mRNA expression profiles between uNK cells isolated from nonpregnant endometrium and early pregnancy decidua have been demonstrated using gene array technology (Kopcow et al., 2010), as well as between NK cells in peripheral blood and early pregnancy decidua (Hanna et al., 2006; Kopcow et al., 2010).

These data suggest that at 8–10 weeks' gestational age, uNK cells are a major producer of angiogenic growth factors, some of which decrease with gestational age. In contrast, at 12–14 weeks' gestational age, uNK cells are a major producer of cytokines, some of which increase with gestational age. The switch that alters the angiogenic growth factor/cytokine secretion profile of uNK cells with gestational age is not clear, although alterations in secretion profile may impact on their *in vivo* function. The change from angiogenic growth factor expression to cytokine expression could reflect alterations in the proportion of uNK cells undergoing *in situ* proliferation and differentiation and those that are trafficked in from the peripheral blood circulation. Alternatively, there is evidence to suggest that uNK cell exposure to HLA-G induces a senescent phenotype characterized by increased IL-6 and IL-8 (reviewed in Rajagopalan, 2014). The function of uNK cells in third-trimester decidua remains unknown.

Trophoblast invasion and spiral artery remodeling both require breakdown of the ECM by proteolytic enzymes such as the matrix metalloproteinases (MMPs) 2 and 9 and the urokinase plasminogen activator (uPA) system. uNK cells secrete MMP-1, MMP-2, MMP-7, MMP-9, MMP-10, tissue inhibitor of metaloproteinase (TIMP)-1, TIMP-2, TIMP-3, uPA, and uPA receptor, although not plasminogen activator inhibitor (PAI)-1 and PAI-2 (Naruse et al., 2009a,b; G.E. Lash, unpublished data). Immunoreactivity of MMP-7 and MMP-9 by leucocytes surrounding spiral arteries during early pregnancy has also been reported (Smith et al., 2009).

18.3.2.3 Regulation of Trophoblast Invasion

EVT cell invasion is tightly regulated, and uNK cells have been proposed to play a role in the control of this process. Hanna et al. (2006) demonstrated that IL-15-stimulated uNK cell supernatants stimulate invasion of isolated CTB cells *in vitro* and that this stimulatory effect can be partially abrogated in the presence of neutralizing antibodies to IL-8 and IP-10 (Hanna et al., 2006). This result is supported in part by Lash et al. (2010b) and De Oliveira et al. (2010), who demonstrated that uNK cell supernatants from 8–10 weeks' gestational age have no effect on *in vitro* EVT invasion from placental explants at the same gestational age. However, when both uNK cells and placenta were from 12–14 weeks' gestational age, uNK cell supernatants stimulated EVT invasion from placental explants (Lash et al., 2010b). This uNK-mediated stimulation of EVT invasion was partially abrogated in the presence of an IL-8 neutralizing antibody (De Oliveira et al., 2010). In contrast, Hu et al. (2006) demonstrated that IL-15-stimulated uNK cell supernatants inhibited migration of EVT in a two-dimensional migration assay via a mechanism dependent on IFN-γ.

18.3.2.4 Spiral Artery Remodelling

Spiral artery remodeling is a key feature of early placental development in human pregnancy, and failure of this process has been linked to several serious pregnancy complications, including preeclampsia, fetal growth restriction, and second-trimester miscarriage (Pijnenborg et al., 2006). Although this process has largely been attributed to the effect of EVT on spiral arteries, with deficient EVT invasion in pathological pregnancy, there is growing support for a "trophoblast-independent" phase of spiral artery remodeling (Pijnenborg et al., 2006) where the initial stages of spiral artery remodeling, including dilatation, some fibrinoid deposition, endothelial swelling and VSMC separation, occur in the absence of EVT (Craven et al., 1998; Kam et al., 1999).

uNK cells are frequently aggregated around the spiral arteries and arterioles in early human pregnancy, and this distribution may reflect a role in mediating vascular changes in pregnancy. Indeed, Smith et al. (2009) demonstrated increased numbers of leucocytes (both uNK cells and macrophages) within 25 μm of the vessel lumen in human decidual spiral arteries showing partial remodeling and an absence of EVT, compared with nonremodeled vessels and those with greater levels of remodeling (including the presence of EVT). In *in vitro* models using either chorionic plate arteries from human term placenta or nonpregnant myometrial arteries, we have shown that uNK cell supernatants from 8–10 weeks' gestation can initiate VSMC separation, while uNK cell supernatants from 12–14 weeks' gestation have a greater effect on dedifferentiation of the VSMCs (Harris et al., 2010; Lash, 2010; Robson et al., 2012). The uNK cell stimulation of EVT invasion at 12–14 weeks' gestational age may play a role in attracting EVT cells toward the spiral arteries for completion of the remodeling process. The uNK cell-derived factors responsible for mediating these effects are still being fully determined but are likely to include Ang-2 (Robson et al., 2012).

18.4 uNK CELL–TROPHOBLAST CELL INTERACTION

EVT and uNK cells are intimately associated within the placental bed and are likely to communicate through the secretion of cytokines and growth factors as well as through ligand–receptor interactions. The key ligand–receptor interactions occur via expression of HLA molecules (particularly HLA-C and HLA-G) by EVT cells and expression of a range of inhibitory and stimulatory HLA molecule receptors (including killer inhibitory receptors [KIRs] and leucocyte immunoglobulin-like receptors [LILRs]).

18.4.1 HLA LIGAND–RECEPTOR INTERACTIONS

One of the distinguishing features of EVTs, compared with villous CTB or syncytiotrophoblast, is their expression of the Class I MHC molecules HLA-C, HLA-E, and HLA-G. However, EVT cells do not express the classic, polymorphic MHC molecules HLA-A and HLA-B. Each of these EVT-expressed molecules interacts with a range of receptors expressed by uNK cells, with differing functional consequences. In particular, HLA-C alleles are recognized by both inhibitory and activating KIRs, including KIR2DL1, KIR2DL2, KIR2DL3, and KIR2DS1. Interestingly, genetic association studies suggest a link between maternal KIR and fetal (paternal) HLA-C haplotypes and reproductive fitness. In particular, a maternal KIR AA haplotype (lacking activating KIR), in combination with a fetal HLA-C2 haplotype, is associated with preeclampsia and recurrent miscarriage (Hiby et al., 2004, 2010), while interaction with KIR BB may confer reproductive protection. In simple terms, HLA-C2 allotypes bind the inhibitory KIR2DL1 and activating KIR2DS1, while HLA-C1 allotypes bind inhibitory KIR2DL2 and KIR2DL3.

HLA-E interacts with the activating CD94/NKG2C and inhibitory CD94/NKG2A heterodimers, the latter interaction conferring protection from killing for the semiallogeneic EVT (Trowsdale and Moffett, 2008). HLA-G receptors include the inhibitory ILT2 (LILRB1) and the activating KIR2DL4. Under normal physiological conditions, HLA-G expression is restricted to EVT cells, leading to the assumption that it was an important molecule for conferring protection on this cell type from uNK cell-mediated cytotoxicity. However, initial studies were performed using peripheral blood mononuclear cells, rather than isolated uNK cells, and it is now becoming clear that the protective effects can be attributed to interactions of HLA-G with T cells and rather than with NK cells (van der Meer et al., 2004, 2007). While HLA-G–uNK cell interactions may not be protective per se, they do result in altered secretion of a range of soluble factors.

18.4.2 EVT–uNK CELL INTERACTIONS—SECRETION OF CYTOKINES AND ANGIOGENIC GROWTH FACTORS

Several studies have investigated EVT–uNK cell interactions in terms of secretion of cytokines and angiogenic growth factors, although many of these have focused on HLA-G. Few studies have been performed with primary isolates of EVT and uNK cells, with most using either HLA-G transfected cell lines or the choriocarcinoma cell lines JEG-3 (HLA-G positive) and JAR (HLA-G negative). In addition, peripheral blood mononuclear cells and uterine mononuclear cells have been used as a proxy for uNK cells. The results of these studies are highly variable and are summarized in Tables 18.1 (cytokines) and 18.2 (angiogenic growth factors). The overall message of these studies will be discussed in further detail below, before the potential functional consequences of these interactions are discussed.

We performed an extensive study of cytokine and angiogenic growth factor secretion after uNK cell coculture with either EVT or CTB, both in direct contact or separated by a 0.4-μm pore filter (Lash et al., 2011). To eliminate any potential allogeneic effects, uNK and EVT cells for coculture were isolated from the same patient. We demonstrated a decrease in secretion of both cytokines and angiogenic growth factors, although whether uNK cells or EVT cells were responsible for this reduction was not determined and the reduction could be due to suppression of secretion by both cell types. Several other observations can be made when studying this data set as a whole. It was interesting to note that, in general, coculture of uNK cells with either EVT or CTB gave similar results; i.e., significant alterations in cytokine or angiogenic growth factor secretion were not restricted to

TABLE 18.1
Summary of Literature on EVT–uNK Cell Interaction Studies—Cytokines

	TNF-α	IFN-γ	GM-CSF	LIF	IL-10	IL-13	IL-4	IL-3	IL-1β	IL-6	IL-8	TGF-β1	CCL3L3	CXCL2
uNK + JEG-3 (Rieger et al., 2001)	=	=	=	=	↑		=							
uNK + JAR (Rieger et al., 2001)	↑	=	=	=	=		=							
Total decidua + JEG-3 (Rieger et al., 2001)	↑	=	=	=	↑		=							
Total decidua + JAR (Rieger et al., 2001)	↑	=	=	=	↑		=							
uNK depleted + JEG-3 (Rieger et al., 2001)	↑	=	=	=	↑		=							
uNK depleted + JAR (Rieger et al., 2001)	↑	=	=	=	↑		=							
uNK + K562-HLA-G (Rieger et al., 2002)	=	↑	↑		↑	↑								
uNK + K562-HLA-E (Rieger et al., 2002)	=	=	=		↑	=	=							
PBMC (NK) + JEG-3 (Ntrivalas et al., 2006)	↓%	=	=		=		=							
PBMC (NK) + JAR (Ntrivalas et al., 2006)	↓%	=			=		=							
PBMC + 721.221-HLA-G (Kanai et al., 2001)	↑	↑					↑							
UMC + 721.221-HLA-G (Kanai et al., 2001)	↑	↑					=							
uNK (NP) + 721.221-HLA-G (van der Meer et al., 2004)		↑		=				=						
UMC (NP) + 721.221-HLA-G (van der Meer et al., 2004)		↑		=				=						
UMC + sHLA-G (van der Meer et al., 2007)	↑	↑												
uNK + EVT (8–10 weeks' GA) (Lash et al., 2011)	=								↓	=	↓	↓		
uNK + CTB (8–10 weeks' GA) (Lash et al., 2011)	=								=	↓	↓	=		
uNK + EVT (12–14 weeks' GA) (Lash et al., 2011)	=								=	↓	↓	↓		
uNK + CTB (12–14 weeks' GA) (Lash et al., 2011)	=								=	↓	↓	↓		
uNK (KIR2DS1sp) + 721.221-HLA-C2 (Xiong et al., 2013)		↑	↑										↑	↑

Note: CCL3L3, chemokine (C–C motif) ligand 3–like 3; CXCL2, chemokine (C–X–C motif) ligand 2; GA, gestational age; NP, nonpregnant; PBMC, peripheral blood mononuclear cells; UMC, uterine mononuclear cells.

TABLE 18.2

Summary of Literature on EVT–uNK Cell Interaction Studies—Angiogenic Growth Factors

	Angiogenin	Ang-1	Ang-2	bFGF	PlGF	VEGF-A	VEGF-C
uNK (NP) + 721.221-HLA-G (van der Meer et al., 2004)		↑		=		↑	
UMC (NP) + 721.221-HLA-G (van der Meer et al., 2004)		↓		=		↑	
uNK + EVT (8–10 weeks' GA) (Lash et al., 2011)	=	↓	=	↓	=	=	↓
uNK + CTB (8–10 weeks' GA) (Lash et al., 2011)	=	↓	=	=	=	=	↓
uNK + EVT (12–14 weeks' GA) (Lash et al., 2011)	↓	↓	=		=	=	↓
uNK + CTB (12–14 weeks' GA) (Lash et al., 2011)	↓	↓	=		=	=	↓

Note: bFGF, basic fibroblast growth factor; GA, gestational age; NP, nonpregnant; UMC, uterine mononuclear cells.

EVT–uNK cell interactions. This suggests that any effects on cytokine or angiogenic growth factor expression were not mediated by HLA molecules, which differ between EVT and CTB, but by other molecules that are shared by both EVT and CTB. In addition, angiogenic growth factor secretion was altered after both direct and indirect coculture, suggesting that these effects were mediated by soluble factors. By contrast, alterations in cytokine secretion were observed only after direct coculture of the two cell types, suggesting that a membrane-bound molecule was required for this response. HLA-C and KIR haplotypes were not determined in this study, and this may account for much of the variation observed, as it now appears that different cytokine and angiogenic growth factor secretion profiles maybe obtained based on the relative haplotype of the EVT and uNK cells present.

Xiong et al. (2013) studied the response of KIR2DL1 or KIR2DS1 uNK cell subsets to coculture with 721.221-parent cells or those transfected with HLA-C2 (221-C2) by microarray analysis. The uNK cell subsets investigated were KIR2DS1⁺KIR2DL1⁻ (KIR2DS1 single positive [sp]), KIR2DS1⁻KIR2DL1⁺ (KIR2DL1sp), KIR2DS1⁺KIR2DL1⁺ (double positive [dp]), or KIR2DS1⁻KIR2DL1⁻ (double negative [dn]). Using cluster analysis, they demonstrated distinct differences in all four uNK cell subsets; 45 transcripts were altered in the KIR2DL1sp group (28 up-regulated, 17 down-regulated), 378 in the KIR2DS1sp group (174 up-regulated, 204 down-regulated), 289 in the dp group (132 up-regulated, 157 down-regulated), and 3 in the dn group (all up-regulated). Interestingly, there was very little overlap among the three positive groups, with only 24 transcripts being altered in common between the KIR2DS1sp and dp groups even though they both expressed KIR2DS1, suggesting that the presence of KIR2DL1 influences the effects of C2 binding to KIR2DS1. Perhaps more surprisingly, there were only six common transcripts between the KIR2DL1sp and dp groups, as well as between the two different sp subsets. It is important to note that within each individual, different subsets of uNK cells exist, which suggests that differential local production of cytokines and growth factors may occur throughout the placental bed where uNK cells and EVT interact. In addition, the described study specifically concentrated on the effect of HLA-C2 on uNK cell transcription. However, EVT cells express a range of ligands that would simultaneously interact with uNK cell-expressed receptors, potentially eliciting very different effects from the ones described here.

18.4.3 Functional Consequence of EVT–uNK Cell Interactions

As shown above, EVT–uNK cell interactions may result in altered cytokine and angiogenic growth factor secretion profiles, and the potential functional consequence of this altered expression will now be discussed.

uNK cells have been shown to stimulate EVT invasion via a mechanism associated with secreted IL-8 and IP-10 (Hanna et al., 2006; De Oliveira et al., 2010; Lash et al., 2010b), but it is likely that other cytokines also play roles in this important process. It is interesting to note that when EVTs are in close association with uNK cells, levels of IL-8 are reduced. It can be speculated that uNK cell-secreted IL-8 (and other cytokines) attracts EVT to different sites within the placental bed, particularly the uterine spiral arteries, and once in contact with the uNK cells around the spiral arteries, interactions between uNK cells and EVT would lead to a reduction in local levels of these important cytokines, which in turn inhibits their onward passage. Recruitment of EVT to the spiral arteries and consequent "transformation" are absolute requirements for an uncomplicated pregnancy. While uNK cells have been shown to initiate this process (through secretion of Ang-1, Ang-2, and VEGF-C) (Robson et al., 2012), EVTs are required to complete this process. Secretion of Ang-1 and VEGF-C is also reduced after EVT–uNK cell coculture, potentially mediating a switch from uNK cell-directed spiral artery remodeling to EVT-directed remodeling.

EVTs are naturally highly invasive yet only invade as far as the inner third of the myometrium. This suggests that external factors limit their invasive properties, possibly by inducing cellular fusion to create the noninvasive terminally differentiated EVT multinucleate giant cells that are a feature of both decidual and myometrial EVT cell populations. Interestingly, in women with focal placenta accreta, the numbers of myometrial multinucleate EVT cells are highly reduced in areas without underlying decidua compared with those areas with decidua underlying the myometrium, suggesting that decidual-derived factors mediate or initiate this fusion process as the cells move toward the myometrium (Hannon et al., 2012). However, it is not known how EVT fusion into multinucleate giant cells is mediated, and at this stage, it is pure speculation that uNK cells may play a role in this process, as other cells within the decidual including decidual stromal cells may be crucial for this process. Nevertheless, since uNK cells are not found in the myometrium, this may be a reasonable assumption.

Therefore, a scenario may be imagined whereby early in gestation, uNK cell-derived angiogenic growth factors initiate spiral artery remodeling and cytokines attract EVT into the decidua and direct their invasion toward the spiral arteries. Once there is interaction (either direct or indirect) between EVT and uNK cells, local production of both cytokines and angiogenic growth factors is altered. While our study suggests that this is in the form of decreased secretion, it is possible that some soluble factors are also increased depending on the type of ligand–receptor interaction and the plethora of cell surface receptors that are expressed by the uNK cells and the EVT that they interact with. This altered local production of cytokines and growth factors would in turn limit further EVT invasion and, at the site of the uterine spiral arteries, switch the vascular remodeling process from being uNK cell mediated to EVT mediated. In interstitial areas away from the spiral arteries, the reduced EVT invasion may allow for the induction of EVT fusion and creation of interstitial EVT giant cells, a terminally differentiated subset of EVTs that are less invasive.

18.5 CONCLUSIONS

It is now clear that EVT–uNK cell interactions are essential for successful pregnancy, not only in terms of conferring tolerance on the semiallogeneic fetus but also for regulation of EVT invasion and remodeling of the uterine spiral arteries. Irrespective of whether fetal tolerance is established, disruption in EVT invasion and uterine spiral artery remodeling are associated with a number of severe pregnancy complications, including placenta accreta (Hannon et al., 2012), late miscarriage (Ball et al., 2006), fetal growth restriction (Khong et al., 1986), and preeclampsia (Pijnenborg et al., 2006). These interactions are highly complex, and the nature of the response is dependent on a range of different factors, including the nature of the ligand–receptor interaction, as well as the EVT and uNK cell phenotype, and likely varies with gestational age. In addition, each individual hosts a number of different uNK cell subsets, thereby meaning that different responses may be occurring in different locations within the placental bed. Because of this high level of complexity, and natural variation, it is unlikely that we will ever fully understand the full extent of these different interactions beyond knowing that they must occur for a successful pregnancy to progress.

REFERENCES

Ball E, Bulmer J, Ayis S, Lyall F, Robson S. 2006. Late sporadic miscarriage is associated with abnormalities in spiral artery transformation and trophoblast invasion. *J Pathol* 208: 535–542.

Bulmer JN, Lash GE. 2005. Human uterine natural killer cells: A reappraisal. *Mol Immunol* 42: 511–521.

Bulmer JN, Morrison L, Longfellow M, Ritson A, Pace D. 1991. Granulated lymphocytes in human endometrium: Histochemical and immunohistochemical studies. *Hum Reprod* 6: 791–798.

Bulmer JN, Williams PJ, Lash GE. 2010. Immune cells in the placental bed. *Int J Dev Biol* 54: 281–294.

Champion H, Innes BA, Robson SC, Lash GE, Bulmer JN. 2012. Effects of interleukin-6 on extravillous trophoblast invasion in early human pregnancy. *Mol Hum Reprod* 18: 391–400.

Chen LJ, Han ZQ, Zhou H, Zou L, Zou P. 2010. Inhibition of HLA-G expression via RNAi abolishes resistance of Extravillous trophoblast cell line TEV-1 to NK lysis. *Placenta* 31: 519–527.

Chumbly G, King A, Robertson K, Holmes N, Loke YW. 1994. Resistance of HLA-G and HLA-A2 transfectants to lysis by decidual NK cells. *Cell Immunol* 155: 312–322.

Craven CM, Morgan T, Ward K. 1998. Decidual spiral artery remodelling begins before cellular interaction with cytotrophoblasts. *Placenta* 19: 241–252.

Damsky CH, Fitzgerald ML, Fisher SJ. 1992. Distribution patterns of extracellular matrix components and adhesion receptors are intricately modulated during first trimester differentiation along the invasive pathway, in vivo. *J Clin Invest* 89: 210–222.

Damsky CH, Librach C, Lim KH, Fitzgerald ML, McMaster MT, Janatpour M, Zhou Y, Logan SK, Fisher SJ. 1994. Integrin switching regulates normal trophoblast invasion. *Development* 120: 3657–3666.

De Oliveira LG, Lash GE, Murray-Dunning C, Bulmer JN, Innes BA, Searle RF, Sass N, Robson SC. 2010. Role of interleukin 8 in uterine natural killer cell regulation of extravillous trophoblast cell invasion. *Placenta* 31: 595–601.

Ellis N, Innes BA, Lash GE, Robson SC, Bulmer JN. 2011. Loss of endothelial cells in spiral artery remodeling: Myths versus facts. *Placenta* 32: A76.

Fitzgerald JS, Poehlmann TG, Schleussner E, Markert UR. 2008. Trophoblast invasion: The role of intracellular cytokine signalling via signal transducer and activator of transcription 3 (STAT3). *Hum Reprod Update* 14: 335–344.

Genbacev O, Joslin R, Damsky CH, Polliotti BM, Fisher SJ. 1996. Hypoxia alters early gestation human cytotrophoblast differentiation/invasion *in vitro* and models the placental defects that occur in preeclampsia. *J Clin Invest* 97: 540–550.

Gude NM, Roberts CT, Kalionis B, King RG. 2004. Growth and function of the normal human placenta. *Thromb Res* 114: 397–407.

Hanna J, Goldman-Wohl D, Hamani Y, Avraham I, Greenfield C, Natanson-Yaron S, Prus D, Cohen-Daniel L, Arnon TI, Manaster I et al. 2006. Decidual NK cell regulate key developmental processes at the human fetal–maternal interface. *Nat Med* 12: 1065–1074.

Hannon T, Innes BA, Lash GE, Bulmer JN, Robson SC. 2012. Effects of local decidua on trophoblast invasion and spiral artery remodeling in focal placenta creta—An immunohistochemical study. *Placenta* 33: 998–1004.

Harris LK, Robson A, Lash GE, Aplin JD, Baker PN, Bulmer JN. 2010. Physiological remodelling of the uterine spiral arteries during human pregnancy: Uterine natural killer cells mediate smooth muscle cell disruption. *Proc Physiol Soc* 19: C42.

Helige C, Ahammer H, Moser G, Hammer A, Dohr G, Huppertz B, Sedlmayr P. 2014. Distribution of decidual natural killer cells and macrophages in the neighbourhood of the trophoblast invasion front: A quantitative evaluation. *Hum Reprod* 29: 8–17.

Hiby SE, Walker JJ, O'Shaughnessy KM, Redman CW, Carrington M, Trowsdale J, Moffett A. 2004. Combinations of maternal KIR and fetal HLA-C genes influence the risk of preeclampsia and reproductive success. *J Exp Med* 200: 957–965.

Hiby SE, Apps R, Sharkey AM, Farrell LE, Gardner L, Mulder A, Claas FH, Walker JJ, Redman CC, Morgan L et al. 2010. Maternal activating KIRs protect against human reproductive failure mediated by fetal HLA-C2. *J Clin Invest* 120: 4102–4110.

Hu Y, Dutz JP, Maccalman CD, Yong P, Tan R, Von Dadelszen P. 2006. Decidual NK cells alter *in vitro* first trimester extravillous cytotrophoblast migration: A role for IFN-gamma. *J Immunol* 177: 8522–8530.

Hustin J, Jauniaux E, Schaaps JP. 1990. Histological study of the materno–embryonic interface in spontaneous abortion. *Placenta* 11: 477–486.

Irving JA, Lysiak JJ, Graham CH, Hearn S, Han VK, Lala PK. 1995. Characteristics of trophoblast cells migrating from first trimester chorionic villus explants and propagated in culture. *Placenta* 16: 413–433.

Jokhi PP, King A, Loke YW. 1994. Production of granulocyte-macrophage colony-stimulating factor by human trophoblast cells and by decidual large granular lymphocytes. *Hum Reprod* 9: 1660–1669.

Kalkunte SS, Mselle TF, Norris WE, Wira CR, Sentman CL, Sharma S. 2009. Vascular endothelial growth factor C facilitates immune tolerance and endovascular activity of human uterine NK cells at the maternal–fetal interface. *J Immunol* 182: 4085–4092.

Kam EP, Gardner L, Loke YW, King A. 1999. The role of trophoblast in the physiological change in decidual spiral arteries. *Hum Reprod* 14: 2131–2138.

Kanai T, Fujii T, Unno N, Yamashita T, Hyodo H, Miki A, Hamai Y, Kozuma S, Taketani Y. 2001. Human leukocyte antigen-G-expressing cells differently modulate the release of cytokines from mononuclear cells present in the decidua versus peripheral blood. *Am J Reprod Immunol* 45: 94–99.

King A, Wellings V, Gardner L, Loke YW. 1989. Immunocytochemical characterization of the unusual large granular lymphocytes in human endometrium throughout the menstrual cycle. *Hum Immunol* 24: 195–205.

Khong TY, Robertson WB. 1987. Placenta creta and placenta praevia creta. *Placenta* 8: 399–409.

Khong TY, De Wolf F, Robertson WB, Brosens I. 1986. Inadequate maternal vascular response to placentation in pregnancies complicated by pre-eclampsia and by small for gestational age infants. *Br J Obstet Gynaecol* 93: 1049–1059.

Khong TY, Liddell HS, Robertson WB. 1987. Defective haemochorial placentation as a cause of miscarriage: A preliminary study. *Br J Obstet Gynaecol* 94: 649–655.

Kim YM, Chaiworapongsa T, Gomez R, Bujold E, Yoon BH, Rotmensch S, Thaler HT, Romero R. 2002. Failure of physiologic transformation of the spiral arteries in the placental bed in preterm premature rupture of membranes. *Am J Obstet Gynecol* 87: 1137–1142.

Kim YM, Bujold E, Chaiworapongsa T, Gomez R, Yoon BH, Thaler HT, Rotmensch S, Romero R. 2003. Failure of physiologic transformation of the spiral arteries in patients with preterm labor and intact membranes. *Am J Obstet Gynecol* 189: 1063–1069.

Knöfler M, Pollheimer J. 2012. IFPA Award in placentology lecture: Molecular regulation of human trophoblast invasion. *Placenta* 33: S55–S62.

Kopcow HD, Allan DS, Chen X, Rybalov B, Andzelm MM, Ge B, Strominger JL. 2005. Human decidual NK cells form immature activating synapses and are not cytotoxic. *Proc Natl Acad Sci* 102: 15563–15568.

Kopcow HD, Eriksson M, Mselle TF, Damrauer SM, Wira CR, Sentman CL, Strominger JL. 2010. Human decidual uNK cells from gravid uteri and NK cells from cycling endometrium are distinct NK cell subsets. *Placenta* 31: 334–338.

Lala PK, Lee BP, Xu G, Chakraborty C. 2002. Human placental trophoblast as an *in vitro* model for tumor progression. *Can J Physiol Pharmacol* 80: 142–149.

Lash GE. 2010. Functional role of uterine natural killer cells in early human pregnancy. *J Reprod Immunol* 86: 14.

Lash GE, Otun HA, Innes BA, Bulmer JN, Searle RF, Robson SC. 2006a. Low oxygen concentrations inhibit trophoblast cell invasion from early gestation placental explants via alterations in levels of the urokinase plasminogen activator system. *Biol Reprod* 74: 403–409.

Lash GE, Otun HA, Innes BA, Kirkley M, De Oliveira L, Searle RF, Robson SC, Bulmer JN. 2006b. Interferon-gamma inhibits extravillous trophoblast cell invasion by a mechanism that involves both changes in apoptosis and protease levels. *FASEB J* 20: 2512–2518.

Lash GE, Schiessl B, Kirkley M, Innes BA, Cooper A, Searle RF, Robson SC, Bulmer JN. 2006c. Expression of angiogenic growth factors by uterine natural killer cells during early pregnancy. *J Leukoc Biol* 80: 572–580.

Lash GE, Robson SC, Bulmer JN. 2010a. Review: Functional role of uterine natural killer (uNK) cells in human early pregnancy decidua. *Placenta* 31: S87–S92.

Lash GE, Otun HA, Innes BA, Percival K, Searle RF, Robson SC, Bulmer JN. 2010b. Regulation of extra-villous trophoblast invasion by uterine natural killer cells is dependent on gestational age. *Hum Reprod* 25: 1137–1145.

Lash GE, Naruse K, Robson A, Innes BA, Searle RF, Robson SC, Bulmer JN. 2011. Interaction between uterine natural killer cells and extravillous trophoblast cells: Effect on cytokine and angiogenic growth factor production. *Hum Reprod* 26: 2289–2295.

Li XF, Charnock-Jones DS, Zhang E, Hiby S, Malik S, Day K, Licence D, Bowen JM, Gardner L, King A et al. 2001. Angiogenic growth factor messenger ribonucleic acids in uterine natural killer cells. *J Clin Endocrinol Metab* 86: 1823–1834.

Manaster I, Mandelboim O. 2008. The unique properties of human NK cells in the uterine mucosa. *Placenta* 29: S60–S66.

Naruse K, Lash GE, Innes BA, Otun HA, Searle RF, Robson SC, Bulmer JN. 2009a. Localization of matrix metalloproteinase (MMP)-2, MMP-9 and tissue inhibitors for MMPs (TIMPs) in uterine natural killer cells in early human pregnancy. *Hum Reprod* 24: 553–561.

Naruse K, Lash GE, Bulmer JN, Innes BA, Otun HA, Searle RF, Robson SC. 2009b. The urokinase plasmino-gen activator (uPA) system in uterine natural killer cells in the placental bed during early pregnancy. *Placenta* 30: 398–404.

Norwitz ER, Schust DJ, Fisher SJ. 2001. Implantation and the survival of early pregnancy. *N Engl J Med* 345: 1400–1408.

Ntrivalas E, Kwak-Kim J, Beaman K, Mantouvalos H, Gilman-Sachs A. 2006. An *in vitro* coculture model to study cytokine profiles of natural killer cells during maternal immune cell-trophoblast interactions. *J Soc Gynecol Investig* 13: 196–202.

Pijnenborg R, Anthony J, Davey DA, Rees A, Tiltman A, Vercruysse L, van Assche A. 1991. Placental bed spiral arteries in the hypertensive disorders of pregnancy. *Br J Obstet Gynaecol* 98: 648–655.

Pijnenborg R, Vercruysse L, Hanssens M. 2006. The uterine spiral arteries in human pregnancy: Facts and controversies. *Placenta* 27: 939–958.

Rajagopalan S. 2014. HLA-G-mediated NK cell senescence promotes vascular remodeling: Implications for reproduction. *Cell Mol Immunol* 11: 460–466.

Rieger L, Kammerer U, Hofmann J, Sutterlin M, Dietl J. 2001. Choriocarcinoma cells modulate the cyto-kine production of decidual large granular lymphocytes in coculture. *Am J Reprod Immunol* 46: 137–143.

Rieger L, Hofmeister V, Probe C, Dietl J, Weiss EH, Steck T, Kammerer U. 2002. Th1- and Th2-like cytokine production by first-trimester decidual large granular lymphocytes is influenced by HLA-G and HLA-E. *Mol Hum Reprod* 8: 255–261.

Ritson A, Bulmer JN. 1989. Isolation and functional studies of granulated lymphocytes in first trimester human decidua. *Clin Exp Immunol* 77: 263–268.

Robson A, Harris LK, Innes BA, Lash GE, Aljunaidy MM, Aplin JD, Baker PN, Robson SC, Bulmer JN. 2012. Uterine natural killer cells initiate spiral artery remodelling in human pregnancy. *FASEB J* 26: 4876–4885.

Rouas-Freiss N, Goncalves RM, Menier C, Dausset J, Carosella ED. 1997. Direct evidence to support the role of HLA-G in protecting the fetus from maternal uterine natural killer cytolysis. *Proc Natl Acad Sci U S A* 94: 11520–11525.

Saito S, Nishikawa K, Morii T, Enomoto M, Narita N, Motooshi K, Ichijo M. 1993. Cytokine produc-tion by CD16⁻CD56^bright natural killer cells in the human early pregnancy decidua. *Int Immunol* 5: 559–563.

Smith SD, Dunk CE, Aplin JD, Harris LK, Jones RL. 2009. Evidence for immune cell involvement in decidual spiral arteriole remodeling in early human pregnancy. *Am J Pathol* 174: 1959–1971.

Spornitz UM. 1992. The functional morphology of the human endometrium and decidua. *Adv Anat Embryol Cell Biol* 124: 1–99.

Trowsdale J, Moffett A. 2008. NK receptor interactions with MHC class I molecules in pregnancy. *Semin Immunol* 20: 317–320.

van der Meer A, Lukassen HGM, van Lierop MJC, Wijnands F, Mosselman S, Braat DDM, Joosten I. 2004. Membrane-bound HLA-G activates proliferation and interferon-γ production by uterine natural killer cells. *Mol Hum Reprod* 10: 189–195.

van der Meer A, Lukassen HG, van Cranenbroek B, Weiss EH, Braat DD, van Lierop MJ, Joosten I. 2007. Soluble HLA-G promotes Th1-type cytokine production by cytokine-activated uterine and peripheral natural killer cells. *Mol Hum Reprod* 13: 123–133.

Williams PJ, Searle RF, Robson SC, Innes BA, Bulmer JN. 2009. Decidual leucocyte populations in early to late gestation normal human pregnancy. *J Reprod Immunol* 82: 24–31.

Xiong S, Sharkey AM, Kennedy PR, Gardner L, Farrell LE, Chazara O, Bauer J, Hiby SE, Colucci F, Moffett A. 2013. Maternal uterine NK cell-activating receptor KIR2DS1 enhances placentation. *J Clin Invest* 123: 4264–4272.

Yagel S. 2009. The developmental role of natural killer cells at the fetal–maternal interface. *Am J Obstet Gynecol* 201: 344–350.

19 Effects of Hyperglycemia on Trophoblast Invasion and Angiogenesis

Sanjay Basak and Asim K. Duttaroy

CONTENTS

ABSTRACT

During pregnancy, the mother supplies multiple nutrients as energy source for fetus growth, including glucose, free fatty acids, amino acids, and ketone bodies. Maternal intakes of both glucose and lipids have been positively associated with infant birth weight. Hyperglycemia during pregnancy profoundly changes the maternal and fetal environment milieu, which are enriched with several growth factors, hormones, and cytokines, those are altered in diabetes. This chapter will evaluate the effects of glucose, free fatty acid, and insulin on the invasion and angiogenesis-related activities of the first-trimester placental trophoblast to understand their effects on early placental development.

KEY WORDS

Angiogenesis, placenta, first trimester trophoblast, hyperglycemia, fatty acid, insulin, gene expression, metabolism, HTR8/SVneo.

19.1 INTRODUCTION

With the onset of global epidemic of diabetes, it is imperative to measure its effect on fetoplacental growth and development. Preeclampsia, a disease of pregnancy with shallow trophoblast invasion of the uterine spiral arterioles, is increased in women with gestational diabetes (Ang and Lumsden 2001; Garner et al. 1990; Ostlund, Haglund, and Hanson 2004). Hyperglycemia during pregnancy profoundly changes maternal and fetal environment milieu that are enriched with growth factors, free fatty acids, hormone, and cytokines (Desoye and Hauguel-de Mouzon 2007). Increased levels of glucose, free fatty acid, and insulin are associated with gestational diabetes mellitus (GDM) (Cvitic, Desoye, and Hiden 2014). Maternal hyperglycemia induces thickening of the placental basement membrane and anticipated to reduce oxygen transport. Optimum oxygen level in the uterus is critical for successful placentation. In normal placental development, maintaining hypoxia condition during early placentation is required for optimum angiogenesis and invasion of the uterine by extravillous trophoblasts (EVTs). During the first trimester, hypoxia condition is critical for a successful pregnancy outcome, as human placenta optimally develops in a hypoxic milieu because of local occlusion of the uterine spiral arterioles by the EVT (Patel et al. 2010). In a low-oxygen environment, hypoxia-inducible factors (HIFs) are the main regulators in the transcription of a number of target genes that can induce anaerobic processes and thus help in reducing oxygen consumption. This hypoxia condition stimulates the expression of proangiogenic factors and establishes optimal vascular environment by promoting angiogenesis (González-Muniesa et al. 2011). Under hypoxia, the global protein synthesis level of the cells is ceased owing to masking of the translation initiation sites of the ribosomal proteins. This confers to allow only specific mRNA that contains alternative, internal ribosomal entry sites (IRESs) to translate preferentially to counteradaptive response to hypoxia stress. These could be the case for IRES of vascular endothelial growth factor (VEGF) and HIF1α (Young et al. 2008).

Diabetic insult during early gestation and its long-term effect on fetoplacental development are not well known. It is not known whether diabetes is influenced by placental hypoxia in first-trimester trophobalst cells. The impact of maternal diabetes on placentation, which includes angiogenesis and invasion of the uterine trophoblast during the first trimester of pregnancy, is being investigated recently. The development of a placental vascular network is essential for trophoblast invasion, angiogenesis, and growth of the developing fetus (Hill 2001). Several factors are involved in these processes, including VEGF, platelet-derived growth factor, angiopoietin-like protein-4 (ANGPTL4), matrix metalloproteinase (MMP), fatty acid binding protein 4 (FABP4), and others (Staun-Ram and Shalev 2005; Torry and Torry 1997). The trophoblast invasion is accompanied by remodeling of the extracellular matrix (ECM) via MMP enzymes that are produced by the cytotrophoblast during the first trimester of pregnancy, and their involvement in the success of EVT functions, such as migration and invasion, is critical. The direct effect of glucose on the first-trimester trophoblast cells, HTR8/SVneo, revealed lower activity of urokinase plasminogen activator and thus implicated reduced invasiveness of the trophoblast (Belkacemi et al. 2005). HTR8-tube-like formation reflects a process that initiates trophoblast migration and differentiation toward an invasive phenotype, a physiologic process that takes place during the first trimester of human pregnancy. The embryonic vasculature is the first system usually developed during placentation and is the most vulnerable to the in utero environmental conditions (Pinter et al. 2001). GDM is associated with fetal macrosomia, which increases the risk of cardiovascular and metabolic disease later in life for both the mother and the offspring. Hyperglycemia, hyperinsulinemia, insulin resistance, hyperleptinemia, and increased inflammation are associated with diabetes and may affect trophoblast growth and metabolism (Vambergue and Fajardy 2011). In this chapter, impact of these factors on placentation will be reviewed and their possible roles on the fetoplacental growth and development will be discussed.

19.2   HYPERGLYCEMIA AND PREGNANCY OUTCOME

GDM is defined as impaired glucose tolerance that can lead to the development of type 2 diabetes mellitus in both the mother and the child. GDM is often associated with increased infant birth weight (macrosomic baby) and adiposity. Unlike GDM, pregestational diabetes refers to the condition that manifests throughout the pregnancy, but hyperglycemia of GDM develops in pregnancy and manifests only in the late second trimester. Thus, GDM may affect more in the angiogenesis and vascular remodeling processes, whereas pregestational diabetes includes also the process of vasculogenesis during initial development. The prevalence of pregestational diabetes has increased tremendously because of increased incidences of type 2 diabetes (Bell et al. 2008). In diabetes, an elevated level of glucose causes an adverse effect on the fetus during pregnancy. Hyperglycemia at conception and during the early stages of pregnancy, particularly in the first trimester, increases the risk of fetal malformation. A similar condition at the later part of the pregnancy increases the risk of macrosomia and metabolic distress. Managing hyperglycemia in pregnancy is the only option for the mother to avoid pregnancy-related complications and fetal abnormalities (Persson, Norman, and Hanson 2009). Data from several studies reported that non-GDM pregnancies should limit fasting glucose levels to 3.9 ± 0.4 mmol/L; 1 hour postprandial, 6.1 ± 0.7 mmol/L; and 2 hours postprandial, 5.5 ± 0.6 mmol/L, with a mean glucose of 4.9 ± 0.6 mmol/L. The Hyperglycemia and Adverse Pregnancy Outcomes study, the largest prospective study of glycemia pattern during pregnancy, reported a mean fasting glucose of 4.5 ± 0.4 mmol/L, derived from 23,316 pregnant women (Metzger et al. 2008). The level of glucose was found slightly higher in non-GDM pregnant obese women than in their lean counterparts. Despite the tight glycemic control of glycated hemoglobin (A1C <7.0%), maternal obesity is independently considered as a risk factor of pregnancy complications (Harmon et al. 2011). The most universal way to screen diabetes during pregnancy is mediated by a 50 g oral glucose challenge test at 24 to 28 weeks of gestation, followed by an oral glucose tolerance test as a diagnostic measure to know the threshold values in the blood.

Pregnancy complications with preexisting diabetes exhibit pronounced effects on fetal sides. Based on glycemia status and its stage, the fetal malformation rate in pregnancies complicated by diabetes is typically 5–10 times more than in pregnancies without diabetes. Late pregnancy complication of the fetus often correlated with the degree of glycemic control and fetal macrosomia. The incidence of polyhydramnios in diabetes is 10%–20% depending on the control of glucose management. Hyperinsulinemia is considered as the cause of fetal hypoxia as this condition increases fetal metabolic rate and oxygen requirement. Macrosomia is the result of altered metabolic environment during pregnancy where the pancreatic islet becomes hyperplasia, and an increase in beta cell mass has been demonstrated in the autopsy of babies from diabetic mothers. These gross structural changes in the growing organs usually start as early as the second trimester of pregnancy. The risk of preterm labor becomes threefold higher in a diabetic mother than in a nondiabetic counterpart. Stillbirth is the most common after the 36th week of gestation in case of type 1 diabetes. Chronic intrauterine hypoxia has been postulated as the primary reason for this event. In cases complicated by vasculopathy, a reduction in uterine blood flow is the possible cause of hypoxia, which results in stillbirth. Frequent random fluctuation in glucose level in the pregnant mother has been associated with stillbirth.

19.3 REGULATION OF PLACENTATION BY THE ACTIVITIES
OF GLUCOSE TRANSPORTERS

The placenta performs a dual role in determining the outcome of the fetus. On one hand, the placenta protects the fetus from toxic xenobiotic compounds by forming an immunological barrier; on the other hand, it forms nutrient transporting corridor to establish the fetal–maternal interactions that are critical for successful human pregnancy. In achieving successful placentation, trophoblast invasion in the uterus is the key event that has been compromised in many pathological pregnancies. Recent data suggest that glucose transporters (GLUTs) could play a role in the process of successful placentation. Glucose is the primary substrate for the oxidative metabolism of fetal growth and development. Glucose transport is concentration dependent across the placenta; however, it is facilitated by a family of GLUTs. So far, 14 isoforms of the membrane-spanning GLUTs are reported, in which GLUT1, GLUT3, and GLUT4 are the key members expressed in the human placental trophoblast (Illsley 2000). The uptake of glucose in the placenta is facilitated by GLUT1 and GLUT 3 proteins. The subcellular location of these transporters is quite contradicting. A recent study with immunohistochemistry of GLUT1, GLUT3, and GLUT4 in tissue sections of first-trimester human placental villous was studied to ascertain their activities in the process of implantation. The negative immunostaining for insulin-sensitive GLUT4 protein in the human feto–maternal interface suggests that this isoform may not express in the first-trimester placenta. Their data support that GLUT1 is the major GLUT in the placenta, especially in the early placentation process (Hahn et al. 1998). GLUT1 protein was positively stained with the syncytial microvillus, which is considered as the primary source of glucose for the fetus. In addition, GLUT1 was found in cytotrophoblast cells and in some of the fetal endothelial cells of first-trimester placental villi, suggesting their requirement to perform different functions associated with implantation (Hahn et al. 2000; Illsley, Sellers, and Wright 1998). The GLUT3 protein is not very prominent in the human placenta (Jansson, Wennergren, and Illsley 1993; Janzen et al. 2013). Since the expression of GLUT3 protein was evidenced in invasive choriocarcinoma cell lines, it is presumed that GLUT3 may be required in the metabolically active dividing first-trimester trophoblast cells (Illsley, Sellers, and Wright 1998). GLUT3 and GLUT1 proteins express in cytotrophoblasts of the first-trimester placental villi. Korgun et al. (2005) suggest that sustained activities of these GLUTs are probably required in providing energy for the proliferation and invasion of EVT during the implantation process. The role of GLUT1 on fetal angiogenesis is predicated since this protein is localized in the capillary tube formation of microvascular connecting tubes formed by one or several angiogenic cells (Demir et al. 2004). GLUT1 and GLUT3 were shown to be expressed in CD45- and CD68-positive cells, suggesting their role in the activation of the decidua leukocytes during implantation and thereby improve immunological tolerance (Korgun et al. 2005).

The effect of maternal hyperglycemia on GLUTs was studied in vitro by immunolabelling using human term placental trophoblast ($n = 5$ placentas) cultured for 48 hours with 25 mmol/L D-glucose. Hyperglycemia down-regulates the GLUT1 glucose transport system of term placental trophoblast by redistribution of the localization of the GLUT1 protein (Hahn et al. 2000). GLUT1 expression was reduced significantly after culture of the cells with 25 mmol/L glucose owing to internalization of plasma membrane GLUT1 that leads to a GLUT1 translocation from the trophoblast surface to intracellular sites. In essence, excess glucose may self-regulate hexose transport in term placental trophoblast by altering GLUT1 partitioning between the plasma membrane and intracellular sites and favor internalization of the GLUT1.

The expression of GLUT proteins in pathological pregnancy such as in intrauterine growth restriction (IUGR) has been contradicted (Jansson, Wennergren, and Illsley 1993; Jansson et al. 2002; Janzen et al. 2013). Hypoxia seems to regulate the expression of GLUT proteins. Many of the in vitro studies demonstrated that reduction in the oxygen tension stimulates the expression of GLUT1 and GLUT3 and thereby increased transepithelial glucose transport, which is mediated by the action of HIF1α (Baumann, Zamudio, and Illsley 2007; Esterman et al. 1997; Hayashi et al. 2004). Under this situation, placental transport of glucose potentially increases the concentration of glucose as an alternate metabolic fuel to both the placenta and fetus as a part of the adaptive response since gluconeogenesis pathways do not operate efficiently in the placenta. Paradoxically, human fetus affected by IUGR demonstrates hypoglycemia; the effect is correlated with severity of growth restriction and decreased blood flow (Economides, Nicolaides, and Campbell 1990). Now, it is widely believed that in conditions of fetal hypoxia leading to IUGR, it is an excess consumption of glucose by the placenta that is responsible for a decreased rate of transplacental transport to the fetus (Zamudio et al. 2010). The stimulation of placental GLUT expression is an adaptive response to decreased uteroplacental perfusion and prolonged exposure to hypoxia, which is associated with late-term IUGR. The general hypothesis is that maternal undernutrition like IUGR cases during pregnancy impairs placental angiogenesis and vascular development. Despite a nutrient-deficient condition, the capillary area density expression of angiogenesis factor in the whole-placenta tissue of ovine adolescent sheep was not affected (Luther et al. 2007). However, reduced uterine blood flow was likely to lead maternal anemia despite induction of angiogenic growth factors.

19.4 EFFECTS OF MATERNAL HYPERGLYCEMIA ON ANGIOGENESIS AND GROWTH OF THE PLACENTA

Although physiological blood glucose level is approximately 5.5 mM, the precise glucose level at the fetal–maternal interface during the first trimester of pregnancy is not known. It was reported that glucose levels are considerably lower in the intervillous fluid of first-trimester placenta than in the maternal serum (Jauniaux et al. 2005). Thus, it is likely that normal placental development takes place under glucose concentrations lower than those present in maternal blood. However, the impact of excess maternal circulatory glucose level as what happens in diabetes on placenta growth, angiogenesis, and metabolism is not known. Maternal diabetes adversely affects embryonic vasculogenesis in mice, which results in embryonic vasculopathy. Under hyperglycemic conditions, vasculogenesis of the blood vessels in the yolk sac is disrupted, and the cellular structures in the vessels are altered with concomitant reduction in the expression of VEGF and HIF1α (Pinter et al. 2001; Yang, Zhao, and Reece 2008). Recent studies in diabetic rats suggest that high glucose blunts VEGF response to hypoxia via the oxidative stress-regulated hypoxia-inducible factor/hypoxia-responsible element pathway (Katavetin et al. 2006). Placenta responds differentially to hyperglycemia at early and late gestation. Diabetic insult at early stages leads to structural changes in the placenta, whereas later stages as in GDM leads to short-term changes for key functions, including gene expression. In case of gestational hyperglycemia, placenta structure is altered by an increase in the number of terminal villi and capillaries to maintain the homeostasis at the maternal–fetal interface. VEGF and its receptor expression were altered in the placenta of hyperglycemic pregnant women. Distinctive morphological appearance of the placenta was revealed by the presence of collagen deposition around large arteries in placenta derived from maternal hyperglycemia. This report clearly indicated that altered glycemia level could be an important indicator for placenta morphology and structure. Moreover, placental response to altered glycemia might have adverse consequences for the fetus. The changes in the placental VEGF:VEGF receptor expression ratio in maternal hyperglycemia suggest hyperangiogenesis in placental tissue, which could lead to hypercapillarization of villi, as observed in these phenotypes (Pietro et al. 2010).

Hyperglycemia results in increased insulin secretion from the fetal pancreas to achieve normoglycemia, and this condition is compensated by increased uptake of glucose into the fetal cells and results in increased adipose mass and macrosomia (Vambergue and Fajardy 2011). During this condition, branching angiogenesis increases, as evidenced in gestational diabetes (GDM), a condition accompanied by elevated fetal insulin levels due to maternal hyperglycemia. The mechanism of the insulin-mediated angiogenesis is not reported in early placentation. However, insulin stimulates angiogenesis in human umbilical venous endothelial cells via the endothelial nitric oxide synthase (eNOS)–HIF1α–VEGF pathway (Yamada et al. 2006). Hyperglycemia can induce a reduction in trophoblast proliferation, which delays placental growth and development during early gestation. In diabetes, placental morphology is altered since surface areas become enlarged because of hypervascularization. The diffusion distance between maternal and fetal circulation increased because of thickening of the trophoblastic membrane with high amounts of collagen deposition (Luo, Qiao, and Yin 2011). Hypervascularization and increased surface area of the placenta lead to alteration in the oxygen diffusion across the placenta and create local hypoxia in the maternal–placenta–fetal axis. The resulting low oxygen level up-regulates the expression of several proangiogenic factors such as VEGF, leptin, fibroblast growth factor, and others. In excess, these factors lead to enhanced vascularization and endothelial cell proliferation and limited trophoblast invasion (Figure 19.1). All these conditions have been linked to higher incidence of spontaneous abortion, preeclampsia, and IUGR associated with diabetes and suggest impaired trophoblast invasion.

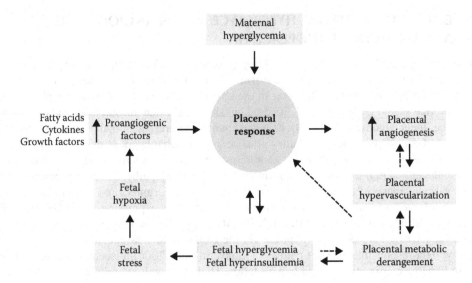

FIGURE 19.1 Hypothetical pathway depicts the effects of maternal hyperglycemia on placental angiogenesis and metabolic activities during pregnancy. Maternal blood flow across the placenta depends largely on placental vascularization. Angiogenesis and vascular systems are regulated by several hormones, growth factors, and cytokines expressed in the placenta. Maternal hyperglycemia often leads to fetal hyperglycemia and fetal hyperinsulinemia conditions that ultimately cause fetal hypoxia, a typical characteristic outcome of a diabetic pregnancy. Hypoxia is a key regulatory factor of the placental angiogenesis since the condition favors expression of several proangiogenic factors. Under this condition, fatty acids, growth factors, and cytokines, by virtue of their proangiogenic action, further increase vascularization and angiogenesis of the placenta, which ultimately leads to hypervascularization of the placenta, alteration in the structure, and growth of the placenta. Placental hypervascularization may lead to altered metabolic response of the placenta.

19.5   EFFECTS OF GLUCOSE AND FATTY ACIDS ON TUBE FORMATION OF THE EXTRAVILLOUS TROPHOBLAST CELLS

The process of placentation begins with implantation of the blastocyst beneath the uterine epithelium and differentiation of trophoblast cell lineage into the embryonic and extra embryonic structures of the conceptus. This invasive behavior follows a precise chronology of vascular events during the first trimester of gestation. These events involve placental tissue angiogenesis, organogenesis, and progressive establishment of the circulations within the placenta in preparation for the second phase of pregnancy fetal growth (Murray and Lessey 1999; Staun-Ram and Shalev 2005). During placentation, MMPs are expressed to facilitate trophoblast invasion into the uterus. MMPs are a family of zinc-containing endopeptidases capable of degrading all components of the ECM, both interstitial matrix and basement membrane. MMP-2 and MMP-9 have a differential expression throughout the gestation, with MMP-2 being the main gelatinase in early first trimester (6–8 weeks) and MMP-9 being dominant in late first trimester (9–12 weeks) (Benaitreau et al. 2010; Jovanović et al. 2010; Lockwood et al. 2008). MMP-2 and MMP-9 are the most important MMP enzymes produced by the cytotrophoblast during the first trimester of pregnancy, and their involvement in the success of EVT functions, such as migration and invasion, has been well documented. MMP-2 has been shown to be located within highly invasive EVT cells and syncytiotrophoblasts, while MMP-9 is found throughout the entire invasive pathway. MMPs are also associated in the implantation process, including regulation of growth factors, cytokines, and angiogenic factors.

We studied the expression of angiogenic factors in first-trimester trophoblast cells in vitro to assess the impact of maternal hyperglycemia on early placentation process using the model of first-trimester trophoblast cells that mimic the condition in vivo. Angiogenesis is scored in terms of cellular capacity to form tube-like structures when cultured in matrigel. Tube-like formation is a two-dimensional measure of angiogenesis process. The first-trimester invasive trophoblast cells, HTR8/SVneo, constitutively form tube-like structure in a matrigel, making these cells an excellent model to study trophoblast invasion and angiogenesis processes in vitro. HTR-tube-like formation reflects trophoblast migration and differentiation toward an invasive phenotype, a physiologic process that takes place during the first trimester of human pregnancy (Johnsen et al. 2011; Waddell et al. 2011). Since fatty acids stimulate tube formation processes in HTR8/SVneo cells, the combined effects of glucose and fatty acids on the tube formation of first-trimester trophoblast cells were evaluated as both of these factors, at higher levels, can contribute to the pathogenesis of GDM. We measured the level of mRNA expression of several proangiogenic factors in first-trimester trophoblast cells in the presence of glucose (5.5 mM vs. 25 mM) in vitro (Table 19.1). Among the proangiogenic factors analyzed in this condition, the mRNA expression of MMP-9 was found to be significantly up regulated in the presence of high glucose condition. In addition, glucose (25 mM) induced tube formation, cellular viability, and proliferation of the first-trimester trophoblast cells, HTR8/SVneo (Basak et al. 2015).

TABLE 19.1

In Vitro mRNA Expression of Angiogenic and Metabolic Growth Factors in the First-Trimester Trophoblast Cells, HTR8/SVneo, After Treatment with Glucose (5.5 mM vs. 25 mM) for 24 hours

Angiogenesis and Metabolic Factors	Gene Name	Gene ID	Fold Expression[a] (Glucose 25 mM/ 5.5 mM)
VEGFA	Vascular endothelial growth factor A	7422	0.74
VEGFB	Vascular endothelial growth factor B	7423	1.27
ANGPTL4	Angiopoietin-like 4	51129	0.45*
KDR	Vascular endothelial growth factor receptor 2	3791	1.14
FGF1	Fibroblast growth factor 1	2246	0.66
FLT1	Vascular endothelial growth factor receptor 1	2321	1.38
MMP-9	Matrix metalloproteinases9/type IV collagen	4318	4.11*
MMP-2	Matrix metalloproteinases2/type IV collagen	4313	1.20
TIMP1	Tissue inhibitor metalloproteinase 1	7076	1.60
TIMP2	Tissue inhibitor metalloproteinase 2	7077	1.23
FABP4	Fatty acid binding protein 4	2167	1.52*
CAV1	Caveolin-1	857	1.66*
FABPpm	Plasma membrane-associated FABP	2806	1.99*
FATP4	Fatty acid transport protein4/SLC27A4	10999	1.34
ACSL5	Acyl-CoA synthetase long-chain family member 5	51703	0.73
ADRP	Adipose differentiation-related protein	123	0.70
COX2	Prostaglandin G/H synthase and cyclooxygenase	5743	1.31
LIPIN1	Phosphatidate phosphatase LPIN1	23175	1.42
GPAT1	Glycerol-3-phosphate acyltransferase 1	57678	1.19
FAT	CD 36 molecule /fatty acid translocase	948	0.51
DGAT1	Diacylglycerol *O*-acyltransferase 1	8694	0.98

[a] Fold expression of each gene was measured at the level of 25 mM glucose after normalizing with endogenous control and calculated over 5.5 mM glucose.

* $p < 0.05$.

It is interesting to note that MMP-9 is a key molecule associated with cellular remodeling that involves trophoblast invasion and angiogenesis of the cells; therefore, selective activation of MMP-9 over MMP-2 without affecting MMP inhibitors was found to be the initial response under hyperglycemia in the first-trimester invasive trophoblast cells, HTR8/SVneo (Basak et al. 2015). These data suggest that increased expression of MMP-9 may contribute a regulatory action in the EVT invasion and remodeling of the decidua during the first trimester of pregnancy, a crucial process for proper functioning of the maternal–fetal interface and trophoblast-mediated spiral artery remodeling of the decidua. Recently, it has been suggested that altered MMP-9 level is a crucial mediator in the development of insulin resistance and inflammation in pregnancies complicated with GDM (Lappas 2014). While hyperglycemia induces MMP-9 expression in first-trimester trophobalst cells, a similar increase in MMP-9 expression was reported in fibroblast cells (Song et al. 2013). High glucose induces epithelial-to-mesenchymal transition of human peritoneal mesothelial cells, and the cellular transition of phenotypic differentiation was regulated by MMP-9 (Li et al. 2012). Available data indicate that MMP-9 is a molecule responsible for cellular remodeling that involves several processes, including migration, differentiation, and cellular invasive activities. Although the mechanism of MMP-9 activation in first-trimester trophoblast cells is not studied yet, excess unmethylated sites of the MMP-9 promoter in the placenta from preeclampsia suggests a possible epigenetic role in MMP-9 activation (Wang et al. 2010). A recent study with 3A-Sub-E trophoblast cells suggested that hyperglycemia induces altered expressions of angiogenesis-associated molecules in trophoblast cells. Hyperglycemia-induced alterations of the cell surface proteoglycans and ECM remodeling on the expressions of angiogenesis-related cytokines and growth factors were reported in these cells (Chang and Vivian Yang 2013).

19.6 INTERPLAY OF GLUCOSE AND FATTY ACID IN METABOLISM AND ANGIOGENESIS OF THE PLACENTA

The direct effect of maternal diabetes during implantation showed increased accumulation of intracellular lipid droplets in blastocysts. Elevated lipid load in embryo was suggested to contribute the adverse effects of maternal diabetes on implantation of embryo development (Schindler et al. 2014). The effect of hyperglycemia and elevated fatty acids and their interactions was reported in trophoblast cells derived from term human placenta. Culture of trophoblasts cells with 250 μM fatty acid inhibited fatty acid oxidation and lipolysis and promoted lipid droplet formation and thereby favored the up-regulation of fatty acid storage and buffering capacity. In contrast to fatty acid, hyperglycemia condition favored intracellular glycogen accumulation and reduced lipid droplet formation but had no other effects on trophoblast metabolism or function. Thus, independent effects of glucose and fatty acid on the trophoblast metabolism of term placenta were suggested (Pathmaperuma et al. 2010). The differential effects of glucose and fatty acids toward tube formation, gene expression, and metabolism of first-trimester trophoblast cells have been reported recently (Basak et al. 2015). We demonstrated earlier that docosahexaenoic acid (DHA) stimulates VEGF secretion in the first-trimester trophoblast cells, HTR8/SVneo. It is not known if this attribute of DHA protects first-trimester trophoblast cells from the disintegration of the capillary tube formation induced by high glucose. The effects mediated by glucose and fatty acid on tube formation of the first-trimester trophoblastic cells were found to be different, as fatty acid increased tube length threefold higher than glucose did at their highest potential dose. VEGF and ANGPTL4 are prominent angiogenic growth factors that are up-regulated by fatty acids in HTR8/SVneo cells (Basak and Duttaroy 2013a,b; Basak, Das, and Duttaroy 2013; Johnsen et al. 2011). Unlike fatty acids, glucose did not alter the expression of VEGF in these cells. VEGF-independent induction was evidenced with leptin- and connective tissue growth factor (CTGF)-induced tube formation of first-trimester trophoblast cells (Basak and Duttaroy 2012; Das et al. 2014). Although the mechanism of DHA-mediated protective effects in vitro is still elusive, several biochemical pathways have been associated with hyperglycemia, including glucose-mediated increases in reactive oxygen species (ROS), diacylglycerol production, and the subsequent activation of the protein kinase C (PKC) pathway flux through the polyol metabolic pathway, accumulation of advanced glycation end products, and cytokine secretion (Leach, Taylor, and Sciota 2009).

To measure hyperglycemic effects on fatty acid metabolic activity in the first trimester, uptake of long chain fatty acid (LCFA) [^{14}C] fatty acids was measured (Basak et al. 2015). In the presence of glucose (25 mM), ^{14}C-EPA (eicosapentaenoic acid, 20:5n-3) uptake was increased significantly as compared with ^{14}C-AA (arachidonic acid, 20:4n-6) and ^{14}C-DHA (22:6n-3) in the first-trimester trophoblast cells, HTR8/SVneo. EPA is the precursor of three series of prostaglandins and an inducer of tube formation in these cells, suggesting that glucose-induced tube formation could be facilitated by an increased ^{14}C-EPA uptake (Johnsen et al. 2011). EPA increases glucose uptake in myotubes (Figueras et al. 2011). Increased uptake of ^{14}C-EPA by glucose was possibly regulated by altered ANGPTL4 expression in these cells, as observed in the presence of 25 mM glucose (Basak et al. 2015). ANGPTL4 is a secreted protein that is involved in dual action as the regulator of angiogenesis and metabolism owing to its differential activities of N-terminal and C-terminal protein. ANGPTL4 is altered by high glucose in retinal epithelial cells (Yokouchi et al. 2013). Since ANGPTL4 inhibits fatty acid uptake by lowering the plasma level of free fatty acid by inhibiting LPL activity, it is possible that the uptake of exogenously added free fatty acids in the cellular system would be increased (Georgiadi et al. 2010). In HTR8/SVneo cells, glucose (25 mM) stimulated the expression of both intracellular (FABP4) and membrane-associated FABPs. FABP4 is being increasingly established to be an intracellular mediator of angiogenesis (Basak and Duttaroy 2013b; Elmasri et al. 2012). Increased expression of FABPs may lead to increased accumulation of fatty acids under high glucose levels. All these data suggest that hyperglycemia in first-trimester trophoblast cells may promote tube-like formation and fatty acid uptake.

19.7 INSULIN RECEPTORS AND BINDING PROTEINS

The peptide hormones insulin, insulin-like growth factor (IGF) 1, and IGF2 mediate a series of metabolic and mitogenic effects by specific binding to the receptor of tyrosine kinase on the surface of the target tissues. Considerable structural homology exists between these two growth factors that often overlaps the binding of these growth factors to the targets. Under physiological level, insulin and IGF1 exclusively bind to their cognate receptors, i.e., the insulin receptor (IR) and the IGF1 receptor (IGF1R), respectively, whereas IGF2 binds to IGF1R especially in rapidly growing tissues such as embryo and cancer (Frasca et al. 1999). Insulin or IGFs regulate fetal and placental growth and development. During maternal diabetes, systemic regulation of insulin, associated growth factors, and binding proteins is altered both in the placenta and/or fetus and in the maternal circulation. The placenta expresses IGF1R both in the apical and the basal surfaces. The expression of IR constantly changes its site during gestation and is regulated by fetal insulin level also. Insulin and IGFs are believed to control the receptor-mediated regulation of placental growth and transport, trophoblast invasion, and placental angiogenesis. Increased placental and fetal growth, observed primarily in diabetes, is causally linked to placental hypervascularization and angiogenesis because of the deregulation of the insulin and growth factors and their receptor-mediated network in these processes. Placental IGF1 and IGF2 expression is regulated differentially by the tissue compartments and stages of the placental development. While IGF1 is expressed throughout gestation in syncytiotrophoblast and cytotrophoblast, IGF2 is not detected in syncytiotrophoblasts. IGF2 is expressed primarily in villous and extravillous cytotrophoblasts of the first trimester, which remain undetected at term, raising its possible involvement in the embryonic development during placentation (Dalcik et al. 2001; Hill et al. 1993; Thomsen et al. 1997).

Insulin-mediated trophobalst action is also regulated by IGF-binding proteins (IGFBPs). IGFBPs are the modulators of the ligand–receptor interaction. There are six IGFBPs reported in the systemic circulation of humans that bind to IGF with superior affinity than their receptors. IGFBPs play a role in sequestering the IGFs from receptor binding (Allan, Flint, and Patel 2001; Hwa, Oh, and Rosenfeld 1999). The interaction improves the survival half-life of IGFs in the circulation and improves their availability for receptor binding by maintaining a local pool of IGFs. The interaction of IGF1 and IGFBP3 is distinct in pregnant and nonpregnant women. In nonpregnant women, IGF1 is bound to form a ternary complex with IGFBP3, while pregnant women have placenta-derived IGFBP3 protease that cleaves the complex and renders the IGFs available for binding to the their receptors in the mother and placenta (Hossenlopp et al. 1990). IGFBP3, which modulates the bio-availability of IGF, has been studied for its potential role in angiogenesis during tissue regeneration and cancer development. IGFBP3 has antiangiogenic activity and demonstrates an independent effect of IGFBP3 on the suppression of VEGF production (Oh et al. 2012). The mRNA expression of six major IGFBPs is reported in the decidua in the second and third trimester, whereas IGFBP1 is the predominant one. In the placenta, IGFBP3 is the predominantly expressed one in extravillous cytotrophoblasts (Hamilton et al. 1998). Epidemiological observation suggests a correlation in the levels of IGF1 and IGFBP3 with birth weight both in the healthy and in the diseased state (Nelson et al. 2008).

19.8   EFFECT OF INSULIN ON ANGIOGENESIS OF THE PLACENTA

Altered vascularization in the placenta is a characteristic morphological change of GDM. However, the impact of maternal diabetes on fetal diabetic environment and their effect on endothelial function of the fetoplacental interface has been highlighted recently (Bulmer et al. 2012). Now, it is being reported that insulin-rich fetal factors in maternal diabetes influence endothelial cell function and, possibly, angiogenesis in vitro. Thus, fetal hyperglycemia and fetal hyperinsulinemia that arise as a result of maternal hyperglycemia in pregnancies complicated with GDM are likely to contribute in the endothelium function of the fetoplacental interface. Insulin-induced angiogenesis is reported to increase the expression of genes associated with angiogenesis and cytoskeleton integrity in these primary endothelial cells. The maintenance or disaggregation of angiogenesis network formation of human umbilical vein endothelial cells (HUVEC) cells was noticeably different in type 1 diabetic pregnancies than in normal ones. In vitro angiogenesis assay demonstrated that insulin increased more branching capillary network formation in HUVEC cells from type 1 diabetic pregnancies after 24 hours of network formation in collagen-1-coated plates, while HUVEC from normal pregnancies showed increased branching at all time points from 2 to 24 hours in the presence of high insulin, followed by a rapid decline in branch formation (Hiden et al. 2012; Leach, Taylor, and Sciota 2009). The placenta shows several alterations in diabetes during pregnancy, with a deregulation of the insulin/IGF homeostasis. IR and IGF1R expression in the placenta is highly regulated, compartmentalized, and gestational specific. Hiden et al. (2006) suggest that the shift in IR expression from the trophoblast to the endothelium represents a shift in regulation of insulin effects from the mother to the fetus. Moreover, it is suggested that placental hyper vascularization in diabetes is the consequence of the proangiogenic action of insulin in the endothelial cells. A recent study showed that insulin enhances two-dimensional networks of tube formation and actin reorganization in third-trimester endothelial cells and activated the phosphatidylinositol 3-kinase–Akt–eNOS pathway (Lassance et al. 2013).

VEGF-induced tube formation was mediated by IGF and its receptor in HUVEC cells, implying direct involvement of IGF1 and its receptor in modulating tube formation of HUVEC cells (Bid et al. 2013). The effects of IGFs on placental trophoblast were studied primarily as growth factors that regulate amino acid transport. Elevated plasma IGF1 and IGF2 level in GDM is correlated with increased levels of fetal amino acid (Cetin et al. 2005). IGFs regulate the proliferation and survival of the cytotrophoblast in human first-trimester placental culture (Forbes and Westwood 2008). The mitogen activated protein kinase (MAPK) and phosphatidylinositol-4,5-bisphosphate 3-kinase

(PI3K) pathways are involved in these processes simultaneously. The subcellular localization of IGF1R in the first-trimester trophoblast is not clear. In the first-trimester trophoblast, these IGFs regulate associated processes that are involved in the trophoblast invasion into the maternal uterus, such as invasiveness (Hamilton et al. 1998), migration (Irving and Lala 1995), MMP-2 production, proliferation (Forbes and Westwood 2008), and membrane-type MMP-1 expression (Hiden et al. 2007). While placental IGFs presumed to regulate fetal insulin level thereby affect fetal growth and development, the other way is also evidenced where placental growth is regulated by fetal insulin. This has been justified by elevated expression of IGF1R in the basal plasma membrane of the syncytiotrophoblast and in endothelial cells. There are studies that suggest that fetal insulin and IGFs control the growth of the placenta.

IGFs are implicated in the receptor-mediated regulation of placental growth and transport, trophoblast invasion, and placental angiogenesis. Dysregulation of growth factors and their receptors may be involved in placental and fetal changes observed in diabetes, i.e., enhanced placental and fetal growth, placental hypervascularization, and higher levels of fetal plasma amino acids. Direct involvement of IGF and its receptor on angiogenesis was recently reported, where targeting both IGF-1 and its ligands could lead to an effective therapeutic strategy to block angiogenesis in IGF-driven tumors. The combination of receptor- and ligand-binding antibodies completely suppressed VEGF-stimulated proliferation of HUVECs in the presence of IGF-I and IGF-2 and suppressed VEGF/IGF-2-driven angiogenesis in vivo (Bid et al. 2013). Insulin enhances VEGF protein expression and secretion. VEGF-induced tube formation was mediated by IGF and its receptor, implying direct involvement of IGF-1 and its receptor in modulating tube formation of HUVEC cells.

Mechanistic studies using different vascular systems have shown that high glucose and insulin levels have profound vascular effects, with elevations in VEGF, nitric oxide (NO), and PKC associated with the alterations in junctional adhesion molecules such as occludin and vascular endothelial-cadherin and vascular leakage of albumin. VEGF and NO appeared to be the main players in the proangiogenic and propermeability aspects of hyperglycemia. This could be the reason why reduced availability of NO in preeclampsia neutralizes the proangiogenic effects of VEGF in this case. The converse may well be true for the diabetic placenta. The study on the direct effects of high glucose on the perfused placental vessels presumably increases in VEGF and increased albumin permeation after hyperglycemic insult. The diabetic changes to NO production and VEGF were reversed by inhibiting the PKC pathway, indicating that insulin stimulates angiogenesis via VEGF–NO–PKC pathways in the endothelial cells (Pietro et al. 2010; Pinter et al. 2001; Siervo et al. 2012; Yang and Reece 2011).

19.9 SUMMARY AND PERSPECTIVE

Maternal hyperglycemia associated with either maternal type 1 diabetes or GDM contributes to several functional changes in the placenta that lead to altered response in mediating placental angiogenesis and vascularization, which are summarized in Table 19.2. The changes in the structure and morphology of the placenta are likely a result of excess collagen deposition in the placenta derived from maternal hyperglycemia. Concurrent with this, glucose (25 mM) treatment in culture stimulated HTR8-tube-like formation, proliferation, and elevated expression of MMP-9; the reduced activity of urokinase-plasminogen activator indicated possible alteration in the invasion and angiogenesis in first-trimester trophobalst cells. Hyperglycemia in first-trimester trophoblast cells promoted contrasting effects mediated by glucose and fatty acid. It is possible that glucose and fatty acid regulate first-trimester trophoblast development in a different manner. Recent study with first-trimester trophoblast cells raises the possibility that inappropriate glucose concentration might contribute to abnormal trophoblast migration and/or invasion, which are associated with major complications of pregnancy.

TABLE 19.2

Functional Changes Attributed to the Effects of Maternal Diabetes (T1D), Gestational Diabetes Mellitus (GDM), and Hyperglycemia Factors on the Angiogenesis and Vascularization of the Placenta

Hyperglycemia Conditions	Characteristics of the Placental Angiogenesis
T1D and GDM	Alteration in the placental vascular structure (Jirkovska et al. 2012; Mayhew 2002; Mayhew et al. 1994; Nelson et al. 2009; Teasdale 1981) ↑Branching capillaries (Jirkovska et al. 2002) ↑Capillary surface area (Teasdale 1981)
GDM	Longer and hypercoiled umbilical cord (Ezimokhai, Rizk, and Thomas 2000)
T1D and GDM	Placental hypervascularization; reduction in the junctional pores ↓Vascular endothelium cadherin (VE-cadherin) (Leach et al. 2004) ↓Occludin and zonula occludin (Babawale et al. 2000)
GDM	Increased in placental angiogenesis ↑FLT-1 (VEGFR1) and KDR (VEGFR2) mRNA expression (Marini et al. 2008) ↑FGF-2 expression and translation (Arany and Hill 1998)
T1D	Vessel maintenance and maturation of sprouting angiogenesis ↑ANG 2 (angiopoietin) mRNA expression (Radaelli et al. 2003) Induces oxidative stress and proinflammatory pathways ↑ROS (Lappas et al. 2011)
Maternal hyperglycemia	Increased expression of proangiogenic inflammatory molecules ↑IL-6 level (Chang and Vivian Yang 2013) ↑Tumor necrosis factor-α level (Moreli et al. 2012)
T1D	Promotes angiogenesis in the placenta
Hyperinsulinemia	↑MT1-MMP (membrane-type matrix metalloproteinase-1) expression (Hiden et al. 2007) ↑e-NOS (nitric oxide synthase) expression (Lassance et al. 2013)
Placental explant Hyperinsulinemia	↑Leptin expression via PI3K- and MAPK-signaling pathways (Perez-Perez et al. 2013)
Glucose (10 mM), first-trimester trophoblast cell line	Reduced invasiveness of the first trimester trophoblast ↓Activity of urokinase-plasminogen activator (Belkacemi et al. 2005)
Glucose (25 mM), first-trimester trophoblast cell line	↑MMP9 mRNA and protein expression (Basak et al. 2015) ↑HTR-tube like formation; ↑Fatty acid uptake
Maternal diabetes and implantation	Increased accumulation of lipid ↑Lipid droplets and increased accumulation of fatty acids (Schindler et al. 2014)
Trophoblast culture, excess fatty acids	↓Fatty acid oxidation (Pathmaperuma et al. 2010) ↑Lipid droplets formation and activity

Note: ↑ indicates elevated levels, ↓ indicates reduced levels.

ACKNOWLEDGMENTS

This work was supported by the Thune Holst Foundation, Norway, and the BOYSCAST visiting fellowship program, India.

REFERENCES

Allan, G. J., D. J. Flint, and K. Patel. 2001. "Insulin-like growth factor axis during embryonic development." *Reproduction* 122 (1):31–9.

Ang, C. and M. A. Lumsden. 2001. "Diabetes and the maternal resistance vasculature." *Clin Sci (Lond)* 101 (6):719–29.

Arany, E. and D. J. Hill. 1998. "Fibroblast growth factor-2 and fibroblast growth factor receptor-1 mRNA expression and peptide localization in placentae from normal and diabetic pregnancies." *Placenta* 19 (2–3):133–42.

Babawale, M. O., S. Lovat, T. M. Mayhew, M. J. Lammiman, D. K. James, and L. Leach. 2000. "Effects of gestational diabetes on junctional adhesion molecules in human term placental vasculature." *Diabetologia* 43 (9):1185–96. doi:10.1007/s001250051511.

Basak, S. and A. K. Duttaroy. 2012. "Leptin induces tube formation in first-trimester extravillous trophoblast cells." *Eur J Obstet Gynecol Reprod Biol* 164 (1):24–9. doi:10.1016/j.ejogrb.2012.05.033.

Basak, S. and A. K. Duttaroy. 2013a. "cis-9,trans-11 conjugated linoleic acid stimulates expression of angiopoietin like-4 in the placental extravillous trophoblast cells." *Biochim Biophys Acta* 1831 (4):834–43. doi:10.1016/j.bbalip.2013.01.012.

Basak, S. and A. K. Duttaroy. 2013b. "Effects of fatty acids on angiogenic activity in the placental extravillious trophoblast cells." *Prostaglandins Leukot Essent Fatty Acids* 88 (2):155–62. doi:10.1016/j.plefa.2012.10.001.

Basak, S., M. K. Das, and A. K. Duttaroy. 2013. "Fatty acid-induced angiogenesis in first trimester placental trophoblast cells: Possible roles of cellular fatty acid-binding proteins." *Life Sci* 93 (21):755–62. doi:10.1016/j.lfs.2013.09.024.

Basak, S., M. K. Das, V. Srinivas, and A. K. Duttaroy. 2015. "The interplay between glucose and fatty acids on tube formation and fatty acid uptake in the first trimester trophoblast cells, HTR8/SVneo." *Mol Cell Biochem* 401 (1–2):11–9. doi:10.1007/s11010-014-2287-9.

Baumann, M. U., S. Zamudio, and N. P. Illsley. 2007. "Hypoxic upregulation of glucose transporters in BeWo choriocarcinoma cells is mediated by hypoxia-inducible factor-1." *Am J Physiol Cell Physiol* 293 (1):C477–85. doi:10.1152/ajpcell.00075.2007.

Belkacemi, L., G. E. Lash, S. K. Macdonald-Goodfellow, J. D. Caldwell, and C. H. Graham. 2005. "Inhibition of human trophoblast invasiveness by high glucose concentrations." *J Clin Endocrinol Metab* 90 (8):4846–51. doi:10.1210/jc.2004-2242.

Bell, R., K. Bailey, T. Cresswell, G. Hawthorne, J. Critchley, and N. Lewis-Barned. 2008. "Trends in prevalence and outcomes of pregnancy in women with pre-existing type I and type II diabetes." *BJOG* 115 (4):445–52. doi:10.1111/j.1471-0528.2007.01644.x.

Benaitreau, D., E. Dos Santos, M. C. Leneveu, N. Alfaidy, J. J. Feige, P. de Mazancourt, R. Pecquery, and M. N. Dieudonne. 2010. "Effects of adiponectin on human trophoblast invasion." *J Endocrinol* 207 (1):45–53. doi:10.1677/JOE-10-0170.

Bid, H. K., C. A. London, J. Gao, H. Zhong, R. E. Hollingsworth, S. Fernandez, X. Mo, and P. J. Houghton. 2013. "Dual targeting of the type 1 insulin-like growth factor receptor and its ligands as an effective antiangiogenic strategy." *Clin Cancer Res* 19:2948–94. doi:10.1158/1078-0432.CCR-12-2008.

Bulmer, J. N., G. J. Burton, S. Collins, T. Cotechini, I. P. Crocker, B. A. Croy, S. Cvitic, M. Desforges, R. Deshpande, M. Gasperowicz, T. Groten, G. Haugen, U. Hiden, A. J. Host, M. Jirkovská, T. Kiserud, J. König, L. Leach, P. Murthi, R. Pijnenborg, O. N. Sadekova, C. M. Salafia, N. Schlabritz-Loutsevitch, J. Stanek, A. E. Wallace, F. Westermeier, J. Zhang, and G. E. Lash. 2012. "IFPA Meeting 2011 workshop report II: Angiogenic signaling and regulation of fetal endothelial function; placental and fetal circulation and growth; spiral artery remodeling." *Placenta* 33:S9–14. doi:10.1016/j.placenta.2011.11.014.

Cetin, I., M. S. de Santis, E. Taricco, T. Radaelli, C. Teng, S. Ronzoni, E. Spada, S. Milani, and G. Pardi. 2005. "Maternal and fetal amino acid concentrations in normal pregnancies and in pregnancies with gestational diabetes mellitus." *Am J Obstet Gynecol* 192 (2):610–7. doi:10.1016/j.ajog.2004.08.011.

Chang, S.-C. and W.-C. Vivian Yang. 2013. "Hyperglycemia induces altered expressions of angiogenesis associated molecules in the trophoblast." *Evid Based Complement Alternat Med* 2013:457971. doi:10.1155/2013/457971.

Cvitic, S., G. Desoye, and U. Hiden. 2014. "Glucose, insulin, and oxygen interplay in placental hypervascularisation in diabetes mellitus." *Biomed Res Int* 2014:145846. doi:10.1155/2014/145846.

Dalcik, H., M. Yardimoglu, B. Vural, C. Dalcik, S. Filiz, S. Gonca, S. Kokturk, and S. Ceylan. 2001. "Expression of insulin-like growth factor in the placenta of intrauterine growth-retarded human fetuses." *Acta Histochem* 103 (2):195–207. doi:10.1078/0065-1281-00580.

Das, M. K., S. Basak, M. S. Ahmed, H. Attramadal, and A. K. Duttaroy. 2014. "Connective tissue growth factor induces tube formation and IL-8 production in first trimester human placental trophoblast cells." *Eur J Obstet Gynecol Reprod Biol* 181C:183–8. doi:10.1016/j.ejogrb.2014.07.045.

Demir, R., U. A. Kayisli, Y. Seval, C. Celik-Ozenci, E. T. Korgun, A. Y. Demir-Weusten, and B. Huppertz. 2004. "Sequential expression of VEGF and its receptors in human placental villi during very early pregnancy: Differences between placental vasculogenesis and angiogenesis." *Placenta* 25 (6):560–72. doi:10.1016/j.placenta.2003.11.011.

Desoye, G. and S. Hauguel-de Mouzon. 2007. "The human placenta in gestational diabetes mellitus: The insulin and cytokine network." *Diabetes Care* 30 (Suppl 2):S120–6. doi:10.2337/dc07-s203.

Economides, D. L., K. H. Nicolaides, and S. Campbell. 1990. "Relation between maternal-to-fetal blood glucose gradient and uterine and umbilical Doppler blood flow measurements." *Br J Obstet Gynaecol* 97 (6):543–4.

Elmasri, H., E. Ghelfi, C.-W. Yu, S. Traphagen, M. Cernadas, H. Cao, G.-P. Shi, J. Plutzky, M. Sahin, G. Hotamisligil, and S. Cataltepe. 2012. "Endothelial cell-fatty acid binding protein 4 promotes angiogenesis: Role of stem cell factor/c-kit pathway." *Angiogenesis* 15 (3):457–68. doi:10.1007/s10456-012-9274-0.

Esterman, A., M. A. Greco, Y. Mitani, T. H. Finlay, F. Ismail-Beigi, and J. Dancis. 1997. "The effect of hypoxia on human trophoblast in culture: Morphology, glucose transport and metabolism." *Placenta* 18 (2–3):129–36.

Ezimokhai, M., D. E. Rizk, and L. Thomas. 2000. "Maternal risk factors for abnormal vascular coiling of the umbilical cord." *Am J Perinatol* 17 (8):441–5. doi:10.1055/s-2000-13452.

Figueras, M., M. Olivan, S. Busquets, F. J. López-Soriano, and J. M. Argilés. 2011. "Effects of eicosapentaenoic acid (EPA) treatment on insulin sensitivity in an animal model of diabetes: Improvement of the inflammatory status." *Obesity (Silver Spring, Md)* 19 (2):362–9. doi:10.1038/oby.2010.194.

Forbes, K. and M. Westwood. 2008. "The IGF axis and placental function. a mini review." *Horm Res* 69 (3):129–37. doi:10.1159/000112585.

Frasca, F., G. Pandini, P. Scalia, L. Sciacca, R. Mineo, A. Costantino, I. D. Goldfine, A. Belfiore, and R. Vigneri. 1999. "Insulin receptor isoform A, a newly recognized, high-affinity insulin-like growth factor II receptor in fetal and cancer cells." *Mol Cell Biol* 19 (5):3278–88.

Garner, P. R., M. E. D'Alton, D. K. Dudley, P. Huard, and M. Hardie. 1990. "Preeclampsia in diabetic pregnancies." *Am J Obstet Gynecol* 163 (2):505–8.

Georgiadi, A., L. Lichtenstein, T. Degenhardt, M. V. Boekschoten, M. van Bilsen, B. Desvergne, M. Müller, and S. Kersten. 2010. "Induction of cardiac Angptl4 by dietary fatty acids is mediated by peroxisome proliferator-activated receptor beta/delta and protects against fatty acid-induced oxidative stress." *Circ Res* 106 (11):1712–21. doi:10.1161/CIRCRESAHA.110.217380.

González-Muniesa, P., C. de Oliveira, F. Pérez de Heredia, M. P. Thompson, and P. Trayhurn. 2011. "Fatty acids and hypoxia stimulate the expression and secretion of the adipokine ANGPTL4 (angiopoietin-like protein 4/ fasting-induced adipose factor) by human adipocytes." *J Nutrigenet Nutrigenomics* 4 (3):146–53. doi:10.1159/000327774.

Hahn, T., S. Barth, U. Weiss, W. Mosgoeller, and G. Desoye. 1998. "Sustained hyperglycemia in vitro down-regulates the GLUT1 glucose transport system of cultured human term placental trophoblast: A mechanism to protect fetal development?" *FASEB J* 12 (12):1221–31.

Hahn, T., D. Hahn, A. Blaschitz, E. T. Korgun, G. Desoye, and G. Dohr. 2000. "Hyperglycaemia-induced subcellular redistribution of GLUT1 glucose transporters in cultured human term placental trophoblast cells." *Diabetologia* 43 (2):173–80. doi:10.1007/s001250050026.

Hamilton, G. S., J. J. Lysiak, V. K. Han, and P. K. Lala. 1998. "Autocrine-paracrine regulation of human trophoblast invasiveness by insulin-like growth factor (IGF)-II and IGF-binding protein (IGFBP)-1." *Exp Cell Res* 244 (1):147–56. doi:10.1006/excr.1998.4195.

Harmon, K. A., L. Gerard, D. R. Jensen, E. H. Kealey, T. L. Hernandez, M. S. Reece, L. A. Barbour, and D. H. Bessesen. 2011. "Continuous glucose profiles in obese and normal-weight pregnant women on a controlled diet: Metabolic determinants of fetal growth." *Diabetes Care* 34 (10):2198–204. doi:10.2337/dc11-0723.

Hayashi, M., M. Sakata, T. Takeda, T. Yamamoto, Y. Okamoto, K. Sawada, A. Kimura, R. Minekawa, M. Tahara, K. Tasaka, and Y. Murata. 2004. "Induction of glucose transporter 1 expression through hypoxia-inducible factor 1alpha under hypoxic conditions in trophoblast-derived cells." *J Endocrinol* 183 (1):145–54. doi:10.1677/joe.1.05599.

Hiden, U., A. Maier, M. Bilban, N. Ghaffari-Tabrizi, C. Wadsack, I. Lang, G. Dohr, and G. Desoye. 2006. "Insulin control of placental gene expression shifts from mother to foetus over the course of pregnancy." *Diabetologia* 49 (1):123–31. doi:10.1007/s00125-005-0054-x.

Hiden, U., E. Glitzner, M. Ivanisevic, J. Djelmis, C. Wadsack, U. Lang, and G. Desoye. 2007. "MT1–MMP expression in first-trimester placental tissue is upregulated in type 1 diabetes as a result of elevated insulin and tumor necrosis factor-levels." *Diabetes* 57 (1):150–7. doi:10.2337/db07-0903.

Hiden, U., L. Lassance, N. Ghaffari Tabrizi, H. Miedl, C. Tam-Amersdorfer, I. Cetin, U. Lang, and G. Desoye. 2012. "Fetal insulin and IGF-II contribute to gestational diabetes mellitus (GDM)-associated up-regulation of membrane-type matrix metalloproteinase 1 (MT1–MMP) in the human fetoplacental endothelium." *J Clin Endocrinol Metab* 97 (10):3613–21. doi:10.1210/jc.2012-1212.

Hill, J. A. 2001. "Maternal–embryonic cross-talk." *Ann N Y Acad Sci* 943:17–25.

Hill, D. J., D. R. Clemmons, S. C. Riley, N. Bassett, and J. R. Challis. 1993. "Immunohistochemical localization of insulin-like growth factors (IGFs) and IGF binding proteins-1, -2 and -3 in human placenta and fetal membranes." *Placenta* 14 (1):1–12.

Hossenlopp, P., B. Segovia, C. Lassarre, M. Roghani, M. Bredon, and M. Binoux. 1990. "Evidence of enzymatic degradation of insulin-like growth factor-binding proteins in the 150K complex during pregnancy." *J Clin Endocrinol Metab* 71 (4):797–805. doi:10.1210/jcem-71-4-797.

Hwa, V., Y. Oh, and R. G. Rosenfeld. 1999. "The insulin-like growth factor-binding protein (IGFBP) superfamily." *Endocr Rev* 20 (6):761–87. doi:10.1210/edrv.20.6.0382.

Illsley, N. P. 2000. "Glucose transporters in the human placenta." *Placenta* 21 (1):14–22. doi:10.1053/plac.1999.0448.

Illsley, N. P., M. C. Sellers, and R. L. Wright. 1998. "Glycaemic regulation of glucose transporter expression and activity in the human placenta." *Placenta* 19 (7):517–24.

Irving, J. A. and P. K. Lala. 1995. "Functional role of cell surface integrins on human trophoblast cell migration: Regulation by TGF-beta, IGF-II, and IGFBP-1." *Exp Cell Res* 217 (2):419–27. doi:10.1006/excr.1995.1105.

Jansson, T., M. Wennergren, and N. P. Illsley. 1993. "Glucose transporter protein expression in human placenta throughout gestation and in intrauterine growth retardation." *J Clin Endocrinol Metab* 77 (6):1554–62. doi:10.1210/jcem.77.6.8263141.

Jansson, T., K. Ylven, M. Wennergren, and T. L. Powell. 2002. "Glucose transport and system A activity in syncytiotrophoblast microvillous and basal plasma membranes in intrauterine growth restriction." *Placenta* 23 (5):392–9. doi:10.1053/plac.2002.0826.

Janzen, C., M. Y. Lei, J. Cho, P. Sullivan, B. C. Shin, and S. U. Devaskar. 2013. "Placental glucose transporter 3 (GLUT3) is up-regulated in human pregnancies complicated by late-onset intrauterine growth restriction." *Placenta* 34 (11):1072–8. doi:10.1016/j.placenta.2013.08.010.

Jauniaux, E., J. Hempstock, C. Teng, F. C. Battaglia, and G. J. Burton. 2005. "Polyol concentrations in the fluid compartments of the human conceptus during the first trimester of pregnancy: Maintenance of redox potential in a low oxygen environment." *J Clin Endocrinol Metab* 90 (2):1171–5. doi:10.1210/jc.2004-1513.

Jirkovska, M., L. Kubinova, J. Janacek, M. Moravcova, V. Krejci, and P. Karen. 2002. "Topological properties and spatial organization of villous capillaries in normal and diabetic placentas." *J Vasc Res* 39 (3):268–78.

Jirkovska, M., T. Kucera, J. Kalab, M. Jadrnicek, V. Niedobova, J. Janacek, L. Kubinova, M. Moravcova, Z. Zizka, and V. Krejci. 2012. "The branching pattern of villous capillaries and structural changes of placental terminal villi in type 1 diabetes mellitus." *Placenta* 33 (5):343–51. doi:10.1016/j.placenta.2012.01.014.

Johnsen, G. M., S. Basak, M. S. Weedon-Fekjaer, A. C. Staff, and A. K. Duttaroy. 2011. "Docosahexaenoic acid stimulates tube formation in first trimester trophoblast cells, HTR8/SVneo." *Placenta* 32:626–32. doi:10.1016/j.placenta.2011.06.009.

Jovanović, M., I. Stefanoska, L. Radojčić, and L. Vićovac. 2010. "Interleukin-8 (CXCL8) stimulates trophoblast cell migration and invasion by increasing levels of matrix metalloproteinase (MMP)2 and MMP9 and integrins α5 and β1." *Reproduction* 139 (4):789–98. doi:10.1530/REP-09-0341.

Katavetin, P., T. Miyata, R. Inagi, T. Tanaka, R. Sassa, J. R. Ingelfinger, T. Fujita, and M. Nangaku. 2006. "High glucose blunts vascular endothelial growth factor response to hypoxia via the oxidative stress-regulated hypoxia-inducible factor/hypoxia-responsible element pathway." *J Am Soc Nephrol* 17 (5):1405–13. doi:10.1681/asn.2005090918.

Korgun, E. T., C. Celik-Ozenci, Y. Seval, G. Desoye, and R. Demir. 2005. "Do glucose transporters have other roles in addition to placental glucose transport during early pregnancy?" *Histochem Cell Biol* 123 (6):621–9. doi:10.1007/s00418-005-0792-3.

Lappas, M. 2014. "NOD1 expression is increased in the adipose tissue of women with gestational diabetes." *J Endocrinol* 222 (1):99–112. doi:10.1530/JOE-14-0179.

Lappas, M., U. Hiden, G. Desoye, J. Froehlich, S. Hauguel-de Mouzon, and A. Jawerbaum. 2011. "The role of oxidative stress in the pathophysiology of gestational diabetes mellitus." *Antioxid Redox Signal* 15 (12):3061–100. doi:10.1089/ars.2010.3765.

Lassance, L., H. Miedl, M. Absenger, F. Diaz-Perez, U. Lang, G. Desoye, and U. Hiden. 2013. "Hyperinsulinemia stimulates angiogenesis of human fetoplacental endothelial cells: A possible role of insulin in placental hypervascularization in diabetes mellitus." *J Clin Endocrinol Metab* 98 (9):E1438–47. doi:10.1210/jc.2013-1210.

Leach, L., C. Gray, S. Staton, M. O. Babawale, A. Gruchy, C. Foster, T. M. Mayhew, and D. K. James. 2004. "Vascular endothelial cadherin and beta-catenin in human fetoplacental vessels of pregnancies complicated by Type 1 diabetes: Associations with angiogenesis and perturbed barrier function." *Diabetologia* 47 (4):695–709. doi:10.1007/s00125-004-1341-7.

Leach, L., A. Taylor, and F. Sciota. 2009. "Vascular dysfunction in the diabetic placenta: Causes and consequences." *J Anat* 215 (1):69–76. doi:10.1111/j.1469-7580.2009.01098.x.

Li, C., Y. Ren, X. Jia, P. Liang, W. Lou, L. He, M. Li, S. Sun, and H. Wang. 2012. "Twist overexpression promoted epithelial-to-mesenchymal transition of human peritoneal mesothelial cells under high glucose." *Nephrol Dial Transplant* 27 (11):4119–24. doi:10.1093/ndt/gfs049.

Lockwood, C. J., C. Oner, Y. H. Uz, U. A. Kayisli, S. J. Huang, L. F. Buchwalder, W. Murk, E. F. Funai, and F. Schatz. 2008. "Matrix metalloproteinase 9 (MMP9) expression in preeclamptic decidua and MMP9 induction by tumor necrosis factor alpha and interleukin 1 beta in human first trimester decidual cells." *Biol Reprod* 78 (6):1064–72. doi:10.1095/biolreprod.107.063743.

Luo, J., F. Qiao, and X. Yin. 2011. "Hypoxia induces FGF2 production by vascular endothelial cells and alters MMP9 and TIMP1 expression in extravillous trophoblasts and their invasiveness in a cocultured model." *J Reprod Dev* 57 (1):84–91.

Luther, J., J. Milne, R. Aitken, M. Matsuzaki, L. Reynolds, D. Redmer, and J. Wallace. 2007. "Placental growth, angiogenic gene expression, and vascular development in undernourished adolescent sheep." *Biol Reprod* 77 (2):351–7. doi:10.1095/biolreprod.107.061457.

Marini, M., D. Vichi, A. Toscano, G. D. Thyrion, L. Bonaccini, E. Parretti, G. Gheri, A. Pacini, and E. Sgambati. 2008. "Effect of impaired glucose tolerance during pregnancy on the expression of VEGF receptors in human placenta." *Reprod Fertil Dev* 20 (7):789–801.

Mayhew, T. M. 2002. "Enhanced fetoplacental angiogenesis in pre-gestational diabetes mellitus: The extra growth is exclusively longitudinal and not accompanied by microvascular remodelling." *Diabetologia* 45 (10):1434–9. doi:10.1007/s00125-002-0927-1.

Mayhew, T. M., F. B. Sorensen, J. G. Klebe, and M. R. Jackson. 1994. "Growth and maturation of villi in placentae from well-controlled diabetic women." *Placenta* 15 (1):57–65.

Metzger, B. E., L. P. Lowe, A. R. Dyer, E. R. Trimble, U. Chaovarindr, D. R. Coustan, D. R. Hadden, D. R. McCance, M. Hod, H. D. McIntyre, J. J. Oats, B. Persson, M. S. Rogers, and D. A. Sacks. 2008. "Hyperglycemia and adverse pregnancy outcomes." *N Engl J Med* 358 (19):1991–2002. doi:10.1056/NEJMoa0707943.

Moreli, J. B., G. Morceli, A. K. De Luca, C. G. Magalhaes, R. A. Costa, D. C. Damasceno, M. V. Rudge, and I. M. Calderon. 2012. "Influence of maternal hyperglycemia on IL-10 and TNF-alpha production: The relationship with perinatal outcomes." *J Clin Immunol* 32 (3):604–10. doi:10.1007/s10875-011-9634-3.

Murray, M. J. and B. A. Lessey. 1999. "Embryo implantation and tumor metastasis: Common pathways of invasion and angiogenesis." *Semin Reprod Endocrinol* 17 (3):275–90. doi:10.1055/s-2007-1016235.

Nelson, S. M., D. J. Freeman, N. Sattar, and R. S. Lindsay. 2008. "Role of adiponectin in matching of fetal and placental weight in mothers with type 1 diabetes." *Diabetes Care* 31 (6):1123–5. doi:10.2337/dc07-2195.

Nelson, S. M., P. M. Coan, G. J. Burton, and R. S. Lindsay. 2009. "Placental structure in type 1 diabetes: Relation to fetal insulin, leptin, and IGF-I." *Diabetes* 58 (11):2634–41. doi:10.2337/db09-0739.

Oh, S.-H., W.-Y. Kim, O.-H. Lee, J.-H. Kang, J.-K. Woo, J.-H. Kim, B. Glisson, and H.-Y. Lee. 2012. "Insulin-like growth factor binding protein-3 suppresses vascular endothelial growth factor expression and tumor angiogenesis in head and neck squamous cell carcinoma." *Cancer Sci* 103 (7):1259–66. doi:10.1111/j.1349-7006.2012.02301.x.

Ostlund, I., B. Haglund, and U. Hanson. 2004. "Gestational diabetes and preeclampsia." *Eur J Obstet Gynecol Reprod Biol* 113 (1):12–6. doi:10.1016/j.ejogrb.2003.07.001.

Patel, J., K. Landers, R. H. Mortimer, and K. Richard. 2010. "Regulation of hypoxia inducible factors (HIF) in hypoxia and normoxia during placental development." *Placenta* 31 (11):951–7. doi:10.1016/j.placenta.2010.08.008.

Pathmaperuma, A. N., P. Mana, S. N. Cheung, K. Kugathas, A. Josiah, M. E. Koina, A. Broomfield, V. Delghingaro-Augusto, D. A. Ellwood, J. E. Dahlstrom, and C. J. Nolan. 2010. "Fatty acids alter glycerolipid metabolism and induce lipid droplet formation, syncytialisation and cytokine production in human trophoblasts with minimal glucose effect or interaction." *Placenta* 31 (3):230–9. doi:10.1016/j.placenta.2009.12.013.

Perez-Perez, A., J. Maymo, Y. Gambino, P. Guadix, J. L. Duenas, C. Varone, and V. Sanchez-Margalet. 2013. "Insulin enhances leptin expression in human trophoblastic cells." *Biol Reprod* 89 (1):20. doi:10.1095/biolreprod.113.109348.

Persson, M., M. Norman, and U. Hanson. 2009. "Obstetric and perinatal outcomes in type 1 diabetic pregnancies: A large, population-based study." *Diabetes Care* 32 (11):2005–9. doi:10.2337/dc09-0656.

Pietro, L., S. Daher, M. V. C. Rudge, I. M. P. Calderon, D. C. Damasceno, Y. K. Sinzato, C. Bandeira, and E. Bevilacqua. 2010. "Vascular endothelial growth factor (VEGF) and VEGF-receptor expression in placenta of hyperglycemic pregnant women." *Placenta* 31 (9):770–80. doi:10.1016/j.placenta.2010.07.003.

Pinter, E., J. Haigh, A. Nagy, and J. A. Madri. 2001. "Hyperglycemia-induced vasculopathy in the murine conceptus is mediated via reductions of VEGF-A expression and VEGF receptor activation." *Am J Pathol* 158 (4):1199–206. doi:10.1016/S0002-9440(10)64069-2.

Radaelli, T., A. Varastehpour, P. Catalano, and S. Hauguel-de Mouzon. 2003. "Gestational diabetes induces placental genes for chronic stress and inflammatory pathways." *Diabetes* 52 (12):2951–8.

Schindler, M., M. Pendzialek, A. Navarrete Santos, T. Plosch, S. Seyring, J. Gurke, E. Haucke, J. M. Knelangen, B. Fischer, and A. N. Santos. 2014. "Maternal diabetes leads to unphysiological high lipid accumulation in rabbit preimplantation embryos." *Endocrinology* 155 (4):1498–509. doi:10.1210/en.2013-1760.

Siervo, M., V. Tomatis, B. C. M. Stephan, M. Feelisch, and L. J. C. Bluck. 2012. "VEGF is indirectly associated with NO production and acutely increases in response to hyperglycaemia(1)." *Eur J Clin Invest* 42 (9):967–73. doi:10.1111/j.1365-2362.2012.02684.x.

Song, S. E., Y.-W. Kim, J.-Y. Kim, D. H. Lee, J.-R. Kim, and S.-Y. Park. 2013. "IGFBP5 mediates high glucose-induced cardiac fibroblast activation." *J Mol Endocrinol* 50 (3):291–303. doi:10.1530/JME-12-0194.

Staun-Ram, E. and E. Shalev. 2005. "Human trophoblast function during the implantation process." *Reprod Biol Endocrinol* 3:56. doi:10.1186/1477-7827-3-56.

Teasdale, F. 1981. "Histomorphometry of the placenta of the diabetic woman: Class A diabetes mellitus." *Placenta* 2 (3):241–251. doi:10.1016/S0143-4004(81)80007-0.

Thomsen, B. M., H. V. Clausen, L. G. Larsen, L. Nurnberg, B. Ottesen, and H. K. Thomsen. 1997. "Patterns in expression of insulin-like growth factor-II and of proliferative activity in the normal human first and third trimester placenta demonstrated by non-isotopic in situ hybridization and immunohistochemical staining for MIB-1." *Placenta* 18 (2–3):145–54.

Torry, D. S. and R. J. Torry. 1997. "Angiogenesis and the expression of vascular endothelial growth factor in endometrium and placenta." *Am J Reprod Immunol* 37 (1):21–9.

Vambergue, A. and I. Fajardy. 2011. "Consequences of gestational and pregestational diabetes on placental function and birth weight." *World J Diabetes* 2 (11):196–203. doi:10.4239/wjd.v2.i11.196.

Waddell, J. M., J. Evans, H. N. Jabbour, and F. C. Denison. 2011. "CTGF expression is up-regulated by PROK1 in early pregnancy and influences HTR-8/Svneo cell adhesion and network formation." *Hum Reprod* 26 (1):67–75. doi:10.1093/humrep/deq294.

Wang, Z., S. Lu, C. Liu, B. Zhao, K. Pei, L. Tian, and X. Ma. 2010. "Expressional and epigenetic alterations of placental matrix metalloproteinase 9 in preeclampsia." *Gynecol Endocrinol* 26 (2):96–102. doi:10.3109/09513590903184100.

Yamada, T., N. Ozaki, Y. Kato, Y. Miura, and Y. Oiso. 2006. "Insulin downregulates angiopoietin-like protein 4 mRNA in 3T3-L1 adipocytes." *Biochem Biophys Res Commun* 347 (4):1138–44. doi:10.1016/j.bbrc.2006.07.032.

Yang, P. and E. A. Reece. 2011. "Role of HIF-1α in maternal hyperglycemia-induced embryonic vasculopathy." *Am J Obstet Gynecol* 204 (4):332.e1–7. doi:10.1016/j.ajog.2011.01.012.

Yang, P., Z. Zhao, and E. A. Reece. 2008. "Blockade of c-Jun N-terminal kinase activation abrogates hyperglycemia-induced yolk sac vasculopathy in vitro." *Am J Obstet Gynecol* 198 (3):321.e1–7. doi:10.1016/j.ajog.2007.09.010.

Yokouchi, H., K. Eto, W. Nishimura, N. Takeda, Y. Kaburagi, S. Yamamoto, and K. Yasuda. 2013. "Angiopoietin-like protein 4 (ANGPTL4) is induced by high glucose in retinal pigment epithelial cells and exhibits potent angiogenic activity on retinal endothelial cells." *Acta Ophthalmol* 91 (4):e289–97. doi:10.1111/aos.12097.

Young, R. M., S. J. Wang, J. D. Gordan, X. Ji, S. A. Liebhaber, and M. C. Simon. 2008. "Hypoxia-mediated selective mRNA translation by an internal ribosome entry site-independent mechanism." *J Biol Chem* 283 (24):16309–19. doi:10.1074/jbc.M710079200.

Zamudio, S., T. Torricos, E. Fik, M. Oyala, L. Echalar, J. Pullockaran, E. Tutino, B. Martin, S. Belliappa, E. Balanza, and N. P. Illsley. 2010. "Hypoglycemia and the origin of hypoxia-induced reduction in human fetal growth." *PLoS One* 5 (1):e8551. doi:10.1371/journal.pone.0008551.

20 Role of Cytokines in Healthy and Pathological Pregnancies

Abhilash D. Pandya, Mrinal K. Das, and Johannes Rolin

CONTENTS

ABSTRACT

From fertilization to child birth, healthy pregnancies undergo various physiological phases. Numerous biochemical changes occur during each of these stages to encounter stress and regulate immune responses. Small proteins secreted mostly by immune cells, called cytokines, are important in countering infectious agents, modulating inflammation, and facilitating growth. In the course of infection, immune cells secrete proinflammatory cytokines and stimulate inflammation. However, pregnancy is a unique condition where anti-inflammatory cytokines are abundantly produced. Maternal and fetal immunological factors play significant roles in maintaining homeostasis during gestation and are determining factors to differentiate healthy versus pathological pregnancy. Several theories and hypotheses have been proposed on the roles of cytokines during pregnancy. This chapter focuses mainly on the cytokine-driven immunological changes in healthy and pathological pregnancies.

KEY WORDS

Immunology, maternal NK cells and trophoblast, cytokines in pregnancy, IL-17, IFN-γ, Th1/Th2 paradigm, preeclampsia.

20.1 INTRODUCTION

The immune system of mammals has evolved different lines of attack to defend the organism against a wide range of potentially infectious pathogens by differentiating self from nonself. Various immunoregulatory proteins play imperative roles in shaping the immune response. To enable allograft (fetus) survival, the immune response allows total immune competence in pregnancy. Consequently, pregnancy reveals two distinctive immunological aspects and raise questions. First, how does a fetus living in a sterile environment develop the essential framework of the immune system? And second, how do fetal and maternal immunological factors work together at the maternal–fetal interface to tolerate the growth of the semiallogeneic fetus? The success or failure of pregnancy depends on cellular immune effectors and their proinflammatory or anti-inflammatory response. The immunological recognition of pregnancy is imperative for the maintenance of gestation and also for modulation of common disorders of pregnancy. Some small soluble proteins like cytokines act as immunomodulators and play a very significant role in this process. Cytokines are small signaling proteins secreted by and acting on a wide array of cells. Through binding of specific receptors, tight regulation of biological processes via secretion and distribution of these potent mediators are achieved. These versatile pluripotent factors are key mediators of reactions ranging from autoimmune diseases, rejection of allografts, and hypersensitivity.

The human immune system is classified into two functional entities, namely, the innate and the adaptive immune systems. Upon invasion by microbes in the body, cells of the innate immune system, such as neutrophils, monocytes, and natural killer (NK) cells, recognize them through a range of receptors specific for molecules broadly expressed among pathogens. Upon activation of such receptors, the innate immune system is activated, and the cells start to produce cytokines. Some of them, the chemokines, attract more innate immune cells, while others, such as interleukin (IL)-1, IL-6, and tumor necrosis factor-α (TNF-α), increase their activity. Monocytes are matured into dendritic cells, which present the foreign material to T cells and B cells. A few days later, the adaptive system launches two sets of responses specifically toward the intruder: cell mediated and humoral immunity. These two responses are fundamentally different in terms of the cytokines they produce.

While vital in the development and regeneration of tissues, cytokines also attract the most attention because of their many essential and easily recognizable effects in inflammation. Considering the potency of the effects of cytokines, a lot of effort has been put into revealing and understanding the mechanisms for the secretion and degradation of the cytokines themselves and their respective receptors. Taking in all these aspects is beyond the scope of this chapter. Rather, we will present here a summary of the current knowledge regarding the effects of various cytokines in the trophoblast microenvironment in early pregnancy. That is, which cells produce specific cytokines, and what implications do the cytokines have on the trophoblasts and their surroundings? Parallels will be drawn to the clinical observations and phenomena caused by the cytokines. Toward the end, pregnancy-related pathological conditions that are related to dysregulation of the cytokine system will be mentioned.

20.2   NK CELLS IN PREGNANCY

It has been proven now that predominant immune interactions in the decidua are between the placental trophoblast and maternal NK cells instead of T cells (Rai, Sacks, and Trew 2005). Aberrant NK cell activation systemically in the maternal blood and locally in the decidua may be the cause of preeclampsia. Among others, uterine NK (uNK) cells are the most abundant and constitute about 70% of the total lymphocytes in early pregnancy. uNK cells secrete different kinds of cytokines and growth factors, including TNF-α, IL-10, granulocyte macrophage colony-stimulating factor (GMCSF), interleukin-1 (IL-1), transforming growth factor beta 1 (TGF-β1), colony stimulating factor 1 (CSF-1), leukemia inhibitory factor (LIF), and interferon (IFN)-γ (Jokhi, King, and Loke 1994, 1997). Cell surface antigens CD16 and CD56 expressed from NK cells require IL-2 for cytotoxic killing. Since CD16 is a low-affinity receptor for immunoglobulin G, it regulates NK-mediated antibody dependent cellular cytotoxicity. Based on the density of expression of CD56 (CD56[bright] versus CD56[dim]), NK cells display preferential function as either primarily cytotoxic cells (CD56[dim]) or cytokine-producing cells of IFN-γ and TNF-α (CD56[bright]). Unlike CD56[dim] NK cells, cytokine-producing CD56[bright] NK cells are mostly agranular. Although uNK cells appear to be primarily of the CD56[bright] subtype and are thus skewed toward cytokine secretion to exhibit immunoregulatory functions, they are highly granular. The peripheral blood CD56[bright]CD16- NK cells secrete proinflammatory granulocyte macrophage (GM)-CSF, TNF-α, and IFN-γ (Saito et al. 1993). Saito et al. also observed m-RNA expression of above cytokines in CD56[bright]CD16- NK cells. *In vitro* culture

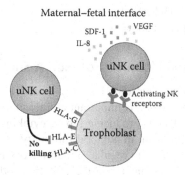

FIGURE 20.1 Immune cross-talk and its interaction between uNK cells and trophoblasts. Because of altered expression of MHC molecules as compared with normal cells, trophoblasts are spared from NK cell lysis despite their foreign gene material. As well as because of their expression of ligands for activating NK cell receptors, they mediate an increase in the secretion of cytokines important for the implantation process. Minor changes in the signals in this interplay may lead to complications such as preeclampsia.

data and transcriptional arrays reveal that human uNK cells are a unique immunomodulatory NK cell subset (Cooper et al. 2001; Koopman et al. 2003).

20.2.1 Role of uNK Cells in Trophoblast Invasion

In early pregnancy, uNK cells play a vital role in stimulating trophoblast growth, differentiation, and invasion (Le Bouteiller and Tabiasco 2006; Moffett and Loke 2006). This takes place mainly via the cytokines and chemokines secreted by NK cells. The trophoblast is the outermost layer of the placenta and is in direct connection with the maternal immune system. During the early stages of pregnancy, the placenta-derived extravillous trophoblast begins to invade the maternal uterus to regulate sufficient blood flow and nutrient supply to the developing fetus. The NK cells might control placentation and trophoblast invasion owing to their close vicinity to trophoblast cells (King et al. 1991; Moffett and Loke 2006).

The trophoblast cells lack expression of classical human leukocyte antigen (HLA) class I and II molecules, thereby preventing recognition by the few maternal T lymphocytes found in the maternal decidua. However, they express other HLA class I molecules, including HLA-C, HLA-G, and HLA-E (Rajagopalan and Long 1999; Moffett and Loke 2006), that protect them from NK cell killing. The trophoblast cells express ligands for major activating NK receptors (Vacca et al. 2008), upon interaction with which uNK cells release elevated amount of IL-8, stromal cell derived factor-1 (SDF-1) and vascular endothelial growth factor (Figure 20.1). Thus, rather than cytotoxic or proinflammatory role, uNK cells seem to stimulate the actions important for building and remodeling of trophoblast and other placental tissues (Sivori et al. 2000; Hanna et al. 2006; Vacca et al. 2008). The few variations of the maternal NK receptor genotype and fetal HLA molecules may result in disproportionate NK cell inhibition and might be linked with larger risk of preeclampsia owing to insufficient spiral artery formation and inappropriate trophoblast and NK cell interactions (Hiby et al. 2004). Consequently, defects in decidual NK cell generation, or incongruous functional interfaces with other cell types, could have major concerns for healthy gestation.

20.3 CYTOKINES IN PREGNANCY

As discussed earlier, cytokines play an imperative role during each phase of pregnancy. Proinflammatory cytokines can induce inflammation and possibly related pathological conditions, whereas anti-inflammatory cytokines play a significant part to regulate the effects of these cytokines. In the early 1990s, Wegmann et al. proposed an interesting hypothesis on cytokine shifts in pregnancy—the T helper (Th) 1/Th2 paradigm. Accordingly, immune response is biased toward Th2 cytokine production during pregnancy.

20.3.1 Th1/Th2 Shifts during Healthy Pregnancy: A Short-Lived Hypothesis

Th1 cells producing type 1 cytokines, including IL-2, IFN-γ, and TNF-β, are central in cell-mediated immunity. This kind of immune reaction is important mainly in removal of cancer cells and intracellular pathogens. Th2 cells or T cells producing type 2 cytokines such as IL-4, IL-5, IL-6, and IL-13, on the other hand, are significant in humoral immunity that involves antibody production. Th2 cytokines play a determining role to regulate inflammatory conditions. These cytokines are anti-inflammatory in nature and thus modulate the effects of other proinflammatory cytokines throughout gestation. This Th1–Th2 shift is very significant and distinguishes a normal pregnancy from a pathological one. During a normal pregnancy, the immune reaction is skewed toward Th2 (Lin et al. 1993) (Figure 20.2). Upon development of preeclampsia, however, the numbers of circulating lymphocytes are affected, as the Th1 cells increase in numbers while the Th2 cells decrease. Both are activated and produce their respective cytokines so that the net effect is a shift toward Th1 (Yoneyama et al. 2002).

A question arising from this observation is what regulates the development of Th1 or Th2 cells in this situation? Sacks et al. has reported that peripheral blood leukocytes from normal pregnant woman produce higher levels of proinflammatory cytokines IL-12, TNF-α, and IL-18 than those from nonpregnant women, where IFN-γ levels are suppressed. On the contrary, in preeclampsia, IFN-γ production is substantially increased, although the levels of IL-12 and TNF-α production by

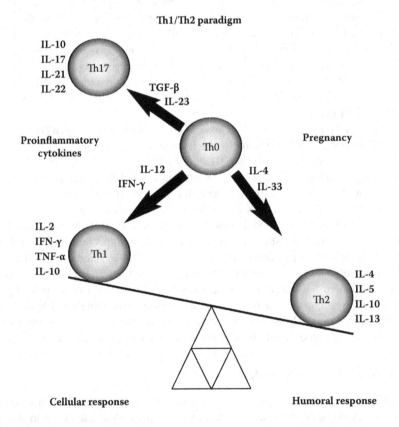

FIGURE 20.2 Th1/Th2 cytokine shift in normal physiological state and during pregnancy. The biased Th2 cytokine shift is observed during pregnancy to avoid maternal T-cell rejection of the fetus.

peripheral blood leukocytes are similar to those seen in normal pregnancy. They have also presented increased cellular production of IL-18 in preeclampsia. IL-18 itself can act as a Th2 cytokine, but it induces Th1 responses when it acts synergistically with IL-12 (Sacks, Redman, and Sargent 2003).

Two cytokines are of special importance when the T cells are directed toward Th1 or Th2 during development, namely, IL-12 and IL-18. Monocytes and dendritic cells are important sources of these cytokines, and their release is determined by the environment around these cells. During a normal pregnancy, IL-10, TGF-β, and prostaglandin E2 (PGE2) are produced by trophoblasts; NK cells and others inhibit the production of IL-12 (Wittmann et al. 1999). A high ratio of IL-18 to IL-12 operates the shift to Th2 during normal pregnancy, and therefore, as there is IL-18 domination, the Th2 type immunity will dominate. Conversely, upon stimulation of monocytes, NK cells, and T cells by the responses to necrotic cell debris in preeclampsia, elevated levels of IFN-γ and GM-CSF are produced, resulting in increased production of IL-12. Thus, a low ratio of IL-18 to IL-12 sets off the Th1 preference and increases IFN-γ production in preeclampsia (Sakai et al. 2004), shifting toward a Th1 response. Consequently, there seems an impetus of focusing on IFN-γ production, influenced by alterations in IL-12 and IL-18 levels during pregnancy and preeclampsia.

For several years, Tom Wegmann's Th1/Th2 hypothesis (Wegmann et al. 1993) has rendered a fruitful framework for studies of the immunology of pregnancy, although recent findings have challenged this concept, which requires reevaluation. Despite the bias toward Th2 cytokine production, no evidence proves the importance of this bias to the success of pregnancy. The bias might simply be a physiological deviation but does not affect pregnancy hormone changes (Rai, Sacks, and Trew 2005). Another strong evidence also indicates that the levels of particular Th1 cytokines are raised, instead of lowered, in normal pregnancy compared with the nonpregnant state (Rai, Sacks, and Trew 2005). However, one of the main disputes with the Th1/Th2 hypothesis in human studies has been the failure of many researchers to differentiate between immunological actions occurring nearby in the uterus and those that occur systemically in the maternal circulation. Several studies on the immunology of human pregnancy are limited to peripheral blood for practical and ethical reasons, but it is difficult to assume that the events in the circulation certainly have any association with those in the decidua (Sargent, Borzychowski, and Redman 2006). However, in pregnancy-related complications such as recurrent miscarriage and preeclampsia, the Th2 bias either cannot develop or moves the shift toward Th1 dominance, which is believed to contribute to these diseases (Parham 2004).

20.3.2 IL-17

The Th1/Th2 paradigm has now been expanded into the Th1/Th2/Th17 and regulatory T-cell paradigm (Peck and Mellins 2010). Th17 cells, which produce the proinflammatory cytokine IL-17, play crucial roles for the induction of inflammation (Crome, Wang, and Levings 2010; Peck and Mellins 2010). IL-17 is abundantly produced in patients with rheumatoid arthritis (RA), and hence, IL-17 has an important role in the pathophysiology of RA (Crome, Wang, and Levings 2010; Peck and Mellins 2010). The symptoms of RA frequently recover during pregnancy (Wegmann et al. 1993), signifying that Th17 cells might be decreased during pregnancy.

Two contradictory reports have been published on the frequency of Th17 cells during pregnancy. Nakashima et al. (2010) reported that the frequency of Th17 cells to Th cells during all stages of pregnancy was similar that in nonpregnant women; however, other reports claim that Th17 cells in the third trimester of pregnancy were lower compared with those in nonpregnant women (Santner-Nanan et al. 2009). Therefore, further studies are required to conclude circulating Th17 cell levels during pregnancy.

20.3.3 IFN-γ

IFN-γ was among the first identified cytokines (Wheelock 1965). IFN-γ plays essential roles in various cellular processes, including inducing apoptosis, inhibiting cell proliferation, and activating innate and adaptive immune responses and, thus, in immune responses against pathogens and immunosurveillance of tumors (Boehm et al. 1997; Szabo et al. 2003; Dunn, Koebel, and Schreiber 2006). IFN-γ is a proinflammatory cytokine and is abundantly produced mostly by uNK cells in maternal endometrium, but in rare cases also by trophoblasts. Since the Th1/Th2 cytokine hypothesis was relevant to pregnancy at the maternal–fetal interface (Lin et al. 1993; Saito et al. 1993), IFN-γ is regularly examined in pregnancy-related research to study differences in normal and healthy gestation.

IFN-γ has been reported to have cytotoxic effects on human trophoblast cells *in vitro* (Yui et al. 1994) and inhibits their proliferation (Berkowitz et al. 1988). As compared with healthy pregnant women, higher proinflammatory cytokine levels have been found in women with recurrent spontaneous miscarriage. Similarly, peripheral blood cells from women who had experienced recurrent miscarriages secreted huge amounts of proinflammatory cytokines (Polgar and Hill 2002). Compared with women with healthy pregnancy, increased levels of IFN-γ were found in women with a history of recurrent spontaneous miscarriage (Marzi et al. 1996), whereas lower levels of IFN-γ were found in healthy pregnancies (Jenkins et al. 2000). Lack of regulation of IFN supposedly contributes to conditions such as cerebral palsy and neonatal brain injury (Patrick and Smith 2002).

A study has shown that IFN therapy as treatment for multiple sclerosis leads to low infant birth weight and higher risks of miscarriage (mentioned in Micallef et al. 2014). As soon as patients stopped IFN therapy, the risk of miscarriage or of developmental malformations was not increased (Waubant and Sadovnick 2005). Recently, Guiddir et al. (2014) reported the adverse effects of anti-cytokine therapy during pregnancy. The neonates were reported to have severe neutropenia. The mothers were receiving anti-TNF-α throughout pregnancy to treat ulcerative colitis and infants born were with abundant CD16 autoantibodies and immature bone marrow (Guiddir et al. 2014). This points out that any alteration in cytokine pathways during pregnancy can result into fetal damage.

20.4 PREECLAMPSIA

Pregnancy is not quite as successful a phenomenon as one may think, since around 20% of pregnancies result in miscarriage in the first 2 weeks, and another 15% of pregnancies fail by the first 14 weeks (Nybo Andersen et al. 2000). An important cause of maternal death worldwide, preeclampsia is a complication of 5%–10% of nulliparous pregnancies (Sibai et al. 1997). Two thirds of the cases are mild; one third are severe (Sibai et al. 1997). It affects primarily nulliparous women, but numerous risk factors such as family history and maternal disease contribute to a substantially increased risk in women with a history of the disease (Dildy, Belfort, and Smulian 2007). Broadly speaking, the risk factors may be grouped in maternal (mainly chronic hypertension, diabetes, nephropathy, and vascular disease) and trophoblastal (increased trophoblast mass and immunological factors). In the following, we will emphasize the factors affecting the trophoblast. Indeed, being the major trophoblast-related disease, preeclampsia is valuable when attempting to delineate the processes involved with deregulation of the placental microenvironment. Numerous theories attempt to describe and explain the pathogenesis and pathophysiology of preeclampsia, and we will give a few examples as to how the cytokine system contributes to the current understanding of this process.

Pregnancy is considered a variable inflammatory state in the mother. In the early first trimester, associated with maternal emesis, trophoblastal invasion of the uterus is involved with considerable breakdown of tissue. Then, as the placenta develops and sequentially starts to break down toward the end of the pregnancy, increasing amounts of cellular debris is released to the maternal circulation. The dominating view of preeclampsia in the literature today is that it is caused by a deregulation of this state of chronic inflammation. Therefore, great emphasis is put on the role of the immune system in the development and potential cure of the disease (Saito et al. 2007). Indeed, it was proposed that preeclampsia occurs when the inflammatory response to placental debris decompensates, either because of an abnormal burden of debris or because of an excessive response (Redman and Sargent 2001).

Numerous factors contribute to this unusually complex inflammatory state. Vitally involved with the processes leading to this situation is the conversion of the spiral arteries of the maternal uterus. During normal placentation, cytotrophoblastic cells invade the arteries, affecting their transformation toward low-resistance vessels without smooth muscle cells in the vessel wall. Thus, blood flow is allowed with low resistance into the intervillous space of the placenta. A characteristic feature of preeclampsia is the absence of such transformation, which is deemed to be instrumental in the pathogenesis of the disease. The result of such flawed development is an ischemic placenta with high-resistance vasculature, leading to inadequate delivery of blood to the fetus, fetal growth deficiency, and preterm delivery.

For the maternal syndrome, dysfunction of the endothelium plays a central role. Dysfunctional endothelial cells produce altered quantities of vasoactive agents, with the balance tilted toward vasoconstrictive or antiangiogenic ones (Levine et al. 2006). Further, as vascular permeability and platelet adhesion are regulated by the endothelium, it is likely that edemas and platelet depletion are also mediated by these cells. Although insufficient conversion of spiral arteries seems to be mediating a lot of the clinically observable features of the disease, its origin and the mechanisms driving the disease is still a matter of much debate—and it possibly involves a complex web of cytokines.

Because of the paternal gene material of the fetus, it is a semiallograft that may be rejected (Erlebacher 2001). However, rejection is very rare because of a multitude of tolerance mechanisms such as reduced expression of major histocompability complex (MHC) class I and II molecules on the syncytiotrophoblast, along with specific expression of HLA-G and HLA-C (Moffett and Loke 2006). Thus, because of the absence of MHC molecules, gene products are not be presented to the maternal immune system as they normally would, and through HLA-G and HLA-C expression, the cytolytic activity of NK cells is prevented. Epidemiological data contribute to the understanding, showing that prolonged exposure to paternal semen or a previous abortion with the same father has a protective effect against preeclampsia (Saito et al. 2007), suggesting that delayed tolerance reactions with the development of memory T cells is of importance. Interestingly, this emphasizes how the immune microenvironment in the placenta is important for the development of preeclampsia and that the immunological properties of the trophoblast cells are important.

20.4.1 IMMUNE SYSTEM ACTIVATION IN PREECLAMPSIA

The innate immune system is involved with housekeeping duties such as the clearance of dying cells and surveillance of the body for tumor cells or infectious agents. Accordingly, as massive amounts of trophoblastic debris are released into the maternal circulation during pregnancy (Huppertz et al. 2003), innate immune cells such as neutrophils and monocytes found in the maternal circulation are activated (Saito et al. 2007). Ingestion of such apoptotic debris is followed by the secretion of cytokines such as IL-10 and TGF-β, resulting in active immunosuppressive and anti-inflammatory responses (Abrahams et al. 2004).

In preeclampsia, because of hypoxia, oxidative stress, and inflammation in the placenta, the debris reaching the maternal blood stream will contain necrotic material (Huppertz et al. 2003). Upon ingestion of such material, macrophages and dendritic cells will respond by producing type 1 cytokines such as TNF-α, IL-12, and IFN-γ that augment inflammation (Huppertz et al. 2003; Abrahams et al. 2004). Endothelial cells are affected in a similar way, as they have phagocytic capacity and can respond to material from necrotic trophoblasts by up-regulating the intercellular adhesion molecule-1 (ICAM-1), which mediates adhesion of leukocytes (Chen et al. 2006). As an indication of the resulting inflammation, T cells and NK cells are found to be activated during preeclampsia, as well as neutrophils and monocytes of the innate immune system, even more so than in a normal or healthy pregnancy (Saito et al. 2007). Hence, it is apparent that pregnancy-related disorders probably involve the actions of both maternal and fetal cells.

Taking everything into account, pregnancy has far more complicated physiology than we yet could comprehend. The fundamental physiological and immunological phenomena do not apply to define changes in pregnancy. Many theories and hypothesis have been suggested to understand the underlying mechanism of gestation. The vast network of cytokines modifies each phase of gestation, ensuring successful pregnancy and fetal growth. Any alteration in cytokine machinery can be detrimental to the mother and fetal health.

20.5 SUMMARY

Taking everything into account, pregnancy has far more complicated physiology than we yet could comprehend. The fundamental physiological and immunological phenomena do not apply to define changes in pregnancy. Many theories and hypotheses have been suggested to understand the underlying mechanism of gestation. In the 1990s, Th1/Th2 model with biased Th2 cytokine shift was suggested to avoid maternal T-cell rejection of fetus. Years later, this paradigm lost its significance when reports came out that uNK cells, and not T cells, interact with trophoblasts in early pregnancy. This cross-talk between uNK cells and trophoblast cells is vital for trophoblast invasion and further fetal growth. The vast network of cytokines modifies each phase of gestation, ensuring successful pregnancy and fetal growth. Any alteration of cytokine machinery can be detrimental to the mother and fetal health.

REFERENCES

Abrahams, V. M., Y. M. Kim, S. L. Straszewski, R. Romero, and G. Mor. 2004. "Macrophages and apoptotic cell clearance during pregnancy." *Am J Reprod Immunol* 51 (4):275–82. doi:10.1111/j.1600-0897.2004.00156.x.

Berkowitz, R. S., J. A. Hill, C. B. Kurtz, and D. J. Anderson. 1988. "Effects of products of activated leukocytes (lymphokines and monokines) on the growth of malignant trophoblast cells *in vitro*." *Am J Obstet Gynecol* 158 (1):199–203.

Boehm, U., T. Klamp, M. Groot, and J. C. Howard. 1997. "Cellular responses to interferon-gamma." *Annu Rev Immunol* 15:749–95. doi:10.1146/annurev.immunol.15.1.749.

Chen, Q., P. R. Stone, L. M. E. McCowan, and L. W. Chamley. 2006. "Phagocytosis of necrotic but not apoptotic trophoblasts induces endothelial cell activation." *Hypertension* 47 (1):116–21.

Cooper, M. A., T. A. Fehniger, S. C. Turner, K. S. Chen, B. A. Ghaheri, T. Ghayur, W. E. Carson, and M. A. Caligiuri. 2001. "Human natural killer cells: A unique innate immunoregulatory role for the CD56(bright) subset." *Blood* 97 (10):3146–51.

Crome, S. Q., A. Y. Wang, and M. K. Levings. 2010. "Translational mini-review series on Th17 cells: Function and regulation of human T helper 17 cells in health and disease." *Clin Exp Immunol* 159 (2):109–19. doi:10.1111/j.1365-2249.2009.04037.x.

Dildy, G. A., 3rd, M. A. Belfort, and J. C. Smulian. 2007. "Preeclampsia recurrence and prevention." *Semin Perinatol* 31 (3):135–41. doi:10.1053/j.semperi.2007.03.005.

Dunn, G. P., C. M. Koebel, and R. D. Schreiber. 2006. "Interferons, immunity and cancer immunoediting." *Nat Rev Immunol* 6 (11):836–48. doi:10.1038/nri1961.

Erlebacher, A. 2001. "Why isn't the fetus rejected?" *Curr Opin Immunol* 13 (5):590–3.

Guiddir, T., M. L. Fremond, T. B. Triki, S. Candon, L. Croisille, T. Leblanc, and L. de Pontual. 2014. "Anti-TNF-alpha therapy may cause neonatal neutropenia." *Pediatrics* 134 (4):e1189–93. doi:10.1542/peds .2014-0054.

Hanna, J., D. Goldman-Wohl, Y. Hamani, I. Avraham, C. Greenfield, S. Natanson-Yaron, D. Prus, L. Cohen-Daniel, T. I. Arnon, I. Manaster, R. Gazit, V. Yutkin, D. Benharroch, A. Porgador, E. Keshet, S. Yagel, and O. Mandelboim. 2006. "Decidual NK cells regulate key developmental processes at the human fetal–maternal interface." *Nat Med* 12 (9):1065–74. doi:10.1038/nm1452.

Hiby, S. E., J. J. Walker, K. M. O'Shaughnessy, C. W. Redman, M. Carrington, J. Trowsdale, and A. Moffett. 2004. "Combinations of maternal KIR and fetal HLA-C genes influence the risk of preeclampsia and reproductive success." *J Exp Med* 200 (8):957–65. doi:10.1084/jem.20041214.

Huppertz, B., J. Kingdom, I. Caniggia, G. Desoye, S. Black, H. Korr, and P. Kaufmann. 2003. "Hypoxia favours necrotic versus apoptotic shedding of placental syncytiotrophoblast into the maternal circulation." *Placenta* 24 (2–3):181–90.

Jenkins, C., J. Roberts, R. Wilson, M. A. MacLean, J. Shilito, and J. J. Walker. 2000. "Evidence of a T(H) 1 type response associated with recurrent miscarriage." *Fertil Steril* 73 (6):1206–8.

Jokhi, P. P., A. King, and Y. W. Loke. 1994. "Production of granulocyte-macrophage colony-stimulating factor by human trophoblast cells and by decidual large granular lymphocytes." *Hum Reprod* 9 (9):1660–9.

Jokhi, P. P., A. King, and Y. W. Loke. 1997. "Cytokine production and cytokine receptor expression by cells of the human first trimester placental–uterine interface." *Cytokine* 9 (2):126–37. doi:10.1006/cyto.1996.0146.

King, A., N. Balendran, P. Wooding, N. P. Carter, and Y. W. Loke. 1991. "CD3-leukocytes present in the human uterus during early placentation: Phenotypic and morphologic characterization of the CD56++ population." *Dev Immunol* 1 (3):169–90.

Koopman, L. A., H. D. Kopcow, B. Rybalov, J. E. Boyson, J. S. Orange, F. Schatz, R. Masch, C. J. Lockwood, A. D. Schachter, P. J. Park, and J. L. Strominger. 2003. "Human decidual natural killer cells are a unique NK cell subset with immunomodulatory potential." *J Exp Med* 198 (8):1201–12. doi:10.1084/jem.20030305.

Le Bouteiller, P. and J. Tabiasco. 2006. "Killers become builders during pregnancy." *Nat Med* 12 (9):991–2. doi:10.1038/nm0906-991.

Levine, R. J., C. Lam, C. Qian, K. F. Yu, S. E. Maynard, B. P. Sachs, B. M. Sibai, F. H. Epstein, R. Romero, R. Thadhani, S. A. Karumanchi, and Cpep Study Group. 2006. "Soluble endoglin and other circulating anti-angiogenic factors in preeclampsia." *N Engl J Med* 355 (10):992–1005. doi:10.1056/NEJMoa055352.

Lin, H., T. R. Mosmann, L. Guilbert, S. Tuntipopipat, and T. G. Wegmann. 1993. "Synthesis of T helper 2-type cytokines at the maternal–fetal interface." *J Immunol* 151 (9):4562–73.

Marzi, M., A. Vigano, D. Trabattoni, M. L. Villa, A. Salvaggio, E. Clerici, and M. Clerici. 1996. "Characterization of type 1 and type 2 cytokine production profile in physiologic and pathologic human pregnancy." *Clin Exp Immunol* 106 (1):127–33.

Micallef, A., N. Grech, F. Farrugia, P. Schembri-Wismayer, and J. Calleja-Agius. 2014. "The role of interferons in early pregnancy." *Gynecol Endocrinol* 30 (1):1–6. doi:10.3109/09513590.2012.743011.

Moffett, A. and C. Loke. 2006. "Immunology of placentation in eutherian mammals." *Nat Rev Immunol* 6 (8):584–94. doi:10.1038/nri1897.

Nakashima, A., M. Ito, S. Yoneda, A. Shiozaki, T. Hidaka, and S. Saito. 2010. "Circulating and decidual Th17 cell levels in healthy pregnancy." *Am J Reprod Immunol* 63 (2):104–9. doi:10.1111/j.1600-0897.2009.00771.x.

Nybo Andersen, A. M., J. Wohlfahrt, P. Christens, J. Olsen, and M. Melbye. 2000. "Maternal age and fetal loss: Population based register linkage study." *BMJ* 320 (7251):1708–12.

Parham, P. 2004. "NK cells and trophoblasts: Partners in pregnancy." *J Exp Med* 200 (8):951–5. doi:10.1084/jem.20041783.

Patrick, L. A. and G. N. Smith. 2002. "Proinflammatory cytokines: A link between chorioamnionitis and fetal brain injury." *J Obstet Gynaecol Can* 24 (9):705–9.

Peck, A. and E. D. Mellins. 2010. "Plasticity of T-cell phenotype and function: The T helper type 17 example." *Immunology* 129 (2):147–53. doi:10.1111/j.1365-2567.2009.03189.x.

Polgar, K. and J. A. Hill. 2002. "Identification of the white blood cell populations responsible for Th1 immunity to trophoblast and the timing of the response in women with recurrent pregnancy loss." *Gynecol Obstet Invest* 53 (1):59–64.

Rai, R., G. Sacks, and G. Trew. 2005. "Natural killer cells and reproductive failure—Theory, practice and prejudice." *Hum Reprod* 20 (5):1123–6. doi:10.1093/humrep/deh804.

Rajagopalan, S. and E. O. Long. 1999. "A human histocompatibility leukocyte antigen (HLA)-G-specific receptor expressed on all natural killer cells." *J Exp Med* 189 (7):1093–100.

Redman, C. W. G. and I. L. Sargent. 2001. "The pathogenesis of pre-eclampsia." *Gynécol Obstét Fertil* 29 (7):518–22.

Sacks, G. P., C. W. Redman, and I. L. Sargent. 2003. "Monocytes are primed to produce the Th1 type cytokine IL-12 in normal human pregnancy: An intracellular flow cytometric analysis of peripheral blood mononuclear cells." *Clin Exp Immunol* 131 (3):490–7.

Saito, S., K. Nishikawa, T. Morii, M. Enomoto, N. Narita, K. Motoyoshi, and M. Ichijo. 1993. "Cytokine production by CD16-CD56bright natural killer cells in the human early pregnancy decidua." *Int Immunol* 5 (5):559–63.

Saito, S., A. Shiozaki, A. Nakashima, M. Sakai, and Y. Sasaki. 2007. "The role of the immune system in pre-eclampsia." *Mol Aspects Med* 28 (2):192–209. doi:10.1016/j.mam.2007.02.006.

Sakai, M., A. Shiozaki, Y. Sasaki, S. Yoneda, and S. Saito. 2004. "The ratio of interleukin (IL)-18 to IL-12 secreted by peripheral blood mononuclear cells is increased in normal pregnant subjects and decreased in pre-eclamptic patients." *J Reprod Immunol* 61 (2):133–43. doi:10.1016/j.jri.2004.01.001.

Santner-Nanan, B., M. J. Peek, R. Khanam, L. Richarts, E. Zhu, B. Fazekas de St Groth, and R. Nanan. 2009. "Systemic increase in the ratio between Foxp3+ and IL-17-producing CD4+ T cells in healthy pregnancy but not in preeclampsia." *J Immunol* 183 (11):7023–30. doi:10.4049/jimmunol.0901154.

Sargent, I. L., A. M. Borzychowski, and C. W. Redman. 2006. "NK cells and human pregnancy—An inflammatory view." *Trends Immunol* 27 (9):399–404. doi:10.1016/j.it.2006.06.009.

Sibai, B. M., M. Ewell, R. J. Levine, M. A. Klebanoff, J. Esterlitz, P. M. Catalano, R. L. Goldenberg, and G. Joffe. 1997. "Risk factors associated with preeclampsia in healthy nulliparous women. The Calcium for Preeclampsia Prevention (CPEP) Study Group." *Am J Obstet Gynecol* 177 (5):1003–10.

Sivori, S., S. Parolini, E. Marcenaro, R. Millo, C. Bottino, and A. Moretta. 2000. "Triggering receptors involved in natural killer cell-mediated cytotoxicity against choriocarcinoma cell lines." *Hum Immunol* 61 (11):1055–8.

Szabo, S. J., B. M. Sullivan, S. L. Peng, and L. H. Glimcher. 2003. "Molecular mechanisms regulating Th1 immune responses." *Annu Rev Immunol* 21:713–58. doi:10.1146/annurev.immunol.21.120601.140942.

Vacca, P., C. Cantoni, C. Prato, E. Fulcheri, A. Moretta, L. Moretta, and M. C. Mingari. 2008. "Regulatory role of NKp44, NKp46, DNAM-1 and NKG2D receptors in the interaction between NK cells and trophoblast cells. Evidence for divergent functional profiles of decidual versus peripheral NK cells." *Int Immunol* 20 (11):1395–405. doi:10.1093/intimm/dxn105.

Waubant, E. and A. D. Sadovnick. 2005. "Interferon beta babies." *Neurology* 65 (6):788–9. doi:10.1212/01.wnl.0000182147.73071.2c.

Wegmann, T. G., H. Lin, L. Guilbert, and T. R. Mosmann. 1993. "Bidirectional cytokine interactions in the maternal–fetal relationship: Is successful pregnancy a TH2 phenomenon?" *Immunol Today* 14 (7):353–6. doi:10.1016/0167-5699(93)90235-D.

Wheelock, E. F. 1965. "Interferon-like virus-inhibitor induced in human leukocytes by phytohemagglutinin." *Science* 149 (3681):310–1.

Wittmann, M., V.-A. Larsson, P. Schmidt, G. Begemann, A. Kapp, and T. Werfel. 1999. "Suppression of interleukin-12 production by human monocytes after preincubation with lipopolysaccharide." *Blood* 94 (5):1717–26.

Yoneyama, Y., S. Suzuki, R. Sawa, K. Yoneyama, G. G. Power, and T. Araki. 2002. "Relation between adenosine and T-helper 1/T-helper 2 imbalance in women with preeclampsia." *Obstet Gynecol* 99 (4):641–6.

Yui, J., M. Garcia-Lloret, T. G. Wegmann, and L. J. Guilbert. 1994. "Cytotoxicity of tumour necrosis factor-alpha and gamma-interferon against primary human placental trophoblasts." *Placenta* 15 (8):819–35.

Section V

Environmental and Lifestyle Factors in Pregnancy

21 Effect of Prepregnancy Body Weight and Pregnancy Outcome

Christine Henriksen

CONTENTS

ABSTRACT

The prevalence of overweight and obesity is increasing among women in reproductive age, and the relationship between maternal prepregnancy body mass index (pBMI) and pregnancy outcome deserves further elucidation. In this chapter, the association between pBMI and birth weight, risk of preterm birth, overweight, obesity, blood pressure, and glucose tolerance in children is discussed. The literature was searched for publications no older than 5 years using the terms *prepregnancy BMI* and *pregnancy outcomes*.

There seems to be an association between high maternal pBMI and birth weight, macrosomia, large for gestational age, risk of preterm birth, as well as overweight and risk factors for metabolic syndrome in children. An association between pBMI and children's neurodevelopment is also suggested as well as an increased risk of fetal loss. Additional research is needed to evaluate potential mechanisms. The state of obesity is associated with increased oxidative stress and inflammation that may mediate the effect on the outcomes. There are several limitations in study design and methods to consider: Maternal prepregnancy weight and height were often self-reported. Most authors adjusted for possible confounding factors such as gestational weight gain, smoking, mother's age, and education but more seldom for the mother's or offspring's physical activity level. Residual confounding cannot be excluded.

The remaining question is if prepregnancy weight reduction will result in health benefit for mother and child. Randomized clinical trials on the clinical effect of prepregnancy weight reduction on pregnancy outcomes are warranted.

KEY WORDS

Prepregnancy BMI, birth weight, preterm birth, adiposity in childhood, neurodevelopment.

21.1 INTRODUCTION

The prevalence of overweight and obesity is increasing among women in reproductive age. Population-based data for the United States show an overall prevalence of 25% overweight and 21%

obesity before pregnancy (Fisher et al. 2013). The most recent data from the general population suggest a slowing or leveling off of these trends, at a prevalence of 35% obesity among adult women. But the prevalence of obesity is still increasing in the non-Hispanic black population (Flegal et al. 2012).

Overweight and obesity among women in reproductive age may have not only consequences for the mother health but also a long-term effect on the health of their children. The relationship between maternal prepregnancy body mass index (pBMI) and pregnancy outcome deserves further elucidation. The association between pBMI and birth weight, risk of preterm birth, overweight, obesity, blood pressure, and glucose tolerance in children will be discussed in this chapter.

21.2   MATERNAL pBMI AND BIRTH WEIGHT

The association between pBMI and birth weight has been recognized for several years, and the Institute of Medicine (IOM) acknowledges both pBMI and gestational weight gain as important for pregnancy outcome. The 2009 guidelines include different recommendations for gestational weigh gain for each pBMI category (IOM 2009).

Several authors have looked further at the association between pBMI and birth weight, especially the risk of infants being born large for gestational age (LGA; birth weight >90th percentile for gestational age) or small for gestational age (SGA; birth weight <10th percentile for gestational age).

Shin and Song (2014) studied the association between pBMI and birth weight using data from the 220,000 women registered in the Pregnancy Risk Assessment Monitoring System (PRAMS) database. Overweight and obesity were associated with higher odds for infants being born LGA (odds ratio [OR] = 1.87; 95% confidence interval [CI]: 1.76–1.99). Prepregnancy underweight (BMI <18.5 kg/m^2) was associated with higher odds for infants being born SGA (OR = 1.36; 95% CI: 1.25–1.49).

Djelantik et al. (2012) estimated the contribution of pBMI to the risk of LGA babies along with other adverse outcomes in the Amsterdam Corn Children and Their Development (ABCD) cohort. The population attributive fraction (PAF) of pBMI >25 kg/m^2 on LGA babies was 15.3%, and the relative contribution of overweight/obesity was higher in non-Western immigrant groups compared with others.

Ng et al. (2014) studied 2230 women from Australia and found that prepregnancy obesity was associated with higher odds of macrosomia (birth weight >4000 g; OR = 2.3; 95% CI: 1.6–3.2).

Heerman et al. (2014) tried to quantify the combined effect of maternal pBMI and gestational weight gain on infant's birth weight and first-year growth. They studied 499 mother-and-child pairs in Tennessee. In contrast to more previous studies, weight was obtained by objective measurement. The results were adjusted for possible confounding factors and showed that the combined effect of pBMI and gestational weight gain resulted in higher birth weight and growth in offsprings. For example, obese mothers with excess gestational weight gain had a significant 13.6% increase in 3-month weight/length percentile compared with overweight mothers with the same weight gain. The effect of gestational weight gain alone did not reach statistical significance in this study.

Dzakpasu et al. (2015) performed the same type of analysis of 5930 women in the Canadian Maternity Experiences Survey and found, on the other hand, that excess gestational weight gain contributed more to LGA than pBMI did (15.9% vs. 6.5%, respectively).

It seems that pBMI is associated with offsping's birth weight, risk of macrosomia, and infant being born LGA, but the relative contribution compared with other risk factors, especially gestational weigh gain, is still being discussed.

21.3   MATERNAL pBMI AND ADIPOSITY IN CHILDHOOD

Gademan et al. (2014) investigated the association between pBMI and obesity among more than 3000 mothers and their children in the ABCD study. Weight and height were measured in children at 5 to 6 years of age. After adjustments for confounders, every unit increase in pBMI was linearly associated with various offspring variables: BMI (β = .10; 95% CI: 0.08–0.12), waist-to-height-ratio

(WHtR) × 100 (β = .13; 95% CI: 0.09–0.17), fat% (β = .21; 95% CI: 0.13–0.29), and increased risk for overweight (OR = 1.15; 95% CI: 1.10–1.20).

21.4 MATERNAL pBMI AND RISK OF PRETERM BIRTH

Lynch et al. (2014) studied the association between pBMI and risk of preterm birth in a cohort of 11,700 ethnically diverse women from Colorado. They found an increased risk of preterm birth in both extremes of BMI. Low pBMI (<17 kg/m^2) was associated with a significantly higher OR of spontaneous preterm labor (OR = 2.4; 95% CI: 1.4–4.2) as well as medically indicated preterm birth (OR = 2.8; 95% CI: 1.4–5.6). Prepregancy obesity class 2 was associated with higher odds of premature rupture of membrane (OR = 1.6; 95% CI: 1.1–2.3) as well as medically indicated preterm birth (OR = 1.5; 95% CI: 1.1–2.2).

These results were confirmed in a case-control study of 4400 preterm births and term babies from the Boston Birth Cohort (Parker et al. 2014). Prepregnancy obesity (>30 kg/m^2) was associated with significantly higher odds of medically induced preterm birth but reduced odds of spontaneous preterm delivery. Hypertension and gestational diabetes seem to explain some of the observed association.

Shaw et al. (2014) looked further into subgroups of preterm deliveries according to ethnicity, gestational age, and parity in a large cohort of nearly a million singleton births in California. Mothers with hypertension and diabetes were excluded in the analyses, and adjustment was made for possible confounders. The results showed, in contrast to Lynch and Parker, that obesity class 1–3 was associated with significantly higher risk of early spontaneous preterm birth among women of parity 1, and this higher risk was not influenced by ethnicity. For non-Hispanic whites, the relative risk of early spontaneous preterm birth was 6.29 (95% CI: 3.06–12.9). A similar but lower risk pattern was observed for women of parity two or more.

Shin and Song (2014), on the other hand, found no significant association between prepregnancy overweight or obesity and risk of preterm birth using data from 220,000 women registered in the PRAMS. Low prepregnancy BMI (<18.5) was associated with preterm birth in this population (OR = 1.25; 95% CI: 1.16–1.36).

Despite some inconsistencies, it can be concluded from the literature that low and high pBMI is associated with all types of preterm birth: both spontaneous and medical induced.

Several authors have tried to estimate the contribution of pBMI to preterm birth compared with other known risk factors such as gestational weight gain and smoking. Djelantik et al. (2012) used data from the ABCD cohort to calculate the PAF of pBMI on extreme preterm birth. The PAF of pBMI >25 kg/m^2 was 22% and higher than for smoking (10.6%). Dzakpasu et al. (2015) performed the same type of analysis of 5930 women in the Canadian Maternity Experiences Survey and found, on the contrary, that excess gestational weight gain contributed more to preterm birth (18.2%) than both pBMI and smoking did.

21.5 MATERNAL pBMI AND OFFSPRING'S METABOLIC PROFILE

Gademan et al. (2013) investigated the association between pBMI and blood pressure at age 5 to 6 years among more than 3000 mothers and their children in the ABCD study. They found a significant, linear association between pBMI and systolic (β = .14 mm Hg) and diastolic (β = .11 mm Hg) pressure after adjusting for confounders. Adding child BMI to the model reduced the effect of pBMI by about 50%, suggesting that environmental factors are also important. Birth weight did not mediate the relationship between pBMI and child's blood pressure in this study.

Elevated blood pressure is a common denominator of all definitions of metabolic syndrome in adults (Alberti et al. 2005). No official definition exists for metabolic syndrome in children, but Oostvogels et al. (2014) has assessed the association between maternal pBMI and offspring's metabolic profile using 1500 mother–children pairs from the ABCD cohort. The authors calculated a score based on waist–height ratio, systolic blood pressure, fasting glucose, triglycerides, and high-density lipoprotein cholesterol. They found that high maternal pBMI was independently associated with adverse metabolic score in early childhood (β = .078) after adjusting for confounders. As expected, early growth rate was also independently associated with adverse metabolic score. A combination of high maternal pBMI and accelerated postnatal growth amplified individual effects.

The results from the Dutch study are confirmed in a smaller study by Derraik et al. (2014) in New Zealand. They studied 70 children at age 9 years, born from healthy mothers with a normal BMI range (mean, 23.2 kg/m^2). Greater pBMI was associated with a higher systolic blood pressure both at day and night time (β = .80). Insulin sensitivity was assessed with a 90-minute intravenous glucose test, and pBMI was inversely associated with insulin sensitivity (β = −.04), meaning that every 1-kg/m^2 increase in BMI results in 4% lower glucose tolerance in the child.

Together, these studies suggest that prepregnancy adiposity might contribute to increased risk of type 2 diabetes and metabolic diseases in the next generation.

21.6 MATERNAL pBMI AND CHILD NEURODEVELOPMENT

Huang et al. (2014) studied the effect of maternal pBMI and children's intelligence quotient (IQ) at 7 years of age using the UU Collaborative Perinatal Project data collected from more than 30,000 women in 1959–1976. There was an inverted U-shaped association between maternal pBMI and their children's IQ, and women with BMI around 20 kg/m^2 had offsprings with the highest IQ. The results remained significant after adjusting for known confounders such as maternal age, education level, race, and socioeconomic status.

The association between pBMI and other neurodevelopmental outcomes were studied using data from the South Carolina Medicaid program (Pan et al. 2014). This cohort included more than 80,000 mother–child pairs, and the results were adjusted for several important confounders. The authors found a significant association between pBMI and offspring cerebral palsy; for every unit increase in pBMI, the OR of cerebral palsy increased by 1.04 (95% CI: 1.01–1.07). There was no association between pBMI and risk of childhood epilepsy.

21.7 SUMMARY AND PERSPECTIVES

There seems to be an association between high maternal pBMI and birth weight, macrosomia, LGA, risk of preterm birth, as well as overweight and risk factors for metabolic syndrome in children (Derraik et al. 2014; Gademan et al. 2013, 2014; Huang et al. 2014; Lynch et al. 2014; Oostvogels et al. 2014; Parker et al. 2014; Shaw et al. 2014). An association between pBMI and children neuro-development is also suggested (Huang et al. 2014; Pan et al. 2014), as well as an increased risk of fetal loss (Gaskins et al. 2014).

Additional research is needed to evaluate potential mechanisms. The state of obesity is associated with increased oxidative stress and inflammation that may mediate the effect on the outcomes.

There are several limitations in study design and methods to consider. In all but one of the cited studies, maternal prepregnancy weight and height were self-reported. People tend to underestimate their weight compared with measured weight, and this will result in an underestimation of BMI. If underestimation of weight is greatest among overweight and obese women, the true effect of pBMI on pregnancy outcome might be even stronger than reported in the literature.

Another challenge in these studies is how to deal with all the confounders that could, at least partly, account for the observed association between prepregnancy BMI and the outcomes. Although it has been adjusted for known confounders in the epidemiological studies (Gademan et al. 2013, 2014; Huang et al. 2014; Lynch et al. 2014; Oostvogels et al. 2014; Pan et al. 2014; Parker et al. 2014; Shaw et al. 2014), residual confounding cannot be excluded, and the observed association may be overestimated.

The remaining question is if prepregnancy weight reduction will result in health benefit for the mother and child. Schummers et al. (2015) has estimated the effect of a 10% weight reduction to be associated with at least a 10% lower risk of several adverse pregnancy outcomes, based on data from a population-based cohort of more than 225,000 Canadian women. Randomized clinical trials on the clinical effect of prepregnancy weight reduction on pregnancy outcomes are warranted.

REFERENCES

Alberti, K. G., P. Zimmet, and J. Shaw. 2005. "The metabolic syndrome—A new worldwide definition." *Lancet* 366 (9491):1059–62. doi:10.1016/s0140-6736(05)67402-8.

Derraik, J. G., A. Ayyavoo, P. L. Hofman, J. B. Biggs, and W. S. Cutfield. 2014. "Increasing maternal pre-pregnancy body mass index is associated with reduced insulin sensitivity and increased blood pressure in their children." *Clin Endocrinol (Oxf)*. doi:10.1111/cen.12665.

Djelantik, A. A., A. E. Kunst, M. F. van der Wal, H. A. Smit, and T. G. Vrijkotte. 2012. "Contribution of over-weight and obesity to the occurrence of adverse pregnancy outcomes in a multi-ethnic cohort: Population attributive fractions for Amsterdam." *BJOG* no. 119 (3):283–90. doi:10.1111/j.1471-0528.2011.03205.x.

Dzakpasu, S., J. Fahey, R. S. Kirby, S. C. Tough, B. Chalmers, M. I. Heaman, S. Bartholomew, A. Biringer, E. K. Darling, L. S. Lee, and S. D. McDonald. 2015. "Contribution of prepregnancy body mass index and gestational weight gain to adverse neonatal outcomes: Population attributable fractions for Canada." *BMC Pregnancy Childbirth* no. 15 (1):21. doi:10.1186/s12884-015-0452-0.

Fisher, S. C., S. Y. Kim, A. J. Sharma, R. Rochat, and B. Morrow. 2013. "Is obesity still increasing among pregnant women? Prepregnancy obesity trends in 20 states, 2003–2009." *Prev Med* 56 (6):372–8. doi:10.1016/j.ypmed.2013.02.015.

Flegal, K. M., M. D. Carroll, B. K. Kit, and C. L. Ogden. 2012. "Prevalence of obesity and trends in the distribution of body mass index among US adults, 1999–2010." *JAMA* no. 307 (5):491–7. doi:10.100/jama.2012.39.

Gademan, M. G., M. van Eijsden, T. J. Roseboom, J. A. van der Post, K. Stronks, and T. G. Vrijkotte. 2013. "Maternal prepregnancy body mass index and their children's blood pressure and resting cardiac autonomic balance at age 5 to 6 years." *Hypertension* no. 62 (3):641–7. doi:10.1161/HYPERTENSIONAHA.113.01511.

Gademan, M. G., M. Vermeulen, A. J. Oostvogels, T. J. Roseboom, T. L. Visscher, M. van Eijsden, M. T. Twickler, and T. G. Vrijkotte. 2014. "Maternal prepregnancy BMI and lipid profile during early preg-nancy are independently associated with offspring's body composition at age 5–6 years: The ABCD study." *PLoS One* no. 9 (4):e94594. doi:10.1371/journal.pone.0094594.

Gaskins, A. J., J. W. Rich-Edwards, D. S. Colaci, M. C. Afeiche, T. L. Toth, M. W. Gillman, S. A. Missmer, and J. E. Chavarro. 2014. "Prepregnancy and early adulthood body mass index and adult weight change in relation to fetal loss." *Obstet Gynecol* no. 124 (4):662–9. doi:10.1097/AOG.0000000000000478.

Heerman, W. J., A. Bian, A. Shintani, and S. L. Barkin. 2014. "Interaction between maternal prepregnancy body mass index and gestational weight gain shapes infant growth." *Acad Pediatr* no. 14 (5):463–70. doi:10.1016/j.acap.2014.05.005.

Huang, L., X. Yu, S. Keim, L. Li, L. Zhang, and J. Zhang. 2014. "Maternal prepregnancy obesity and child neuro-development in the Collaborative Perinatal Project." *Int J Epidemiol* no. 43 (3):783–92. doi:10.1093/ije/dyu030.

Institute of Medicine (IOM). 2009. *Weight Gain during Pregnancy: Reexamining the Guidelines*. Wshington, DC: National Research Council.

Lynch, A. M., J. E. Hart, O. C. Agwu, B. M. Fisher, N. A. West, and R. S. Gibbs. 2014. "Association of extremes of prepregnancy BMI with the clinical presentations of preterm birth." *Am J Obstet Gynecol* no. 210 (5):428.e1–9. doi:10.1016/j.ajog.2013.12.011.

Ng, S. K., C. M. Cameron, A. P. Hills, R. J. McClure, and P. A. Scuffham. 2014. "Socioeconomic dispari-ties in prepregnancy BMI and impact on maternal and neonatal outcomes and postpartum weight retention: The EFHL longitudinal birth cohort study." *BMC Pregnancy Childbirth* no. 14:314. doi:10.1186/1471-2393-14-314.

Oostvogels, A. J., K. Stronks, T. J. Roseboom, J. A. van der Post, M. van Eijsden, and T. G. Vrijkotte. 2014. "Maternal prepregnancy BMI, offspring's early postnatal growth, and metabolic profile at age 5–6 years: The ABCD Study." *J Clin Endocrinol Metab* no. 99 (10):3845–54. doi:10.1210/jc.2014-1561.

Pan, C., C. B. Deroche, J. R. Mann, S. McDermott, and J. W. Hardin. 2014. "Is prepregnancy obesity associated with risk of cerebral palsy and epilepsy in children?" *J Child Neurol* no. 29 (12):NP196–201.
doi:10.1177/0883073813510971.

Parker, M. G., F. Ouyang, C. Pearson, M. W. Gillman, M. B. Belfort, X. Hong, G. Wang, L. Heffner, B. Zuckerman,
and X. Wang. 2014. "Prepregnancy body mass index and risk of preterm birth: Association heterogeneity by preterm subgroups." *BMC Pregnancy Childbirth* no. 14:153. doi:10.1186/1471-2393-14-153.

Schummers, L., J. A. Hutcheon, L. M. Bodnar, E. Lieberman, and K. P. Himes. 2015. "Risk of adverse pregnancy outcomes by prepregnancy body mass index: A population-based study to inform prepregnancy
weight loss counseling." *Obstet Gynecol* no. 125 (1):133–43. doi:10.1097/AOG.0000000000000591.

Shaw, G. M., P. H. Wise, J. Mayo, S. L. Carmichael, C. Ley, D. J. Lyell, B. Z. Shachar, K. Melsop, C. S.
Phibbs, D. K. Stevenson, J. Parsonnet, J. B. Gould, and March of Dimes Prematurity Research Center
at Stanford University School of Medicine. 2014. "Maternal prepregnancy body mass index and risk
of spontaneous preterm birth." *Paediatr Perinat Epidemiol* no. 28 (4):302–11. doi:10.1111/ppe.12125.

Shin, D. and W. O. Song. 2014. "Prepregnancy body mass index is an independent risk factor for gestational
hypertension, gestational diabetes, preterm labor, and small- and large-for-gestational-age infants."
J Matern Fetal Neonatal Med 29:1–8. doi:10.3109/14767058.2014.964675.

22 The Aryl Hydrocarbon Receptor in the Human Placental Trophoblast
The Impact of Nutraceuticals and Natural Products

Petr Pavek and Tomas Smutny

CONTENTS

ABSTRACT

The aryl hydrocarbon receptor (AHR) and its heterodimer AHR nuclear translocator (ARNT) form a ligand-activated transcription complex that regulates the expression of numerous target genes involved in the biotransformation of both xenobiotic and endogenous compounds, including cytochrome P450 enzymes CYP1A1, CYP1A2, and CYP1B1; glutathione S-transferase GST1; UDP-glucuronosyltransferases UGT1A1 and UGT1A6; NAD(P)H-dependent quinone dehydrogenase NQO1; aldehyde dehydrogenase ALDH3A1; and breast cancer resistance protein. Placental expression, as well as the ontogeny of AHR, has been recently described both in human or rat placenta, and the regulation of its target genes has been studied in the placental trophoblast. Interestingly, of the AHR target genes, only cytochrome P450 CYP1A1 has been found to be significantly inducible in the human placental trophoblast, with significant enzymatic activities having been described. Herein, we summarize recent findings related to the toxicological consequences of AHR activation and CYP1A1 induction during human gestation via natural compounds, as well as the consequences of this induction for prenatal toxicology.

KEY WORDS

Placenta, trophoblast, CYP1A1, aryl hydrocarbon receptor, pregnancy, natural compounds, DNA adducts.

22.1 INTRODUCTION

22.1.1 Placenta

The placenta is the primary exchange organ between the mother and the fetus, serving as a temporary respiratory, metabolic, excretory, and endocrine organ during intrauterine development. Via the placenta, the fetus is supplied with oxygen and nutrients from the mother, and its endocrine function is necessary for the maintenance of pregnancy. At the same time, metabolic waste products are cleared from fetal blood across the placenta into the maternal circulation.

The human placenta is of the hemochorial type, in which the fetal trophoblast is in direct contact with the maternal blood. The so-called placental barrier separating maternal and fetal circulations consists of the endothelium of the fetal capillaries, a discontinuous cytotrophoblast layer, and the syncytiotrophoblast. During the second and third trimesters, the cytotrophoblast layer becomes discontinuous. The syncytiotrophoblast layer then remains as the critical anatomical, physiological, and metabolic component of the placental exchange "barrier."

22.1.1.1 Metabolic Function of the Placenta

The placental metabolic capacity is directed mainly toward the synthesis of endogenous substances and hormones that are important for the maintenance of fetus development (Pasqualini 2005). In addition to the synthesis of endogenous compounds, placental enzymes also metabolize a number of both exogenous and endogenous compounds and hormones to less toxic or inactive chemicals that are further eliminated. Several enzymes of the cytochrome P450 (CYP) superfamily that are involved in phase I xenobiotic metabolism are expressed in the placental trophoblast or placental fetal capillaries. However, most of the enzymes are expressed at very low levels, and there is a general absence of appropriate catalytic activities for the proteins. Therefore, placental metabolism is relatively minor in comparison with the maternal hepatic biotransformation, and it is thus not a significant factor in limiting the transplacental passage of xenobiotics. Among placental xenobiotic-metabolizing enzymes, the activity of CYP1A1 enzyme is significant throughout the pregnancy, although the expression of the enzyme should be induced by ligands of the aryl hydrocarbon receptor (AHR), which essentially controls the enzyme's gene expression (Stejskalova and Pavek 2011). Although placental enzyme activities are not significant for overall detoxification, xenobiotic compounds may be activated by placental enzymes to reactive toxicants that have an adverse effect on the fetus. The oxygenation of carcinogens/procarcinogens such as polycyclic aromatic hydrocarbons (PAHs) or heterocyclic amines (HAs) via CYP1 enzymes forms arene oxide or other electrophilic reactive moieties that create DNA and protein adducts, resulting in tumor initiation and genotoxicity (Ma and Lu 2007).

22.2 THE AHR

The AHR is a member of the basic helix-loop-helix (bHLH)-PAS superfamily of transcriptional factors (Fujii-Kuriyama and Kawajiri 2010; Barouki et al. 2012). bHLH-PAS proteins play important roles in developmental and physiological events, including neurogenesis, tracheal and salivary duct formation, toxin metabolism, circadian rhythms, response to hypoxia, and hormone receptor function (Fujii-Kuriyama and Kawajiri 2010; Barouki et al. 2012; Murray, Patterson, and Perdew 2014). bHLH-PAS proteins form heterodimers, and AHR was found to heterodimerize with AHR nuclear translocator (ARNT) to a functional transcription complex (Crews 1998; Fujii-Kuriyama and Kawajiri 2010). The AHR was first identified in mouse liver by the use of a binding assay with radiolabeled 2,3,7,8-tetrachlorodibenzo-*p*-dioxin (TCDD) (Poland, Glover, and Kende 1976). This was the first ligand-activated transcription factor discovered that induces the expression of enzymes involved in drug detoxification (Greenlee and Poland 1979).

Localization of the human AHR gene is assigned to chromosome 7p15 (Micka et al. 1997); that of ARNT gene is assigned to chromosome 1q21 (Johnson et al. 1993). The AHR gene encodes a 96-kDa protein (Dolwick et al. 1993; Bennett, Ramsden, and Williams 1996). AHR is formed by several domains critical for its function. The bHLH domain is required for specific DNA binding, and the ligand-binding domain forms a pocket to harbor ligands (Reisz-Porszasz et al. 1994; Fukunaga et al. 1995). The unliganded form of AHR is found in cytosol in a complex with chaperone heat shock protein 90 (Hsp90), AHR interacting protein (AIP), and p23 (Ma and Whitlock 1997; Carver et al. 1998; Meyer et al. 1998). Ligand binding to AHR changes the conformation of the AHR/Hsp90 complex, leading to translocation of the complex to the nucleus, where it dissociates from the Hsp90 and dimerizes with its heterodimerization partner ARNT (Lees and Whitelaw 1999). The AHR/ARNT complex binds to specific xenobiotic response elements (XREs) or dioxin response elements (DREs) in the gene promoter. The subsequent recruitment of coactivators and general transcription factors such as ERAP140, RIP140, CBP/P300, BRG-1, NCOA1 (SRC-1), NCOA2 (GRIP-1 or TIF-2), and NCOA3 (AIB-1, p/CIP, and ACTR) results in transactivation of the target gene. The XRE/DRE consensus response element is composed of a core pentanucleotide sequence 5'-GCGTG-3' (Safe 2001; Ishimura et al. 2009; Fujii-Kuriyama and Kawajiri 2010).

AHR target genes are involved in xenobiotic handling and xenobiotic metabolism, including phase I metabolizing enzymes of the CYP family, namely, CYP1A1, CYP1A2, and CYP1B1, along with phase II metabolizing enzymes, such as glutathione S-transferases (GST1), UDP-glucuronosyltransferases (UGT1A1, UGT1A6), NAD(P)H-dependent dehydrogenase quinone 1 (NQO1), and the aldehyde dehydrogenase (ALDH3A1) (Tirona and Kim 2005; Puga, Ma, and Marlowe 2009) (Figure 22.1).

Over the past two decades many papers have reported on AHR; in addition to its function as a regulator of xenobiotic metabolism, its numerous functions in cell biology, development, and physiology have been explored (Fujii-Kuriyama and Kawajiri 2010). Ablation of the *Ahr* gene in mice leads to cardiovascular diseases, hepatic fibrosis, reduced liver size, spleen T-cell deficiency, dermal fibrosis, liver retinoid accumulation, and generally a shortened life span.

In the placenta, exogenous AHR ligand-mediated AHR activation (such as using TCDD) is involved in vascular remodeling in the placenta, accompanied by a proposed decrease in the diameter of maternal sinusoids, reduced maternal blood flow, suppressed development of sinusoids and trophoblast cells, apoptosis of trophoblast cells, and subsequent the intrauterine fetal restriction and death (Ishimura et al. 2009; Wu et al. 2014). AHR activation is also connected with choriocarcinoma BeWo cell line differentiation (Le Vee et al. 2014). In addition, maternal T regulatory cells, which critically regulate immunological tolerance at the feto–maternal interface, have been also hypothesized to be under the control of AHR signaling (Hao et al. 2013).

Significantly, AHR activation resulting in increased the invasion of cytotrophoblast cells has been proposed as protection against preeclampsia (Wang et al. 2011).

In contrast to its detoxification function, the AHR has been shown as a mediator of toxicity via the CYP1-induced metabolism of particular xenobiotics such as dioxin, PAHs, and halogenated biphenyls, which are involved in events such as tumor initiation, promotion, and progression (Gasiewicz, Henry, and Collins 2008). AHR ligands also act as endocrine disruptors, which cause reproductive and developmental defects, immunosuppression, etc. (Swedenborg and Pongratz 2009).

AHR ligands

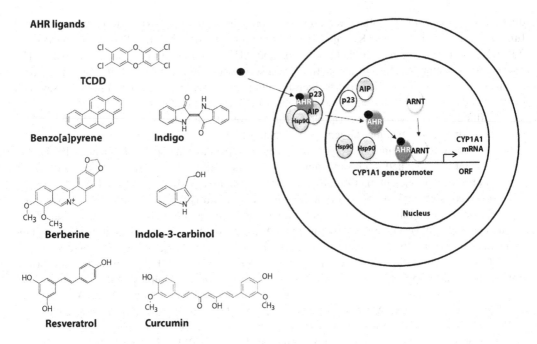

TCDD

Benzo[a]pyrene   **Indigo**

Berberine   **Indole-3-carbinol**

Resveratrol   **Curcumin**

FIGURE 22.1 Activation of AHR with its ligands. Schematic of the ligand-activated AHR in CYP1A1 gene transcription regulation. An AHR ligand enters the cell and binds to the cytosolic complex of AHR, composed of chaperones Hsp90, cochaperone p23, and the AIP. Liganded AHR complex then translocates into the nucleus, where AHR forms a heterodimer with the ARNT. The heterodimer binds responsive elements in the CYP1A1 gene promoter. The AHR/ARNT heterocomplex recruits coactivators and several TBP-associated factors, which start the general transcriptional machinery with RNA polymerase II (RNA pol II) and the transcriptional activation of target genes.

22.2.1 PLACENTAL LOCALIZATION OF AHR

It has been found that AHR and ARNT genes are highly expressed in the placenta, lung, liver, and kidney (Manchester et al. 1987; Dolwick et al. 1993; Yamamoto et al. 2004). AHR and ARNT mRNAs have been detected at high levels in first-trimester and term human and rodent placental tissues (Manchester et al. 1987; Dolwick et al. 1993; Carver, Hogenesch, and Bradfield 1994; Hakkola et al. 1997; Tscheudschilsuren et al. 1999; Kitajima et al. 2004; Yamamoto et al. 2004). In a recent report, we localized AHR/*Ahr* and ARNT/*Arnt* in rat placental trophoblasts throughout gestation and in first-trimester and term human placental trophoblast (Stejskalova et al. 2011). We described AHR expression in the trophoblast cells of secondary villi in first-trimester placenta. Staining was detected in the nuclei of outer layer cells (syncytiotrophoblast) rather than in the cytotrophoblast cells (inner layer). ARNT was also localized in the cytoplasm of first-trimester placenta trophoblast cells. Nuclear AHR and ARNT localization was detected in syncytiotrophoblast layer in fetal villi in term placentas (Stejskalova et al. 2011). These data correlate with previous reports in which AHR immunoreactivity was reported primarily in the syncytiotrophoblasts of human term placentas (Jiang et al. 2010).

The ARNT protein has been detected in the first and second trimesters using Western blotting; immunohistochemistry has been employed to show nuclear localization in placental trophoblasts (Ietta et al. 2006). On the other hand, the human placental AHR has a lower affinity for its ligand and is less stable than the receptor in rodent tissues (Manchester et al. 1987). Hakkola et al. (1997) have shown a large interindividual variation in AHR expression, while no such difference was seen in ARNT in the human placenta. Gestation time did not modulate the expression of these factors in human placental samples (Hakkola et al. 1997). Exposure to choriocarcinoma JEG-3 cells did not significantly affect the expression of AHR or ARNT (Hakkola et al. 1997). No significant difference was detected between normal placentas and placentas with intrauterine growth retardation (IUGR) in the concentration of AHR sites and in its affinity to bind AHR ligand [³H]TCDD (Okey et al. 1997).

22.3 CYTOCHROME CYP1A1

CYP is a superfamily of hemoproteins that catalyze the monooxygenase reaction both of endogenous (hormones, eicosanoids, steroids) and exogenous (Hasler 1999; Anzenbacher and Anzenbacherova 2001) substrates. In the reaction catalyzed by CYP enzymes, molecular dioxygen is cleaved by the sequential input of two reducing equivalents, supplied by nicotinamide adenine dinucleotide 2'-phosphate (NADPH) or nicotinamide adenine dinucleotide (NADH). Thus, a single oxygen atom is inserted into the substrate to produce an oxygenated metabolite, alcohol (ROH), with concomitant generation of water from the second oxygen atom (Guengerich 2007).

CYP1A1, also known as aryl hydrocarbon hydroxylase, is a member of the CYP1A subfamily of enzymes. Human CYP1A1 is localized on chromosome 15 (15q22-q24). Together with CYP1A2, which is oriented in the opposite direction, it shares the 5'flanking region of the DNA. The CYP1A1 gene consists of 6069 basis (beginning at 72,798,936 bp, ending at 72,805,004 bp) and codes a protein of 512 amino acids (58,165 Da). Cytochrome CYP1A1 plays an important role in the metabolism of many exogenous and endogenous compounds, including steroids, fatty acids, and xenobiotics (Anzenbacher and Anzenbacherova 2001; Guengerich 2007; Stejskalova, Dvorak, and Pavek 2011). It is also considered to be a hallmark for the initiation of carcinogenesis through the formation of reactive species that interact with DNA (Androutsopoulos, Tsatsakis, and Spandidos 2009).

The primary localization of CYP1A1 is in extrahepatic tissues such as in lungs, skin, kidney, the small intestine, and placenta (Pavek and Dvorak 2008). In fact, CYP1A1 has a low expression in these organs, but via ligand-dependent AHR-mediated induction, its activity can be substantially increased.

Like CYP1B1 and CYP1A2, CYP1A1 also belongs to the CYP1 family. Although they are involved in the same cytochrome family and have several similar properties such as regulation through the ligand-activated AHR and overlapped substrate specifities, each has specific tissue distribution and different catalytic properties (Don et al. 2003; Nebert et al. 2004; Neve and Ingelman-Sundberg 2008). Generally, cytochromes CYP1A1 and CYP1B1 are involved in the metabolism of PAHs, whereas CYP1A2 substrates are mostly N-heterocyclics and arylamines (Dragin et al. 2006; Ma and Lu 2007).

The gene expression of CYP1A1 can be strongly induced by exposure to AHR ligands such as PAHs (benzo[a]pyrene, 3-methylcholanthrene [3MC], β-naphthoflavone), polychlorobiphenyls (PCBs), TCDD, and other agents (Westerink, Stevenson, and Schoonen 2008). There are 13 AHR binding site (XRE response element) sequences in the CYP1A1 gene promoter that participate in CYP1A1 induction following the activation of the AHR/ARNT transcription complex (Galijatovic et al. 2004).

Studies have also shown that the drugs omeprazole, lansoprazole, and primaquine induce human cytochrome CYP1A1 without its direct binding to AHR, in contrast to typical AHR ligands (Curi-Pedrosa et al. 1994; Werlinder et al. 2001; Yoshinari et al. 2008).

22.3.1 EXPRESSION CYP1A1 IN PLACENTAL TISSUE

CYP1A1 is the only CYP xenobiotic-metabolizing enzyme for which substantial expression has been demonstrated in the human placental trophoblast (Stejskalova and Pavek 2011; Storvik et al. 2014). Recently, we demonstrated that only CYP1A1 mRNA, but not CYP1A2, CYP1B1, UGT1A1, breast cancer resistance protein (BCRP), AHR, ARNT, or aryl-hydrocarbon receptor repressor (AHRR) mRNAs, is significantly induced in human term placental trophoblast cultures after exposure to prototype AHR ligands/activators TCDD, 3MC, omeprazole, and β-naphthoflavone (Stejskalova et al. 2011). These data indicate that only CYP1A1, but not other AHR target genes, may be regulated in the human placental trophoblast.

CYP1A1 has been detected in human placentas in first-trimester and in some full-term placenta samples (Hakkola, Pasanen et al. 1996; Czekaj et al. 2005). Microsomes prepared from human cyto-trophoblast isolated from the placentas of nonsmokers grown in primary culture also retained low ethoxyresorufin-O-deethylase (EROD) activity (Avery, Meek, and Audus 2003). The expression of cytochrome CYP1A1 has been localized to the syncytium of the placental villi at the maternal–fetal interface and it was not observed in the fetal endometrium (Collier et al. 2002).

CYP1A2 mRNA was identified in first-trimester placentas but was not detected in full-term placentas. CYP1B1 mRNA was constitutively detected at a low level in first-trimester and full-term placentas, but CYP1B1 mRNA was not induced in the placentas of smokers (Hakkola, Pasanen et al. 1996; Hakkola, Raunio et al. 1996; Hakkola et al. 1997).

22.3.2 Biotransformation of Exogenous Compounds by CYP1A1

CYP1A1 is responsible for the biotransformation of numerous drugs and xenobiotics, including dietary and natural compounds. However, the oxygenation of carcinogens/procarcinogens such as PAHs and HAs gives rise to arene oxide, dioloxide and other electrophilic reactive species that form DNA adducts which contribute to mutagenesis and, ultimately, tumor formation (Ma and Lu 2007). One well-known procarcinogen that is metabolized by CYP1A1 to its reactive metabolites is benzo[a]pyrene (BaP), a PAH. At the same time, BaP is a ligand of AHR and a substrate of CYP1A1. Other PAHs that are metabolized by CYP1A1 include benz[a]anthracene, benzo[b]fluoranthene, benzo[c]phenanthrene, chrysene, benzo[g]chrysene, and 5,6-dimethylchrysene (Schwarz et al. 2001; Shimada and Fujii-Kuriyama 2004; Murray, Patterson, and Perdew 2014). PAHs are present in various petroleum and combustion products. PAHs are also produced by the pyrolysis of organic matters such as during tobacco smoking and in grilled food (Jernstrom and Graslund 1994). CYP1A1 has been shown to be involved in the activation of the tobacco-related carcinogenic compounds N-nitrosamines, such as 4-(methylnitrosamino)-1-(3-pyridyl)-1-butanone, N-nitrosonornicotine, N-nitrosodimethylamine, along with CYP1A2, CYP2A6, and other CYP isoforms (Fujita and Kamataki 2001; Arranz et al. 2007; Androutsopoulos, Tsatsakis, and Spandidos 2009), although CYP1A1 prefers the biotransformation of planar aromatic hydrocarbons. In addition, CYP1A1 also catalyzes the metabolite activation of the well-known heterocyclic carcinogen PhIP (2-amino-1-methyl-6-phenylimidazo[4,5-b]pyridine) (Crofts, Sutter, and Strickland 1998; Thomas et al. 2006).

Among drugs, caffeine, a major constituent of coffee, tea, and cola beverages, is also metabolized by CYP1A2 and CYP1A1 enzymes (Goasduff et al. 1996). Warfarin racemate is prescribed for the treatment of deep venous thrombosis and pulmonary embolism and also prophylactically for the prevention of thromboembolic events (Caldwell et al. 2007). R-warfarin is metabolized mainly via CYP3A4 with involvement of CYP1A1, CYP1A2, CYP2C8, CYP2C9, CYP2C18, and CYP2C19 (Zhang et al. 1995; Kaminsky and Zhang 1997). Other drugs such as erlotinib, defitinib, and imatinib are metabolized by the CYP1A1 enzyme.

22.3.3 Biotransformation of Endogenous Compound by CYP1A1

Many endogenous substrates of CYP1A1 are hormones or endocrine active compounds (such as 17β-estradiol, arachidonic acid [AA], and eicosapentaenoic acid [EPA]) that are essential for placental functions, maintenance of pregnancy, as well as proper parturition (Schwarz et al. 2004; Pasqualini 2005; Murphy et al. 2006).

17β-estradiol (E_2) (a biologically active form of estrogen) has an important role in placental growth, implantation, and embryo development (Rama, Petrusz, and Rao 2004; Pasqualini 2005).

Dehydroepiandrosterone sulfate produced by the fetus acts as a precursor of placental estradiol synthesis that is desulfonated and further metabolized to the final E_2 (Pasqualini 2005; Samson, Labrie, and Luu-The 2009). 17β-estradiol (E_2) and estrone (E_1) undergo oxidative metabolism to various hydroxylated metabolites catalyzed by CYP1A1 and other CYP isoforms. In the human placenta, CYP1A1 is involved in the biotransformation of E_2 to numerous 2-, 4-, 6α, and 15α hydroxylated metabolites, with 2-OH-E_2 being the main catalyzed metabolite, followed by 15α-, 6α-, and 4-hydroxylation. Consistent with the up-regulation of CYP1A1 by cigarette smoke, which contains numerous AHR ligands, the 15α-, 7α-, and 4α-hydroxylation of E_2 was markedly elevated in the placentas of smokers (Zhu et al. 2002; Zhu and Lee 2005). Significantly, 4-OH E_2 has been found to interact with DNA and to have mutagenic properties (Cavalieri et al. 2000).

AAs and EPAs are substrates hydroxylated by CYP1A1 to form 19-OH-AA, the major metabolite of AA, and to other hydroxymetabolites (16-, 17-, and 18-OH-AA metabolites) or to 19-OH-EPA, the major EPA metabolite (Schwarz et al. 2004).

Human CYP1A1s also metabolize retinal to retinoic acids (Zhang, Dunbar, and Kaminsky 2000).

22.3.4 INHIBITION OF CYP1A1

Among natural compounds, rhapontigenin and resveratrol have been shown as potent inhibitors of human CYP1A1. Rhapontigenin (3, 3',5-trihydroxy-4'-methoxystilbene), isolated from the Asian medical plant *Rheum undulatum*, exhibits potent and selective inhibition of human cytochrome CYP1A1 (Chun et al. 2001). Resveratrol (trans 3,4',5-trihydroxystilbene) is a phytoalexin compound found mainly in wine produced from dark-skinned grape cultivars. Resveratrol is a selective human CYP1A1 inhibitor and is often considered for use as a strong cancer chemopreventive agent in humans (Chun, Kim, and Guengerich 1999).

Similarly, flavonoids such as 7-hydroxyflavone, chrysin, and apigenin inhibit enzymes CYP1A1 and CYP1A2 (Zhai et al. 1998; Lautraite et al. 2002).

22.3.5 SMOKING AND PLACENTAL CYP1A1

Cigarette smoke is a mixture of CYP1A1 inducers and AHR ligands including HA, PAH, and pyridine alkaloids nicotine (Czekaj et al. 2005). Exposure to cigarette smoke is known to affect diverse reproductive and developmental processes. Epidemiological studies have shown that smoke may be associated with preterm birth, low birth weight, premature rupture of the amniotic membrane, IUGR, low birth length, congenital anomalies, immature lung developments, sudden infant death of neonates, and other conditions. (Sanyal, Li, and Belanger 1994; Okey et al. 1997; Wang et al. 2002). Maternal smoking during pregnancy is also known to be associated with placental abruption, ectopic pregnancy, and spontaneous abortion (Shiverick and Salafia 1999).

The first studies performed on the effect of maternal smoking on placental enzymatic activities have reported that CYP1 activities are poorly elevated by inducers during the first trimester (Juchau 1971). A more recent study, however, showed that placental CYP1A1 activity is inducible by maternal cigarette smoking as early as gestation age 8–11 weeks (Sanyal et al. 1993; Hakkola, Raunio et al. 1996).

Significant placental upregulation of CYP1A1 has been found in smoking or ex-smoking mothers at the level of mRNA (Pasanen et al. 1990; Whyatt et al. 1995, 1998; Hakkola, Pasanen et al. 1996; Huuskonen et al. 2008; Bruchova et al. 2010) and at the level of protein or its catalytic activity (Kaelin and Cummings 1983; Boden et al. 1995; Hakkola et al. 1997; Okey et al. 1997; Collier et al. 2002; Czekaj et al. 2005). Nevertheless, contradictive data have also been reported (Sanyal and Li 2007). Notably, in ex-smokers who quit smoking before pregnancy, placental CYP1A1 mRNA levels remained significantly increased likely because of PAH accumulation in body lipid deposits (Whyatt et al. 1995).

22.3.6 ENVIRONMENTAL CONTAMINANTS

The effects of environmental contaminants that interact with AHR have also been reported in pregnant women. Inuit women from Quebec exposed to organochlorine in their diet had significantly alleviated placental EROD activity and formed PAH-related DNA adducts in placentas, although contradictory data have been reported as well in the same population (Lagueux et al. 1999; Pereg et al. 2002). Consistently, exposure of pregnant women to PCBs and polychlorinated dibenzofurans has been reported, and significant up-regulation of CYP1A1 in human placenta has been found (Lucier, Sunahara, and Wong 1990; Gallagher et al. 1994).

CYP1A1 inducibility by AHR ligands has also been studied in placental choriocarcinoma JEG-3 and BeWo cell lines, although the lines have a relatively low expression of AHR mRNA (Hakkola et al. 1997; Avery, Meek, and Audus 2003; Stejskalova et al. 2011; Wojtowicz et al. 2011).

22.4 NATURAL OR DIETARY LIGANDS OF AHR

Over the years, a number of AHR ligands, both synthetic and natural, have been discovered. The ligands of AHR (or rodent Ahr) can be classified into two classes. The first category includes ligands that are formed from anthropogenic activities (synthetic exogenous chemicals), which are formed in biological systems as a result of natural processes. The second category can be further divided into two subgroups: dietary AHR ligands and endogenous physiological ligands (Denison et al. 2002; Nguyen and Bradfield 2008; Fujii-Kuriyama and Kawajiri 2010; Stejskalova, Dvorak, and Pavek 2011). Diet is a key source of the naturally occurring ligands of AHR. There are numerous reports on naturally occurring dietary chemicals, e.g., flavonoids (Ashida et al. 2000), carotenoids (β-apo-8′carotenal, canthaxanthin, and astaxanthin) (Gradelet et al. 1997), berberine (Vrzal et al. 2005), and others (Gradelet et al. 1997; Ciolino, Wang, and Yeh 1998; Ciolino et al. 1998; Allen et al. 2001), that activate or antagonize the AHR. Many natural sources of traditional remedies are used regularly, meaning that humans in developed countries are exposed to AHR ligands every day. Flavonoids, naturally occurring polyphenols present in many fruits and vegetables consumed in an average diet, are the most abundant natural compounds and ligands of AHR. The most important AHR ligands in the average diet as well as in drug supplements and traditional remedies are summarized in Table 22.1. The precise effect of these natural AHR ligands on the placental AHR needs to be carefully evaluated and their effects further explored to eliminate their toxic potential via placental AHR interactions.

22.5 CROSS-TALK FROM AHR TO OTHER SIGNALING PATHWAYS IN THE FETOPLACENTAL UNIT

AHR interacts with other signaling pathways such as those mediated by the estrogen receptor (ER) and other steroid hormone receptors, hypoxia (Gradin et al. 1996), nuclear factor-κB (Tian 2009), and retinoblastoma protein (Rb) (Elferink, Ge, and Levine 2001). AHR interactions with ERs as well as with the androgen receptor (AR), thyroid hormone receptor, and glucocorticoid receptor pathways have been recently comprehensively reviewed (Monostory et al. 2009; Swedenborg and Pongratz 2009; Stejskalova et al. 2011).

It was also demonstrated that in utero exposure to TCDD or cigarette smoke that contains AHR ligands affects vasculogenesis and vascular remodeling in the rat placenta via AHR signaling by interacting with the hypoxia-inducible factor 1-alpha (HIF-1α) pathway. Ishimura et al. (2009) have found that in utero exposure to TCDD markedly suppressed the development of sinusoids and trophoblast cells and the apoptosis of trophoblast cells under hypoxic conditions, resulting in a higher incidence of fetal death.

There is extensive evidence showing that cross-talk between the ER and AHR pathways results in the inhibition of estrogenic signaling (Ohtake, Fujii-Kuriyama, and Kato 2009; Swedenborg and

TABLE 22.1

Natural Activators or Antagonists of AHR

Types	Source	Agonist/Antagonist	References
Flavonoids (e.g., chrysin, tectochrysin, galangin, baicalein, genistein, apigenin quercetin, kaempferol, 5,7, dimethoxyflavone)	Fruits, vegetables, whole grains, red wine, and tea soy	Agonist/antagonist	Amakura et al. 2003; Van der Heiden et al. 2009; Powell and Ghotbaddini 2014
Flavonol Quercetin (3,3',4',5,7-pentahydrozyflavone)	Numerous vegetables, fruits, seeds, nuts, tea, and red wine	Antagonist	Busbee et al. 2013
Daidzein, glycitein	Soy	Agonist	Amakura et al. 2011
Indoles Indole-3-carbinol (I3C)	Cruciferous vegetables such as broccoli, cauliflower, cabbage, and Brussels sprouts	Agonist	Wattenberg and Loub 1978; Denison et al. 2002
Catechins are (-)-epigallocatechin gallate (EGCG), (-)-epigallocatechin (EGC), (-)-epicatechin gallate (ECG) and (-)-epicatechin (EC)	Green tea	Antagonist	Palermo et al. 2003; Fukuda et al. 2015
Stilbenes Resveratrol (3,5,4'-trihydroxystilbene)	A variety of dietary sources, including grape seeds, peanuts and mulberries, red wine	Competitive inhibitor of AHR	Powell and Ghotbaddini 2014
Isoquinoline alkaloid Berberin	Plants, e.g., *Berveris vulgaris*, *Hydrastis canadensis*	Activates AHR	Vrzal et al. 2005
Curcumin	Rhizome of the plant *Curcuma longa* (turmeric), Zingeberaceae	Antagonist of AHR	Nishiumi, Yoshida, and Ashida 2007; Powell and Ghotbaddini 2014
Harman (1-methyl-9H-pyrido-[3,4-*b*] indole), an aromatic β-carbolines	Tobacco smoke, coffee	Weak ligand of AHR	El Gendy and El-Kadi 2010
Indigoids Indigo, indirubin	Dried leaves of the flowering plant *Isatis tinctoria*	Agonist	Busbee et al. 2013

Pongratz 2009; Fujii-Kuriyama and Kawajiri 2010). The mechanism of the cross-talk was found to be the fact that AHR is contained in an E3 ubiquitin ligase complex that catalyzes the ubiquitylation of ERα, ERβ, and ARs (Fujii-Kuriyama and Kawajiri 2010).

Vice versa, some AHR ligands have estrogenic effects and activate ER signaling (such as of 3MC) (Shipley and Waxman 2006).

It has also been proposed that progesterone can function as an AHR ligand and induces CYP1A1 expression in an AHR-dependent manner. In addition, progesterone has been proposed to be a potential substrate for CYP1A enzymes (Eugster et al. 1993). On the contrary, the antagonistic effect of TCDD on progesterone has also been demonstrated by the TCDD exposure of luteal cells isolated from mature porcine *corpora lutea*, resulting in decreases in progesterone secretion and in a decrease in uterine and hepatic progesterone receptors proteins in rats (Romkes and Safe 1988; Gregoraszczuk et al. 2000).

Recently, we have shown that glucocorticoids alone had no effect on the activity and protein/ mRNA expression of CYP1A1; on the other hand, glucocorticoids significantly stimulated *CYP1A1* mRNA, but not CYP1A2, CYP1B1, UGT1A1, or *BCRP* mRNAs, with AHR-mediated induction in the primary human placental trophoblast. Dexamethasone did not influence AHR and ARNT in the human trophoblast (Stejskalová et al. 2013).

22.6 CONCLUSION

Placental CYP1A1, the only high-activity placental xenobiotic metabolizing enzyme, is responsible for the oxygenation of carcinogens/procarcinogens such as PAH and HAs that form reactive species and DNA adducts. Moreover, there are numerous association studies demonstrating correlations between CYP1A1 induction in smoking women by AHR ligands and pregnancy-related complications such as premature birth, risk of low birth weight and low birth length structural abnormalities, IUGR, fetal death, and placenta abruption. Moreover, clinical studies also indicate that pregnancy outcomes may be affected by environmental toxins binding to the AHR and show a deteriorate effect of AHR activation in the placenta during pregnancy by cigarette smoking. There is therefore an urgent need for investigations as to whether natural compounds contained in traditional remedies or in dietary supplements interact with the AHR. In addition, the intake of natural medicines should be reconsidered during pregnancy because of the risk of placental AHR activation and CYP1A1 induction with toxicological consequences for the developing fetus.

ACKNOWLEDGMENT

This manuscript was supported by the Czech Scientific Foundation (GACR 303/12/G163).

REFERENCES

Allen, S. W., L. Mueller, S. N. Williams, L. C. Quattrochi, and J. Raucy. 2001. "The use of a high-volume screening procedure to assess the effects of dietary flavonoids on human cyp1a1 expression." *Drug Metab Dispos* 29 (8):1074–9.

Amakura, Y., T. Tsutsumi, M. Nakamura, H. Kitagawa, J. Fujino, K. Sasaki, M. Toyoda, T. Yoshida, and T. Maitani. 2003. "Activation of the aryl hydrocarbon receptor by some vegetable constituents determined using in vitro reporter gene assay." *Biol Pharm Bull* 26 (4):532–9.

Amakura, Y., T. Tsutsumi, M. Nakamura, H. Handa, M. Yoshimura, R. Matsuda, and T. Yoshida. 2011. "Aryl hydrocarbon receptor ligand activity of commercial health foods." *Food Chem* 126 (4):1515–20. doi:10.1016/j.foodchem.2010.12.034.

Androutsopoulos, V. P., A. M. Tsatsakis, and D. A. Spandidos. 2009. "Cytochrome P450 CYP1A1: Wider roles in cancer progression and prevention." *BMC Cancer* 9:187.

Anzenbacher, P. and E. Anzenbacherova. 2001. "Cytochromes P450 and metabolism of xenobiotics." *Cell Mol Life Sci* 58 (5–6):737–47.

Arranz, N., A. I. Haza, A. Garcia, J. Rafter, and P. Morales. 2007. "Protective effect of vitamin C towards N-nitrosamine-induced DNA damage in the single-cell gel electrophoresis (SCGE)/HepG2 assay." *Toxicol In Vitro* 21 (7):1311–7.

Ashida, H., I. Fukuda, T. Yamashita, and K. Kanazawa. 2000. "Flavones and flavonols at dietary levels inhibit a transformation of aryl hydrocarbon receptor induced by dioxin." *FEBS Lett* 476 (3):213–7.

Avery, M. L., C. E. Meek, and K. L. Audus. 2003. "The presence of inducible cytochrome P450 types 1A1 and 1A2 in the BeWo cell line." *Placenta* 24 (1):45–52.

Barouki, R., M. Aggerbeck, L. Aggerbeck, and X. Coumoul. 2012. "The aryl hydrocarbon receptor system." *Drug Metabol Drug Interact* 27 (1):3–8.

Bennett, P., D. B. Ramsden, and A. C. Williams. 1996. "Complete structural characterisation of the human aryl hydrocarbon receptor gene." *Clin Mol Pathol* 49 (1):M12–6.

Boden, A. G., P. G. Bush, M. D. Burke, D. R. Abramovich, P. Aggett, T. M. Mayhew, and K. R. Page. 1995. "Human placental cytochrome P450 and quinone reductase enzyme induction in relation to maternal smoking." *Reprod Fertil Dev* 7 (6):1521–4.

Bruchova, H., A. Vasikova, M. Merkerova, A. Milcova, J. Topinka, I. Balascak, A. Pastorkova, R. J. Sram, and R. Brdicka. 2010. "Effect of maternal tobacco smoke exposure on the placental transcriptome." *Placenta* 31 (3):186–91.

Busbee, P. B., M. Rouse, M. Nagarkatti, and P. S. Nagarkatti. 2013. "Use of natural AhR ligands as potential therapeutic modalities against inflammatory disorders." *Nutr Rev* 71 (6):353–69. doi:10.1111/nure.12024.

Caldwell, M. D., R. L. Berg, K. Q. Zhang, I. Glurich, J. R. Schmelzer, S. H. Yale, H. J. Vidaillet, and J. K. Burmester. 2007. "Evaluation of genetic factors for warfarin dose prediction." *Clin Med Res* 5 (1):8–16.

Carver, L. A., J. B. Hogenesch, and C. A. Bradfield. 1994. "Tissue specific expression of the rat Ah-receptor and ARNT mRNAs." *Nucleic Acids Res* 22 (15):3038–44.

Carver, L. A., J. J. LaPres, S. Jain, E. E. Dunham, and C. A. Bradfield. 1998. "Characterization of the Ah receptor-associated protein, ARA9." *J Biol Chem* 273 (50):33580–7.

Cavalieri, E., K. Frenkel, J. G. Liehr, E. Rogan, and D. Roy. 2000. "Estrogens as endogenous genotoxic agents—DNA adducts and mutations." *J Natl Cancer Inst Monogr* (27):75–93.

Chun, Y. J., M. Y. Kim, and F. P. Guengerich. 1999. "Resveratrol is a selective human cytochrome P450 1A1 inhibitor." *Biochem Biophys Res Commun* 262 (1):20–4.

Chun, Y. J., S. Y. Ryu, T. C. Jeong, and M. Y. Kim. 2001. "Mechanism-based inhibition of human cytochrome P450 1A1 by rhapontigenin." *Drug Metab Dispos* 29 (4 Pt 1):389–93.

Ciolino, H. P., P. J. Daschner, T. T. Wang, and G. C. Yeh. 1998. "Effect of curcumin on the aryl hydrocarbon receptor and cytochrome P450 1A1 in MCF-7 human breast carcinoma cells." *Biochem Pharmacol* 56 (2):197–206.

Ciolino, H. P., T. T. Wang, and G. C. Yeh. 1998. "Diosmin and diosmetin are agonists of the aryl hydrocarbon receptor that differentially affect cytochrome P450 1A1 activity." *Cancer Res* 58 (13):2754–60.

Collier, A. C., M. D. Tingle, J. W. Paxton, M. D. Mitchell, and J. A. Keelan. 2002. "Metabolizing enzyme localization and activities in the first trimester human placenta: The effect of maternal and gestational age, smoking and alcohol consumption." *Hum Reprod* 17 (10):2564–72.

Crews, S. T. 1998. "Control of cell lineage-specific development and transcription by bHLH-PAS proteins." *Genes Dev* 12 (5):607–20.

Crofts, F. G., T. R. Sutter, and P. T. Strickland. 1998. "Metabolism of 2-amino-1-methyl-6-phenylimidazo[4,5-b]pyridine by human cytochrome P4501A1, P4501A2 and P4501B1." *Carcinogenesis* 19 (11):1969–73.

Curi-Pedrosa, R., M. Daujat, L. Pichard, J. C. Ourlin, P. Clair, L. Gervot, P. Lesca, J. Domergue, H. Joyeux, G. Fourtanier et al. 1994. "Omeprazole and lansoprazole are mixed inducers of CYP1A and CYP3A in human hepatocytes in primary culture." *J Pharmacol Exp Ther* 269 (1):384–92.

Czekaj, P., A. Wiaderkiewicz, E. Florek, and R. Wiaderkiewicz. 2005. "Tobacco smoke-dependent changes in cytochrome P450 1A1, 1A2, and 2E1 protein expressions in fetuses, newborns, pregnant rats, and human placenta." *Arch Toxicol* 79 (1):13–24.

Denison, M. S., A. Pandini, S. R. Nagy, E. P. Baldwin, and L. Bonati. 2002. "Ligand binding and activation of the Ah receptor." *Chem Biol Interact* 141 (1–2):3–24.

Dolwick, K. M., J. V. Schmidt, L. A. Carver, H. I. Swanson, and C. A. Bradfield. 1993. "Cloning and expression of a human Ah receptor cDNA." *Mol Pharmacol* 44 (5):911–7.

Don, M. J., D. F. Lewis, S. Y. Wang, M. W. Tsai, and Y. F. Ueng. 2003. "Effect of structural modification on the inhibitory selectivity of rutaecarpine derivatives on human CYP1A1, CYP1A2, and CYP1B1." *Bioorg Med Chem Lett* 13 (15):2535–8.

Dragin, N., T. P. Dalton, M. L. Miller, H. G. Shertzer, and D. W. Nebert. 2006. "For dioxin-induced birth defects, mouse or human CYP1A2 in maternal liver protects whereas mouse CYP1A1 and CYP1B1 are inconsequential." *J Biol Chem* 281 (27):18591–600.

El Gendy, M. A. and A. O. El-Kadi. 2010. "Harman induces CYP1A1 enzyme through an aryl hydrocarbon receptor mechanism." *Toxicol Appl Pharmacol* 249 (1):55–64.

Elferink, C. J., N. L. Ge, and A. Levine. 2001. "Maximal aryl hydrocarbon receptor activity depends on an interaction with the retinoblastoma protein." *Mol Pharmacol* 59 (4):664–73.

Eugster, H. P., M. Probst, F. E. Wurgler, and C. Sengstag. 1993. "Caffeine, estradiol, and progesterone interact with human CYP1A1 and CYP1A2. Evidence from cDNA-directed expression in Saccharomyces cerevisiae." *Drug Metab Dispos* 21 (1):43–9.

Fujii-Kuriyama, Y. and K. Kawajiri. 2010. "Molecular mechanisms of the physiological functions of the aryl hydrocarbon (dioxin) receptor, a multifunctional regulator that senses and responds to environmental stimuli." *Proc Jpn Acad Ser B Phys Biol Sci* 86 (1):40–53.

Fujita, K. and T. Kamataki. 2001. "Predicting the mutagenicity of tobacco-related N-nitrosamines in humans using 11 strains of Salmonella typhimurium YG7108, each coexpressing a form of human cytochrome P450 along with NADPH-cytochrome P450 reductase." *Environ Mol Mutagen* 38 (4):339–46.

Fukuda, I., S. Nishiumi, R. Mukai, K. I. Yoshida, and H. Ashida. 2015. "Catechins in tea suppress the activity of cytochrome P450 1A1 through the aryl hydrocarbon receptor activation pathway in rat livers." *Int J Food Sci Nutr* 66 (3):300–7. doi:10.3109/09637486.2014.992007.

Fukunaga, B. N., M. R. Probst, S. Reisz-Porszasz, and O. Hankinson. 1995. "Identification of functional domains of the aryl hydrocarbon receptor." *J Biol Chem* 270 (49):29270–8.

Galijatovic, A., N. Beaton, N. Nguyen, S. Chen, J. Bonzo, R. Johnson, S. Maeda, M. Karin, F. P. Guengerich, and R. H. Tukey. 2004. "The human CYP1A1 gene is regulated in a developmental and tissue-specific fashion in transgenic mice." *J Biol Chem* 279 (23):23969–76.

Gallagher, J. E., R. B. Everson, J. Lewtas, M. George, and G. W. Lucier. 1994. "Comparison of DNA adduct levels in human placenta from polychlorinated biphenyl exposed women and smokers in which CYP 1A1 levels are similarly elevated." *Teratog Carcinog Mutagen* 14 (4):183–92.

Gasiewicz, T. A., E. C. Henry, and L. L. Collins. 2008. "Expression and activity of aryl hydrocarbon receptors in development and cancer." *Crit Rev Eukaryot Gene Expr* 18 (4):279–321.

Goasduff, T., Y. Dreano, B. Guillois, J. F. Menez, and F. Berthou. 1996. "Induction of liver and kidney CYP1A1/1A2 by caffeine in rat." *Biochem Pharmacol* 52 (12):1915–9.

Gradelet, S., P. Astorg, T. Pineau, M. C. Canivenc, M. H. Siess, J. Leclerc, and P. Lesca. 1997. "Ah receptor-dependent CYP1A induction by two carotenoids, canthaxanthin and beta-apo-8'-carotenal, with no affinity for the TCDD binding site." *Biochem Pharmacol* 54 (2):307–15.

Gradin, K., J. McGuire, R. H. Wenger, I. Kvietikova, M. L. Fhitelaw, R. Toftgard, L. Tora, M. Gassmann, and L. Poellinger. 1996. "Functional interference between hypoxia and dioxin signal transduction pathways: Competition for recruitment of the Arnt transcription factor." *Mol Cell Biol* 16 (10):5221–31.

Greenlee, W. F. and A. Poland. 1979. "Nuclear uptake of 2,3,7,8-tetrachlorodibenzo-p-dioxin in C57BL/6J and DBA/2J mice. Role of the hepatic cytosol receptor protein." *J Biol Chem* 254 (19):9814–21.

Gregoraszczuk, E. L., A. K. Wojtowicz, E. Zabielny, and A. Grochowalski. 2000. "Dose-and-time dependent effect of 2,3,7,8-tetrachlorodibenzo-P-dioxin (TCDD) on progesterone secretion by porcine luteal cells cultured in vitro." *J Physiol Pharmacol* 51 (1):127–35.

Guengerich, F. P. 2007. "Mechanisms of cytochrome P450 substrate oxidation: MiniReview." *J Biochem Mol Toxicol* 21 (4):163–8.

Hakkola, J., M. Pasanen, J. Hukkanen, O. Pelkonen, J. Maenpaa, R. J. Edwards, A. R. Boobis, and H. Raunio. 1996. "Expression of xenobiotic-metabolizing cytochrome P450 forms in human full-term placenta." *Biochem Pharmacol* 51 (4):403–11.

Hakkola, J., H. Raunio, R. Purkunen, O. Pelkonen, S. Saarikoski, T. Cresteil, and M. Pasanen. 1996. "Detection of cytochrome P450 gene expression in human placenta in first trimester of pregnancy." *Biochem Pharmacol* 52 (2):379–83.

Hakkola, J., M. Pasanen, O. Pelkonen, J. Hukkanen, S. Evisalmi, S. Anttila, A. Rane, M. Mantyla, R. Purkunen, S. Saarikoski, M. Tooming, and H. Raunio. 1997. "Expression of CYP1B1 in human adult and fetal tissues and differential inducibility of CYP1B1 and CYP1A1 by Ah receptor ligands in human placenta and cultured cells." *Carcinogenesis* 18 (2):391–7.

Hao, K., Q. Zhou, W. Chen, W. Jia, J. Zheng, J. Kang, K. Wang, and T. Duan. 2013. "Possible role of the 'IDO-AhR axis' in maternal–foetal tolerance." *Cell Biol Int* 37 (2):105–8. doi:10.1002/cbin.10023.

Hasler, J. A. 1999. "Pharmacogenetics of cytochromes P450." *Mol Aspects Med* 20 (1–2):12–24, 25–137.

Huuskonen, P., M. Storvik, M. Reinisalo, P. Honkakoski, J. Rysa, J. Hakkola, and M. Pasanen. 2008. "Microarray analysis of the global alterations in the gene expression in the placentas from cigarette-smoking mothers." *Clin Pharmacol Ther* 83 (4):542–50.

Ietta, F., Y. Wu, J. Winter, J. Xu, J. Wang, M. Post, and I. Caniggia. 2006. "Dynamic HIF1A regulation during human placental development." *Biol Reprod* 75 (1):112–21.

Ishimura, R., T. Kawakami, S. Ohsako, and C. Tohyama. 2009. "Dioxin-induced toxicity on vascular remodeling of the placenta." *Biochem Pharmacol* 77 (4):660–9. doi:10.1016/j.bcp.2008.10.030.

Jernstrom, B. and A. Graslund. 1994. "Covalent binding of benzo[a]pyrene 7,8-dihydrodiol 9,10-epoxides to DNA: Molecular structures, induced mutations and biological consequences." *Biophys Chem* 49 (3):185–99.

Jiang, Y. Z., K. Wang, R. Fang, and J. Zheng. 2010. "Expression of aryl hydrocarbon receptor in human placentas and fetal tissues." *J Histochem Cytochem* 58 (8):679–85.

Johnson, B., B. A. Brooks, C. Heinzmann, A. Diep, T. Mohandas, R. S. Sparkes, H. Reyes, E. Hoffman, E. Lange, R. A. Gatti et al. 1993. "The Ah receptor nuclear translocator gene (ARNT) is located on q21 of human chromosome 1 and on mouse chromosome 3 near Cf-3." *Genomics* 17 (3):592–8.

Juchau, M. R. 1971. "Human placental hydroxylation of 3,4-benzpyrene during early gestation and at term." *Toxicol Appl Pharmacol* 18 (3):665–75.

Kaelin, A. C. and A. J. Cummings. 1983. "A survey of aryl hydrocarbon hydroxylase activity in human placental homogenates." *Placenta* 4 Spec No:471–8.

Kaminsky, L. S. and Z. Y. Zhang. 1997. "Human P450 metabolism of warfarin." *Pharmacol Ther* 73 (1):67–74.

Kitajima, M., K. N. Khan, A. Fujishita, M. Masuzaki, T. Koji, and T. Ishimaru. 2004. "Expression of the arylhydrocarbon receptor in the peri-implantation period of the mouse uterus and the impact of dioxin on mouse implantation." *Arch Histol Cytol* 67 (5):465–74.

Lagueux, J., D. Pereg, P. Ayotte, E. Dewailly, and G. G. Poirier. 1999. "Cytochrome P450 CYP1A1 enzyme activity and DNA adducts in placenta of women environmentally exposed to organochlorines." *Environ Res* 80 (4):369–82.

Lautraite, S., A. C. Musonda, J. Doehmer, G. O. Edwards, and J. K. Chipman. 2002. "Flavonoids inhibit genetic toxicity produced by carcinogens in cells expressing CYP1A2 and CYP1A1." *Mutagenesis* 17 (1):45–53.

Le Vee, M., E. Kolasa, E. Jouan, N. Collet, and O. Fardel. 2014. "Differentiation of human placental BeWo cells by the environmental contaminant benzo(a)pyrene." *Chem Biol Interact* 210:1–11. doi:10.1016/j.cbi.2013.12.004.

Lees, M. J. and M. L. Whitelaw. 1999. "Multiple roles of ligand in transforming the dioxin receptor to an active basic helix–loop–helix/PAS transcription factor complex with the nuclear protein Arnt." *Mol Cell Biol* 19 (8):5811–22.

Lucier, G. W., G. I. Sunahara, and T. K. Wong. 1990. "Placental markers of human exposure to polychlori-nated dibenzofurans and polychlorinated biphenyls: Implications for risk assessment." *IARC Sci Publ* 104:55–62.

Ma, Q. and J. P. Whitlock Jr. 1997. "A novel cytoplasmic protein that interacts with the Ah receptor, contains tetratricopeptide repeat motifs, and augments the transcriptional response to 2,3,7,8-tetrachlorodibenzo-p-dioxin." *J Biol Chem* 272 (14):8878–84.

Ma, Q. and A. Y. Lu. 2007. "CYP1A induction and human risk assessment: An evolving tale of in vitro and in vivo studies." *Drug Metab Dispos* 35 (7):1009–16.

Manchester, D. K., S. K. Gordon, C. L. Golas, E. A. Roberts, and A. B. Okey. 1987. "Ah receptor in human pla-centa: Stabilization by molybdate and characterization of binding of 2,3,7,8-tetrachlorodibenzo-p-dioxin, 3-methylcholanthrene, and benzo(a)pyrene." *Cancer Res* 47 (18):4861–8.

Meyer, B. K., M. G. Pray-Grant, J. P. Vanden Heuvel, and G. H. Perdew. 1998. "Hepatitis B virus X-associated protein 2 is a subunit of the unliganded aryl hydrocarbon receptor core complex and exhibits transcrip-tional enhancer activity." *Mol Cell Biol* 18 (2):978–88.

Micka, J., A. Milatovich, A. Menon, G. A. Grabowski, A. Puga, and D. W. Nebert. 1997. "Human Ah receptor (AHR) gene: Localization to 7p15 and suggestive correlation of polymorphism with CYP1A1 inducibil-ity." *Pharmacogenetics* 7 (2):95–101.

Monostory, K., J. M. Pascussi, L. Kobori, and Z. Dvorak. 2009. "Hormonal regulation of CYP1A expression." *Drug Metab Rev* 41 (4):547–72.

Murphy, V. E., R. Smith, W. B. Giles, and V. L. Clifton. 2006. "Endocrine regulation of human fetal growth: The role of the mother, placenta, and fetus." *Endocr Rev* 27 (2):141–69.

Murray, I. A., A. D. Patterson, and G. H. Perdew. 2014. "Aryl hydrocarbon receptor ligands in cancer: Friend and foe." *Nat Rev Cancer* 14 (12):801–14. doi:10.1038/nrc3846.

Nebert, D. W., T. P. Dalton, A. B. Okey, and F. J. Gonzalez. 2004. "Role of aryl hydrocarbon receptor-mediated induction of the CYP1 enzymes in environmental toxicity and cancer." *J Biol Chem* 279 (23):23847–50.

Neve, E. P. and M. Ingelman-Sundberg. 2008. "Intracellular transport and localization of microsomal cyto-chrome P450." *Anal Bioanal Chem* 392 (6):1075–84.

Nguyen, L. P. and C. A. Bradfield. 2008. "The search for endogenous activators of the aryl hydrocarbon recep-tor." *Chem Res Toxicol* 21 (1):102–16.

Nishiumi, S., K. Yoshida, and H. Ashida. 2007. "Curcumin suppresses the transformation of an aryl hydrocar-bon receptor through its phosphorylation." *Arch Biochem Biophys* 466 (2):267–73.

Ohtake, F., Y. Fujii-Kuriyama, and S. Kato. 2009. "AhR acts as an E3 ubiquitin ligase to modulate steroid recep-tor functions." *Biochem Pharmacol* 77 (4):474–84.

Okey, A. B., J. V. Giannone, W. Smart, J. M. Wong, D. K. Manchester, N. B. Parker, M. M. Feeley, D. L. Grant, and A. Gilman. 1997. "Binding of 2,3,7,8-tetrachlorodibenzo-p-dioxin to AH receptor in placentas from normal versus abnormal pregnancy outcomes." *Chemosphere* 34 (5–7):1535–47.

Palermo, C. M., J. I. Hernando, S. D. Dertinger, A. S. Kende, and T. A. Gasiewicz. 2003. "Identification of potential aryl hydrocarbon receptor antagonists in green tea." *Chem Res Toxicol* 16 (7):865–72. doi:10.1021/tx025672c.

Pasanen, M., T. Haaparanta, M. Sundin, P. Sivonen, K. Vakakangas, H. Raunio, R. Hines, J. A. Gustafsson, and O. Pelkonen. 1990. "Immunochemical and molecular biological studies on human placental cigarette smoke-inducible cytochrome P-450-dependent monooxygenase activities." *Toxicology* 62 (2):175–87.

Pasqualini, J. R. 2005. "Enzymes involved in the formation and transformation of steroid hormones in the fetal and placental compartments." *J Steroid Biochem Mol Biol* 97 (5):401–15.

Pavek, P. and Z. Dvorak. 2008. "Xenobiotic-induced transcriptional regulation of xenobiotic metaboliz-ing enzymes of the cytochrome P450 superfamily in human extrahepatic tissues." *Curr Drug Metab* 9 (2):129–43.

Pereg, D., E. Dewailly, G. G. Poirier, and P. Ayotte. 2002. "Environmental exposure to polychlorinated biphe-nyls and placental CYP1A1 activity in Inuit women from northern Quebec." *Environ Health Perspect* 110 (6):607–12.

Poland, A., E. Glover, and A. S. Kende. 1976. "Stereospecific, high affinity binding of 2,3,7,8-tetrachlorodibenzo-p-dioxin by hepatic cytosol. Evidence that the binding species is receptor for induction of aryl hydrocarbon hydroxylase." *J Biol Chem* 251 (16):4936–46.

Powell, J. B. and M. Ghotbaddini. 2014. "Cancer-promoting and inhibiting effects of dietary compounds: Role of the aryl hydrocarbon receptor (AhR)." *Biochem Pharmacol (Los Angel)* 3 (1). doi:10.4172/2167-0501.1000131.

Puga, A., C. Ma, and J. L. Marlowe. 2009. "The aryl hydrocarbon receptor cross-talks with multiple signal transduction pathways." *Biochem Pharmacol* 77 (4):713–22.

Rama, S., P. Petrusz, and A. J. Rao. 2004. "Hormonal regulation of human trophoblast differentiation: A possible role for 17beta-estradiol and GnRH." *Mol Cell Endocrinol* 218 (1–2):79–94.

Reisz-Porszasz, S., M. R. Probst, B. N. Fukunaga, and O. Hankinson. 1994. "Identification of functional domains of the aryl hydrocarbon receptor nuclear translocator protein (ARNT)." *Mol Cell Biol* 14 (9):6075–86.

Romkes, M. and S. Safe. 1988. "Comparative activities of 2,3,7,8-tetrachlorodibenzo-p-dioxin and progesterone as antiestrogens in the female rat uterus." *Toxicol Appl Pharmacol* 92 (3):368–80.

Safe, S. 2001. "Molecular biology of the Ah receptor and its role in carcinogenesis." *Toxicol Lett* 120 (1–3):1–7.

Samson, M., F. Labrie, and V. Luu-The. 2009. "Specific estradiol biosynthetic pathway in choriocarcinoma (JEG-3) cell line." *J Steroid Biochem Mol Biol* 116 (3–5):154–9.

Sanyal, M. K. and Y. L. Li. 2007. "Differential metabolism of benzo[alpha]pyrene in vitro by human placental tissues exposed to active maternal cigarette smoke." *Birth Defects Res B Dev Reprod Toxicol* 80 (1):49–56.

Sanyal, M. K., Y. L. Li, W. J. Biggers, J. Satish, and E. R. Barnea. 1993. "Augmentation of polynuclear aromatic hydrocarbon metabolism of human placental tissues of first-trimester pregnancy by cigarette smoke exposure." *Am J Obstet Gynecol* 168 (5):1587–97.

Sanyal, M. K., Y. L. Li, and K. Belanger. 1994. "Metabolism of polynuclear aromatic hydrocarbon in human term placenta influenced by cigarette smoke exposure." *Reprod Toxicol* 8 (5):411–8.

Schwarz, D., P. Kisselev, I. Cascorbi, W. H. Schunck, and I. Roots. 2001. "Differential metabolism of benzo[a]pyrene and benzo[a]pyrene-7,8-dihydrodiol by human CYP1A1 variants." *Carcinogenesis* 22 (3):453–9.

Schwarz, D., P. Kisselev, S. S. Ericksen, G. D. Szklarz, A. Chernogolov, H. Honeck, W. H. Schunck, and I. Roots. 2004. "Arachidonic and eicosapentaenoic acid metabolism by human CYP1A1: Highly stereoselective formation of 17(R),18(S)-epoxyeicosatetraenoic acid." *Biochem Pharmacol* 67 (8):1445–57. doi:10.1016/j.bcp.2003.12.023.

Shimada, T. and Y. Fujii-Kuriyama. 2004. "Metabolic activation of polycyclic aromatic hydrocarbons to carcinogens by cytochromes P450 1A1 and 1B1." *Cancer Sci* 95 (1):1–6.

Shipley, J. M. and D. J. Waxman. 2006. "Aryl hydrocarbon receptor-independent activation of estrogen receptor-dependent transcription by 3-methylcholanthrene." *Toxicol Appl Pharmacol* 213 (2):87–97.

Shiverick, K. T. and C. Salafia. 1999. "Cigarette smoking and pregnancy I: Ovarian, uterine and placental effects." *Placenta* 20 (4):265–72.

Stejskalova, L. and P. Pavek. 2011. "The function of cytochrome P450 1A1 enzyme (CYP1A1) and aryl hydrocarbon receptor (AhR) in the placenta." *Curr Pharm Biotechnol* 12 (5):715–30.

Stejskalova, L., Z. Dvorak, and P. Pavek. 2011. "Endogenous and exogenous ligands of aryl hydrocarbon receptor: Current state of art." *Curr Drug Metab* 12 (2):198–212.

Stejskalova, L., L. Vecerova, L. M. Perez, R. Vrzal, Z. Dvorak, P. Nachtigal, and P. Pavek. 2011. "Aryl hydrocarbon receptor and aryl hydrocarbon nuclear translocator expression in human and rat placentas and transcription activity in human trophoblast cultures." *Toxicol Sci* 123 (1):26–36. doi:10.1093/toxsci/kfr150.

Stejskalová, L., R. Vrzal, A. Rulcova, Z. Dvorak, and P. Pavek. 2013. "Effects of glucocorticoids on cytochrome P450 1A1 (CYP1A1) expression in isolated human placental trophoblast." *J Appl Biomed.* 11 (3):163–72. doi:10.2478/v10136-012-0022-y (in press).

Storvik, M., P. Huuskonen, P. Pehkonen, and M. Pasanen. 2014. "The unique characteristics of the placental transcriptome and the hormonal metabolism enzymes in placenta." *Reprod Toxicol* 47:9–14. doi:10.1016/j.reprotox.2014.04.010.

Swedenborg, E. and I. Pongratz. 2009. "AhR and ARNT modulate ER signaling." *Toxicology.* 268 (3):132–8. doi: 10.1016/j.tox.2009.09.007.

Thomas, R. D., M. R. Green, C. Wilson, A. L. Weckle, Z. Duanmu, T. A. Kocarek, and M. Runge-Morris. 2006. "Cytochrome P450 expression and metabolic activation of cooked food mutagen 2-amino-1-methyl-6-phenylimidazo[4,5-b]pyridine (PhIP) in MCF10A breast epithelial cells." *Chem Biol Interact* 160 (3):204–16.

Tian, Y. 2009. "Ah receptor and NF-kappaB interplay on the stage of epigenome." *Biochem Pharmacol* 77 (4):670–80.

Tirona, R. G. and R. B. Kim. 2005. "Nuclear receptors and drug disposition gene regulation." *J Pharm Sci* 94 (6):1169–86.

Tscheudschilsuren, G., S. Hombach-Klonisch, A. Kuchenhoff, B. Fischer, and T. Klonisch. 1999. "Expression of the arylhydrocarbon receptor and the arylhydrocarbon receptor nuclear translocator during early gestation in the rabbit uterus." *Toxicol Appl Pharmacol* 160 (3):231–7.

Van der Heiden, E., N. Bechoux, M. Muller, T. Sergent, Y. J. Schneider, Y. Larondelle, G. Maghuin-Rogister, and M. L. Scippo. 2009. "Food flavonoid aryl hydrocarbon receptor-mediated agonistic/antagonistic/synergic activities in human and rat reporter gene assays." *Anal Chim Acta* 637 (1–2):337–45.

Vrzal, R., A. Zdarilova, J. Ulrichova, L. Blaha, J. P. Giesy, and Z. Dvorak. 2005. "Activation of the aryl hydrocarbon receptor by berberine in HepG2 and H4IIE cells: Biphasic effect on CYP1A1." *Biochem Pharmacol* 70 (6):925–36.

Wang, X., B. Zuckerman, C. Pearson, G. Kaufman, C. Chen, G. Wang, T. Niu, P. H. Wise, H. Bauchner, and X. Xu. 2002. "Maternal cigarette smoking, metabolic gene polymorphism, and infant birth weight." *JAMA* 287 (2):195–202.

Wang, K., Q. Zhou, Q. He, G. Tong, Z. Zhao, and T. Duan. 2011. "The possible role of AhR in the protective effects of cigarette smoke on preeclampsia." *Med Hypotheses* 77 (5):872–4. doi:10.1016/j.mehy.2011.07.061.

Wattenberg, L. W. and W. D. Loub. 1978. "Inhibition of polycyclic aromatic hydrocarbon-induced neoplasia by naturally occurring indoles." *Cancer Res* 38 (5):1410–3.

Werlinder, V., M. Backlund, A. Zhukov, and M. Ingelman-Sundberg. 2001. "Transcriptional and post-translational regulation of CYP1A1 by primaquine." *J Pharmacol Exp Ther* 297 (1):206–14.

Westerink, W. M., J. C. Stevenson, and W. G. Schoonen. 2008. "Pharmacologic profiling of human and rat cytochrome P450 1A1 and 1A2 induction and competition." *Arch Toxicol* 82 (12):909–21.

Whyatt, R. M., S. J. Garte, G. Cosma, D. A. Bell, W. Jedrychowski, J. Wahrendorf, M. C. Randall, T. B. Cooper, R. Ottman, D. Tang et al. 1995. "CYP1A1 messenger RNA levels in placental tissue as a biomarker of environmental exposure." *Cancer Epidemiol Biomarkers Prev* 4 (2):147–53.

Whyatt, R. M., D. A. Bell, W. Jedrychowski, R. M. Santella, S. J. Garte, G. Cosma, D. K. Manchester, T. L. Young, T. B. Cooper, R. Ottman, and F. P. Perera. 1998. "Polycyclic aromatic hydrocarbon–DNA adducts in human placenta and modulation by CYP1A1 induction and genotype." *Carcinogenesis* 19 (8):1389–92.

Wojtowicz, A. K., E. Honkisz, D. Zieba-Przybylska, T. Milewicz, and M. Kajta. 2011. "Effects of two isomers of DDT and their metabolite DDE on CYP1A1 and AhR function in human placental cells." *Pharmacol Rep* 63 (6):1460–8.

Wu, Y., X. Chen, Q. Zhou, Q. He, J. Kang, J. Zheng, K. Wang, and T. Duan. 2014. "ITE and TCDD differentially regulate the vascular remodeling of rat placenta via the activation of AhR." *PLoS One* 9 (1):e86549. doi:10.1371/journal.pone.0086549.

Yamamoto, J., K. Ihara, H. Nakayama, S. Hikino, K. Satoh, N. Kubo, T. Iida, Y. Fujii, and T. Hara. 2004. "Characteristic expression of aryl hydrocarbon receptor repressor gene in human tissues: Organ-specific distribution and variable induction patterns in mononuclear cells." *Life Sci* 74 (8):1039–49.

Yoshinari, K., R. Ueda, K. Kusano, T. Yoshimura, K. Nagata, and Y. Yamazoe. 2008. "Omeprazole transactivates human CYP1A1 and CYP1A2 expression through the common regulatory region containing multiple xenobiotic-responsive elements." *Biochem Pharmacol* 76 (1):139–45.

Zhai, S., R. Dai, F. K. Friedman, and R. E. Vestal. 1998. "Comparative inhibition of human cytochromes P450 1A1 and 1A2 by flavonoids." *Drug Metab Dispos* 26 (10):989–92.

Zhang, Z., M. J. Fasco, Z. Huang, F. P. Guengerich, and L. S. Kaminsky. 1995. "Human cytochromes P4501A1 and P4501A2: R-warfarin metabolism as a probe." *Drug Metab Dispos* 23 (12):1339–46.

Zhang, Q. Y., D. Dunbar, and L. Kaminsky. 2000. "Human cytochrome P-450 metabolism of retinals to retinoic acids." *Drug Metab Dispos* 28 (3):292–7.

Zhu, B. T. and A. J. Lee. 2005. "NADPH-dependent metabolism of 17beta-estradiol and estrone to polar and nonpolar metabolites by human tissues and cytochrome P450 isoforms." *Steroids* 70 (4):225–44.

Zhu, B. T., M. X. Cai, D. C. Spink, M. M. Hussain, C. M. Busch, A. C. Ranzini, Y. L. Lai, G. H. Lambert, P. E. Thomas, and A. H. Conney. 2002. "Stimulatory effect of cigarette smoking on the 15 alpha-hydroxylation of estradiol by human term placenta." *Clin Pharmacol Ther* 71 (5):311–24.

23 Impact of Environmental Pollutants on Placentation

Nur Duale, Kristine Bjerve Gutzkow, Tim Hofer, and Birgitte Lindeman

CONTENTS

ABSTRACT

Exposure to environmental pollutants has been associated with implantation failure and with impaired placentation, which again may result in reduced fertility, intrauterine growth restriction, and increased disease susceptibility in offspring. However, the impact of environmental pollutants on placentation is not well understood. Gaining more knowledge on how chemicals in our environment affect the placenta is important for adequate chemical risk management activities aimed at promoting female fertility and child health.

Proper trophoblast cells proliferation and differentiation are essential for embryo implantation and placentation. Experiments using cultured human trophoblasts and animals have shown that several common pollutants may affect the viability, differentiation, and function of placental trophoblast cells. Among cellular signaling pathways known to be perturbed by environmental pollutants are pathways regulated by estrogen-related receptors and peroxisome proliferator-activated receptors. Furthermore, the placenta ensures proper regulation of the fetal environment, and ATP-binding cassette (ABC) transporters contribute to this important function. Environmental pollutants may impair the placental barrier function by inhibiting ABC transporter levels or activities. More recently, the importance of potential epigenetic changes in the placenta has become an area of focus. Studies of cultured human trophoblasts and placentas have shown associations between exposures to environmental pollutants and epigenetic changes. The potential consequences for fetal adaptation and later disease susceptibility are not known.

In this chapter, data on selected environmental pollutants representing different substance groups are discussed. Our hope is that the increased interest in the impact of environmental exposures on the placenta will close some of the knowledge gaps in the near future.

KEY WORDS

Placenta, trophoblast, heavy metals, organotin, xenoestrogens, bisphenol A, PAHs, PFAS, environmental pollutants, endocrine disruptors.

23.1   INTRODUCTION

The significance of exposure to environmental stressors during development for health and disease risk later in life is becoming increasingly clear. The concept, now known as developmental origins of health and disease, was inspired by the early work of David Barker (Barker and Osmond 1986) showing an association between low birth weight and subsequent risk of metabolic and cardiovascular disease in adult life. The mechanisms underlying the effects of environmental stressors during the critical phases of development on disease susceptibility later in life are unclear. However, it is considered likely that epigenetic modifications play an important role in the developmental plasticity that allows adaptive regulation of the developing fetus in response to environmental perturbations.

Proper placentation is essential for healthy fetal development, and the effect of environmental pollutants on placental function is gaining increased interest. The placenta is an active interface between maternal and fetal blood circulation and is responsible for exchange of gas and nutrients, fetal waste disposal, and hormone production, and the placenta also represents an immunologic barrier. Transfer of environmental pollutants across the placenta is dependent on, e.g., molecular size, lipophilicity, and placental efflux pumps (Syme et al. 2004). The so-called barrier function of the placenta is important for proper regulation of the fetal environment, but it is a potential target for environmental pollutants such as the perfluoroalkyl and polyfluoroalkyl substances (PFASs). In addition to the barrier function, environmental pollutants may affect the placental structure and function both as a consequence of parental preconceptional exposures and as a result of maternal exposures during pregnancy, thus influencing implantation and fetal development.

The trophoblast is the main functional cell in the early placenta and is present from the blastocyst stage onward. Trophoblasts are required for attachment of the embryo to the uterus and for invasion of the maternal vasculature. A correct placentation depends on adequate trophoblast proliferation, differentiation, and invasion. Relatively few studies have so far examined the role of environmental pollutants in placental modifications, but evidence suggests that exposure to at least some xenobiotics during pregnancy can contribute to incomplete placentation and functional changes. Several of these studies have been performed in mice or rats that, like humans, have a hemochorial placenta, where the maternal blood comes directly into contact with the trophoblast (Soncin et al. 2015). The mouse placenta is divided into two morphologically and functionally distinct regions, the junctional (basal) and labyrinth zones. The junctional zone is composed of trophoblast giant cells, spongiotrophoblast, and trophoblast glycogen cells. The junctional zone forms the maternal interface and secretes multiple hormones and metalloproteinases, which facilitate their locally invasive potential. The interhemal region of the mouse placenta, the labyrinth zone, is the site of gas and nutrient transfer between the maternal and fetal blood spaces (Soncin et al. 2015).

The deleterious effects of common metal pollutants such as cadmium (Cd), tin (Sn), mercury (Hg), and arsenic on placental function are recognized, and there is currently a focus on the potential placental effects of exposure to endocrine disruptors (EDs) via the environment. Both heavy metals and EDs have been shown to modify epigenetic processes, even at lower exposure levels (Bernal and Jirtle 2010; Fragou et al. 2011), and such modifications may occur at the placenta level

(Susiarjo et al. 2013); however, the possible consequences for placental function and, subsequently, the developing fetus are uncertain.

This review concerns the effects of environmental pollutants on trophoblast integrity and placentation. The data are derived primarily from experimental rodent studies and from studies using cultured human trophoblasts.

23.2 IMPACT OF ENVIRONMENTAL POLLUTANTS ON PLACENTATION

In the following chapters, data from studies of selected environmental pollutants on trophoblast integrity and their effects on placentation are discussed.

23.2.1 XENOESTROGENS

A variety of environmental pollutants have been found to have effects on the endocrine system of experimental and wildlife animals. There are concerns that exposure to EDs at vulnerable stages of development may contribute to the increasing incidences of several endocrine related diseases in the human population (WHO/UNEP 2013).

Early to midgestational exposure to higher doses of xenoestrogens has been shown to cause embryo/fetal loss, increased neonatal mortality, decidual hypoplasia, and decreased placental blood flow in rodents (Furukawa et al. 2013; Matsuura et al. 2004; Scott and Adejokun 1980). At physiological doses, trophoblast degeneration and disturbed placentation have been reported in rats (Matsuura et al. 2004). These *in vivo* studies suggest that early xenoestrogen exposure could limit trophoblast invasion of the endometrium, placing the fetus at risk of intrauterine growth restriction (IUGR) or prenatal and neonatal mortality. The importance of the peri-implantation exposure window for disruption of placental development is illustrated by studies showing impaired trophoblast development (Tremblay et al. 2001) and placental epigenetic changes (Susiarjo et al. 2013) after exposure to xenoestrogens.

In the following, we briefly describe studies on the classic xenoestrogen diethylstilbestrol (DES) to illustrate the mechanisms of placental effects of DES, although DES is not per se an environmental pollutant. In addition, we discuss the reported effects of bisphenol A (BPA) on the placenta as this substance is ubiquitous in our environment and is one of the best studied substances with respect to effects on placentation.

23.2.1.1 Diethylstilbestrol

DES is a synthetic estrogen that was prescribed to pregnant women to prevent miscarriage, premature labor, and related complications of pregnancy from the 1940s to the 1970s. The use of DES declined after studies in the 1950s showed that the drug was not effective in preventing these problems. Later, increased incidences of cancer and other health problems were revealed in children of women who were given DES during pregnancy.

A few experimental studies have shown that administration of DES during the early and midstages of pregnancy may induce placental toxicity (Nagao et al. 2013; Scott and Adejokun 1980).

Scott and Adejokun (1980) reported a dose-dependent reduction in placental size of DES-treated pregnant animals associated with thinning of the labyrinth zone and an apparent inhibition of trophoblast maturation and development of fetal blood vessels. More recently, Nagao and coworkers have shown that DES at doses associated with increased fetal mortality induces decidual hypoplasia and placental hemorrhage. In addition, impaired development of the labyrinth zone was reported and there were structural changes of the rough-surfaced endoplasmic reticulum of trophoblast giant cells (Nagao et al. 2013).

Tremblay et al. (2001) examined the effect of DES exposure on trophoblast development *in vitro* and *in utero* and specifically the effect of exposure on estrogen-related receptor (ERR) activities. ERRs are a subfamily of orphan nuclear receptors closely related to the classic estrogen receptors

(ERs). The authors reported that DES interacts with ERRα, ERRβ, and ERRγ and inhibits transcription from a reporter gene, presumably by suppressing coactivator binding. Furthermore, treatment of trophoblast stem cells with DES led to their differentiation toward the polyploid giant-cell lineage. DES-treated pregnant mice were reported to exhibit abnormal development of the early placenta associated with a marked reduction or absence of the labyrinth zone and spongiotrophoblast layer with a concomitant increase in the trophoblast giant cell layer and an absence of diploid trophoblasts. β-estradiol treatment did not induce similar changes in this experiment.

ERRs seem to play important roles in early placentation. The absence of ERRβ is associated with an increased number of trophoblast giant cells and a severe deficiency of diploid trophoblast (Luo et al. 1997), whereas ERRγ is highly expressed in metabolically active tissues, including the placenta, and is likely to be involved in control of cellular energy metabolism. Thus, down-regulation of ERRβ and ERRγ activities by DES may contribute to disturbed placental development and function.

23.2.1.2 Bisphenol A

There is widespread human exposure to BPA owing to its use as a monomer in the manufacture of polycarbonates and epoxy resins and as an additive in plastics. Detectable concentrations of BPA have been measured in follicular fluid, amniotic fluid, placental tissue, and cord serum in humans (Cantonwine et al. 2013), giving rise to concern for potential health effects. Human BPA exposure levels, toxicity, and mode of action have been extensively studied and debated during the last decade. BPA is recognized as being toxic to development and reproduction. Whether lower exposure levels approaching the human situation may cause such toxicity is subject to evaluation (EFSA 2015). Several epidemiological studies have shown an association between maternal BPA exposure and fetal growth, but the results from such studies are conflicting (Cantonwine et al. 2013). One obvious challenge in epidemiological studies of BPA-related toxicity has been obtaining an appropriate estimate of actual maternal exposure during critical developmental periods. Rodent studies, on the other hand, have demonstrated negative effects of BPA exposure on female reproduction (EFSA 2015; Shelby 2008). In a series of mouse studies (Berger et al. 2008, 2010), early gestational exposure to BPA was reported to induce reduced blastocyst implantation and decreased litter size. Further studies suggest that effects on both the level of the oocyte (Cabaton et al. 2011; Susiarjo et al. 2007) and on uterus receptivity as a consequence of neonatal exposure (Varayoud et al. 2014) may contribute to reduced female reproductive capacity in response to BPA exposure.

Placentation was examined at days 10 and 12 of gestation in mice exposed during early gestation to BPA by subcutaneous administration (Tachibana et al. 2007). In this study, BPA treatment was associated with embryo loss and reduced uterus weight. Furthermore, the labyrinth zone of the placenta was reduced, the intervillous spaces were narrower, and degenerative changes in the trophoblastic giant cells and the spongiotrophoblast layer were reported.

A few studies report the effects of BPA exposure on cultured human trophoblasts. These studies show that BPA exposure at concentrations relevant for humans may induce apoptosis in a human placental choriocarcinoma cell line (JEG-3) and in primary cytotrophoblasts isolated from human placentas (Benachour and Aris 2009; Morice et al. 2011). In addition, the ability of a low concentration of BPA to increase the secretion of the pregnancy hormone human chorionic gonadotropin (hCG) from placental explants has been shown (Morck et al. 2010). Similar findings were reported in a recent study (Mannelli et al. 2014), which also showed that if placental explants were exposed to conditioned media from BPA-exposed endometrial stromal cells, the BPA-induced increase in hCG was abolished. The authors of this latter paper underlined the importance of considering also maternal effects in *in vitro* models, including retention or metabolism of BPA by endometrial cells.

A few studies have explored epigenetic changes in placental cells as a potential consequence of BPA exposure, which may have implications for placental function. Avissar-Whiting et al. (2010) investigated the effect of BPA exposure on microRNA (miRNA) expression in three immortalized cytotrophoblast cell lines representing two stages of placental development (3A, first-trimester villous cells; TCl-1, an EVT cell line; HTR-8, first trimester extravillous cell line). They found that a total of 25 miRNAs were significantly altered in response to BPA treatment, in both of the two first trimester cell lines (3A and HTR-8). miR-146a was significantly induced by the highest concentration of BPA (25 ng/μL) in both 3A and HTR-8 cells. 3A cells transfected to overexpress miR-146a showed an altered rate of proliferation as well as higher sensitivity to the DNA damaging agent bleomycin. Several additional studies have been performed suggesting that BPA may disturb the epigenome (Kim et al. 2014; Mileva et al. 2014; Susiarjo et al. 2013). Susiarjo and coworkers exposed F1 hybrid mice to a low and a high dose of dietary BPA from the premating phase until embryonic day 9.5 and examined the placental expression of imprinted genes and DNA methylation changes. The study showed that *in utero* exposure to both a high dose of BPA and to a lower but physiologically relevant dose may disrupt the parental-specific, monoallelic expression of imprinted genes in the placenta (Susiarjo et al. 2013). Exposure at a later embryonic stage (embryonic day 5.5 to 12.5) did not induce similar alterations in imprinted gene expression. Further analysis of DNA methylation revealed that some of the gene transcription changes were associated with altered methylation at differentially methylated regions.

Unconjugated BPA is regarded as the endocrine active form of BPA, which acts as a weak estrogen with a significantly lower affinity for the nuclear forms of ERα and ERβ than endogenous estrogen (EFSA 2015). However, BPA has more recently been shown to bind with higher affinity to other estrogen binding receptors, including membrane-bound forms of ERs (membrane bound estrogen receptor α [mERα], membrane bound estrogen receptor β [mERβ], and G protein-coupled estrogen-binding receptor [GPER]/GPR30ERα) and also to the orphan receptor ERRγ. ERRγ is involved in cellular metabolism and is constitutively active (Liu et al. 2014). Binding of BPA to ERRγ does not seem to alter the structure or the activity of ERRγ, implying that the physiological importance of this interaction is uncertain.

23.2.2 Polycyclic Aromatic Hydrocarbons

Polycyclic aromatic hydrocarbons (PAHs) such as benzo(a)pyrene (BaP) are ubiquitous environmental toxicants, generated by incomplete combustion of organic material. The major natural sources are forest fires and volcanic eruptions. Anthropogenic sources include heating, car outlet, car tire and asphalt wear, wood burning, and industrial applications (Bostrom et al. 2002). Occupational exposure also represents a source of high exposure, e.g., in coal industries, offshore, and smelter industries. The nonsmoking general population is exposed to PAHs through the diet, soil, water, and air, but the main exposure route is through the diet, accounting for over 90% of the daily intake (Hattemer-Frey and Travis 1991). PAHs are also found in ambient outdoor and indoor air. Tobacco smoke is one of the important sources of exposure to PAHs. BaP is the most studied PAH, and it is commonly used as a model PAH in many experimental studies. In the following section, the effects of BaP on trophoblast and placental function will be discussed.

23.2.2.1 Benzo(a)pyrene

BaP is classified as carcinogenic to humans (International Agency for Research on Cancer [IARC], group 1) (Straif et al. 2005). BaP is metabolized in humans and animals to form a number of metabolites that may elicit toxicity, and the reactive intermediate metabolites are capable of forming DNA adducts that can lead to cancer or inflammatory responses. BaP is metabolized to its carcinogen metabolite, 7,8-dihydro-9,10-epoxy-7,8,9,10tetrahydrobenzo(a)pyrene by phase I enzymes CYP1A1 or CYP1B1. Recently, a high amount of DNA damage in sperm from smokers was found, which may be a result of BaP exposure (Sipinen et al. 2010), and there are evidences of transmission of DNA adducts from spermatozoa to embryos (Zenzes et al. 1999). Humans are continuously exposed to BaP, and it is of importance to establish the contribution of this PAH to adverse altered placental function and pregnancy outcomes. BaP has received much attention because of its ubiquitous distribution, its carcinogenic and mutagenic potential, endocrine disrupting properties, and modulation of the epigenetic machineries (Maccani et al. 2010).

There are several reports investigating the effects of BaP exposure on placentation and embryo development. Maternal cigarette smoking during pregnancy is associated with adverse pregnancy outcomes. Maccani et al. (2010) have observed changes in the expression level of three miRNAs (miR-16, miR-21, and miR-146a) in cigarette smoke-exposed immortalized placental cell lines, and the expression level of miR-146a decreased in a BaP dose-dependent manner in the human trophoblast cell line, TCL-1. Further, Xie and coworkers have evaluated methylation status of the interferon-γ (IFNγ) promoter in cord white blood cells from 53 participants in the Columbia Center for Children's Environmental Health cohort. Maternal PAH exposure was estimated by personal air monitoring during pregnancy. They observed an association between maternal PAH exposure and DNA hypermethylation of the IFNγ promoter in cord blood DNA from cohort children, indicating a potential link between PAH exposure and epigenetic reprogramming in the fetus (Xie et al. 2010). IUGR has been associated with decreased cord blood concentrations of immunoreactive insulin-like growth factor 1 (IGF-1) and development disorders. The potential mechanisms of PAH-induced IUGR were investigated by exposing human placental trophoblast cells in culture with BaP (Fadiel et al. 2013). BaP exposure of human placental trophoblast cells resulted in a reduction in IGF-1 expression and an increase in base pair mutations, indicating that BaP may not need to cross the placenta to cause adverse effects (Fadiel et al. 2013). Furthermore, the exposure of human placental choriocarcinoma JEG-3 cell line to BaP inhibits cell proliferation and modulates the expression levels of transforming growth factor beta 1 (TGF-β1) and c-myc genes, two important genes in the regulation of trophoblast growth (Zhang and and Shiverick 1997). Further, both basal and epidermal growth factor (EGF)-stimulated secretion of hCG was reduced significantly by BaP exposure in human trophoblast cell line, BeWo, indicating altered trophoblast proliferation and endocrine function (Zhang et al. 1995). Recently, we observed that paternal BaP exposure altered the expression of numerous genes and miRNAs in the developing embryo, especially at the blastocyst stage and delayed embryo division. The target genes for some of the dysregulated miRNAs were enriched in pathways that are likely to be relevant for the developing mouse embryo (Brevik et al. 2012a,b). Genes related to DNA methylation, histone acetylation, and embryo development were affected by paternal BaP exposure at the blastocyst stage (Brevik et al. 2012b). The dysregulated miRNAs may provide valuable knowledge about potential trophoblast effects of sublethal exposure to chemicals. Mouse blastocysts exposed with both caffeine and BaP show increased embryotoxicity and sister chromatid exchange frequency (Spindle and Wu 1985). Embryonic gene and miRNA expression studies seem useful to identify perturbations of signaling pathways resulting from exposure to contaminants and can be used to address mechanisms of parental effects on embryo development.

23.2.3 Persistent Organic Pollutants

Persistent organic pollutants (POPs) (such as PFAS, decaBDE, dioxins, and certain pesticides) are chemical substances that are resistant to environmental degradation and therefore persistent in nature. Many POPs are resistant to metabolism, are able to bioaccumulate in human and animal tissue, and are subject to long-range transport. They are found in food, water, textiles, and many different household products and are shown to have negative impact on human health and the environment. Most of them can cross the placenta and cause harm to the developing fetus. In the following section, we will discuss the effects of the fluorinated compounds (PFAS) such as perfluorooctanesulfonic acid (PFOS) and perfluorooctanoic acid (PFOA) and their potential effect on placentation.

23.2.3.1 PFAS

Several studies, both animal and human, have investigated the association between different PFAS exposures and fetal growth. Animal studies report early pregnancy loss and reduced birth weight or fetal growth in offspring with increasing levels of PFOA or PFOS exposure *in utero* (Lau et al. 2006; Luebker et al. 2005). Several human studies have shown an association between reduced birth weight and relatively low serum concentrations of PFOA and PFOS (Bach et al. 2015; Darrow et al. 2013; Johnson et al. 2014). The mechanism behind these effects has not yet been established.

However, the results from animal studies and the fact that exposure is ubiquitous for humans indicate a potential human health risk.

Because of their oil- and water-repellent properties, PFASs are used in many different household products such as carpets, nonstick cookware, shoes, all-weather jackets, shampoo, and food packaging. Since PFASs are persistent, are not metabolized, and bioaccumulate, they can be found in different wildlife species in the Arctic as well as in human serum and breast milk. Food is generally the major source of exposure, although other sources such as drinking water, inhalation of air, ingestion of dust, as well as dermal exposure may lead to an increased PFAS-serum concentration (Haug et al. 2011). The fetus is exposed to PFAS through transport across the placental barrier (Gutzkow et al. 2012), and breastfed children are also exposed through breast milk (Thomsen et al. 2010). It has been demonstrated that, e.g., fluorotelomer alcohols (FTOHs) and polyfluoroalkyl phosphates found in many different consumer products can be biodegraded to PFOA (Butt et al. 2014; Nabb et al. 2007), thus potentially contributing to the overall exposure. The most widely studied PFASs are PFOA and PFOS. They have serum half-lives in humans of approximately 3.5 and 5.5 years, respectively (Olsen et al. 2007). PFASs are distributed mainly to plasma, bound to albumin, and to tissues with high perfusion such as liver, and kidney as well as placenta. The National Health and Nutrition Examination Survey (NHANES) showed that the median concentration in human serum from the US general population in 2003 to 2008 was approximately 12 ng/mL for PFOS and 3 ng/mL for PFOA, which is similar to European levels (Bach et al. 2015).

Increasing levels of maternal serum PFOA or PFOS during gestation are associated with reduced fetal growth and litter loss in several mouse studies (Lau et al. 2006; Lee et al. 2015; Suh et al. 2011). Recent human and nonhuman meta-analyses concluded that there is sufficient evidence to conclude that exposure to PFOA leads to reduced fetal growth (Johnson et al. 2014; Koustas et al. 2014).

Exposure levels used in experimental studies are more than 1000 times higher than the general human background exposure levels illustrated by NHANES data (Olsen et al. 2009). Furthermore, differences in half-lives and metabolism of PFASs across species complicate the interpretation of animal studies in relation to human health. In addition, it has been suggested that the observed PFOA-mediated birth weight reduction in humans is caused by a reverse causality effect due to reduced glomerular filtration and reduced expansion of plasma volume in mothers giving birth to smaller babies, which could lead to an increased plasma concentration of PFAS (Morken et al. 2014). However, a systematic review concluded that the evidence was insufficient and makes it less likely that there is a reverse causality between environmental contaminants and birth weight (Vesterinen et al. 2014). In light of the above discussion, there is a need for a mechanistic understanding for the observed reduced birth weight and whole litter loss with increasing PFOA or PFOS exposure. Different pathways for the biological effects of PFASs have been suggested, and several studies indicate a hormone disruptive effect. PFASs influence the expression of estrogen-responsive genes in animal studies (Benninghoff et al. 2011; Wei et al. 2007) and have been shown to interfere with the ER in human cell lines and by direct binding to trout liver ER *in vitro* to exert estrogen-like activity. It was also shown that PFOA and PFOS have antiestrogenic effects and that mixtures of PFAS are more potent (Benninghoff et al. 2011; Henry and Fair 2013; Kjeldsen and Bonefeld-Jorgensen 2013).

PFASs have been shown to inhibit CYP19 aromatase activity in the human placental choriocarcinoma cell line (JEG-3) (Gorrochategui et al. 2014). Inhibition of CYP19 may affect the androgen:estrogen balance. In the same study, a mixture of eight PFASs was reported to affect membrane lipid patterns.

Interestingly, a few publications speculate whether placentation is affected by the endocrine disruptive properties of PFOA (Suh et al. 2011) and PFOS (Lee et al. 2015). The study by Suh et al. (2011) indicates a possible mode of action for PFOA. The observed reduced pup weight in this study seems to involve reduced placental efficiency (fetal weight/placental weight). They demonstrate that PFOA has an indirect inhibitory effect on the expression of the placental prolactin-family hormone genes (PRL-family genes) in mice. PRL-family hormones have a vital role in adaptation to physiological stressors and for maintaining pregnancy in mammals (Soares et al. 2007). In the placenta, most PRL-family genes are expressed in trophoblasts, and estradiol and progesterone stimulate the proliferation of these cells in mice (Roby and Soares 1993). Suh and coworkers found a PFOA-mediated reduction in trophoblast cell frequency in the mouse placenta. A significant dose-dependent decrease in trophoblast cell frequency was observed in the placental junctional zone, and a decrease in frequency was observed in the labyrinth zone when exposed to high doses of PFOA. Placental weight was reduced by PFOA in a dose-dependent manner in this study. Northern blot analysis, together with *in situ* hybridization of placental tissue from PFOA-treated mice, revealed a dose-dependent significant reduction of several PRL-family genes, such as mPL-II, m-PLP-E, and m-PLP-F mRNA, possibly reflecting reduced numbers of trophoblasts. In addition, real-time PCR (RT-PCR) analyses revealed a PFOA-dose-dependent decrease in Pit-1α and β transcription factors activating PRL and growth hormone genes. Estrogen may act as a positive transcriptional activator for the Pit-1 gene, and the authors suggest accordingly that PFOA disrupts estrogen-induced activation of Pit-1 gene transcription, which leads to a decrease in PRL-family mRNA levels in mouse placenta. Finally, reduced placental efficiency partly contributed to fetal growth retardation in the mouse, indicating a mode of action for reduced pup weight. A recent study by the same group showed similar results after PFOS exposure (Lee et al. 2015). The molecular mechanism for PFOS toxicity was also similar, although the degrees of severity were different.

Placental function also depends on a set of active transporters to transport substances across a concentration barrier in the placenta. These transporters are called the ATP-binding cassette (ABC) transporters, a family of transmembrane proteins. In the placenta, these transporters are involved in, e.g., maternal–fetal cholesterol delivery (Aye et al. 2010). PFASs such as PFOA and PFOS are shown in several studies to target and inhibit the ABC transporters or influence their mRNA expression level, although these observations were performed in testis cells (Dankers et al. 2013; Lindeman et al. 2012). Thus, there is a possibility that PFAS may affect the ABC-transporters in placenta as well, either through direct or indirect mechanisms.

It is well known that PFAS resembles fatty acids and binds peroxisome proliferator-activated receptors (PPARs) affecting lipid metabolism and adipogenesis. Studies in PPARα knockout mice demonstrated that the reduced developmental effects of PFOA, but not PFOS, depended partly on the expression of PPARα (Abbott 2009). PPARγ is also expressed in the placenta, and PFOA has been shown to bind to this receptor as well. Activation of PPARγ stimulates the production and secretion of hormones required during pregnancy and fetal development, including human placental growth hormone and leptin essential for the maturation of a functional placenta (Tarrade et al. 2001).

A few studies have shown a PFAS-mediated inhibition of 11β-hydroxysteroid dehydrogenase type 2 (11β-HSD2), which is important for converting cortisol to cortisone and lower active glucocorticoid levels (Ye et al. 2012; Zhao et al. 2011). The placental 11β-HSD2 plays a key role in pregnancy maintenance and fetal maturation and protects the fetus from overexposure to maternal cortisol (Seckl and Holmes 2007). Inhibition of 11β-HSD2 activity may thus lead to increased fetal cortisol levels. In the placenta, 11β-HSD2 activity seems to play a role in placental function and fetal development (Nacharaju et al. 2004). Fetal body weight and placental weight were significantly reduced in 11β-HSD2 knockout mouse. This was partially mediated by altered placental transport of nutrients and reduction in placental blood system (Wyrwoll et al. 2009).

Taken together, PFASs such as PFOA and PFOS have been shown to act as EDs and seem to affect normal placental development through various mechanisms. Further elucidation of these mechanisms may help to explain the observed reduced birth weight and fetal growth both in animal studies and humans. In addition, other health effects may also be attributed to reduced placental function, which is not discussed here and also warrant further mechanistic studies for better understanding.

23.2.4 HEAVY METALS

Heavy metals (such as Cd, lead, arsenic, Sn and Hg) present in the environment can affect human health, and they are often categorized as industrial pollutants. These heavy metals are resistant to metabolism and may bioaccumulate in tissues and body fluids. Most of them can cross the placenta and cause harm to the developing fetus. In the following sections, the effects of Cd, Sn, and Hg on placentation function will be discussed.

23.2.4.1 Cadmium

Cd is a common environmental pollutant and a major constituent of tobacco smoke, and it is classified as a group 1 carcinogen by IARC (1993). Natural sources of Cd to the environment include volcanic activity, forest fires, and windblown transport of soil particles. Cd can also be released from heavy metal mines, metallurgy, and industrial use (e.g., manufacturing of nickel-Cd batteries, pigments, plastic-stabilizers, and anticorrosives products) as a byproduct. The nonsmoking general population is exposed to Cd primarily via ingestion of contaminated food (e.g., food crop grown on Cd-containing soils or on soils naturally rich in Cd) and water, to a lesser extent, via inhalation of ambient air. Cigarette smoking is considered to be the most significant source of human Cd exposure. The absorption of Cd varies depending on route of exposure. Once absorbed, Cd is transported throughout the body usually bound to metallothionein (MT) and is distributed mainly to the liver and kidney.

Cd exposure induces a wide range of harmful effects on several organ systems, including on the reproduction system. The toxic and carcinogenic mechanisms of Cd is not yet fully understood but has been linked to several properties, such as inhibition of DNA repair mechanisms, induction of reactive oxygen species, reduction of glutathione levels, interfering with mitochondrial function, and alteration of the epigenetic machinery. Further, Cd's metalloestrogen and endocrine-disrupting properties in reproductive tissues and during fetal development have been reported (Henson and Chedrese 2004; Stasenko et al. 2010).

Cd has been shown to be a developmental toxicant in animals, resulting in reduced fetal or pup weights, fetal abnormalities, and impaired neurobehavioral development (Nagymajtenyi et al. 1997). Cd can partially cross the placenta, and it has been detected in umbilical cord blood (Iyengar and Rapp 2001; Tian et al. 2009). Cd accumulates in the placenta with advancing gestation, disrupting the synthesis and release of hormones produced by the trophoblast (Henson and Chedrese 2004; Piasek et al. 2002).

Cd exposure of pregnant women has been shown to have a negative influence on pregnancy outcome and neonatal birth weight. A negative association between high Cd levels in umbilical cord blood and thyroid hormone status at birth or birth weight (Lin et al. 2011; Zhang et al. 2004) was observed. The metalloestrogenic or endocrine disrupting property of Cd has been demonstrated in several human trophoblast cells. Stasenko et al. (2010) have observed that the expression of leptin mRNA level declined in human trophoblast cells exposed to Cd for 96 hours. Furthermore, Cd exposure has been linked to interfere with progesterone biosynthesis by decreasing the mRNA expression levels of P450-cholesterol side-chain cleavage (P450(scc)) gene and its enzymatic activity in cultured trophoblast cells (Henson and Chedrese 2004). In addition, placental low-density lipoprotein receptor mRNA declines upon Cd exposure, suggesting an inhibition in the pathway that provides cholesterol precursor from the maternal peripheral circulation (Henson and Chedrese 2004). Depending on the stage of exposure and dose given, Cd exposure causes a wide range of abnormalities in the developing embryos. Cd exposure has been shown to affect the preimplantation embryos, and particularly, Cd accumulates in embryos from the four-cell stage onward (De et al. 1993), and high Cd doses inhibit progression to the blastocyst stage and may cause blastocysts degeneration (De et al. 1993). Possible mechanisms by which Cd may affect placental function include perturbation of steroid hormone biosynthesis, disruption of the actions of endogenous estrogens, or interfering with the DNA binding zinc-finger motifs.

23.2.4.2 Hg and Organomercury Compounds

Metallic mercury (Hg [l or g]) and organic Hg compounds (e.g., methylmercury [CH_3Hg]$^+$ [meHg], ethylmercury [C_2H_5Hg]$^+$, and phenylmercury [C_6H_5Hg]$^+$) readily cross the placenta and are toxic to the developing fetus (Clarkson 2002). Concentrations of meHg in the fetal blood are slightly higher than in the maternal blood (Inouye and Kajiwara 1988), and meHg is concentrated to a level in fetal brain at least 5–7 times that of maternal blood (Clarkson 2002). Inorganic Hg salts (e.g., mercury chloride [$HgCl_2$]), however, do not cross the placenta easily (Inouye and Kajiwara 1988). Hg is more readily oxidized to divalent mercuric Hg (Hg^{2+}) than is meHg, and once either of them becomes oxidized into Hg^{2+} in the fetus (or tissue), it is trapped because of the low lipophilicity of this divalent ion. Autoradiographic studies suggest that Hg oxidation also occurs in the placenta and fetus, although the extent of oxidation is not known.

Most of the studies on Hg/meHg are on placental transfer, and there are only few studies on placental effects. The effects of Hg/meHg on carnitine acetyltransferase (CRAT) activity in trophoblast cells were investigated (Shoaf et al. 1986). CRATs are a large family of enzymes in the metabolic pathway in mitochondria, peroxisomes, and endoplasmic reticulum, which play a main role in cellular energy metabolism, i.e., fatty acid oxidation, and dysregulation of CRATs is linked to serious human diseases. CRATs catalyze the reversible exchange of acyl groups between coenzyme A and carnitine. The acetylating activity of membranous CRAT in membrane vesicles from the maternal surface of human placental syncytiotrophoblast has been shown to be inhibited by Hg and meHg (Shoaf et al. 1986). Hg and meHg may inhibit the CRAT enzyme by binding to the sulfhydryl group of the enzyme, which may contribute to the Hg-induced fetotoxicity (Shoaf et al. 1986).

23.2.4.3 Sn and Organotins

Because of ubiquitous environmental contamination, humans are exposed to various organotins through the food chain, particularly through seafood. Organotin compounds are used in a broad variety of products, and Sn^{IV} compounds dominate. Tetrabutyltin (Bu_4Sn) is the starting material for synthesis of tributyltin (TBT; contains a Bu_3Sn group), dibutyltin (DBT; contains a Bu_2Sn group), and monobutyltin (MBT; contains a BuSn group), all Sn^{IV} compounds (Davies 2004). TBTs were previously used as biocides (anti-biofouling agents in ship bottom paint, antifungal agents in textiles, paper, wood pulp, and paper mill systems) but are now banned according to the Rotterdam convention as they caused masculinization in female marine snails presumably as a result of testosterone buildup by inhibiting the enzymatic activity of cytochrome P450 aromatase (CYP19A1) (Matthiessen and Gibbs 1998). DBTs are still widely used, particularly as stabilizers and catalysts in plastics and paint (Davies 2004). TBT has generally been considered a more potent toxicant than DBT, although some studies have found the opposite. MBT, on the other hand, appears to be relatively nontoxic. Organotins are subject to biotransformation reactions; they may hydrolyze in the stomach to become chlorine salts; for instance, dibutyltin dilaurate hydrolyzes into dibutyltin dichloride (DBTC; the toxicophore is DBT [Bu_2Sn^{2+}]) at low pH, and in vivo, dealkylation reactions can transform the TBT moiety into DBT, and then further into MBT.

Animal studies have shown that both inorganic Sn (Theuer et al. 1971) and organotin compounds (Moser et al. 2009) can cross the placenta and reach the fetus. Whereas inorganic tins are thought to pose little health concern, rodent studies have demonstrated that already very low levels of organotins can cause teratogenic toxicity in the embryo, possibly as a result of endocrine disruptive effects in the placenta. In monkeys, however, the organotin DBTC was embryo lethal, but not teratogenic (Ema et al. 2009), which may be related to placental differences among rodents and primates.

The mechanism responsible for the teratogenic activity of organotins is not fully understood and could result from placental endocrine disruption or other mechanisms, such as direct effects in differentiating stem cells in the embryo. One suggested reproduction toxicity mechanism is through inhibition of placental aromatase enzyme (CYP19) that catalyzes androgen-to-estrogen conversions. Whereas human placental tissue expresses high levels of aromatase, the rat placenta lacks aromatase, and estrogen is produced during pregnancy by the ovary. Using human term placenta as source of enzymes, Heidrich et al. (2001) evaluated the aromatase activity in response to exposure to a series of organotins. TBT was a partial competitive inhibitor of aromatase activity and DBT was a less potent inhibitor, but DBT's inhibition was at least half that of TBT, whereas tetrabutyltin and

MBT had no significant effect. Cooke (2002) also found that TBT and DBT (but not MBT) inhibited aromatase activity, with TBT being the most potent organotin.

Organotins (particularly TBT, but also triphenyltin [TPT]) are high-affinity ligands (agonist) for both the retinoid X receptor (RXR) and PPARγ (Nakanishi 2008). RXR/PPARγ or RXR/RXR receptor dimers regulate gene expression, and dependent on cell type, aromatase may be down-regulated (as in trophoblast derived choriocarcinoma cells, e.g., JEG-3) or up-regulated (as in ovarian granulosa-like tumor cell line, designated KGN) already at very low organotin concentrations, suggesting that aromatase mRNA regulating effects could better explain ED effects rather than aromatase enzymatic inhibition that seems to occur at higher dose levels (Nakanishi 2008).

Moreover, the placenta protects the fetus from glucocorticoid toxicity through placental 11β-HSD2, an enzyme converting active 11β-hydroxyglucocorticoids into inactive 11-ketoglucocorticoids. Atanasov et al. (2005) found that DBT, TBT, and diphenyltin and TPT can inhibit 11β-HSD2 activity. 11β-HSD2 inhibition may lead to increased fetal glucocorticoid concentrations causing reduced birth weight.

23.3 CONCLUDING REMARK

Understanding how environmental pollutants interfere with early stages of human development may provide innovative preventive strategies promoting female fertility and child health. The possible mechanisms by which environmental pollutants may affect placental function include disruption of placental hormonal signaling, impairment of the placental barrier function, or epigenetic modifications, which may ultimately lead to altered expression of genes important for placental integrity and fetal development. Currently, there is a markedly increased interest in the effects of environmental stressors on placental function, so hopefully, several of the knowledge gaps will be approached in the near future.

Among the endocrine receptors shown to be targeted by at least some xenoestrogens are the ERRs that are expressed in trophoblasts and are important for placentation. Whereas BPA binds to ERRγ apparently without influencing its activity, other xenoestrogens, like DES, have been shown to inhibit the activity of the ERRs and may thus influence placental development.

The placenta, in addition to its other roles, provides an active barrier that ensures proper regulation of the fetal environment. ABC transporters contribute to this important barrier function, but their activity has been shown to be influenced by environmental pollutants, including PFAS such as PFOA and PFOS, and the xenoestrogen BPA. One potential concern is whether environmental pollutants may impair the placental regulation of fetal thyroid hormone status. Before 16 weeks of gestation, the human fetus relies solely on transplacental delivery of maternal thyroxine (T4), and any reduction in T4 levels could cause neurodevelopmental toxicity. The placenta has a critical role in transferring maternal T4 to the fetus, a process regulated by trophoblast ABC transporters.

The importance of the peri-implantation exposure window for disruption of placental development is illustrated by studies showing epigenetic changes and impaired trophoblast development after exposure to xenoextrogens. In addition, parental preconceptional exposures have been shown to influence preimplantation development, and even paternal exposure may affect blastocyst mRNA and miRNA expression. To what degree preconceptional and periconceptional exposures to human relevant levels of environmental pollutants may impair placental development and function is currently not known. This is an intriguing question that clearly deserves further attention.

REFERENCES

Abbott, B. D. 2009. Review of the expression of peroxisome proliferator-activated receptors alpha (PPAR alpha), beta (PPAR beta), and gamma (PPAR gamma) in rodent and human development. *Reprod Toxicol*, no. 27 (3–4):246–57.

Atanasov, A. G., L. G. Nashev, S. Tam, M. E. Baker, and A. Odermatt. 2005. Organotins disrupt the 11beta-hydroxysteroid dehydrogenase type 2-dependent local inactivation of glucocorticoids. *Environ Health Perspect*, no. 113 (11):1600–6.

Avissar-Whiting, M., K. R. Veiga, K. M. Uhl et al. 2010. Bisphenol A exposure leads to specific microRNA alterations in placental cells. *Reprod Toxicol*, no. 29 (4):401–6.

Aye, I. L., B. J. Waddell, P. J. Mark, and J. A. Keelan. 2010. Placental ABCA1 and ABCG1 transporters efflux cholesterol and protect trophoblasts from oxysterol induced toxicity. *Biochim Biophys Acta*, no. 1801 (9):1013–24.

Bach, C. C., B. H. Bech, N. Brix et al. 2015. Perfluoroalkyl and polyfluoroalkyl substances and human fetal growth: A systematic review. *Crit Rev Toxicol*, 1–15.

Barker, D. J. and C. Osmond. 1986. Infant mortality, childhood nutrition, and ischaemic heart disease in England and Wales. *Lancet*, no. 1 (8489):1077–81.

Benachour, N. and A. Aris. 2009. Toxic effects of low doses of Bisphenol-A on human placental cells. *Toxicol Appl Pharmacol*, no. 241 (3):322–8.

Benninghoff, A. D., W. H. Bisson, D. C. Koch et al. 2011. Estrogen-like activity of perfluoroalkyl acids *in vivo* and interaction with human and rainbow trout estrogen receptors *in vitro*. *Toxicol Sci*, no. 120 (1):42–58.

Berger, R. G., J. Shaw, and D. deCatanzaro. 2008. Impact of acute bisphenol-A exposure upon intrauterine implantation of fertilized ova and urinary levels of progesterone and 17beta-estradiol. *Reprod Toxicol*, no. 26 (2):94–9.

Berger, R. G., W. G. Foster, and D. deCatanzaro. 2010. Bisphenol-A exposure during the period of blastocyst implantation alters uterine morphology and perturbs measures of estrogen and progesterone receptor expression in mice. *Reprod Toxicol*, no. 30 (3):393–400.

Bernal, A. J. and R. L. Jirtle. 2010. Epigenomic disruption: The effects of early developmental exposures. *Birth Defects Res A Clin Mol Teratol*, no. 88 (10):938–44.

Bostrom, C. E., P. Gerde, A. Hanberg et al. 2002. Cancer risk assessment, indicators, and guidelines for polycyclic aromatic hydrocarbons in the ambient air. *Environ Health Perspect*, no. 110 Suppl 3:451–88.

Brevik, A., B. Lindeman, G. Brunborg, and N. Duale. 2012a. Paternal benzo[a]pyrene exposure modulates microRNA expression patterns in the developing mouse embryo. *Int J Cell Biol*, no. 2012:407431.

Brevik, A., B. Lindeman, V. Rusnakova et al. 2012b. Paternal benzo[a]pyrene exposure affects gene expression in the early developing mouse embryo. *Toxicol Sci*, no. 129 (1):157–65.

Butt, C. M., D. C. Muir, and S. A. Mabury. 2014. Biotransformation pathways of fluorotelomer-based polyfluoroalkyl substances: A review. *Environ Toxicol Chem*, no. 33 (2):243–67.

Cabaton, N. J., P. R. Wadia, B. S. Rubin et al. 2011. Perinatal exposure to environmentally relevant levels of bisphenol A decreases fertility and fecundity in CD-1 mice. *Environ Health Perspect*, no. 119 (4):547–52.

Cantonwine, D. E., R. Hauser, and J. D. Meeker. 2013. Bisphenol A and human reproductive health. *Expert Rev Obstet Gynecol*, no. 8 (4):329–35.

Clarkson, T. W. 2002. The three modern faces of mercury. *Environ Health Perspect*, no. 110 Suppl 1:11–23.

Cooke, G. M. 2002. Effect of organotins on human aromatase activity *in vitro*. *Toxicol Lett*, no. 126 (2):121–30.

Dankers, A. C., M. J. Roelofs, A. H. Piersma et al. 2013. Endocrine disruptors differentially target ATP-binding cassette transporters in the blood–testis barrier and affect Leydig cell testosterone secretion *in vitro*. *Toxicol Sci*, no. 136 (2):382–91.

Darrow, L. A., C. R. Stein, and K. Steenland. 2013. Serum perfluorooctanoic acid and perfluorooctane sulfonate concentrations in relation to birth outcomes in the Mid-Ohio Valley, 2005–2010. *Environ Health Perspect*, no. 121 (10):1207–13.

Davies, A. G. 2004. *Organotin Chemistry*. Weinheim: Wiley–VCH, 2nd ed., 438 pp. Copyright © 2004 John Wiley & Sons, Ltd.

De, S. K., B. C. Paria, S. K. Dey, and G. K. Andrews. 1993. Stage-specific effects of cadmium on preimplantation embryo development and implantation in the mouse. *Toxicology*, no. 80 (1):13–25.

EFSA. 2015. Panel on Food Contact Materials Enzymes Flavourings and Processing Aids (CEF). Scientific Opinion on the risks to public health related to the presence of bisphenol A (BPA) in foodstuffs (to be published February 2015).

Ema, M., A. Arima, K. Fukunishi et al. 2009. Developmental toxicity of dibutyltin dichloride given on three consecutive days during organogenesis in cynomolgus monkeys. *Drug Chem Toxicol*, no. 32 (2):150–7.

Fadiel, A., B. Epperson, M. I. Shaw et al. 2013. Bioinformatic analysis of benzo-alpha-pyrene-induced damage to the human placental insulin-like growth factor-1 gene. *Reprod Sci*, no. 20 (8):917–28.

Fragou, D., A. Fragou, S. Kouidou, S. Njau, and L. Kovatsi. 2011. Epigenetic mechanisms in metal toxicity. *Toxicol Mech Methods*, no. 21 (4):343–52.

Furukawa, S., S. Hayashi, K. Usuda et al. 2013. Effect of estrogen on rat placental development depending on gestation stage. *Exp Toxicol Pathol*, no. 65 (5):695–702.

Gorrochategui, E., E. Perez-Albaladejo, J. Casas, S. Lacorte, and C. Porte. 2014. Perfluorinated chemicals: Differential toxicity, inhibition of aromatase activity and alteration of cellular lipids in human placental cells. *Toxicol Appl Pharmacol*, no. 277 (2):124–30.

Gutzkow, K. B., L. S. Haug, C. Thomsen et al. 2012. Placental transfer of perfluorinated compounds is selective—A Norwegian Mother and Child sub-cohort study. *Int J Hyg Environ Health*, no. 215 (2):216–9.

Hattemer-Frey, H. A. and C. C. Travis. 1991. Benzo-a-pyrene: Environmental partitioning and human exposure. *Toxicol Ind Health*, no. 7 (3):141–57.

Haug, L. S., S. Huber, M. Schlabach, G. Becher, and C. Thomsen. 2011. Investigation on per- and polyfluorinated compounds in paired samples of house dust and indoor air from Norwegian homes. *Environ Sci Technol*, no. 45 (19):7991–8.

Heidrich, D. D., S. Steckelbroeck, and D. Klingmuller. 2001. Inhibition of human cytochrome P450 aromatase activity by butyltins. *Steroids*, no. 66 (10):763–9.

Henry, N. D. and P. A. Fair. 2013. Comparison of *in vitro* cytotoxicity, estrogenicity and anti-estrogenicity of triclosan, perfluorooctane sulfonate and perfluorooctanoic acid. *J Appl Toxicol*, no. 33 (4):265–72.

Henson, M. C. and P. J. Chedrese. 2004. Endocrine disruption by cadmium, a common environmental toxicant with paradoxical effects on reproduction. *Exp Biol Med (Maywood)*, no. 229 (5):383–92.

Inouye, M. and Y. Kajiwara. 1988. Developmental disturbances of the fetal brain in guinea-pigs caused by methylmercury. *Arch Toxicol*, no. 62 (1):15–21.

International Agency for Research on Cancer (IARC). 1993. Cadmium and cadmium compounds. In: *Beryllium, Cadmium, Mercury, and Exposures in the Glass Manufacturing Industry*. Working Group Views and Expert Opinions, Lyon, 9–16 February 1993. IARC Monogr. Eval. Carcinog. Risks Hum. 58: 41–117.

Iyengar, G. V. and A. Rapp. 2001. Human placenta as a "dual" biomarker for monitoring fetal and maternal environment with special reference to potentially toxic trace elements. Part 1: Physiology, function and sampling of placenta for elemental characterisation. *Sci Total Environ*, no. 280 (1–3):195–206.

Johnson, P. I., P. Sutton, D. S. Atchley et al. 2014. The Navigation Guide—Evidence-based medicine meets environmental health: Systematic review of human evidence for PFOA effects on fetal growth. *Environ Health Perspect*, no. 122 (10):1028–39.

Kim, J. H., M. A. Sartor, L. S. Rozek et al. 2014. Perinatal bisphenol A exposure promotes dose-dependent alterations of the mouse methylome. *BMC Genomics*, no. 15:30.

Kjeldsen, L. S. and E. C. Bonefeld-Jorgensen. 2013. Perfluorinated compounds affect the function of sex hormone receptors. *Environ Sci Pollut Res Int*, no. 20 (11):8031–44.

Koustas, E., J. Lam, P. Sutton et al. 2014. The Navigation Guide—Evidence-based medicine meets environmental health: Systematic review of nonhuman evidence for PFOA effects on fetal growth. *Environ Health Perspect*, no. 122 (10):1015–27.

Lau, C., J. R. Thibodeaux, R. G. Hanson et al. 2006. Effects of perfluorooctanoic acid exposure during pregnancy in the mouse. *Toxicol Sci*, no. 90 (2):510–8.

Lee, C. K., S. G. Kang, J. T. Lee et al. 2015. Effects of perfluorooctane sulfuric acid on placental PRL-family hormone production and fetal growth retardation in mice. *Mol Cell Endocrinol*, 401:165–72.

Lin, C. M., P. Doyle, D. Wang, Y. H. Hwang, and P. C. Chen. 2011. Does prenatal cadmium exposure affect fetal and child growth? *Occup Environ Med*, no. 68 (9):641–6.

Lindeman, B., C. Maass, N. Duale et al. 2012. Effects of per- and polyfluorinated compounds on adult rat testicular cells following *in vitro* exposure. *Reprod Toxicol*, no. 33 (4):531–7.

Liu, X., A. Matsushima, M. Shimohigashi, and Y. Shimohigashi. 2014. A characteristic back support structure in the bisphenol A-binding pocket in the human nuclear receptor ERRgamma. *PLoS One*, no. 9 (6):e101252.

Luebker, D. J., R. G. York, K. J. Hansen, J. A. Moore, and J. L. Butenhoff. 2005. Neonatal mortality from *in utero* exposure to perfluorooctanesulfonate (PFOS) in Sprague-Dawley rats: Dose–response, and biochemical and pharamacokinetic parameters. *Toxicology*, no. 215 (1–2):149–69.

Luo, J., R. Sladek, J. A. Bader et al. 1997. Placental abnormalities in mouse embryos lacking the orphan nuclear receptor ERR-beta. *Nature*, no. 388 (6644):778–82.

Maccani, M. A., M. Avissar-Whiting, C. E. Banister et al. 2010. Maternal cigarette smoking during pregnancy is associated with downregulation of miR-16, miR-21, and miR-146a in the placenta. *Epigenetics*, no. 5 (7):583–9.

Mannelli, C., F. Ietta, C. Carotenuto et al. 2014. Bisphenol A alters beta-hCG and MIF release by human placenta: An *in vitro* study to understand the role of endometrial cells. *Mediators Inflamm*, no. 2014: 635364.

Matsuura, S., A. Itakura, Y. Ohno et al. 2004. Effects of estradiol administration on fetoplacental growth in rat. *Early Hum Dev*, no. 77 (1–2):47–56.

Matthiessen, P. and P. E. Gibbs. 1998. Critical appraisal of the evidence for tributyltin-mediated endocrine disruption in mollusks. *Environ Toxicol Chem*, no. 17 (1):37–43.

Mileva, G., S. L. Baker, A. T. Konkle, and C. Bielajew. 2014. Bisphenol-A: Epigenetic reprogramming and effects on reproduction and behavior. *Int J Environ Res Public Health*, no. 11 (7):7537–61.

Morck, T. J., G. Sorda, N. Bechi et al. 2010. Placental transport and *in vitro* effects of Bisphenol A. *Reprod Toxicol*, no. 30 (1):131–7.

Morice, L., D. Benaitreau, M. N. Dieudonne et al. 2011. Antiproliferative and proapoptotic effects of bisphenol A on human trophoblastic JEG-3 cells. *Reprod Toxicol*, no. 32 (1):69–76.

Morken, N. H., G. S. Travlos, R. E. Wilson, M. Eggesbo, and M. P. Longnecker. 2014. Maternal glomerular filtration rate in pregnancy and fetal size. *PLoS One*, no. 9 (7):e101897.

Moser, V. C., J. K. McGee, and K. D. Ehman. 2009. Concentration and persistence of tin in rat brain and blood following dibutyltin exposure during development. *J Toxicol Environ Health A*, no. 72 (1):47–52.

Nabb, D. L., B. Szostek, M. W. Himmelstein et al. 2007. *In vitro* metabolism of 8-2 fluorotelomer alcohol: Interspecies comparisons and metabolic pathway refinement. *Toxicol Sci*, no. 100 (2):333–44.

Nacharaju, V. L., A. Divald, C. O. McCalla, L. Yang, and O. Muneyyirci-Delale. 2004. 11beta-hydroxysteroid dehydrogenase inhibitor carbenoxolone stimulates chorionic gonadotropin secretion from human term cytotrophoblast cells differentiated *in vitro*. *Am J Reprod Immunol*, no. 52 (2):133–8.

Nagao, T., N. Kagawa, Y. Saito, and M. Komada. 2013. Developmental effects of oral exposure to diethylstilbestrol on mouse placenta. *J Appl Toxicol*, no. 33 (11):1213–21.

Nagymajtenyi, L., H. Schulz, and I. Desi. 1997. Behavioural and functional neurotoxicological changes caused by cadmium in a three-generational study in rats. *Hum Exp Toxicol*, no. 16 (12):691–9.

Nakanishi, T. 2008. Endocrine disruption induced by organotin compounds: Organotins function as a powerful agonist for nuclear receptors rather than an aromatase inhibitor. *J Toxicol Sci*, no. 33 (3):269–76.

Olsen, G. W., J. M. Burris, D. J. Ehresman et al. 2007. Half-life of serum elimination of perfluorooctanesulfonate, perfluorohexanesulfonate, and perfluorooctanoate in retired fluorochemical production workers. *Environ Health Perspect*, no. 115 (9):1298–305.

Olsen, G. W., J. L. Butenhoff, and L. R. Zobel. 2009. Perfluoroalkyl chemicals and human fetal development: An epidemiologic review with clinical and toxicological perspectives. *Reprod Toxicol*, no. 27 (3–4): 212–30.

Piasek, M., J. W. Laskey, K. Kostial, and M. Blanusa. 2002. Assessment of steroid disruption using cultures of whole ovary and/or placenta in rat and in human placental tissue. *Int Arch Occup Environ Health*, no. 75 Suppl:S36–44.

Roby, K. F. and M. J. Soares. 1993. Trophoblast cell differentiation and organization: Role of fetal and ovarian signals. *Placenta*, no. 14 (5):529–45.

Scott, J. N. and F. Adejokun. 1980. Placental changes due to administration of diethylstilbestrol (DES). *Virchows Arch B Cell Pathol Incl Mol Pathol*, no. 34 (3):261–7.

Seckl, J. R. and M. C. Holmes. 2007. Mechanisms of disease: Glucocorticoids, their placental metabolism and fetal 'programming' of adult pathophysiology. *Nat Clin Pract Endocrinol Metab*, no. 3 (6):479–88.

Shelby, M. D. 2008. NTP-CERHR monograph on the potential human reproductive and developmental effects of bisphenol A. *NTP CERHR MON* (22):v, vii–ix, 1–64 passim.

Shoaf, A. R., S. Jarmer, and R. D. Harbison. 1986. Heavy metal inhibition of carnitine acetyltransferase activity in human placental syncytiotrophoblast: Possible site of action of HgCl2, CH3HgCl, and CdCl2. *Teratog Carcinog Mutagen*, no. 6 (5):351–60.

Sipinen, V., J. Laubenthal, A. Baumgartner et al. 2010. *In vitro* evaluation of baseline and induced DNA damage in human sperm exposed to benzo[a]pyrene or its metabolite benzo[a]pyrene-7,8-diol-9,10-epoxide, using the comet assay. *Mutagenesis*, no. 25 (4):417–25.

Soares, M. J., T. Konno, and S. M. Alam. 2007. The prolactin family: Effectors of pregnancy-dependent adaptations. *Trends Endocrinol Metab*, no. 18 (3):114–21.

Soncin, F., D. Natale, and M. M. Parast. 2015. Signaling pathways in mouse and human trophoblast differentiation: A comparative review. *Cell Mol Life Sci*, no. 72 (7):1291–302. doi:10.1007/s00018-014-1794-x.

Spindle, A. and K. Wu. 1985. Developmental and cytogenetic effects of caffeine on mouse blastocysts, alone or in combination with benzo(a)pyrene. *Teratology*, no. 32 (2):213–8.

Stasenko, S., E. M. Bradford, M. Piasek et al. 2010. Metals in human placenta: Focus on the effects of cadmium on steroid hormones and leptin. *J Appl Toxicol*, no. 30 (3):242–53.

Straif, K., R. Baan, Y. Grosse et al. 2005. Carcinogenicity of polycyclic aromatic hydrocarbons. *Lancet Oncol*, no. 6 (12):931–2.

Suh, C. H., N. K. Cho, C. K. Lee et al. 2011. Perfluorooctanoic acid-induced inhibition of placental prolactin-family hormone and fetal growth retardation in mice. *Mol Cell Endocrinol*, no. 337 (1–2):7–15.

Susiarjo, M., T. J. Hassold, E. Freeman, and P. A. Hunt. 2007. Bisphenol A exposure *in utero* disrupts early oogenesis in the mouse. *PLoS Genet*, no. 3 (1):e5.

Susiarjo, M., I. Sasson, C. Mesaros, and M. S. Bartolomei. 2013. Bisphenol a exposure disrupts genomic imprinting in the mouse. *PLoS Genet*, no. 9 (4):e1003401.

Syme, M. R., J. W. Paxton, and J. A. Keelan. 2004. Drug transfer and metabolism by the human placenta. *Clin Pharmacokinet*, no. 43 (8):487–514.

Tachibana, T., Y. Wakimoto, N. Nakamuta et al. 2007. Effects of bisphenol A (BPA) on placentation and survival of the neonates in mice. *J Reprod Dev*, no. 53 (3):509–14.

Tarrade, A., K. Schoonjans, J. Guibourdenche et al. 2001. PPAR gamma/RXR alpha heterodimers are involved in human CG beta synthesis and human trophoblast differentiation. *Endocrinology*, no. 142 (10):4504–14.

Theuer, R. C., A. W. Mahoney, and H. P. Sarett. 1971. Placental transfer of fluoride and tin in rats given various fluoride and tin salts. *J Nutr*, no. 101 (4):525–32.

Thomsen, C., L. S. Haug, H. Stigum et al. 2010. Changes in concentrations of perfluorinated compounds, polybrominated diphenyl ethers, and polychlorinated biphenyls in Norwegian breast-milk during twelve months of lactation. *Environ Sci Technol*, no. 44 (24):9550–6.

Tian, L. L., Y. C. Zhao, X. C. Wang et al. 2009. Effects of gestational cadmium exposure on pregnancy outcome and development in the offspring at age 4.5 years. *Biol Trace Elem Res*, no. 132 (1–3):51–9.

Tremblay, G. B., T. Kunath, D. Bergeron et al. 2001. Diethylstilbestrol regulates trophoblast stem cell differentiation as a ligand of orphan nuclear receptor ERR beta. *Genes Dev*, no. 15 (7):833–8.

Varayoud, J., J. G. Ramos, M. Munoz-de-Toro, and E. H. Luque. 2014. Long-lasting effects of neonatal bisphenol a exposure on the implantation process. *Vitam Horm*, no. 94:253–75.

Vesterinen, H. M., P. I. Johnson, D. S. Atchley et al. 2014. Fetal growth and maternal glomerular filtration rate: A systematic review. *J Matern Fetal Neonatal Med*, 1–6.

Wei, Y., J. Dai, M. Liu et al. 2007. Estrogen-like properties of perfluorooctanoic acid as revealed by expressing hepatic estrogen-responsive genes in rare minnows (Gobiocypris rarus). *Environ Toxicol Chem*, no. 26 (11):2440–7.

WHO/UNEP. 2013. *State of the Science of Endocrine Disrupting Chemicals—2012*. Edited by A. Bergman, J. J. Heindel, S. Jobling, K. A. Kidd and R. Thomas Zoeller. United Nations Environment Programme and the World Health Organization.

Wyrwoll, C. S., J. R. Seckl, and M. C. Holmes. 2009. Altered placental function of 11beta-hydroxysteroid dehydrogenase 2 knockout mice. *Endocrinology*, no. 150 (3):1287–93.

Xie, Y., M. E. Abdallah, A. O. Awonuga et al. 2010. Benzo(a)pyrene causes PRKAA1/2-dependent ID2 loss in trophoblast stem cells. *Mol Reprod Dev*, no. 77 (6):533–9.

Ye, L., B. Zhao, X. H. Cai et al. 2012. The inhibitory effects of perfluoroalkyl substances on human and rat 11beta-hydroxysteroid dehydrogenase 1. *Chem Biol Interact*, no. 195 (2):114–8.

Zenzes, M. T., L. A. Puy, R. Bielecki, and T. E. Reed. 1999. Detection of benzo[a]pyrene diol epoxide-DNA adducts in embryos from smoking couples: Evidence for transmission by spermatozoa. *Mol Hum Reprod*, no. 5 (2):125–31.

Zhang, L. and K. T. Shiverick. 1997. Benzo(a)pyrene, but not 2,3,7,8-tetrachlorodibenzo-p-dioxin, alters cell proliferation and c-myc and growth factor expression in human placental choriocarcinoma JEG-3 cells. *Biochem Biophys Res Commun*, no. 231 (1):117–20.

Zhang, L., E. E. Connor, N. Chegini, and K. T. Shiverick. 1995. Modulation by benzo[a]pyrene of epidermal growth factor receptors, cell proliferation, and secretion of human chorionic gonadotropin in human placental cell lines. *Biochem Pharmacol*, no. 50 (8):1171–80.

Zhang, Y. L., Y. C. Zhao, J. X. Wang et al. 2004. Effect of environmental exposure to cadmium on pregnancy outcome and fetal growth: A study on healthy pregnant women in China. *J Environ Sci Health A Tox Hazard Subst Environ Eng*, no. 39 (9):2507–15.

Zhao, B., Q. Lian, Y. Chu et al. 2011. The inhibition of human and rat 11beta-hydroxysteroid dehydrogenase 2 by perfluoroalkylated substances. *J Steroid Biochem Mol Biol*, no. 125 (1–2):143–7.

Section VI

Epigenetics, microRNA,
and Placental Gene Expression

24 Differential Gene Expression of the Placenta in Normal and Pathological Human Pregnancy

Vasilis Sitras and Ganesh Acharya

CONTENTS

ABSTRACT

The placenta is a major organ during the intrauterine life that largely determines fetal development and well-being. Being a dynamic structure that is rapidly growing and maturing, its gene expression profile, as well as structure and function, changes throughout the pregnancy. As a temporary organ, its role of sustaining life *in utero* ceases after 9 months, and it is readily available for investigation after delivery. A genomic approach to investigation can be applied to study the pathophysiological processes associated with placenta-specific disorders, understand their etiologies, and identify screening, diagnostic, and prognostic markers. The aim of this chapter is to provide an overview of differential gene expression of the placenta in physiological pregnancy and in pregnancies complicated by placenta-specific disorders. In the future, studying placental gene expression profile may become a routine screening procedure that may be used to assess and predict each individual's risk of developing diseases later in life, individualize health monitoring programs, and provide appropriate advice on health-promoting activities, diet, and lifestyle.

KEY WORDS

Placenta, gene expression, microarrays, transcriptome, genome, pregnancy complications, placental disorders, placental biomarkers.

24.1   INTRODUCTION

The placenta is a temporary organ that sustains life *in utero*. The placenta plays a central role in human embryonic/fetal development and largely determines pregnancy outcome. Human placental development is a complex biological process that is regulated at molecular level. Cells in this dynamic tissue divide, differentiate, migrate, and grow simultaneously, and these biological processes are controlled by a large number of genes. The expression of genetic codes that coordinate all cellular processes and ultimately determine the phenotype of an individual is tightly regulated in time and space at the transcriptional, posttranscriptional, and posttranslational levels. Genetic variations that affect the function of genes at any level may result in abnormal phenotypes, often leading to diseases. Understanding how the spectrum of genetic variations in the placenta affects phenotype in interaction with the environment is important, as it may allow predictive modeling of phenotypic outcomes based on individual genomes. Recent advances in microarray technology have allowed biologists and clinical scientists to perform genomic studies, which are hypothesis generating rather than hypothesis testing. However, large amount of data are generated in such experiments, making them complex to analyze and draw appropriate conclusions. Use of suitable biological samples based on the study objectives is therefore crucial. A genomic approach to investigation can be applied to study pathophysiological processes, understand the etiology of diseases, and identify screening, diagnostic, and prognostic markers. In recent years, genomic research in obstetrics has focused mainly on using the technology to develop placental biomarkers of pregnancy complications.

24.2   GENE EXPRESSION

The human genome, i.e., the complete DNA sequence containing all genetic information, is grossly estimated to contain 30,000 genes. Gene expression is the process by which a gene's coded information is converted into the structures present and operating in the cell, which ultimately define the phenotype of a cell or an organism. Expressed genes include those that are transcribed into mRNA and then translated into protein and those that are transcribed into RNA but not translated into protein (e.g., transfer, ribosomal, micro, small interfering RNAs). In fact, protein-coding genes comprise only about 2% of the human genome; the remainder consists of noncoding intergenic regions that provide chromosomal structural integrity and regulate where, when, and in what quantity proteins are produced. Indeed, the estimated number of human gene products is in the range of 1 million. In other words, gene expression is a complex process that "brings genes to life." It is carefully regulated in time and space, depending on the cell's developmental stage or function, and determines the cell's response to external stimuli. For a comprehensive overview on the issues regarding gene expression, we recommend reading *Molecular Biology, Principles of Genome Function, Second Edition*, by Craig N. et al., Oxford University Press, 2014.

It is believed that RNA molecules in modern organisms play a central role in RNA processing, protein synthesis, and regulation of gene expression. Transcription is the key step in gene expression and is carefully regulated in all cells. There are several methods to investigate the expression of an individual gene, a set of specific genes, or the entire population of mRNAs in a given tissue at a given time or condition. Most of the methodologies rely on hybridization techniques to specific probes. Northern blot analysis and quantitative reverse transcription polymerase chain reaction are used to investigate the expression of selected genes, while DNA microarray technology is used to investigate genome-wide expression profiles. The founding report on microarray technique was based on the genome of the flowering plant *Arabidopsis thaliana* containing the smallest genome of any higher eukaryote examined to date (Schena et al. 1995). It was a pioneering study demonstrating a novel high-capacity system that could monitor the expression of 45 genes in parallel. Later, the Human Genome Project was established as an international effort with the aim to identify the chromosomal position and genomic organization of all human genes (IHGSC 2004). A microarray is a small (approximately 1.3 × 1.3 cm) glass, silicon slide, or chip upon the surface of which a large number of known human genes (usually from 500 to 35,000) are fixed in defined positions in a matrix-fashion. There are two types of microarrays: (i) cDNA microarrays, where individual DNA sequences are spotted on the array and (ii) oligonucleotide arrays, where oligonucleotide chains (usually 70-mers) are built on the array. The potential of microarray studies is to analyze the expression state (i.e., transcript abundance) of each gene of the whole genome in a single experiment. Yet, it is impossible to quantify the absolute expression level of a gene in units. It is thus necessary to perform comparative studies, for example, normal versus diseased tissue samples, to obtain the relative gene expression profile of a given sample. Taking these facts in account, for the purpose of this chapter, we are going to selectively review the existing literature regarding differential gene expression profiles between normal and compromised human placentas.

24.3 DIFFERENTIAL PLACENTAL GENE EXPRESSION IN NORMAL PREGNANCY

24.3.1 EFFECT OF GESTATIONAL AGE

Human placentation is a process of continuous evolution of the fetal–placental and maternal interface during pregnancy, aiming to satisfy the changing needs of the fetus in the adapting maternal environment. Therefore, it is natural to hypothesize that gene expression profile of the placenta changes throughout gestation. Investigation of the molecular evolution of the human placenta is difficult owing to ethical and methodological constrains. A time course microarray analysis of murine placentas showed a gene switch in midtrimester by the same cellular populations without any major morphological changes (Knox and Baker 2008). Some efforts have been made to investigate differential gene expression in pregnancy in human placentas. The transcription profile of villous tissues obtained from first-, second-, and third-trimester normal placentas showed activation of genes related to cell cycle, DNA, amino acid, and carbohydrate metabolism during the first trimester, suggesting significant proliferative activity during that period (Mikheev et al. 2008). On the contrary, genes related to signal transduction and cell communication were underexpressed in first-trimester versus term placentas. Similar results were found when basal plate specimens of placentas obtained during midgestation and term pregnancies, indicating dramatic changes also in the maternal–fetal interface (Winn et al. 2007). We performed a similar study on villous tissues, showing that there are profound differences in global gene expression profile between first- and third-trimester placentas, reflecting the temporal changes in placental structure and function (Sitras et al. 2012).

24.3.2 PLACENTAL SAMPLING SITE

The human placenta is composed of numerous and diverse cellular populations of maternal and fetal origin. The majority of the studies investigating placental gene expression profiles are based on biopsies including several cell types. It has been shown that global gene expression profile varies within the normal placenta, depending on the sample site (Sood et al. 2006). It appears that hypoxia-related genes are up-regulated in sites distant to the umbilical cord insertion and toward the basal and chorionic plates, reflecting reduced blood perfusion in these sites. In fact, increased villous maturation, syncytial knots, and fibrin deposition, which are all histological features of reduced perfusion, are shown to be more frequent in the subchorionic lateral border of the placenta and correlate with increased hypoxia-related transcripts (Wyatt et al. 2005).

24.3.3 MODE OF DELIVERY

In general, complex interactions between fetal, placental, and maternal factors are thought to trigger labor at term gestation. A disturbance in the finely tuned interplay of these factors might be responsible for preterm labor. The role of the placenta in human parturition is not completely clarified.

We found that global placental gene expression profile is not significantly altered by normal labor near term, indicating that the placenta plays an intermediary role in the communication between mother and fetus (Sitras et al. 2008). On the contrary, several other genomic studies have indicated that genes involved in prostaglandin synthesis and inflammatory response are differentially expressed in the myometrium, cervix, and chorio-amniotic membranes in laboring compared with nonlaboring women (Romero et al. 2006). These findings are supported by another study showing that genes involved in oxidative stress, inflammation, and angiogenic factors were up-regulated in women undergoing prolonged labor, probably because of hypoxia re-perfusion events during uterine contractions (Cindrova-Davies et al. 2007). The role of matrix metalloproteinase has also been advocated in the initiation of parturition in a microarray study comparing placentas from laboring and from nonlaboring women (Vu et al. 2008).

24.3.4 Environmental Factors

The fetoplacental unit develops within the uterine milieu, which in turn is influenced by the environment the mother lives in. For example, placentas obtained from women living at high altitudes show histopathological features of hypoxia, such as increased villous vascularization, thinning of the villous membranes, proliferation of the villous cytotrophoblast, and reduced perisyncytial fibrin deposition (Zamudio 2003). It fact, it is shown that the gene expression profile of placentas obtained from high-altitude pregnancies is similar to that of trophoblast explants cultured in low-oxygen tension and of preeclamptic placentas (Soleymanlou et al. 2005). Low birth weight and impaired placental development are also associated with maternal smoking. Several transcriptomic studies showed increased levels of genes encoding for xenobiotic- and steroid-metabolizing enzymes in placentas obtained from women smoking during pregnancy (Bruchova et al. 2010; Huuskonen et al. 2008; Sitras et al. 2012). Similarly, maternal alcohol consumption is shown to effect placental gene expression in rats, involving genes associated with central nervous system development, organ morphogenesis, placental endocrine function, and immunological response (Rosenberg et al. 2010). Maternal diet is another determining factor of placental development and fetal well-being. The availability of nutrients from the mother to the fetus, across the placenta, can cause a wide range of conditions, from intrauterine growth restriction (IUGR) to macrosomia. Again, most of the studies investigating the effect of maternal diet on placental gene expression are performed on animals (Brett et al. 2014). A human transcriptomic study showed that maternal choline intake influenced a wide range of placental genes, including genes associated with angiogenesis (Jiang et al. 2013).

24.4 PATHOLOGICAL PREGNANCY

24.4.1 Preeclampsia

Preeclampsia is a pregnancy-specific disorder characterized by hypertension and proteinuria after 20 weeks' gestation in a previously normotensive woman. Definitive resolution of the symptoms occurs only after delivery of the placenta. Therefore, it is believed that the placenta plays a crucial role in the pathophysiology of preeclampsia. The possibility to study differential gene expression between healthy and preeclamptic placentas has been advocated in the early 2000s (Bilban et al. 2000). Several studies have been published since, and the results are summarized in a narrative review (Louwen et al. 2012) and a meta-analysis (Kleinrouweler et al. 2013). In general, these studies show several genes involved in angiogenesis, immune response, apoptosis, and metabolism to be deregulated in preeclamptic placentas. In particular, genes like fms-like tyrosine kinase 1 (FLT1), endoglin, vascular endothelial growth factor with its receptors, and placental growth factor (PlGF) are consistently deregulated in the majority of the studies. This is not surprising if one considers the fact that the placenta is a highly vascularized organ, with the main function to mediate oxygen and nutrients from the mother to the demanding fetus. Many of these gene products are found in the maternal circulation and might be used to identify women that are destined to develop pre-eclampsia. For example, it has been shown that circulating levels of sFLT1 are increased (Maynard et al. 2003) and of PlGF are decreased (Levine et al. 2006) in the serum of women with preeclampsia compared with controls. Furthermore, microarray studies have shown the importance of genes involved in immune response and defense to be involved in the pathogenesis of preeclampsia. This is also a somewhat expected phenomenon, since the placenta is the physiological link between the immune system of the mother and the fetal semiallograft. Immunity-related genes that are shown to be differentially expressed between preeclamptic and healthy placentas are sialic acid binding Ig-like lectin 6, sialic acid acetyl esterase, ST6 beta-galactosamide alpha-2,6-sialytransferase1, and Epstein–Barr virus induced gene 3. Apoptosis, cell survival, and differentiation related genes are also shown to be altered in preeclampsia, underlying the degenerative events occurring in the developing placenta, which might lead to placental insufficiency and fetal growth restriction. Finally, a gene that is consistently reported as highly up-regulated in preeclamptic placentas and its gene product increased in the serum of preeclamptic mothers is leptin (LEP). LEP has multiple metabolic, inflammatory, and angiogenic effects (Park and Ahima 2014) that could explain its importance in the pathophysiology of preeclampsia.

However, the majority of these studies were performed during the third trimester of pregnancy. Early-onset preeclampsia (i.e., manifesting before 34 weeks of gestation) has more deleterious effects especially for the fetus, owing to prematurity and higher rates of IUGR. Therefore, its prediction would have a larger clinical impact as appropriate strategies for prevention, monitoring, and treatment could be timely employed. Interestingly, so far, only two microarray studies have performed subgroup analysis between early- and late-onset preeclampsia (Junus et al. 2012; Sitras et al. 2009) and one study investigated the gene expression profile of first-trimester placentas in women who later developed preeclampsia (Founds et al. 2009). These studies have shown that early- and late-onset preeclampsia might have a different pathophysiology with inflammation, immune response, and cell motility mainly involved in early-stage disease. Similarly, severity of the disease also appears to have an effect, as placental genes are shown to be differentially up- or down-regulated in moderate and severe preeclampsia compared with controls (Trifonova et al. 2014). However, hemolysis, elevated liver enzymes, and low platelet syndrome appears to have an overlapping placental gene expression profile as that of early-onset preeclampsia, indicating a common pathophysiology (Várkonyi et al. 2011). Ethnicity also seems to affect the differences in placental gene expression profile observed in preeclampsia compared with normal pregnancy, as different genes have been shown to be up- or down-regulated in preeclampsia depending on the populations studied.

Recently, a bioinformatic analysis of seven microarray data sets across multiple platforms revealed three subsets of preeclampsia based on gene expression profiles (Leavey et al. 2015). Whether classification of preeclampsia based on molecular/genomic diversity could yield more robust stratification leading to better management and improved outcomes remains to be seen.

24.4.2 Intrauterine Growth Restriction

IUGR may be caused by several factors but is generally associated with placental dysfunction. Genetic component in the etiology of IUGR caused by placental insufficiency may be significant. Placental gene expression profile in IUGR was found to be quite similar to that of early-onset preeclampsia, with up-regulation of genes involved in inflammatory pathways, and only a few genes were differentially expressed between placentas obtained from IUGR pregnancies with and without preeclampsia (Sitras et al. 2009). Up-regulation of imprinted genes, such as CDKN1C, H19, IGF2, KCNQ1, and PHLDA2, in IUGR placentas has also been reported (Cordeiro et al. 2014). Altered expression of genes involved in steroid metabolism (Sitras et al. 2009), mitochondrial function, and oxidative phosphorylation (Madeleneau et al. 2015) has been reported. LEP, insulin-like growth factor binding protein 1, and retinol binding protein 4 genes are among the most induced (Madeleneau et al. 2015) that may have a clear role in the pathophysiology of IUGR.

24.4.3 GESTATIONAL DIABETES MELLITUS

Maternal gestational diabetes mellitus (GDM) is another gestational disorder that is associated with increased perinatal morbidity and mortality mainly because of complications related to macrosomia. Placental size is also large in GDM pregnancies. The prevalence of GDM is on the rise, and obese women are more at risk. Universal or risk-factor-based screening of pregnant women for GDM is practiced in most countries. Altered expression of genes related to placental apoptosis and inflammatory response may be a cause of macrosomia in GDM (Magee et al. 2014). Global gene expression profile was studied on placental samples obtained from 19 GDM cases and 21 controls, which showed that 66 genes involved in cell activation, immune response, organ development, and regulation of cell death were differentially expressed (up-regulated) in GDM placentas (Enquobahrie et al. 2009). Moreover, preferential activation of genes involved in placental lipid metabolism has been observed in GDM compared with type I diabetes (Radaelli et al. 2009). The gene expression profile of placenta may be important in determining the incidence and recurrence of GDM.

24.5 CONCLUSION

Placental gene expression studies may help to understand the normal development of pregnancy and the mechanisms involved in the pathophysiology of placenta-specific pregnancy disorders. They may help to generate hypotheses, stratify disease, and identify DNA/RNA-based biomarkers that have direct predictive or diagnostic value. However, several limitations, including diversity of phenotype, challenges related to appropriate selection and description of patient populations of interest, and choosing correct sampling time (gestational age), tissue type, and sample site, are important to take into consideration when designing and conducting such studies. Placental gene expression profile may be used in future to predict individual risk of developing diseases in adulthood, individualize health monitoring programs, and provide appropriate advice on health promoting activities, diet and life style.

REFERENCES

Bilban M, Head S, Desoye G, and Quaranta V. 2000. DNA microarrays: A novel approach to investigate genomics in trophoblast invasion—A review. *Placenta* 21 Suppl A: S99–S105.

Brett KE, Ferraro ZM, Yockell-Lelievre J, Gruslin A, and Adamo KB. 2014. Maternal–fetal nutrient transport in pregnancy pathologies: The role of the placenta. *Int. J. Mol. Sci.* 15 (9): 16153–16185.

Bruchova H, Vasikova A, Merkerova M, Milcova A, Topinka J, Balascak I, Pastorkova A, Sram RJ, and Brdicka R. 2010. Effect of maternal tobacco smoke exposure on the placental transcriptome. *Placenta* 31 (3): 186–191.

Cindrova-Davies T, Yung HW, Johns J, Spasic-Boskovic O, Korolchuk S, Jauniaux E, Burton GJ, and Charnock-Jones DS. 2007. Oxidative stress, gene expression, and protein changes induced in the human placenta during labor. *Am. J. Pathol.* 171 (4): 1168–1179.

Cordeiro A, Neto AP, Carvalho F, Ramalho C, and Dória S. 2014. Relevance of genomic imprinting in intrauterine human growth expression of CDKN1C, H19, IGF2, KCNQ1 and PHLDA2 imprinted genes. *J. Assist. Reprod. Genet.* 31 (10): 1361–1368.

Enquobahrie DA, Williams MA, Qiu C, Meller M, and Sorensen TK. 2009. Global placental gene expression in gestational diabetes mellitus. *Am. J. Obstet. Gynecol.* 200 (2): 206.e1–206.e13.

Founds SA, Conley YP, Lyons-Weiler JF, Jeyabalan A, Hogge WA, and Conrad KP. 2009. Altered global gene expression in first trimester placentas of women destined to develop preeclampsia. *Placenta* 30 (1): 15–24.

Huuskonen P, Storvik M, Reinisalo M, Honkakoski P, Rysa J, Hakkola J, and Pasanen M. 2008. Microarray analysis of the global alterations in the gene expression in the placentas from cigarette-smoking mothers. *Clin. Pharmacol. Ther.* 83 (4): 542–550.

IHGSC. 2004. Finishing the euchromatic sequence of the human genome. *Nature* 431 (7011): 931–945.

Jiang X, Bar HY, Yan J, Jones S, Brannon PM, West AA, Perry CA, Ganti A, Pressman E, Devapatla S, Vermeylen F, Wells MT, and Caudill MA. 2013. A higher maternal choline intake among third-trimester pregnant women lowers placental and circulating concentrations of the antiangiogenic factor fms-like tyrosine kinase-1 (sFLT1). *FASEB J.* 27 (3): 1245–1253.

Junus K, Centlow M, Wikstrom AK, Larsson I, Hansson SR, and Olovsson M. 2012. Gene expression profiling of placentae from women with early- and late-onset pre-eclampsia: Down-regulation of the angiogenenis-related genes ACVRL1and EGFL7 in early-onset disease. *Mol. Hum. Reprod.* 18 (3): 146–155.

Kleinrouweler CE, van UM, Moerland PD, Ris-Stalpers C, van der Post JA, and Afink GB. 2013. Differentially expressed genes in the pre-eclamptic placenta: A systematic review and meta analysis. *PLoS One* 8 (7): e68991.

Knox K and Baker JC. 2008. Genomic evolution of the placenta using co-option and duplication and divergence. *Genome Res.* 18 (5): 695–705.

Leavey K, Bainbridge SA, and Cox BJ. 2015. Large scale aggregate microarray analysis reveals three distinct molecular subclasses of human preeclampsia. *PLoS One* 10 (2): e0116508.

Levine RJ, Lam C, Qian C, Yu KF, Maynard SE, Sachs BP, Sibai BM, Epstein FH, Romero R, Thadhani R, and Karumanchi SA. 2006. Soluble endoglin and other circulating antiangiogenic factors in preeclampsia. *N. Engl. J. Med.* 355 (10): 992–1005.

Louwen F, Muschol-Steinmetz C, Reinhard J, Reitter A, and Yuan J. 2012. A lesson for cancer research: Placental microarray gene analysis in preeclampsia. *Oncotarget* 3 (8): 759–773.

Madeleneau D, Buffat C, Mondon F, Grimault H, Rigourd V, Tsatsaris V, Letourneur F, Vaiman D, Barbaux S, and Gascoin G. 2015. Transcriptomic analysis of human placenta in Intra-Uterine Growth Restriction. *Pediatr. Res.* 77 (6): 799–807.

Magee TR, Ross MG, Wedekind L, Desai M, Kjos S, and Belkacemi L. 2014. Gestational diabetes mellitus alters apoptotic and inflammatory gene expression of trophoblasts from human term placenta. *J. Diabetes Complications* 28 (4): 448–459.

Maynard SE, Min JY, Merchan J, Lim KH, Li J, Mondal S, Libermann TA, Morgan JP, Sellke FW, Stillman IE, Epstein FH, Sukhatme VP, and Karumanchi SA. 2003. Excess placental soluble fms-like tyrosine kinase 1 (sFlt1) may contribute to endothelial dysfunction, hypertension, and proteinuria in preeclampsia. *J. Clin. Invest.* 111 (5): 649–658.

Mikheev AM, Nabekura T, Kaddoumi A, Bammler TK, Govindarajan R, Hebert MF, and Unadkat JD. 2008. Profiling gene expression in human placentae of different gestational ages: An OPRU Network and UW SCOR Study. *Reprod. Sci.* 15 (9): 866–877.

Park HK and Ahima RS. 2014. Leptin signaling. *F1000Prime. Rep.* 6: 73.

Radaelli T, Lepercq J, Varastehpour A, Basu S, Catalano PM, and Hauguel-De Mouzon S. 2009. Differential regulation of genes for fetoplacental lipid pathways in pregnancy with gestational and type 1 diabetes mellitus. *Am. J. Obstet. Gynecol.* 201 (2): 209.e1–209.e10.

Romero R, Espinoza J, Gotsch F, Kusanovic JP, Friel LA, Erez O, Mazaki-Tovi S, Than NG, Hassan S, and Tromp G. 2006. The use of high-dimensional biology (genomics, transcriptomics, proteomics, and metabolomics) to understand the preterm parturition syndrome. *BJOG* 113 Suppl 3: 118–135.

Rosenberg MJ, Wolff CR, El-Emawy A, Staples MC, Perrone-Bizzozero NI, and Savage DD. 2010. Effects of moderate drinking during pregnancy on placental gene expression. *Alcohol* 44 (7–8): 673–690.

Schena M, Shalon D, Davis RW, and Brown PO. 1995. Quantitative monitoring of gene expression patterns with a complementary DNA microarray. *Science* 270 (5235): 467–470.

Sitras V, Paulssen RH, Gronaas H, Vartun A, and Acharya G. 2008. Gene expression profile in labouring and non-labouring human placenta near term. *Mol. Hum. Reprod.* 14 (1): 61–65.

Sitras V, Paulssen RH, Gronaas H, Leirvik J, Hanssen TA, Vartun A, and Acharya G. 2009. Differential placental gene expression in severe preeclampsia. *Placenta* 30 (5): 424–433.

Sitras V, Fenton C, Paulssen R, Vartun A, and Acharya G. 2012. Differences in gene expression between first and third trimester human placenta: A microarray study. *PLoS One* 7 (3): e33294.

Soleymanlou N, Jurisica I, Nevo O, Ietta F, Zhang X, Zamudio S, Post M, and Caniggia I. 2005. Molecular evidence of placental hypoxia in preeclampsia. *J. Clin. Endocrinol. Metab.* 90 (7): 4299–4308.

Sood R, Zehnder JL, Druzin ML, and Brown PO. 2006. Gene expression patterns in human placenta. *Proc. Natl. Acad. Sci. U.S.A.* 103 (14): 5478–5483.

Trifonova EA, Gabidulina TV, Ershov NI, Serebrova VN, Vorozhishcheva AY, and Stepanov VA. 2014. Analysis of the placental tissue transcriptome of normal and preeclampsia complicated pregnancies. *ACTA Naturae* 6 (2): 71–83.

Várkonyi T, Nagy B, Füle T, Tarca AL, Karászi K, Schönléber J, Hupuczi P, Mihalik N, Kovalszky I, Rigó J Jr, Meiri H, Papp Z, Romero R, and Than NG. 2011. Microarray profiling reveals that placental transcriptomes of early-onset HELLP syndrome and preeclampsia are similar. *Placenta* 32 Suppl: S21–S29.

Vu TD, Yun F, Placido J, and Reznik SE. 2008. Placental matrix metalloproteinase-1 expression is increased in labor. *Reprod. Sci.* 15 (4): 420–424.

Winn VD, Haimov-Kochman R, Paquet AC, Yang YJ, Madhusudhan MS, Gormley M, Feng KT, Bernlohr DA, McDonagh S, Pereira L, Sali A, and Fisher SJ. 2007. Gene expression profiling of the human maternal–fetal interface reveals dramatic changes between midgestation and term. *Endocrinology* 148 (3): 1059–1079.

Wyatt SM, Kraus FT, Roh CR, Elchalal U, Nelson DM, and Sadovsky Y. 2005. The correlation between sampling site and gene expression in the term human placenta. *Placenta* 26 (5): 372–379.

Zamudio S. 2003. The placenta at high altitude. *High Alt. Med. Biol.* 4 (2): 171–191.

25 Placental Gene Expression in Pathological Pregnancies

Saumitra Chakravarty

CONTENTS

ABSTRACT

The heterogeneity of placental gene expression profile, both spatially and temporally having potential implications in the development and propagation of different pregnancy-related pathologies, has been reported. In addition, changes in DNA methylation may contribute to the altered expression of genes linked to pathological pregnancies. In fact, epigenetics provides an important gene expression regulatory mechanism in placenta. Therefore, it is reasonable to look for the potential association of placental insufficiency (e.g., preeclampsia and miscarriage) with the genes regulating those processes. Placental immunology may be considered herewith while discussing the genetic background of the disorders of placental insufficiency. Application of gene expression profiles and knowledge of epigenetic anomalies may become integral parts of diagnostic procedures and assisted reproductive technologies in the near future. This chapter deals only with placental gene expression in pathological pregnancies.

KEY WORDS

Preeclampsia, miscarriage, intrauterine growth restriction, placental insufficiency, hypoxia, stress, gene expression, epigenetics, microRNA, nutrition, immunology, assisted reproductive technologies.

25.1 INTRODUCTION

Normal fetal growth is determined by genetically predetermined growth potential and is further modulated by maternal, fetal, placental, dietary, and environmental factors. The placenta provides critical transport functions between the maternal and fetal circulations during intrauterine development. Formation of this interface is controlled by several growth factors, cytokines, and transcription factors. Identification of genes differentially expressed in placenta in healthy and pathologic pregnancies is therefore essential to understand the molecular mechanisms involved in the etiology of pathological pregnancies. Changes in DNA methylation may contribute to the altered expression of genes linked to pathological pregnancies and exclude this mechanism as an important regulatory factor in other related pregnancy complications. In addition, we highlight previously uncharacterized genes involved in placental steroidogenesis as differentially methylated in preeclampsia. Additional functional characterization of these genes is required to further assess the relationship between DNA methylation and gene expression in the human placenta and will form the basis of future experiments. Unraveling which genetic pathways are susceptible to epigenetic modification in the placenta may provide a clearer etiological perspective in disease cases and basis for targeted intervention. Epigenetics is defined as the study of heritable chemical modification of DNA or chromatin that does not alter the DNA sequence itself (Kumar et al. 2010, p. 180). The study of epigenetics provides us with testable mechanisms for the evidence of environmental influence on heritable factors, i.e., genes. Just as adding methyl group to (or removing it from) DNA nucleotides may alter gene expression, modifying the other principal structural component of the chromosome, i.e., histone, by adding or removing different chemical groups, i.e., acetyl, phosphate, methyl, adenosine diphosphate (ADP) ribosyl, ubiquitin, etc., also plays regulatory roles over the expression of genes. Some authors even speculate that there might exist a "histone code": similar to the triplets of nucleotides corresponding to a particular amino acid (or stop codon), binding of specific chemical groups at specific amino acid residues of specific histone proteins in certain specific combinations (or alone) could actually code for on/off switches of specific genes, although the code itself, if it exists at all, is yet to be found. Besides the three classic types of RNAs (messenger, transfer, and ribosomal), there are other types of noncoding RNAs (microRNA, small nuclear RNA, etc.), grouped together as "interference RNA," which have recently been attributed regulatory role in gene expression, hence the name of the group because they mostly "interfere" with mRNAs to suppress their translation into proteins. Certain information regarding the density of chromatin (heterochromatin vs. euchromatin) and relative intranuclear position (3D coordinate) may also regulate gene expression. The mechanisms described above involving non-DNA regulation on DNA are among the current arsenals of epigenetics. There are evidences that these epigenetic tags or marks can be modified (epimutation) by environmental factors (Chason et al. 2011; Lee and Ding 2012). Epigenetic tags are shown to be heritable as well (Hughes 2014), exerting their effects over more than one generation (Jimenez-Chillaron et al. 2009). When the inheritance of epigenetic tags is parent specific, resulting in monoallelic expression of a gene in the offspring, it is known as "imprinting." Now, if environment can influence genes via epigenetic marks and those marks can be inherited, it may be argued reasonably that "acquired" traits could transmit across generations, just like its "genetic" counterpart. Such argument blurs the distinction between the two seemingly mutually exclusive classes of traits and also brings about potential resurrection of Lamarckism (or at least some form of it). But it must be noted that, because genomic imprinting is wiped out at least twice during a complete mammalian life cycle, and because of some other observed facts pointing to gaps in the current mechanistic models of epigenetics, recently, some authors are beginning to doubt the extent of trans-generational inheritance of epigenetic tags in humans (Heard and Martienssen 2014).

25.2 PLACENTAL GENE EXPRESSION

To date, there are at least 720 genes identified as having "statistically significant" differences in expression between embryo and placenta, and among them, at least 300 genes are more strongly expressed in the placenta (Winstead 2000). Interestingly, the number of unique, truly placenta-specific genes that have been discovered to date is very small (Rawn and Cross 2008). According to Cross, Werb, and Fisher (1994), the number is merely 30, although Tanaka et al. (2000) has proposed another 259 potential candidates in mouse placenta. Placenta-specific genes like *Gcml*, *Mash2*, and *Peg10* play important roles in the development and maintenance of placental morphology and function (Cross et al. 2003). But that does not mean that genes not expressed exclusively in placenta have any less importance. For instance, fibroblast growth factor (FGF) has been found essential in controlling the growth of placental precursors (Rappolee 1999), and several members of the epidermal growth factor (EFG) ligand and receptor families are implicated in genetic regulation during the peri-implantation period as a prelude to placentation (Cross et al. 2003). Certain genes may be expressed differentially in the placenta when there are some associated disorders. For instance, the serum ADAM12 level (mainly secreted form) of pre-eclamptic mothers have been found to be reduced (Laigaard et al. 2005), while placental expression of *Adam12* (determined by mRNA assay) increases significantly in preeclampsia (Enquobahrie et al. 2012) compared with normotensive controls. One must be careful during sampling placental tissue to measure gene expression levels because sampling from an inadequate number of sites from a single placenta has been attributed as a possible cause of the observed lack of reproducibility of several gene expression studies. For example, Surmon et al. (2014) has found that, to obtain representative sample for *Flt1* expression, sampling has to be done from at least 10 and 11 sites, respectively, in case of normal and preeclamptic placentae. Some peculiarities regarding gene expression do not seem to be conserved when one tries to extrapolate findings from mouse study to predict and compare with its human analogue. For example, murine *Igf2* gene is found to possess a unique promoter sequence available only in the placenta, designated as P0, and at least three other promoter sequences of the same gene designated as P1–P3 were found both in placenta and fetus. It turned out that knocking out P0 (and not the other three) from mouse placenta results in deleterious effects almost similar in extent and magnitude as knocking out the whole of the *Igf2* gene, highlighting the crucial role of *Igf2P0* transcript (Reik et al. 2003). But that is not the case for humans (Frost and Moore 2010). However, altered expression of *Igf2* does have dire consequences in humans as well (discussed later), although it seems to have no placenta-specific transcript in particular. We must be cautious about the existence of human-placenta-specific epipolymorphisms associated placental pathologies (e.g., association of *Tusc3* promoter methylation with preeclampsia), for which primary data from other species would be of little help (Yuen et al. 2010). For comprehensive meta-analysis of differentially expressed placental genes in preeclampsia, the reader may refer to Kleinrouweler et al. (2013).

25.3 EVOLUTIONARY TUG OF WAR BETWEEN MATERNAL AND PATERNAL GENES IN THE PLACENTA

This section highlights an epigenetic mechanism known as imprinting, where certain genes in an offspring express monoallelically in a consistent parent-of-origin manner (Chason et al. 2011). A classic example of this is illustrated by a pair of syndromes: Prader–Willi syndrome (PWS) and Angelman syndrome (AS). Both result from the deletion or mutation of the 15q12 region, the only difference being which chromosome is affected: if paternal, then PWS occurs, and if maternal, then AS, because normally, the genes required to avoid PWS are active only in paternally derived chromosome and silenced by imprinting in maternally derived one, and vice versa in case of AS (Kumar et al. 2010, p. 172). Probably, the most popular notion explaining the evolutionary origins of imprinting is the conflict hypothesis, which postulates that paternal genes increase their fitness by directing more resources to the developing fetus, and on the other hand, maternal genes increase their fitness by restricting resource allocation to the fetus and thus preserving the precious resources for future reproductions (Diplas et al. 2009; Frost and Moore 2010). Although this hypothesis was first conceived to explain imprinting in eutherian placental mammals and marsupials, later, it was extrapolated to include plants and insects. Whatever might be the case, this hypothesis is supported by findings such as the association of disorders presented as increased birth weight (i.e., Beckwith-Wiedemann syndrome [BWS] and transient neonatal diabetes mellitus [TNDM]) with loss of maternally expressed imprinted genes (i.e., *H19* and *Phlda2*) as well as biallelic expression of imprinted genes (i.e., *Igf2*) normally expressed in paternal chromosome only and/or the associa-tion of disorders presented as decreased birth weight (i.e., Silver-Russel syndrome [SRS], subsets of intrauterine growth restriction [IUGR]) with loss of paternally expressed imprinted genes (i.e., *Igf2* and *Plagl1*) as well as biallelic expression of imprinted genes (i.e., *H19*) normally expressed in maternal chromosome only (Frost and Moore 2010). Paternally expressed imprinted genes may also exert their growth-enhancing effects on the fetus by promoting the growth of extraembryonic tissues and placenta, besides directly stimulating fetal growth, which is demonstrated by aberrant and excessive growth of trophoblastic tissues in case of complete hydatidiform mole resulting from paternal uniparental disomy (Wen and den Veyver 2011, p. 92), and another contrasting example could be the insufficient or "shallow" trophoblastic invasion in case of preeclampsia, where mater-nally expressed imprinted genes are overexpressed (Oudejans et al. 2004). Chason et al. (2011) describes two main purposes served by imprinting in development: to activate or deactivate the *right* gene at *right* place at *right* time and to ensure the *right* dosage of gene expression. Given the usefulness of imprinting from genetic to population levels of organization, one might expect a lot many genes to be imprinted. But surprisingly, only about 90 genes in mouse and less so in humans have been found imprinted to date and most imprinted genes are expressed in placenta (Wen and den Veyver 2011, p. 87). This lack of imprinted human genes means that imprinting is relatively incompletely conserved in humans from an evolutionary point of view. For instance, although the murine or bovine genes coding Igf2 and its receptor Igf2r are both imprinted and expressed in paternal and maternal chromosomes, respectively, illustrating the "most convincing" example of evolutionary tug of war between mother and father, the imprinting of *Igf2r* is not found in humans. Incomplete conservation of imprinting means not only fewer genes to be imprinted but also less tis-sue specificity or restriction for the expression of imprinted genes. For example, unlike in mice, the expression of human ortholog of murine *Igf2P0* transcript is not restricted to the placenta, although in both the species, the transcripts are imprinted and paternally expressed. Morison, Ramsay, and Spencer (2005) have catalogued many examples of incomplete conservation of imprinted genes in humans compared with mouse. The probable cause behind the observed lack of phylogenetic con-servation of imprinting in humans might include neotenic as well as singleton pregnancies where a smaller pelvis is associated with the evolution on bipedalism, resulting in a smaller newborn requir-ing less maternal resources in the first place (Diplas et al. 2009; Frost and Moore 2010). This could also explain the predominance of maternally expressed (and paternally silenced) imprinting pattern in humans, consistent with the resource-restricting role of maternal genes predicted by the conflict hypothesis. However, as with most generalizations of biological sciences, the conflict hypothesis has its pitfalls, too. For instance, imprinting defects not only cause perturbations of placental devel-opment or birth weight but also result in neurological deficits (i.e., PWS and AS) and condition pertaining to the lack of expression of imprinted paternal gene with the unrestricted expression of imprinted maternal gene has also been associated with "big baby" (i.e., PWS), although the opposite was to be expected. Likewise, certain subsets of IUGR have been associated with upregulation of imprinted genes (i.e., *Nnat* and *Peg10*) expressed paternally, which seems paradoxical in the light of conflict hypothesis. These discrepancies have led to extensions of the conflict hypothesis (Haig and Wharton 2003) or some alternate hypotheses (Wolf and Hager 2006). Even those are not without some degree of inconsistencies, although those competing hypotheses are nevertheless useful for explaining the evolutionary origins of imprinting of at least some loci (Spencer and Clark 2014).

25.4   GENES INVOLVED IN PLACENTATION

Placentation is a multistep process and requires complex interactions among many events at the cellu-lar, molecular, genetic, and epigenetic levels of organization. It has been observed that blastocyst wan-ders away from its original implantation site before and during the course of placental development, suggesting that placenta tends to develop toward the direction of better blood supply, analogous to the tendency of plants to grow toward light. This concept is known as dynamic placentation and may help explain many phenomena, including trophotropism, the apparent migration of normal placenta from the lower to the upper uterine segment as pregnancy progresses. Because placental size and shape are ultimately determined by its vascular growth patterns, it is reasonable to assume that there are correlations between placental morphology and the conditions arising from derangement of placental vascularization. A computer-generated model that simulates vascular endothelial growth factor (VEGF)-A/VEGFR2-mediated signaling of placental vascular growth gives three distinct types of placental shapes (round, multilobed, and star shaped) as outputs, depending on when (early or late) the rate of branching is reduced and how responsive the vascular tips are to follow growth stimuli in course of placentation, consistent with the corresponding real-life observations of placental insufficiency being associated with malformed placentae resulting from abnormal vasculogenic as well as angiogenic signaling (Yampolsky et al. 2008). Regulators of *Vegf* expression in placenta are of particular interest when we consider the pathophysiology of preeclampsia. *In vitro* experiments with *Sema3b*, a gene that is found excessively expressed in preeclamptic placenta, suggest that some hitherto unknown *in vivo* factors might dysregulate cytotrophoblast differentiation, crippling its ability to invade the decidua by down-regulating VEGF signaling through the phophatidyl-inositol-3-kinase (PI3K) serine/threonine-specific protein kinase (AKT) and glycogen synthase kinase-3 (GSK3) pathways, culminating into preeclampsia (Zhou et al. 2013). In a related note, placental expression of *Sema4d* and its receptors, along with *Ptprc*, is found dysregulated in miscarriage, especially around the 10th week of gestation, when progesterone production switches from the corpus luteum to the placenta (Lorenzi et al. 2012). Similar trophoblastic invasion-inhibitory effect as *Sema3b* is seen in case of *Kiss1*, a highly expressed gene in preeclamptic placenta (especially early-onset type), which is also associated with reduced matrix metalloproteinase (MMP) activity (especially of MMP-2 and -9), restricting the extent of placentation (Zhang et al. 2011). Interestingly, GPR54, a G-protein-coupled receptor implicated in the development of sexual behavior and genitalia, happens to maintain a stable level in fetus and placenta regardless of the expression of placental *Kiss1*, although one of its products, metastin, is a ligand for GPR54 (Qiao et al. 2012). Prolonged hypoxic milieu as in preeclamptic placenta might diminish VEGF itself, perpetuating a vicious positive feedback loop of placentation defect, exemplified by the findings that the expression of *Dusp9*, a gene essential for placental function, but maybe not so important for normal embryonic development (Christie et al. 2005) and is increased in placenta exposed to prolonged hypoxic stress and therefore down-regulates *Vegf* probably through some non-extracellular signal regulated kinase (ERK) signaling pathways that are yet to be revealed (Czikk et al. 2013), thus setting the stage for severe preeclampsia. Such disruptions in placentation may also have epigenetic entailment exemplified by observations like the blockade of expression of VEGF-B, another proangiogenic factor, by miR-182*, which is expressed in excess in preeclamptic placenta (Yang et al. 2005). Epidemiological data showed that miR-195, a microRNA with hitherto unknown function, is elevated in preeclamptic placenta. Then, bioinformatic searching algorithms identified its potential target, *Acvr2a*, a gene that is expressed excessively in preeclamptic placenta, and driven by this result, several "wet-lab" techniques confirmed that *Acvr2a* is indeed a direct target of miR-195, followed by the finding that *Acvr2a* acts to inhibit trophoblastic invasion through Activin/Nodal signaling, thus interfering with the dynamics of normal placentation. Therefore, it may be inferred that *Acvr2a* probably serves some sort of physiological purpose by preventing the cells to become invasive (e.g., as in malignancies), but this inhibitory function is normally suppressed in placental trophoblasts by miR-195 through the repression of *Acvr2a* so that those cells can invade, properly ensuring adequate placentation. A decrease in placental miR-195 removes epigenetic repression of *Acvr2a* expression, therefore leading to inadequate placentation and its dire sequels like preeclampsia (Bai et al. 2012).

25.5 PLACENTAL GENES REGULATING ITS NUTRIENT TRANSPORT

In Section 25.2, we have seen that placental genes are differentially imprinted compared with the fetus. Now, we will try to see how that affects nutrient transport through placenta as well as fetal growth. Just like the evolutionary tug of war between maternally and paternally imprinted genes suggested by the conflict hypothesis, there is another tug of war between imprinted genes in the placenta and fetal compartment. The former seems to be in control of supply, while the latter controls the demand of nutrients (Reik et al. 2003). For example, the observation that IGF2 is found to have different and distinctive classes of receptors in the placenta (insulin-like growth factor 1 receptor [IGF-IR] and insulin receptor [INS-R]) compared with that of the fetus (Efstratiadis 1998), combined with another observation that chimeric murine conceptus with Igf2 levels normal in placenta but decreased in fetal compartment are found to develop small placentae (Gardner et al. 1999), might suggest that Igf2 is growth promoting for the placenta, underscoring the supply-enhancing role of *Igf2*, which is known to be imprinted in placenta. This inference is further strengthened by the observations where overexpressions of *Igf2* are associated with abnormally large placentae (Eggenschwiler et al. 1997). Interestingly, if imprinted paternally expressed gene *Igf2* is knocked out specifically in the placenta, another imprinted paternally expressed gene, *Ata3*, comes to the rescue, which encodes a component of the system A amino acid transport system (Mizunoa et al. 2002) in the fetus (and also in placenta), but even its up-regulation may not ultimately compensate for fetal growth restriction resulting from the placental loss of *Igf2*, although the compensation seems to be effective until late gestation (Constância et al. 2002). This result may be interpreted as a compensatory increase in fetal demand (and also some increase in placental supply) in response to a decrease in placental supply, leading to a supply–demand mismatch and, ultimately, a failed or decompensated response aimed toward acquiring normal fetal growth. The above speculation is supported by the finding that mice lacking *Igf2* in both the placenta and fetus has no such compensatory placental increase in amino acid transport at all even in early gestation because they have not only less supply (placental *Igf2* knockout) but also less demand (fetal *Igf2* knockout) of nutrient in the first place (Reik et al. 2003). Another instance of supply–demand linkage may be inferred from the finding that the expression of *Htra1*, a gene that encodes a serine protease that may increase the availability of IGF2 by cleaving it from its binding protein as well as remodel placenta along with its vasculature, is significantly elevated in preeclamptic placentae compared with normotensive controls (Enquobahrie et al. 2012), which might be due to a feedback response secondary to supply–demand mismatch of placental insufficiency, albeit the confirmation of such claims needs to be verified by further research. Placental transport of nutrient molecules not requiring direct involvement of transporters or channel proteins might also fit in this supply–demand model (Constância et al. 2002). Some findings seemingly paradoxical in the light of conflict hypothesis may be explained efficiently by this model. For example, maternally expressed murine imprinted gene *Ipl* knockouts are expected to have larger fetus, but in reality, they produce larger placentae with normal-sized fetus (Frank et al. 2002), although it is consistent with the interpretation that knocking out a maternally expressed imprinted placental gene from the placenta increases the nutrient supply (thus placentomegaly) without any corresponding increase in fetal demand for nutrient, resulting in a normal-sized fetus (Reik et al. 2003). Therefore, the supply–demand model of imprinted genes can be regarded as an extended alternative to the conflict hypothesis. Keeping in mind the fetal–placental supply–demand relationship on the background of epigenetics, it is intriguing to stumble upon new causal relations between previously known causes and effects. For instance, because mammalian one-carbon metabolism pathways are sole contributors of methyl groups for almost all methylation reactions known to date, a deficiency of methyl donors and cofactors (e.g., folate) in maternal diet may be interpreted by placental epigenetic machinery as decreased supply of methyl group relative to fetal demand. This lack of supply signal may be responsible for the observed down-regulation of one-carbon pathway genes (e.g., *Dnmt1*) leading to a lack of global DNA methylation (Lillycropa et al. 2007) in the placenta, which would normally commence in mammals during the preimplantation period to reestablish appropriate epigenetic tags and imprinting (Chason et al. 2011). Despite the doubtful role of human *Dnmt1* silencing in global hypomethylation (Novakovic and Saffery 2013), such genome-wide disruption of methylation is quite likely to ramify toward several pathologies; e.g., hypomethylation of *Cullins* genes may lead to inadequate placental vascular differentiation, remodeling, and shallow invasion, thus increasing the susceptibility to develop preeclampsia, and *Mthfr* mutation (e.g., 677C/T) in either the mother or the father is associated with suboptimal DNA methylation as well as higher miscarriage rates (Gascoin-Lachambre et al. 2010). In a related note, the same mutation, along with few others, including *Fvl* 1691G/A (Leiden mutation) and *F2* 20210G/A mutation, is found associated with miscarriages related to antiphospholoipid antibody syndrome, a condition where autoantibodies against different phospholipids (especially membrane components like phosphatidylinositol and phosphatidylserine) play key role in its pathogenesis. Such placentation defects may be accentuated by promoter hypomethylation of cytochrome P450 encoding genes (e.g., *Cyp1A1*), which elevates reactive oxygen species (ROS) levels especially if the mother is smoking (Huuskonen et al. 2008). Additionally, dietary lack of folate, vitamin B_{12}, and ω-3 fatty acids in pregnant women has been linked to homocysteinemia, resulting in an increased susceptibility of placental abruption and spontaneous abortion (Dasarathy et al. 2010). Moreover, associations have been found between the lack of global DNA methylation in the placenta and inadequate and abnormal vascularization of the placenta and fetal organs (Rexhaj et al. 2011), superadded by the direct effects of maternal micronutrient deficiency, contributing to induce fetal neurodevelopmental anomalies, e.g., neural tube defect. These observations are consistent with the Barker hypothesis of developmental origins of health and disease (Barker 2004), underscoring the importance and far-reaching epigenetic effects of derangements in placental nutrient handling programs. Odent (2014) argued that because of the association of preeclampsia with both increased and decreased birth weight, the disease process is to be seen from a whole new perspective where placental insufficiency may result from a conflict between mother and fetus for their competing demands and contradictory priorities, which is best demonstrated from a nutritional point of view. He proposed that in the face of a fierce competition for docosahexaenoic acid (DHA) between the fetus and the mother for the purpose of brain development and maintenance of eicosanoids level (especially PGI_2), respectively, necessary for placental sufficiency, the fetal brain wins most of the resources, leaving the mother susceptible to preeclampsia, which accounts for normal or elevated serum DHA level along with a steep decrease in its precursor eicosapentaenoic acid in preeclamptic mothers and preeclampsia risk reduction associated with nutritional supplements (e.g., ω-3 fatty acids such as DHA) that boost up maternal DHA repertoire. The genetic (or epigenetic) basis of such conflict hypotheses is not well understood; nevertheless, these are consistent with many other observations as well as the evolutionary theory. In a similar note, dehydroepiandrosterone (DHEA) supplementation seems to improve pregnancy outcomes in women having recurrent miscarriage (Gleicher et al. 2009) despite the findings that many women with recurrent spontaneous abortion (RSA) have elevated levels of DHEA sulfate (Gürbüz et al. 2003) and supposed oxidative, antiprogesterone, and/or implantation-inhibitory roles of DHEA in mice probably because of its ability to down-regulate *Pibf1* expression, up-regulate *Cox2* expression, elevate interleukin (IL) 2 level, and diminish IL6 level (Sander et al. 2005).

25.6 PLACENTAL INSUFFICIENCY: GENES INVOLVED

Simply put, placental insufficiency means any inadequacy of placental supply relative to fetal demand leading to clinically recognizable patterns of abnormalities. Although it may result from both decreased supply capacity of the placenta or increased demand of the fetus, we confined the discussion in this section primarily to the scenarios resulting from placental factors only. Shallow trophoblastic invasion and relatively hypoxic intrauterine environment are regarded as important causes of placental insufficiency (Figure 25.1) that manifests itself clinically as conditions like preeclampsia and IUGR (Brosens et al. 2011). Epigenetic perturbations seem to be associated with placental insufficiency, especially if the perturbation happens during early gestation. For instance, early intrauterine hypoxia, being a necessary signal for adequate placental trophoblastic invasion, might trigger abnormal stress response in placenta if O_2 level somehow reduces below a certain limit, resulting in hypomethylation of certain genes as well as expression of certain trophoblastic miRNAs, leading to preeclampsia (Mouillet al. 2010). This dose-dependent role of hypoxia as "friend-to-fiend," which is discussed in detail later in this chapter, can be equally applicable to at least few

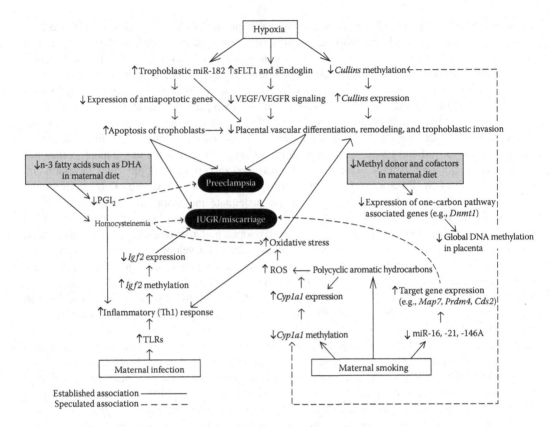

FIGURE 25.1 Simplified representation of the associations between some important environmental factors including maternal diet and disorders of placental insufficiency, acting through epigenetic interface. Note that the factors depicted in the figure are but a small portion of a much bigger and complex picture. DHA, docosahexaenoic acid; IUGR, intrauterine growth restriction; PGI$_2$, prostaglandin I$_2$ or prostacyclin; ROS, reactive oxygen species; TLR, toll-like receptor. (Based on data compiled from Lee, S.-A. and C. Ding, *Epigenomics*, 4, 561–569, 2012; Chason, R.J. et al., *Trends in Endocrinology and Metabolism*, 22, 412–420, 2011; Frost, J.M. and G.E. Moore, *PLoS Genetics*, 6, e1001015, 2010; Hansson, S.R. et al., *Molecular Human Reproduction*, 12, 169–179, 2006; and Reik, W. et al., *The Journal of Physiology*, 547, 35–44, 2003.)

other stresses associated with placentation. Again, there are many microRNAs (e.g., miR-181a, -182, -182*, -210) suspected to interfere epigenetically with normal placentation regardless of hypoxia, thus contributing to the development of preeclampsia and other placental insufficiency disorders as well (Mayor-Lynn et al. 2011). Maternal smoking, another potential risk factor for placental insufficiency (Figure 25.1), probably exerts its effects via down-regulating several microRNAs (e.g., miR-16, -21, and -146a) (Maccania et al. 2010), thus removing the epigenetic barrier for the expression (or overexpression) of their target genes (e.g., *Map7*, *Prdm4*, and *Cds2*), contributing to induce the insufficiency. However, the placenta has been shown to have remarkable resilience to withstand many genetic as well as environmental insults otherwise lethal to the fetus. Even if the conceptus can survive the initial insult or stress and the intrauterine environment is no longer stressful, the epigenetic alterations might still persist and predispose the fetus to lasting consequences. For example, placental-insufficiency-associated promoter hypomethylation of genes affecting neurobehavioral and neuroendocrine regulation in the developing fetus (e.g., *Hsd11b2* and *Cdkn1c*) (Lee and Ding 2012) may increase postnatal susceptibility of the offspring to develop mood disorders and schizophrenia (Potter and Hollister 2007, p. 458) as well as diabetes mellitus (Peña, Monk, and Champagne 2012) by means of disrupting the fetal–placental barrier to maternal glucocorticoid, causing fetal overexposure to maternal stress, leading to abnormality in serotonin- and catecholamine-driven hypothalamic programming of the hypothalamic–pituitary–adrenal (HPA) axis (Wyrwoll and Holmes 2012) and/ or by abnormally up-regulating dopaminergic machineries (Vucetic et al. 2010). The scenario might be complicated further by elevated levels of glucocorticoid receptors along with the proteins responsible for their phosphorylation in the hippocampus of the developing fetus owing to placental-insufficiency-associated histone modifications of the genes encoding those proteins (Ke et al. 2006). It is noteworthy that such epigenetic mechanisms and their dysregulations provide us with more and more compelling evidences for the Barker hypothesis (Barker 2004), thus underscoring the need to change the attitude toward placental epigenetics because of its potential effects not only during pregnancy but also far beyond postnatal period, even into adulthood of the offspring.

25.7 GENES INVOLVED IN PLACENTAL IMMUNOLOGY

Certain specific genes are found to be involved in miscarriages than others. For example, if extravillous trophoblast expresses human leukocyte antigen (HLA)-C2 (one of the two main variants of human HLA-C) on its surface and maternal uterine natural killer (uNK) cell is homozygous for killer-cell immunoglobulin-like receptor (KIR) haplotype-A (the other one is B), which is a surface receptor for the HLA, then there is a significantly higher rate of placental insufficiency compared with the rest of the HLA-C–KIR combinations (Carter 2011). Several polymorphisms of *Hla-g* in at least three different ethnic populations and of *Foxp3* in Han Chinese women were epidemiologically linked to an increased chance of having miscarriage and preeclampsia, respectively, although these findings are still to be vindicated by further research. Elevated expression of antigen-presenting genes (e.g., *Hla-b*) might be associated with down-regulation of chemotaxis-inducing genes and the nuclear factor-κB signaling pathway, thereby protecting "notch-only" placentae (i.e., high placental vascular resistance without preeclamptic manifestations) from developing full-blown preeclampsia (Centlow et al. 2011). While it is predictable that the proinflammatory cytokines (e.g., IL-2, interferon-γ) of Th1 response would create a more hostile milieu for the conceptus than would the noninflammatory cytokines (e.g., IL-4, IL-5, IL-6, IL-9, IL-10, and IL-13) of Th2, the real question is how this balance is shifted in the first place. There is a strong possibility that certain hormones (e.g., progesterone, human placental growth hormone, human pituitary growth hormone, or simply growth hormone) and secreted factors (e.g., leukemia inhibitory factor [LIF]), along with their receptors (e.g., LIF-R), might hold the key to answering the question (Thellin et al. 2000). Overall, immunological discourse is still one of the murkiest realms of placentology. Given that the effects of maternal T cells and antibodies on trophoblasts have not been convincingly demonstrated until now, potential causal connections between disorders of placental insufficiency (e.g., IUGR, preeclampsia, and RSA) and graft rejection cannot be entirely excluded. Concordant with the speculations of Kumar and Malhotra (2008), it has been confirmed that, normally, there are anti-idiotypic antibodies in maternal sera that specifically blocks autologous T-cell receptors (TCRs), which have the capability to recognize paternal HLA-DR; MHC class II cell surface receptor haplotypes, and this provides yet another explanation for maternal tolerance of fetal graft as well as a scientific basis for immunotherapy of RSA patients. The inhibitory effects of tryptophan depleting enzyme indoleamine 2,3-dioxygenase elaborated by syncytotrophoblast on maternal immune response (Mellor and Munn 2003), death receptor (CD95/CD95-L), and/ or tumor necrosis factor/tumor necrosis factor receptor (TNF/TNF-R) apoptotic signaling pathways operating in between surfaces of placental cells and maternal lymphocytes, resulting mostly in the death of the latter (Thellin et al. 2000), anti-inflammatory role of suppressor aka "alternatively activated" macrophage (M2) in placenta (Goerdt and Orfanos 1999), and maternal regulatory T cells in both placenta and systemic circulation (Sasaki et al. 2004), may be more crucial players in the delicate game of fetal survival versus miscarriage. Novel factors like Annexin-II and *Crry* (complement receptor 1-related gene) may provide novel insights into mechanisms like reduction of maternal antibodies and complements in placenta aiding fetal survival in the face of maternal immunity (Thellin et al. 2000). Certain aspects of placental physiology (e.g., normal placentation) and pathology (e.g., RSA) can be modeled approximately as immune responses resulting from the interplay between a graft which is both invasive and allogenic (i.e., conceptus) and a not-necessarily immunocompromised host (i.e., mother), but taking these immunological models as general rules is far from reality.

25.8   PLACENTAL GENES IN IMPLANTATION

Events leading to normal placentation show remarkable temporal precision as a testament of the strong selection pressure on the entire process at every step because it is tied too strongly with reproductive success. Decidual milieu is so dynamic that parameters essential for one such step might be detrimental if applied to another step, even if the two steps are in close temporal proximity. Phenomenon pertaining to developmental timing, especially in early pregnancy, has been studied quite extensively in mice, from which we will attempt to extrapolate a few findings in case of humans. In preimplantation mouse embryo, active demethylation of paternal genes occurs up to 2-cell stage (E1), followed by passive demethylation of the whole genome (including maternal genes) occurring in between 2-cell and 8-cell stage (E1–E3), while imprinting is maintained the whole time chiefly by *Dnmt1* (Chason et al. 2011). Studies show a lower level of *Dnmt1* expression in spontaneous abortus compared with medically terminated ones at the villi in early pregnancy (Yin et al. 2012), indicating that normalcy might not ensue even if adequate *Dnmt1* dosage is established at a later time probably because preimplantation deficit of *Dnmt1* could set into motion a domino effect of cascading failure in the following sequential steps associated with zygote genome activation. Although imprinting in humans is less conserved compared with mice, and unlike mice, the *Dnmt1* promoter itself is monoallelically methylated, thus the gene is partially silenced (i.e., imprinted, maybe maternally) in primate placenta (Das et al. 2013), epigenetic disorders are by no means less important or infrequent in humans compared with disorders without epigenetic entailment. Another example of temporal disruption would be in relation to the timing of functional maturity of definitive placenta, which is normally attained in mice within a brief window of E10.5–E12.5 (Georgiades, Ferguson-Smith, and Burton 2002). Sooner than E10.5 and pregnancy is at risk due to the high oxygen tension provided by increased blood flow because either the conceptus is not ready to handle elevated ROS associated with the tension as the zygote's mitochondria as well as antioxidant genes may not be fully activated yet (Chason et al. 2011) or there is a lack of hypoxic stress signal that may be necessary for that particular stage of development, or maybe a bit of both. Later than E12.5 and there is greater chance of mismatched oxygen and nutrient supply relative to increased fetal demand resulting in placental insufficiency. These predictions are vindicated by the findings that mouse embryo with normal yolk sac but without functional definitive placenta (i.e., lack of labyrinthine vascular invasion) die *in utero* and/or abort spontaneously within that exact time frame of E10.5–E12.5 (Gnarra et al. 1997). It should be noted that effective maternal circulation is not established until around the 12th week of gestation in humans, and murine E10.5–E12.5 corresponds to about the end of first trimester in humans in terms of fetal development when organogenesis takes place (Kaufman 1990, pp. 81–92), warranting a statuary warning for us!

25.9   CLINICO-GENETIC CORRELATIONS OF TWO IMPORTANT CONDITIONS: BRIDGING THE GAP

25.9.1   PREECLAMPSIA

For day-to-day clinical practice, the notion of preeclampsia as a constellation of features including hypertension and proteinuria in pregnant women after 20 weeks of gestation usually suffices for a working definition. Despite this arbitrary threshold of 20 weeks, current trends regard preeclampsia as at least a two-stage disease (Hahn, Huppertz, and Holzgreve 2005) where the initial asymptomatic stage begins well before 20 weeks and the subsequent stage of clinical manifestation after 20 weeks makes the second stage, "preeclampsia proper." We can answer some of the clinical questions regarding preeclampsia from a morphophysiological standpoint alone. Those answers are fine as long as we are content with current clinical practices, but a better way to approach the condition requires a better understanding, which is not attainable solely with morphophysiology. The pair of questions "Why are some women more prone to develop preeclampsia?" and "Is it heritable?" are actually two sides of the same coin. The easy as well as misleading answer to both is "...because it is genetic," but the hard part is to find answers to the questions that follow, like "Which genes?" or "How?" Some genes are found to be convincingly involved in the pathogenesis of preeclampsia as well as other disorders of placental insufficiency (Table 25.1). Maybe most of the dilemmas and confusions regarding understanding preeclampsia (and its sequels) lie in the possibility that it might be in fact a heterogeneous disorder forced under a single label (Cross 2003).

25.9.2 Miscarriage

The term *miscarriage* denotes "spontaneous abortion," i.e., abortion without any medical (or criminal or accidental) intervention; the two terms being used interchangeably. It is well known that most spontaneous abortions are actually nature's way to negatively select "unfit" offsprings, evidenced by high prevalence of chromosomal as well as genetic anomalies in abortus. It might not be surprising that at least some cases of secondary recurrent miscarriage (predominantly of male conceptus) can be explained at a population level by Fisher hypothesis that the sex ratio of 1:1 usually gives maximum evolutionary advantage to an individual in a population in the long run, which is supported by the role of H-Y gene (Nielsen 2011). However, in this section, we will limit our discussion mainly to euploid miscarriages, where changes, however subtle, at the genetic and/or epigenetic

TABLE 25.1
Some Genes Associated with Preeclampsia and Their Potential Clinical Implications

Genes	Molecular Anomalies	Placental Pathophysiology	Clinical Correlations	References
Hif2α, glycogen phosphorylases (*Pygm, Pygb, Pygl*), and *Ldha4*	Global overexpression	Induction of hypoxia	Precursor of placental insufficiency	Rajakumar and Conrad (2000); Tsoi et al. (2003)
Flt1, endoglin	Hypoxia-induced increased expression producing decoy receptors for VEGFs, PlGF, TGFβ, etc.	Perpetuation of hypoxia by positive feedback	Decreased angiogenesis; small placenta	Tal et al. (2010); Elhawary, El-Bendary, and Demerdash (2012)
miR-182	Overexpression leading to downregulation of anti-apoptotic genes	Abnormally increased rate of trophoblast apoptosis and reduced trophoblastic invasion	Shallow placentation	Kim et al. (2012)
Gadd45a	Stress-induced overexpression and maintenance by positive feedback	Perpetual elevation of stress level	Preeclampsia, once initiated, soon becomes a self-propagating calamity as long as the preeclamptic pregnancy persists	Geifman-Holtzman, Xiong, and Holtzman (2013)

TABLE 25.2

Some Genes Associated with Miscarriage and Their Potential Clinical Implications

Genes	Molecular Anomalies	Placental Pathophysiology	Clinical Correlations	References
Igf2	Hypermethylation-induced epigenetic silencing	Supply/demand mismatch and/or aberration of immune response	Placental insufficiency	Bobetsis et al. (2007)
Mbl, Tnf, Lta	Certain allelic variations and several polymorphisms	Higher infection susceptibility and severity	Greater risk of recurrent miscarriage	Baxter et al. (2001)
Pai1, Fvl	Certain polymorphisms and mutations	Defects in insulin metabolism and hemodynamics	Thrombophilic complications and miscarriage in PCOS	Essah, Cheang, and Nestler (2004); Nawaz et al. (2008)
11β-HSD1/ 11β-HSD2	Down-regulation of anti-inflammatory eicosanoid LXA4 with a decrease in the expression ratio	Promotion of Th1 milieu	Greater risk of miscarriage	Xu et al. (2013)
Hla-g	Homozygosity for G*0105N allele (a null variant) or transmission of high-risk alleles (including G*0105N) from either parent	Reduction/loss of maternal immune tolerance to the conceptus	Greater risk of miscarriage	Moffett-King (2002); Ober et al. (2003)

Note: LXA4, lipoxin A4; PCOS, polycystic ovary syndrome.

level might trigger such a mishap (Table 25.2). The molecular and genetic background of different environmental factors potentially related to miscarriage (e.g., alcohol, smoking, and caffeine) has not been revealed to considerable detail.

25.10　NOVEL DIAGNOSTICS: PROMISES AND PROSPECTS

Besides biophysical tests for indirect assessment of placental adequacy (e.g., Doppler ultrasonogram of uterine artery), maternal serum soluble endoglin (sEndoglin) level at the 13th gestational week could be a predictive marker for preeclampsia (Elhawary, El-Bendary, and Demerdash 2012) and several biochemical analytes (e.g., pregnancy associated plasma protein-A [PAPP-A], placental growth factor [PlGF], placental protein 13 [PP13], Inhibin-A, Activin-A, Pentraxin 3, and P-Selectin) have been found to be potential candidates for screening and early detection of different pregnancy-related disorders (Akolekar et al. 2011), not singly but when combined with clinical history and physical examination. In a similar manner, the fact that fetal cells and cell-free fetal nucleic acids are released into maternal circulation, as well as their observed association with different pathological pregnancies, gives us an opportunity to look into, and even predict, those pathologies using methods no more invasive than drawing blood from the mother's antecubital vein. We are not only talking about prenatal detection of fetal anomalies (e.g., trisomy 21 and trisomy 18) here, which are already in clinical practice, but also emphasizing on predicting maternal complications of pregnancy. For example, placental trophoblasts, along with fetal hematopoietic cells and DNA, are found at a higher-than-normal level in mother's blood as a prelude to preeclampsia, while preterm labor patients show higher levels of fetal nucleic acids with normal frequency of fetoplacental cell trafficking or deportation in maternal circulation. The main difficulty with the detection of fetoplacental cells in maternal circulation is the very low yield of those cells even when it is magnitudes higher than normal count (Hahn and Holzgreve 2002). Detection of fetal nucleic acid by polymerase chain reaction (PCR) is relatively straightforward and very sensitive too, but its specificity is still suboptimal, probably except for detection of fetal gender (e.g., *Sry* for male) or Rh immunization (e.g., presence of *Rhd*), i.e., those genes that are present in conceptus but absent in the mother. Attempts have been made to improve specificity for detecting fetal nucleic acids in maternal circulation, with considerable success, through focusing on detection of genes (both DNA fragments and their mRNA transcripts) having placenta-specific expression profile, e.g., *Hla-g*, *Crh*, *Cg*, and *Hpl* (Tsui et al. 2004). It seems within our grasp to develop a standardized battery of nucleic acid PCR panel that would forecast preeclampsia well before it is symptomatic, giving us a therapeutic window for necessary intervention to ensure proper placentation or at least to keep the suspected cases under close observation. The same goes for many other pathological pregnancies like preterm labor, hemolysis, elevated liver enzymes and low platelet count (HELLP), IUGR, polyhydramnios, hyperemesis gravidarum, and (over-)invasive placenta (Hahn, Huppertz, and Holzgreve 2005). Then again, can we stratify risk even before one conceives? In other words, what about individual variation? That also seems plausible because of the advancements in the field of genomics and the detection of different mutations and polymorphisms associated with certain pregnancy-related pathologies (Table 25.2); e.g., women with polycystic ovary syndrome having certain polymorphic genotypes (reference sequences 1799941 and 727428) may be at additionally higher risk of miscarriage because of the diabetes-independent association of those genotypes with low *Shbg* expression (Wickham et al. 2011). This kind of "molecular horoscope" would enable future physicians to provide preconception genetic counseling regarding pregnancy-associated risks, just like it is done today in case of Mendelian disorders, not only to genetically high-risk women but also to high-risk couples who bear potentially unfavorable genetic combinations.

25.11   ASSISTED REPRODUCTIVE TECHNOLOGY: IMPRINTING ANOMALIES AND MORE

Imitating *in vivo* biology *in vitro* is the essence of most of the assisted reproductive technologies (ARTs). But simply inserting or replacing genetic materials into a cell (as in *in vitro* fertilization) is far from sufficient to get the desired results; instead, one has to find a way to mimic the regulatory machineries as well as spatiotemporally control the readout of genetic information contained in the materials, i.e., *in vitro* regulation of gene expression. Since we are still somewhat lagging behind in this aspect to understand the gene expression regulatory mechanisms, it is not surprising that imprinting anomalies (e.g., BWS, AS, SRS, and TNDM) are relatively more common in conceptus conceived by ART; rest assured, such anomalies are themselves quite rare (Wen and den Veyver 2011, p. 93). The higher incidence of preeclampsia associated with ART, especially in case of multiple gestations, underscores the possibility of imprinting defects in the placenta, leading to placental insufficiency (Tandberg et al. 2014). In the light of such evidences, Thomopoulos et al. (2013) has proposed the implementation of single embryo technique in ART to reduce pregnancy-associated hypertensive complications like preeclampsia. Nevertheless, it is not yet confirmed whether imprinting anomalies associated with ART are the result of the technology itself or if it is caused by the indication (e.g., infertility) that prompted the use of ART in the first place, or both. Although it is still a matter of debate whether ART can improve pregnancy outcomes in RSA patients, ART has the potential to become the frontline option for a portion of "incurably" infertile couples with RSA in the near future if it is possible to categorize ART-failure RSA cases into at least three functionally as well as therapeutically distinct categories: (1) miscarriage due to poor embryo quality produced by ART, (2) miscarriage due to inadequate endometrial receptivity, and (3) miscarriage due to problems with embryo transfer (Pérez-Peña et al. 2006, p. 180). Despite the slight but significant above-normal risk of epigenetic disorders in ART, chromosomal abnormalities are not more prevalent compared with "natural" conception (Bettio, Venci, and Levi Setti 2008), which may primarily be a result of advancement of medical science leading to the betterment of category 1 defect mentioned above. Category 3 defect also seems manageable for the same reason. But regarding category 2, no clear consensus is yet reached and may be the main source of the scientific controversy surrounding the application of ART in RSA. Although it is possible to evaluate the endometrium for receptivity with our current diagnostic arsenals (e.g., cervical smear cytology, endometrial curettage histology, and hormonal assays), clearly, those are not enough to satisfactorily ensure ART success in RSA patients right now, warranting workups at genetic levels discussed previously in this chapter. However, once endometrial unreceptiveness (category 2) is identified, an easy solution could be surrogacy, but that is not always feasible for various ethical, sociocultural, economic, and legal reasons. Nevertheless, one must keep in mind that several of the treatments to improve one category of defect in ART might come with the cost of deteriorating another. For example, DHEA supplementation in ART may help to improve embryo quality (category 1) by helping the production of healthy oocyte (Mamas and Mamas 2009) but, on the other hand, may decrease endometrial receptiveness (category 2) at the same time (Frolova et al. 2011). The genetic and epigenetic basis of such counterbalancing effects may be a fertile ground for further research on ART.

25.12 SUMMARY

Environmental factors, including maternal nutrition, stress, smoking, and infection, have impacts on pregnancy itself as well as its outcome, not directly but through epigenetic interface, affecting the gene expression. Genes expressed in the placenta, such as, *Igf2*, have multifaceted role in determining pregnancy outcomes because they are linked to many pathways of gene regulatory machineries, including methylation pathways. Several environmental parameters, including nutritional factors (e.g., DHA, folate, vitamin B_{12}, and ω-3 fatty acids), may likewise influence the outcomes. Genes related to immunological processes and stress (e.g., *Gadd45a*, *Hla* genes, and *Cullins* genes) set the background for such interactions in many cases (Tables 25.1 and 25.2). Hypoxia, a key player in determining placental health and disease, is amenable to the effects of nutrition and stress, which act upon different genes associated with placental angiogenesis and trophoblast apoptosis (e.g., *Hif2α*, *Flt1*, *Endoglin*, *Vegf*, and *Vegfr* genes). The role of microRNAs (e.g., miR-181a, -182, -182*, -210, -195, and -146a) is recently being elucidated in a number of pathological pregnancies, including preeclampsia and miscarriage. Batteries of gene profiling are gradually being standardized and optimized as the next generation of diagnostics. The success of ARTs is also more and more dependent on how well we understand fertilization and implantation at its molecular genetic level within a milieu that is no longer considered an innocent bystander.

REFERENCES

Akolekar, R., A. Syngelaki, R. Sarquis, M. Zvanca, and K. H. Nicolaides. 2011. "Prediction of early, intermediate and late pre-eclampsia from maternal factors, biophysical and biochemical markers at 11–13 weeks." *Prenatal Diagnosis* 31 (1): 66–74. doi:10.1002/pd.2660.

Bai, Y., W. Yang, H.-X. Yang, Q. Liao, G. Ye, G. Fu, L. Ji et al. 2012. "Downregulated miR-195 detected in preeclamptic placenta affects trophoblast cell invasion via modulating ActRIIA expression." *PLoS One* 7 (6): e38875. doi:10.1371/journal.pone.0038875.

Barker, D. J. P. 2004. "Developmental origins of adult health and disease." *Journal of Epidemiology and Community Health* 58 (2): 114–115. doi:10.1136/jech.58.2.114.

Baxter, N., M. Sumiya, S. Cheng, H. Erlich, L. Regan, A. Simons, and J. A. Summerfield. 2001. Recurrent miscarriage and variant alleles of mannose binding lectin, tumour necrosis factor and lymphotoxin alpha genes. *Clinical and Experimental Immunology* 126 (3): 529–534. doi:10.1046/j.1365-2249.2001.01663.x.

Bettio, D., A. Venci, and P. E. Levi Setti. 2008. "Chromosomal abnormalities in miscarriages after different assisted reproduction procedures." *Placenta* 29 (2): 126–128. doi:10.1016/j.placenta.2008.08.015.

Bobetsis, Y. A., S. P. Barros, D. M. Lin, J. R. Weidman, D. C. Dolinoy, R. L. Jirtle, K. A. Boggess, J. D. Beck, and S. Offenbacher. 2007. "Bacterial infection promotes DNA hypermethylation." *Journal of Dental Research* 86 (2): 169–174. doi:10.1177/154405910708600212.

Brosens, I., R. Pijnenborg, L. Vercruysse, and R. Romero. 2011. "The 'great obstetrical syndromes' are associated with disorders of deep placentation." *American Journal of Obstetrics and Gynecology* 204 (3): 193–201. doi:10.1016/j.ajog.2010.08.009.

Carter, A. M. 2011. "Comparative studies of placentation and immunology in non-human primates suggest a scenario for the evolution of deep trophoblast invasion and an explanation for human pregnancy disorders." *Reproduction* 141: 391–396. doi:10.1530/REP-10-0530.

Centlow, M., C. Wingren, C. Borrebaeck, M. J. Brownstein, and S. R. Hansson. 2011. Differential gene expression analysis of placentas with increased vascular resistance and pre-eclampsia using whole-genome microarrays. *Journal of Pregnancy* 2011: 472354. doi:10.1155/2011/472354.

Chason, R. J., J. Csokmay, J. H. Segars, A. H. DeCherney, and D. R. Armant. 2011. "Environmental and epigenetic effects upon preimplantation embryo metabolism and development." *Trends in Endocrinology and Metabolism* 22 (10): 412–420. doi:10.1016/j.tem.2011.05.005.

Christie, G. R., D. J. Williams, F. Macisaac, R. J. Dickinson, I. Rosewell, and S. M. Keyse. 2005. "The dual-specificity protein phosphatase DUSP9/MKP-4 is essential for placental function but is not required for normal embryonic development." *Molecular and Cellular Biology* 25 (18): 8323–8333. doi:10.1128/MCB.25.18.8323-8333.2005.

Constância, M., M. Hemberger, J. Hughes, W. Dean, A. Ferguson-Smith, R. Fundele, F. Stewart et al. 2002. "Placental-specific IGF-II is a major modulator of placental and fetal growth." *Nature* 417: 945–948. doi:10.1038/nature00819.

Cross, J. C. 2003. "The genetics of pre-eclampsia: A fetoplacental or maternal problem?" *Clinical Genetics* 64 (2): 96–103. doi:10.1034/j.1399-0004.2003.00127.x.

Cross, J. C., D. Baczyk, N. Dobric, M. Hemberger, M. Hughes, D. G. Simmons, H. Yamamoto, and J. C. Kingdom. 2003. "Genes, development and evolution of the placenta." *Placenta* 24 (2–3): 123–130.

Cross, J. C., Z. Werb, and S. J. Fisher. 1994. "Implantation and the placenta: Key pieces of the developing puzzle." *Science* 266 (5190): 1508–1518. doi:10.1126/science.7985020.

Czikk, M. J., S. Drewlo, D. Baczyk, S. L. Adamson, and J. Kingdom. 2013. "Dual specificity phosphatase 9 (DUSP9) expression is down-regulated in the severe pre-eclamptic placenta." *Placenta* 34 (2): 174–181. doi:10.1016/j.placenta.2012.11.029.

Das, R., Y. K. Lee, R. Strogantsev, S. Jin, Y. C. Lim, P. Y. Ng, and X. M. Lin et al. 2013. "DNMT1 and AIM1 Imprinting in human placenta revealed through a genome-wide screen for allele-specific DNA methylation." *BMC Genomics* 14: 685. doi:10.1186/1471-2164-14-685.

Dasarathy, J., L. L. Gruca, C. Bennett, P. S. Parimi, C. Duenas, S. Marczewski, J. L. Fierro, and S. C. Kalhan. 2010. "Methionine metabolism in human pregnancy." *The American Journal of Clinical Nutrition* 91 (2): 357–365. doi:10.3945/ajcn.2009.28457.

Diplas, A. I., L. Lambertini, M.-J. Lee, R. Sperling, Y. L. Lee, J. Wetmur, and J. Chen. 2009. "Differential expression of imprinted genes in normal and IUGR human placentas." *Epigenetics* 4 (4): 235–240. doi:10.4161/epi.9019.

Efstratiadis, A. 1998. "Genetics of mouse growth." *The International Journal of Developmental Biology* 42: 955–976.

Eggenschwiler, J., T. Ludwig, P. Fisher, P. A. Leighton, S. M. Tilghman, and A. Efstratiadis. 1997. "Mouse mutant embryos overexpressing IGF-II exhibit phenotypic features of the Beckwith-Wiedemann and Simpson-Golabi-Behmel syndromes." *Genes and Development* 11: 3128–3142. doi:10.1101/gad.11.23.3128.

Elhawary, T. M., A. S. El-Bendary, and H. Demerdash. 2012. "Maternal serum endoglin as an early marker of pre-eclampsia in high-risk patients." *International Journal of Womens Health* 2012 (4): 521–525. doi:10.2147/IJWH.S35318.

Enquobahrie, D. A., K. Hevner, C. Qiu, D. F. Abetew, T. K. Sorensen, and M. A. Williams. 2012. "Differential expression of HtrA1 and ADAM12 in placentas from preeclamptic and normotensive pregnancies." *Reproductive System and Sexual Disorders* 1 (3): 1000110. doi:10.4172/2161-038X.1000110.

Essah, P. A., K. I. Cheang, and J. E. Nestler. 2004. "The pathophysiology of miscarriage in women with polycystic ovary syndrome. Review and proposed hypothesis of mechanisms involved." *Hormones (Athens)* 3 (4): 221–227. doi:10.14310/horm.2002.11130.

Frank, D., W. Fortino, L. Clark, R. Musalo, W. Wang, A. Saxena, C.-M. Li, W. Reik, T. Ludwig, and B. Tycko. 2002. "Placental overgrowth in mice lacking the imprinted gene Ipl." *Proceedings of the National Academy of Sciences of the United States of America* 99: 7490–7495. doi:10.1073/pnas.122039999.

Frolova, A., K. E. O'Neill, and K. H. Moley. 2011. "Dehydroepiandrosterone inhibits glucose flux through the pentose phosphate pathway in human and mouse endometrial stromal cells, preventing decidualization and implantation." *Molecular Endocrinology* 25 (8): 1444–1455. doi:10.1210/me.2011-0026.

Frost, J. M. and G. E. Moore. 2010. "The importance of imprinting in the human placenta." *PLoS Genetics* 6 (7): e1001015. doi:10.1371/journal.pgen.1001015.

Gardner, R. L., S. Squire, S. Zaina, S. Hills, and C. F. Graham. 1999. "Insulin like growth factor-2 regulation of conceptus composition: Effects of the trophectoderm and inner cell mass genotypes in the mouse." *Biology of Reproduction* 60: 190–195. doi:10.1095/biolreprod60.1.190.

Gascoin-Lachambre, G., C. Buffat, R. Rebourcet, S. T. Chelbi, V. Rigourd, F. Mondon, T.-M. Mignot et al. 2010. "Cullins in human intra-uterine growth restriction: Expressional and epigenetic alterations." *Placenta* 31 (2): 151–157. doi:10.1016/j.placenta.2009.11.008.

Geifman-Holtzman, O., Y. Xiong, and E. J. Holtzman. 2013. "Gadd45 stress sensors in preeclampsia." *Advances in Experimental Medicine and Biology* 793: 121–129. doi:10.1007/978-1-4614-8289-5_7.

Georgiades, P., A. C. Ferguson-Smith, and G. J. Burton. 2002. "Comparative developmental anatomy of the murine and human definitive placentae." *Placenta* 23 (1): 3–19. doi:10.1053/plac.2001.0738.

Gleicher, N., E. Ryan, A. Weghofer, S. Blanco-Mejia, and D. H. Barad. 2009. "Miscarriage rates after dehydroepiandrosterone (DHEA) supplementation in women with diminished ovarian reserve: A case control study." *Reproductive Biology and Endocrinology* 7: 108. doi:10.1186/1477-7827-7-108.

Gnarra, J. R., J. M. Ward, F. D. Porter, J. R. Wagner, D. E. Devor, A. Grinberg, M. R. Emmert-Buck, H. Westphal, R. D. Klausner, and W. M. Linehan. 1997. "Defective placental vasculogenesis causes embryonic lethality in VHL-deficient mice." *Proceedings of the National Academy of Sciences of the United States of America* 94 (17): 9102–9107.

Goerdt, S. and C. E. Orfanos. 1999. "Other functions, other genes: Alternative activation of antigen-presenting cells." *Immunity* 10: 137–142. doi:10.1016/S1074-7613(00)80014-X.

Gürbüz, B., S. Yalti, C. Fiçicioğlu, S. Özden, G. Yildirim, and C. Sayar. 2003. "Basal hormone levels in women with recurrent pregnancy loss." *Gynecological Endocrinology* 17 (4): 317–321. doi:10.1080/gye.17.4.317.321.

Hahn, S. and W. Holzgreve. 2002. "Prenatal diagnosis using fetal cells and cell-free fetal DNA in maternal blood: What is currently feasible?" *Clinical Obstetrics and Gynecology* 45 (3):649–656; discussion 730-2.

Hahn, S., B. Huppertz, and W. Holzgreve. 2005. "Fetal cells and cell free fetal nucleic acids in maternal blood: New tools to study abnormal placentation?" *Placenta* 26 (7): 515–526. doi:10.1016/j.placenta.2004.10.017.

Haig, D. and R. Wharton. 2003. "Prader-Willi syndrome and the evolution of human childhood." *American Journal of Human Biology* 15: 320–329. doi:10.1002/ajhb.10150.

Hansson, S. R., Y. Chen, J. Brodszki, M. Chen, E. Hernandez-Andrade, J. M. Inman, O. A. Kozhich et al. 2006. "Gene expression profiling of human placentas from preeclamptic and normotensive pregnancies." *Molecular Human Reproduction* 12 (3): 169–179. doi:10.1093/molehr/gal011.

Heard, E. and R. A. Martienssen. 2014. "Transgenerational epigenetic inheritance: Myths and mechanisms." *Cell* 157 (1): 95–109. doi:10.1016/j.cell.2014.02.045.

Hughes, V. 2014. "Epigenetics: The sins of the father." *Nature* 507: 22–24. doi:10.1038/507022a.

Huuskonen, P., M. Storvik, M. Reinisalo, P. Honkakoski, J. Rysä, J. Hakkola, and M. Pasanen. 2008. "Microarray analysis of the global alterations in the gene expression in the placentas from cigarette-smoking mothers." *Clinical Pharmacology and Therapeutics* 83: 542–550. doi:10.1038/sj.clpt.6100376.

Jimenez-Chillaron, J. C., E. Isganaitis, M. Charalambous, S. Gesta, T. Pentinat-Pelegrin, R. R. Faucette, J. P. Otis et al. 2009. "Intergenerational transmission of glucose intolerance and obesity by *in utero* undernutrition in mice." *Diabetes* 58: 460–468. doi:10.2337/db08-0490.

Kaufman, M. 1990. "Morphological stages of postimplantation embryonic development." In *Postimplantation Mammalian Embryos: A Practical Approach*, edited by A. J. Copp and D. L. Cockroft. Oxford, England: IRL Press.

Ke, X., Q. Lei, S. J. James, S. Kelleher, S. Melnyk, S. Jernigan, X. Yu et al. 2006. "Uteroplacental insufficiency affects epigenetic determinants of chromatin structure in brains of neonatal and juvenile IUGR rats." *Physiological Genomics* 25 (1): 16–28. doi:10.1152/physiolgenomics.00093.2005.

Kim, K. M., S. J. Park, S.-H. Jung, E. J. Kim, G. Jogeswar, J. Ajita, Y. Rhee, C.-H. Kim, and S.-K. Lim. 2012. "miR-182 is a negative regulator of osteoblast proliferation, differentiation, and skeletogenesis through targeting FoxO1." *Journal of Bone and Mineral Research* 27 (8): 1669–1679. doi:10.1002/jbmr.1604.

Kleinrouweler, C. E., M. van Uitert, P. D. Moerland, C. Ris-Stalpers, J. A. M. van der Post, and G. B. Afink. 2013. "Differentially expressed genes in the pre-eclamptic placenta: A systematic review and meta-analysis." *PLoS One* 8 (7): e68991. doi:10.1371/journal.pone.0068991.

Kumar, P. and N. Malhotra, eds. 2008. *Jeffcoate's Principles of Gynaecology*, 7th Ed. India: Jaypee.

Kumar, V., A. K. Abbas, N. Fausto, and J. Aster, eds. 2010. *Robbins & Cotran Pathologic Basis of Disease*, 8th Ed. Philadelphia, PA: Saunders Elsevier.

Laigaard, J., T. Sørensen, S. Placing, P. Holck, C. Fröhlich, K. R. Wøjdemann, K. Sundberg et al. 2005. "Reduction of the disintegrin and metalloprotease ADAM12 in preeclampsia." *Obstetrics and Gynecology* 106 (1): 144–149. doi:10.1097/01.AOG.0000165829.65319.65.

Lee, S.-A. and C. Ding. 2012. "The dysfunctional placenta epigenome: Causes and consequences." *Epigenomics* 4 (5): 561–569. doi:10.2217/epi.12.49.

Lillycropa, K. A., J. L. Slater-Jefferiesa, M. A. Hansona, K. M. Godfreya, A. A. Jacksona, and G. C. Burdge. 2007. "Induction of altered epigenetic regulation of the hepatic glucocorticoid receptor in the offspring of rats fed a protein-restricted diet during pregnancy suggests that reduced DNA methyltransferase-1 expression is involved in impaired DNA methylation and changes in histone modifications." *The British Journal of Nutrition* 97 (6): 1064–1073. doi:10.1017/S000711450769196X.

Lorenzi, T., A. Turi, M. Lorenzi, F. Paolinelli, F. Mancioli, L. La Sala, M. Morroni et al. 2012. "Placental expression of CD100, CD72 and CD45 is dysregulated in human miscarriage." *PLoS One* 7 (5): e35232. doi:10.1371/journal.pone.0035232.

Maccania, M. A., M. Avissar-Whitinga, C. E. Banistera, B. McGonnigalb, J. F. Padburyb, and C. J. Marsit. 2010. "Maternal cigarette smoking during pregnancy is associated with downregulation of miR-16, miR-21, and miR-146a in the placenta." *Epigenetics* 5 (7): 583–589. doi:10.4161/epi.5.7.12762.

Mamas, L. and E. Mamas. 2009. "Dehydroepiandrosterone supplementation in assisted reproduction: Rationale and results." *Current Opinion in Obstetrics and Gynecology* 21 (4): 306–308. doi:10.1097/GCO.0b013e32832e0785.

Mayor-Lynn, K., T. Toloubeydokhti, A. C. Cruz, and N. Chegini. 2011. "Expression profile of microRNAs and mRNAs in human placentas from pregnancies complicated by preeclampsia and preterm labor." *Reproductive Science* 18 (1): 46–56. doi:10.1177/1933719110374115.

Mellor, A. L. and D. H. Munn. 2003. "Tryptophan catabolism and regulation of adaptive immunity." *The Journal of Immunology* 170: 5809–5813. doi:10.4049/jimmunol.170.12.5809.

Mizunoa, Y., Y. Sotomarud, Y. Katsuzawad, T. Konod, M. Meguroe, M. Oshimurae, J. Kawai et al. 2002. "Asb4, Ata3, and Dcn are novel imprinted genes identified by high-throughput screening using RIKEN cDNA microarray." *Biochemical and Biophysical Research Communications* 290: 1499–1505. doi:10.1006/bbrc.2002.6370.

Moffett-King, A. 2002. "Natural killer cells and pregnancy." *Nature Reviews Immunology* 2 (9): 656–663. doi:10.1038/nri886.

Morison, I. M., J. P. Ramsay, and H. G. Spencer. 2005. "A census of mammalian imprinting." *Trends in Genetics* 21 (8): 457–465. doi:10.1016/j.tig.2005.06.008.

Mouillet, J.-F., T. Chu, C. A. Hubel, D. M. Nelson, W. A. Parks, and Y. Sadovsky. 2010. "The levels of hypoxia-regulated microRNAs in plasma of pregnant women with fetal growth restriction." *Placenta* 31 (9): 781–784. doi:10.1016/j.placenta.2010.07.001.

Nawaz, F. H., R. Khalid, T. Naru, and J. Rizvi. 2008. "Does continuous use of metformin throughout pregnancy improve pregnancy outcomes in women with polycystic ovarian syndrome?" *Journal of Obstetrics and Gynaecology Research* 34 (5): 832–837. doi:10.1111/j.1447-0756.2008.00856.x.

Nielsen, H. S. 2011. "Secondary recurrent miscarriage and H-Y immunity." *Human Reproduction Update* 17 (4): 558–574. doi:10.1093/humupd/dmr005.

Novakovic, B. and R. Saffery. 2013. "Placental pseudo-malignancy from a DNA methylation perspective: Unanswered questions and future directions." *Frontiers in Genetics* 4: 285. doi:10.3389/fgene.2013.00285.

Ober, C., C. L. Aldrich, I. Chervoneva, C. Billstrand, F. Rahimov, H. L. Gray, and T. Hyslop. 2003. "Variation in the *HLA-G* promoter region influences miscarriage rates." *American Journal of Human Genetics* 72 (6): 1425–1435. doi:10.1086/375501.

Odent, M. 2014. "Preeclampsia as a maternal–fetal conflict." *Medscape*. Accessed December 25. Available at http://www.medscape.com/viewarticle/429966_1.

Oudejans, C. B. M., J. Mulders, A. M. A. Lachmeijer, M. van Dijk, A. A. M. Könst, B. A. Westerman, I. J. van Wijk et al. 2004. "The parent-of-origin effect of 10q22 in pre-eclamptic females coincides with two regions clustered for genes with down-regulated expression in androgenetic placentas." *Molecular Human Reproduction* 10 (8): 589–598. doi:10.1093/molehr/gah080.

Peña, C. J., C. Monk, and F. A. Champagne. 2012. "Epigenetic effects of prenatal stress on 11β-hydroxysteroid dehydrogenase-2 in the placenta and fetal brain." *PLoS One* 7 (6): e39791. doi:10.1371/journal.pone.0039791.

Pérez-Peña, E., A. Gutiérrez-Gutiérrez, and A. Garza-Morales. 2006. "Endometrial morphology, uterine contractions, and blood flow: All influence implantation." In *Contemporary Perspectives on Assisted Reproductive Technology*, edited by G. Allahbadia and R. Merchant. India: Elsevier.

Potter, W. Z. and L. E. Hollister. 2007. "Antipsychotic agents and lithium." In *Basic & Clinical Pharmacology*, 10th Ed., edited by B. G. Katzung. New York: McGraw-Hill.

Qiao, C., C. Wang, J. Zhao, C. Liu, and T. Shang. 2012. "Elevated expression of KiSS-1 in placenta of Chinese women with early-onset preeclampsia." *PLoS One* 7 (11): e48937. doi:10.1371/journal.pone.0048937.

Rajakumar, A. and K. P. Conrad. 2000. "Expression, ontogeny, and regulation of hypoxia-inducible transcription factors in the human placenta." *Biology of Reproduction* 63 (2): 559–569. doi:10.1095/biolreprod63.2.559.

Rappolee, D. A. 1999. "It's not just baby's babble/babel: Recent progress in understanding the language of early mammalian development: A mini review." *Molecular Reproduction and Development* 52: 234–240.

Rawn, S. M. and J. C. Cross. 2008. "The evolution, regulation, and function of placenta-specific genes." *Annual Review of Cell and Developmental Biology* 24: 159–181. doi:10.1146/annurev.cellbio.24.110707.175418.

Reik, W., M. Constância, A. Fowden, N. Anderson, W. Dean, A. Ferguson-Smith, B. Tycko, and C. Sibley. 2003. "Regulation of supply and demand for maternal nutrients in mammals by imprinted genes." *The Journal of Physiology* 547 (1): 35–44. doi:10.1113/jphysiol.2002.033274.

Rexhaj, E., J. Bloch, P.-Y. Jayet, S. F. Rimoldi, P. Dessen, C. Mathieu, J.-F. Tolsa, P. Nicod, U. Scherrer, and C. Sartori. 2011. "Fetal programming of pulmonary vascular dysfunction in mice: Role of epigenetic mechanisms." *American Journal of Physiology. Heart and Circulatory Physiology* 301 (1): H247–H252. doi:10.1152/ajpheart.01309.2010.

Sander, V., M. E. Solano, E. Elia, C. G. Luchetti, G. Di Girolamo, C. Gonzalez, and A. B. Motta. 2005. "The influence of dehydroepiandrosterone on early pregnancy in mice." *Neuroimmunomodulation* 12 (5): 285–292. doi:10.1159/000087106.

Sasaki, Y., M. Sakai, S. Miyazaki, S. Higuma, A. Shiozaki, and S. Saito. 2004. "Decidual and peripheral blood CD4+CD25+ regulatory T cells in early pregnancy subjects and spontaneous abortion cases." *Molecular Human Reproduction* 10: 347–353. doi:10.1093/molehr/gah044.

Spencer, H. G. and A. G. Clark. 2014. "Non-conflict theories for the evolution of genomic imprinting." *Heredity* 113 (2): 112–118. doi: 10.1038/hdy.2013.129.

Surmon, L., G. Bobek, A. Makris, C. L. Chiu, C. A. Lind, J. M. Lind, and A. Hennessy. 2014. "Variability in mRNA expression of *Fms-like tyrosine kinase-1* variants in normal and preeclamptic placenta." *BMC Research Notes* 7: 154. doi:10.1186/1756-0500-7-154.

Tal, R., A. Shaish, I. Barshack, S. Polak-Charcon, A. Afek, A. Volkov, B. Feldman, C. Avivi, and D. Harats. 2010. "Effects of hypoxia-inducible factor-1α overexpression in pregnant mice: Possible implications for preeclampsia and intrauterine growth restriction." *The American Journal of Pathology* 177 (6): 2950–2962. doi:10.2353/ajpath.2010.090800.

Tanaka, T. S., S. A. Jaradat, M. K. Lim, G. J. Kargul, X. Wang, M. J. Grahovac, S. Pantano et al. 2000. "Genome-wide expression profiling of mid-gestation placenta and embryo using a 15,000 mouse developmental cDNA microarray." *Proceedings of the National Academy of Sciences of the United States of America* 97 (16): 9127–9132.

Tandberg, A., K. Klungsøyr, L. B. Romundstad, and R. Skjærven. 2014. "Pre-eclampsia and assisted reproductive technologies: Consequences of advanced maternal age, interbirth intervals, new partner and smoking habits." *BJOG* 122 (7): 915–922. doi:10.1111/1471-0528.13051. [Epub ahead of print].

Thellin, O., B. Coumans, W. Zorzi, A. Igout, and E. Heinen. 2000. "Tolerance to the foeto-placental 'graft': Ten ways to support a child for nine months." *Current Opinion in Immunology* 12 (6): 731–737. doi:10.1016/S0952-7915(00)00170-9.

Thomopoulos, C., C. Tsioufis, H. Michalopoulou, T. Makris, V. Papademetriou, and C. Stefanadis. 2013. "Assisted reproductive technology and pregnancy-related hypertensive complications: A systematic review." *Journal of Human Hypertension* 27 (3): 148–157. doi:10.1038/jhh.2012.13.

Tsoi, S. C. M., J. M. Cale, I. M. Bird, and H. H. Kay. 2003. "cDNA microarray analysis of gene expression profiles in human placenta: Up-regulation of the transcript encoding muscle subunit of glycogenphosphorylase in preeclampsia." *Journal of the Society for Gynecology Investigation* 10 (8): 496–502. doi:10.1016/S1071-5576(03)00154-0.

Tsui, N. B. Y., S. S. Chim, R. W. K. Chiu, T. K. Lau, E. K. O. Ng, T. N. Leung, Y. K. Tong, K. C. A. Chan, and Y. M. D. Lo. 2004. "Systematic micro-array based identification of placental mRNA in maternal plasma: Towards non-invasive prenatal gene expression profiling." *Journal of Medical Genetics* 41 (6): 461–467. doi:10.1136/jmg.2003.016881.

Vucetic, Z., K. Totoki, H. Schoch, K. W. Whitaker, T. Hill-Smith, I. Lucki, and T. M. Reyes. 2010. "Early life protein restriction alters dopamine circuitry." *Neuroscience* 168 (2): 359–370. doi:10.1016/j.neuroscience.2010.04.010.

Wen, S. and I. B. V. den Veyver. 2011. "Imprinting in the human placenta." In *The Placenta: From Development to Disease*, edited by H. Kay, D. M. Nelson, and Y. Wang. West Sussex, UK, Wiley-Blackwell.

Wickham, E. P. 3rd, K. G. Ewens, R. S. Legro, A. Dunaif, J. E. Nestler, and J. F. Strauss 3rd. 2011. "Polymorphisms in the SHBG gene influence serum SHBG levels in women with polycystic ovary syndrome." *Journal of Clinical Endocrinology and Metabolism* 96 (4): E719–E727. doi:10.1210/jc.2010-1842.

Winstead, E. R. 2000. "Profiling the placenta: Gene expression in mouse embryonic and placental tissues." *Genome News Network*. Available at http://www.genomenewsnetwork.org/articles/08_00/profiling_placenta.shtml.

Wolf, J. B. and R. Hager. 2006. "A maternal–offspring coadaptation theory for the evolution of genomic imprinting." *PLoS Biology* 4 (12): e380. doi:10.1371/journal.pbio.0040380.

Wyrwoll, C. S. and M. C. Holmes. 2012. "Prenatal excess glucocorticoid exposure and adult affective disorders: A role for serotonergic and catecholamine pathways." *Neuroendocrinology* 95 (1): 47–55. doi:10.1159/000331345.

Xu, Z., J. Zhao, H. Zhang, T. Ke, P. Xu, W. Cai, F. Katirai, D. Ye, Y. Huang, and B. Huang. 2013. "Spontaneous miscarriages are explained by the stress/glucocorticoid/lipoxin A4 axis." *The Journal of Immunology* 190 (12): 6051–6058. doi:10.4049/jimmunol.1202807.

Yampolsky, M., C. M. Salafia, O. Shlakhter, D. Haas, B. Eucker, and J. Thorp. 2008. "Modeling the variability of shapes of human placenta." *Placenta* 29 (9): 790–797. doi:10.1016/j.placenta.2008.06.005.

Yang, W. J., D. D. Yang, S. Na, G. E. Sandusky, Q. Zhang, and G. Zhao. 2005. "Dicer is required for embryonic angiogenesis during mouse development." *Journal of Biological Chemistry* 280 (10): 9330–9335. doi:10.1074/jbc.M413394200.

Yin, L.-J., Y. Zhang, P.-P. Lv, W.-H. He, Y.-T. Wu, A.-X. Liu, G.-L. Ding et al. 2012. "Insufficient maintenance DNA methylation is associated with abnormal embryonic development." *BMC Medicine* 10: (26). doi:10.1186/1741-7015-10-26.

Yuen, R. K. C., M. S. Peñaherrera, P. von Dadelszen, D. E. McFadden, and W. P. Robinson. 2010. "DNA methylation profiling of human placentas reveals promoter hypomethylation of multiple genes in early-onset preeclampsia." *European Journal of Human Genetics* 18 (9): 1006–1012. doi:10.1038/ejhg.2010.63.

Zhang, H., Q. Long, L. Ling, A. Gao, H. Li, and Q. Lin. 2011. "Elevated expression of KiSS-1 in placenta of preeclampsia and its effect on trophoblast." *Reproductive Biology* 11 (2): 99–115. doi:10.1016/S1642-431X(12)60048-5.

Zhou, Y., M. J. Gormley, N. M. Hunkapiller, M. Kapidzic, Y. Stolyarov, V. Feng, M. Nishida et al. 2013. "Reversal of gene dysregulation in cultured cytotrophoblasts reveals possible causes of preeclampsia." *The Journal of Clinical Investigation* 123 (7): 2862–2872. doi:10.1172/JCI66966.

26 Regulation of microRNA Expression and Function of First-Trimester and Term Placentas in Humans

Yuping Wang

CONTENTS

ABSTRACT

microRNAs (miRNAs) are short endogenous noncoding RNA molecules (~22 nucleotides) that regulate gene expression at the posttranscription level. miRNAs are thought to be a vital and evolutionary component of genetic regulation. They are enriched in the placenta. Recent findings have demonstrated that miRNAs are emerging as major players in gene regulation, not only contributing to diverse biological processes in the placental development but also modulating maternal immune tolerance during pregnancy. In this chapter, current knowledge of miRNA clusters associated with placental development and function, trophoblast specific exosome miRNAs and maternal immunomodulation, and miRNAs related to epithelial–mesenchymal transition in placenta development will be discussed.

KEY WORDS

Placenta, trophoblast, miRNA, miRNA cluster, C14MC, C19MC, exosome, epithelial–mesenchymal transition (EMT).

26.1 INTRODUCTION

microRNAs (miRNAs) are endogenously expressed small noncoding RNA molecules about 21–25 nucleotides in length. miRNAs were first described in the early 1990s (Lee, Feinbaum, and Ambros 1993), but they were not recognized as a distinct class of biological regulators until the early 2000s. To date, thousands of miRNAs have been identified, and the expression and production of subset of miRNAs are found to be cell type, tissue, and organ specific (Lagos-Quintana et al. 2002). miRNA biogenesis is regulated at multiple levels by two RNase III proteins: Drosha in the nucleus and Dicer in cytoplasm (Bartel 2004; Cullen 2004). The main function of miRNAs is to regulate gene expression through mechanisms of translational repression, messenger RNA (mRNA) cleavage, and deadenylation by binding to complementary sequences of untranslated regions (UTRs) on the target mRNA transcripts. Given the large number of miRNAs annotated in the human genome, it is expected that miRNAs regulate up to 60% of all mammalian genes, which virtually control almost all cellular events from stem cell differentiation (Houbaviy, Murray, and Sharp 2003; Chen et al. 2004) to organ development and formation (Boettger and Braun 2012; Cochella and Hobert 2012), aging (Inukai et al. 2012), etc. miRNAs are well conserved in both animals and plants and are thought to be a vital and evolutionary component of genetic regulation and play essential roles during development. This has been demonstrated by the knockout of the Dicer gene in animal models, since Dicer knockout inhibits the production of nearly all miRNAs and Dicer-deficient embryos die at an early embryonic stage, which indicates the essential role of miRNAs in embryogenesis and stem cell development (Bernstein et al. 2003; Yang et al. 2005).

The placenta is the first organ formed during pregnancy. It connects the developing fetus to the mother's uterine wall and influences almost every aspect of fetal development and growth such as gas exchange, nutrient uptake, waste elimination, and hormone production. The placenta produces miRNAs. Evolving evidence has shown that placental miRNA expression/ production not only plays critical roles in placental development but also mediates maternal immune tolerance during pregnancy. First, the finding of differential miRNA expression profiles between first-trimester and term placentas demonstrates spatial and temporal miRNA synthesis and regulation during placental development (Gu et al. 2013; Farrokhnia et al. 2014). Second, identification of placental-specific miRNAs, chromosome 14 miRNA cluster (C14MC) miRNAs imprinted from maternal chromosome (Seitz et al. 2004), and chromosome 19 miRNA cluster (C19MC) miRNAs imprinted from paternal chromosome (Noguer-Dance et al. 2010) emphasizes inherited genetic regulation during placenta development and their potential role in immunomodulation during pregnancy. Third, demonstration of altered miRNA expression in placentas in miscarriage, preeclampsia, intrauterine growth restriction, etc., provides evidence that deregulation of placental miRNAs is associated with placental disorders (Pineles et al. 2007; Mayor-Lynn et al. 2011; Ventura et al. 2013). Moreover, detection of trophoblast-derived miRNAs in the maternal circulation and findings of different patterns of circulating miRNAs at different gestational age and pregnancy disorders (Gilad et al. 2008; Luo et al. 2009) further indicate that placental miRNAs could serve as valuable biomarkers of placental function and the likelihood of molecular regulators acting on the maternal systemic vasculature and immune systems during pregnancy.

A recent study conducted by Gu et al. analyzed miRNA expression profiles in the human placenta. They found that among the 1105 miRNA transcripts examined, approximately 17% of the miRNAs were differentially expressed between first-trimester and term placentas (Gu et al. 2013). Further analysis revealed that a large portion (>40%) of miRNAs that are either up-regulated in the first-trimester placentas or up-regulated in the term placentas appear to be clustered. miRNAs that are up-regulated in the first-trimester placentas belong to four miRNA clusters, which are localized mainly on chromosomes 13, 14, and 19. They are the miR17-92 cluster on chromosome 13q31.3, C14MC on chromosome 14q32, and the miR-371 cluster and C19MC on chromosome 19q13.42 (Table 26.1). In comparison, miRNA families and clusters that are up-regulated in the

TABLE 26.1

miRNA Clusters or Families That Are Differentially Expressed in First-Trimester and Term Placentas in Humans[a]

Cluster	Chromosome Location	miRNAs	Functions	References
Clusters of miRNAs That Are Up-Regulated in First-Trimester vs. Term Placentas				
miR-17-92 cluster	13q31.3	miR-17, miR-18a, miR-19a	Immune tolerance, oncogenic	Bouillet et al. 2002
		miR-19b-1*, miR-20a, miR-20b	Angiogenic, proliferation, antiapoptotic	Xiao et al. 2008; Dews et al. 2010
		miR-92a, miR-92a-1*	Modulate TGF-β signaling	Osada and Takahashi 2011
miR-106a cluster	Xq26.2	miR-106a, miR-18b, miR-20b	Antiproliferative, angiogenic, immunoregulator	Khuu et al. 2014
miR-106b cluster	7q22.1	miR-25, miR-93	Modulate TGF-β signaling, oncogenic, antiapoptotic	Petrocca et al. 2008; Dews et al. 2010
C14MC cluster	4q32.2	miR-127, miR-345, miR-370, miR-431	Immune suppressive	Tay et al. 2008
		miR-665	Anti-inflammatory response	Aguado-Fraile et al. 2012
			Protect ischemic/hypoxia injury	
	14q32.31	miR-134, miR-323, miR-409, miR-412	Immune suppressive, lipid metabolism	Tay et al. 2008; Kagami et al. 2012
		miR-654, miR-758	Protect ischemic/hypoxia injury	Zhang et al. 2012
			Angiogenic associated with neuron function	
miR-371 cluster	19q13.42	miR-371, miR-372, miR-373	Stem cell signature, oncogenic	Belair et al. 2011; Voorhoeve et al. 2007
			Immune suppressive	Qi et al. 2009
C19MC cluster	19q13.42	miR-498, miR-518b, miR-518c, miR-518d	Immune suppressive	Donker et al. 2012
		miR-518e, miR-518f, miR-519a*, miR-519b	Innate/adaptive immune responses	Keklikoglou et al. 2012
		miR-519c, miR-520a, miR-520c, miR-520d miR-520f, miR-520g, miR-520h, miR-522 miR-523, miR-525, miR-526a	Antivirus	Delorme-Axford et al. 2013 Miao et al. 2014
Clusters or Families of miRNAs That Are Up-Regulated in Term vs. First-Trimester Placentas				
miR-29 family	7q32.3	miR-29a, miR-29b	Tumor suppressor, differentiation	Cui et al. 2011; Nguyen et al. 2011
	1q32.2	miR-29c	Innate/adaptive immune responses	Liston et al. 2012; Li et al. 2013
			ECM regulation	

(Continued)

TABLE 26.1 (CONTINUED)
miRNA Clusters or Families That Are Differentially Expressed in First-Trimester and Term Placentas in Humans[a]

Cluster	Chromosome Location	miRNAs	Functions	References
miR-34 family	1p36.22	miR-34a	Tumor suppressor, anti-apoptosis	Hermeking 2010; Misso et al. 2014
	11q23.1	miR-34b, miR-34c	Onco-immunology	
miR-195 cluster	17q13.1	miR-195, miR-497	Cell cycle control, tumor suppressor	Flavin et al. 2009
			Differentiation, lymph genic	
miR-181c cluster	19p13.13	miR-181c, miR-181d	Differentiation, tumor suppressor	Río et al. 2012
			Autoimmunity, hematopoietic	Schonrock et al. 2012
miR-188 cluster	Xp11.23	miR-188, miR-660, miR-362	Tumor suppressor, cardiovascular	Lee et al. 2012; Wu et al. 2014
			Development, insulin-signaling pathway	
let-7 family	11q24.1	*let-7a*	Promote differentiation	Jérôme et al. 2007
	22q13.31	*let-7b*	Tumor suppressor	Johnson et al. 2007
21q21.1		*let-7c*		Roush and Slack 2008
	9q22.32	*let-7d*		Liu et al. 2012
	19q13.41	*let-7e*		
	9q22.32 (Xp11.22)	*let-7f-1 (7f-2)*		
	3p21.1	*let-7g*		
	12q14.1	*let-7i*		
let-7a cluster	11q24.1	*let-7a*, miR-100, miR-125b	Tumor suppressor, differentiation	Jérôme et al. 2007
let-7c cluster	21q21.1	*let-7c*, miR-99a	Tumor suppressor, differentiation	Roush and Slack 2008
let-7f-2 cluster	Xp11.22	*let-7f-2*, miR98		Nadiminty et al. 2012
let-7d cluster	9q22.32	*let-7d*, *let-7f-1*		

Note: miRNA with asterisk (*) is the star-form partner miRNA.

[a] Data are cited from Gu, Y. et al., *Am. J. Physiol. Endocrinol. Metab.* 304, E836–E843, 2013.

term placentas are different. They are the miR-29 cluster on chromosome 7q32.3, the miR-188 cluster on chromosome Xp11.23, and the miR-34 family and *let-7* family/cluster miRNAs, etc. (Table 26.1). The observation of different miRNA cluster patterns in the placenta supports the notion that nearly 40% of the known human miRNA genes are highly clustered and have typical conservative patterns (Altuvia et al. 2005). In fact, organ-specific miRNA clusters associated with organ-specific functionality have been reported in animals (Xu et al. 2007). It is speculated that the biological functions and targets of miRNA cluster genes are also highly related (Altuvia et al. 2005). This chapter will discuss current knowledge of miRNA clusters that are relevant to placental function. Trophoblast-specific exosome miRNAs and miRNAs that are associated with the epithelial–mesenchymal transition (EMT) in placental development will also be discussed.

26.2 miRNA CLUSTERS AND THEIR FUNCTION IN FIRST-TRIMESTER AND TERM PLACENTAS

26.2.1 MiR-17-92 CLUSTER

The miR-17-92 cluster is probably among the most studied miRNA clusters in the literature. The miR-17-92 cluster is located on chromosome 13q31.3 and is composed of six miRNAs, including miR-17, miR-18a, miR-19a, miR-19b-1, miR-20a, and miR-92-1. The miR-17-92 cluster miRNAs are expressed in placentas throughout pregnancy, but higher expression levels were noticed in first-trimester placentas than in placentas at term (Table 26.1) (Gu et al. 2013). The miRNA cluster has two paralog clusters, which were identified through duplication and deletion studies (Lindsay 2008), i.e., miR-106a-363 cluster (miR-106a, miR-18b, miR-20b, miR-19b-2, miR-92-2, and miR-363) localized on chromosome Xq26.2 and miR-106b-25 cluster (miR-106b, miR-93, and miR-25) localized on chromosome 7q22.1. Interestingly, all members of the miR-17-92 cluster miRNAs and several members of miRNAs in the paralog clusters are up-regulated in first-trimester placentas (Table 26.1). These observations indicate the importance of miR-17-92 cluster miRNAs in placental development during early pregnancy.

Studies have shown that miR-17-92 cluster miRNAs target a number of critical molecules involved in the regulation of cell proliferation, differentiation, migration, and cell cycle control processes. These miRNAs also play antiapoptotic roles in resisting cell death (Xiao et al. 2008). Among the predicted gene targets of miR-17-92, gene codes for transcription factor (E2Fs; E2F1, E2F2, and E2F3), phosphatase, and tensin homolog (PETN), and transforming growth factor beta (TGF-β) receptor II (TGFBR II) signaling pathway molecules are probably the most being reported (Woods, Thomson, and Hammond 2007; Ventura et al. 2008; Dews et al. 2010). E2Fs are transcription factors essential to the regulation of the cell cycle and apoptosis. E2Fs act on tumor suppressor proteins by targeting the transforming proteins of small DNA tumor viruses. Both miR-17 and miR-20a regulate E2F1 expression. miR-20a could also modulate the translation of E2F2 and E2F3 through binding to their 3'-UTRs (Sylvestre et al. 2007). In fibroblasts, inhibition of miR-17 and miR-20a was found to lead to G1 checkpoint activation due to an accumulation of DNA double-stranded breaks, resulting from premature temporal accumulation of the E2F1 transcription factor (Pickering, Stadler, and Kowalik 2009). This provides a mechanistic view of miRNA-based regulation of E2F1 in the context of miRNA coordination to the timing of cell cycle progression.

PETN, another target of miR-17-92, is a tumor suppressor gene through the action of its phosphatase products. PETN plays multiple roles in a wide range of cellular processes, including cell growth, proliferation, and migration, which are achieved by antagonizing phosphatidylinositol 3-kinase, regulating cell cycle, and coordinating cell growth through prevention of cells from proliferation and division. PTEN specifically catalyzes the dephosporylation of the 3'phosphate of the inositol ring in phosphatidylinositol (3,4,5)-trisphosphate (PIP$_3$), which results in inhibition of the serine/threonine-specific protein kinase (AKT) pathway signaling. Targeting of PTEN's 3'UTR by miR-19a and miR-19b-1 has also been reported (Liang et al. 2011). The miR-17-92 cluster could also mediate human fibroblast reprogramming through transcriptional factors (Oct4, Sox2, and Klf4, or 3F). One study has shown that miR-19a/b exhibits the most potent effect on stimulating fibroblast reprogramming to induction of pluripotent stem cells (He et al. 2014). In early pregnancy loss, placental expression of miR-17 and miR-19b was found to be down-regulated and PETN expression was significantly up-regulated (Ventura et al. 2013). These findings evoke the importance of miR-17-92 cluster miRNAs in placental development, especially during early pregnancy. The higher expression levels of miR-17-92 cluster miRNAs and its paraloga cluster miRNAs in first-trimester placentas suggest that they probably regulate the cell survival of both trophoblasts and nontrophoblast cells. This notion is supported by findings of miR-17-92 and miR-106a-363 clusters inhibiting trophoblast differentiation through repressing hGCM1 and aromatase hCYP19A1 expressions (Kumar et al. 2013).

Promotion of placental cell survival and placental development by miR-17-92 cluster miRNAs could also be achieved through targeting TGF-β signaling pathway molecules. miR-17-92 miRNAs are potent inhibitors of TGF-β acting on multiple levels in the TGF-β signaling cascade (O'Connor et al. 1998; Bouillet et al. 2002). miR-17 and miR-20a directly target TGFBR II. miR-18a targets Smad2 and Smad4. Both of them are TGF-β signaling pathway members. TGF-β is a major repressor of cytotrophoblast outgrowth, and different TGF-β isoforms are found at the maternal–fetal interface (Graham et al. 1992; Schilling and Yeh 2000; Jones et al. 2006). TGF-β is a vital regulator of placental development and functions and exerts several modulatory effects on trophoblast cells, such as inhibition of proliferation and invasiveness and stimulation of differentiation by inducing cytotrophoblast syncytiolization. Although the specific role of miR-17-92 miRNAs on TGF-β in placental cells is largely unknown, the finding of deregulation of miR-17 and miR-92a expression in placentas from early spontaneous miscarriage (Ventura et al. 2013) provides a link that altered miR-17-92 expression is associated with abnormal placental development in humans.

26.2.2 Chromosome 14 miRNA Cluster

The chromosome 14 miRNA cluster (C14MC) is located on chromosome 14q32, which hosts one of the largest miRNA clusters (C14MC) in the human genome, with 12 miRNAs located in 14q32.2 and 38 miRNAs located in 14q32.31. As shown in Table 26.1, several miRNAs in the C14MC are up-regulated in first-trimester placentas compared with term placentas (Gu et al. 2013). C14MC is the largest imprinted, maternally expressed human miRNA cluster in the placenta (Seitz et al. 2004). The chromosome 14q32.2 region also carries a cluster of imprinted genes, the DLK1-DIO3 genomic region. This region contains paternally expressed genes such as DLK1 and RTL1 and maternally expressed genes such as GTL2 (alias, MEG3), RTL1as (RTL1 antisense), and MEG8 (Ogata and Kagami 2008). Since parent-of-origin-specific monoallelic expression patterns of imprinted genes are highly related to the methylation status of differentially methylated regions (Murphy, Huang, and Hoyo 2012; Das et al. 2013), it is believed that the production and function of C14MC miRNAs are likely controlled through epigenetic regulation.

Imprinted genes are required for the formation of the placenta as well as the development of cellular lineages such as those derived from the mesoderm and ectoderm (Hernandez et al. 2002). C14MC miRNAs play an essential role in the regulation of genomic imprinting gene expression in a parent-of-origin-specific manner. For example, miR-127 (14q32.2) is located near Cytosine-phosphate-Guanine dinucleotide (CpG) islands in the imprinted region encoding RTL1 and is normally transcribed in an antisense orientation to the gene. RTL1 is a key gene in placenta formation, and the loss or overexpression of RTL1 could lead to late-fetal or neonatal lethality in mice (Sekita et al. 2008). The role of miR-134 (14q32.31) in the regulation of stem cell growth and differentiation has also been reported (Tay et al. 2008). miR-134 expression was found to be increased in mouse embryonic stem cells (mESCs) after being stimulated with retinoic acid (Tay et al. 2008), which is essential in mediating the functions of vitamin A required for neural and retinal cell growth and development (Duester 2008). An animal model study also revealed that the elevation of miR-134 levels alone in mESCs could enhance differentiation toward ectodermal lineages (Tay et al. 2008). Promotion of mESC differentiation by miR-134 is believed to be due, in part, to its direct translational attenuation of Nanog and LRH1; both are positive regulators of Oct4/POU5F1 and mESC growth. In CD34+ cells derived from umbilical cord blood, deregulation of miR-136 (14q32.2) expression was found throughout erythropoiesis showing lineage commitment (Choong, Yang, and McNiece 2007), indicating that C14MC miRNAs are also involved in erythropoiesis. It is very likely that C14MC miRNAs may be involved in differentiation and maturation of placental cells, including trophoblasts, villous core endothelial cells, pericytes, and stromal cells. C14MC miRNAs also regulate erythroid commitment during fetal growth since C14MC miRNAs and associated imprinted genes, specially RTL1, play a pivotal role in the development of vascular endothelial cells and pericytes (Kagami et al. 2012).

miR-379/miR-410 (14q32.2), members of C14MC, were also reported to be central for metabolic adaptation in early postnatal life. A target disruption study of the miR-379/miR-410 in a mouse model showed that miR-379/miR-410-deficient pups had difficulties maintaining energy homeostasis, which was associated with profound changes in the hepatic gene expression at the transition from fetal to postnatal life (Labialle et al. 2014). This phenotype suggests a pivotal role for C14MC miRNAs in neonatal survival, at least in part by controlling metabolic adaptation at birth. Whether C14MC miRNAs are involved in energy metabolism in placental trophoblasts warrants further investigation.

26.2.3 CHROMOSOME 19 MIRNA CLUSTER

The chromosome 19 miRNA cluster (C19MC) is a primate-specific and paternal imprinted miRNA cluster (Noguer-Dance et al. 2010). It is the largest miRNA gene cluster in humans. It consists of 46 miRNAs in encoding and produces a total of 56 mature miRNAs (Bortolin-Cavaillé et al. 2009). C19MC miRNAs are predominantly expressed in the human placenta throughout pregnancy. Studies have shown that the expression pattern of C19MC miRNAs and the distribution of C19MC miRNAs are spatial and temporal during placental development. On one hand, the expression of a subset of C19MC miRNAs, including miR-518b, miR-519a, miR-520a, miR-520c, miR-520h, and miR-526a, etc., was found to be higher in early-gestation placentas than in term placentas (Hromadnikova et al. 2012; Gu et al. 2013). On the other hand, the expression of a subset of C19MC miRNAs, including miR-526b, was found to be higher in term placentas than in early-pregnancy placentas (Gu et al. 2013). A difference in the production of C19MC miRNAs in cultured placental trophoblasts was also noticed by Donker et al. They found that differentiation of cultured primary placental trophoblast cells was associated with a reduction in C19MC miRNAs among the total cellular miRNAs expressed in the differentiated trophoblast cells (Donker et al. 2012). Their data suggest that the production of C19MC miRNAs is likely associated with differentiation state in trophoblasts (Donker et al. 2012). Xie et al. (2014) also uncovered differences in C19MC miRNA expression between villous trophoblasts and extravillous trophoblasts, in which the expression of miR-517-3p, miR-518b, miR-519d, miR-520g, miR-515-5p, and miR-1323 was significantly higher in villous trophoblasts than in extravillous trophoblasts. Their study also revealed that miR-519d was able to directly regulate the extravillous trophoblast invasive phenotype by targeting CXCL6, NR4A2, and FOXL2 transcripts through a 3'UTR miRNA-responsive element (Xie et al. 2014). These findings infer that C19MC miRNAs play a diverse role in phenotypic and functional differences between villous and extravillous trophoblasts. Similar to C14MC, epigenetic regulation is also considered to play an essential role in the activation of C19MC miRNAs. The C19MC miRNA expression pattern is highly correlated with the methylation state of a distal CpG-rich region. This has been demonstrated in cultured placental-derived mesenchymal stromal cells and in nonplacental cancer cells, in which up-regulation of C19MC miRNA expression can be induced by the demethylating agent 5-aza-2'-deoxycytidine (Tsai et al. 2009; Flor et al. 2012).

The functional diversity of different C19MC miRNAs has been intensively studied in various cancers and tumor cells. Some members are considered oncogenic, whereas others are considered tumor suppressing, based on different cell types and are regulated through different signaling pathways. For example, miR-517a is considered an oncogenic miRNA. It is able to increase proliferation, migration, and invasion in cultured hepatocellular carcinoma cells in vitro and to promote tumor genesis and metastatic dissemination in vivo (Toffanin et al. 2011). In contrast, miR-520 family miRNAs exert tumor suppressor functions. By targeting eukaryotic translation initiation factor 4 gamma 2 (eIF4GII), miR-520c-3p is able to repress diffuse large B-cell lymphoma development (Mazan-Mamczarz et al. 2014). miR-520c-3p also has the ability to inhibit hepatocellular carcinoma cell proliferation and invasion through induction of cell apoptosis by targeting glypican-3, a membrane-associated heparan sulfate proteoglycan (Miao et al. 2014). Moreover, miR-520/373 was also found to be a tumor suppressor in estrogen receptor-negative breast cancer by targeting nuclear factor-κB and TGF-β signaling pathway molecules (Keklikoglou et al. 2012).

C19MC miRNAs could be detected in maternal blood from first-trimester pregnancies. and these are a major group of miRNAs found in the maternal circulation in pregnant women (Miura et al. 2010). The fact that C19MC miRNA levels are reduced after delivery suggests that placental tropho-blasts could be the major source of C19MC miRNAs shed into the maternal circulation. This notion is supported by the findings that a large amount of miRNAs packed into trophoblast-derived exo-somes consists of C19MC miRNAs (Donker et al. 2012). Abundant expression and hemimethylation of C19MC miRNAs were also noticed in cultured stromal cells derived from human placenta (Flor et al. 2012). Recently, antiviral effects of C19MC miRNAs were also reported by Delorme-Axford et al. (2013). These investigators tested several viruses, including coxsackievirus B3, poliovirus, vesicular stomatitis virus, vaccinia virus, herpes simplex virus-1, and human cytomegalovirus, and found that cultured primary human placental trophoblasts with C19MC mimics (miR-517-3p, -516b-5p, and -512-3p) are highly resistant to viral infection. They further noticed that C19MC miRNAs in exosomes derived from primary isolated trophoblasts could protect nontrophoblast cells from viral infection by induction of autophagy in recipient cells (Delorme-Axford et al. 2013). The anti-viral effect by trophoblast C19MC miRNAs provides further evidence of the defense mechanism of placental-derived C19MC in the protection of the developing embryo and fetus from antigen attack during pregnancy. C19MC-miRNA-induced suppression of T-cell signaling offers another mechanism of placental-derived exosomes (C19MC) in the regulation of maternal innate immune response. The exosome-carrying C19MC miRNAs derived from syncytiotrophoblasts would be a unique molecular system to mediate placenta–maternal communication during pregnancy (see below).

26.2.4 miRNA-371-3 Cluster

Both C19MC and miR-371-3 miRNA clusters are considered stem cell miRNA gene clusters. The miRNA-371-3 cluster miRNAs (miR-371, miR-372, and miR-373) are also located on chromosome 19q13.42, in close proximity to C19MC miRNAs. Several recent studies have linked the expression of members of the miR-371-3 cluster and the C19MC with the miRNA signature characteristics for human embryonic stem cells (Laurent et al. 2008; Li et al. 2009a; Rosenbluth et al. 2013). miR-371-3 is expressed in the placenta throughout pregnancy, but the level of miRNA-371-3 expression is sig-nificantly higher during the first trimester than at term (Table 26.1). Results from the in situ hybrid-ization study further confirmed that miRNA-371-5p is predominantly expressed in cytotrophoblasts in first-trimester placentas (Gu et al. 2013), thus supporting the concept that miR-371-3 expression is closely linked to the undifferentiated phenotype. This concept is further supported by the findings of miR-371-3 expression in many germ and nongerm tumor and cancer cells, including testicular germ cell tumors (Voorhoeve et al. 2007).

The miR-371-3 expression appears to have both a predictive and a functional role in determi-nation of neurogenic differentiation behavior in human pluripotent stem cells (Kim et al. 2011). Kim et al. found that transient transfection of Kruppel-like factor 4 (KLF4, transcription factor) into human embryonic stem cells up-regulated miR-371-3 expression along with altered neurogenic behavior and pluripotency marker expression. Conversely, suppression of miR-371-3 expression in KLF4-transduced cells rescued neural differentiation propensity (Kim et al. 2011). In addition, miR-371-3 miRNAs are also considered oncomiRs. They could promote tumor cell invasion and metastasis through several mechanisms including stimulation of cell proliferation, blockage of cell cycle progression, regulation of tumor suppressor genes, and suppression of CD44, a cell-surface glycoprotein involved in cell–cell interactions, etc. (Qi et al. 2009; Belair et al. 2011).

26.2.5 miR-29 Family

The miR-29 family consists of three members: miR-29a, miR-29b, and miR-29c. miR-29a and miR-29b are located on chromosome 7q32.3 and miR-29c is located on chromosome 1q32.2. miR-29 family miRNAs have significant impact on cell biology related to cell proliferation, differentiation, and apoptosis. Regulation of extracellular matrix (ECM) is an important function of the miR-29 family miRNAs. Studies have shown that miR-29 family members target at least 16 genes that encode ECM proteins, including matrix metalloproteinase-2 (MMP-2), integrin β1, elastin, laminin, etc. (Li et al. 2009b; Liu et al. 2010). Interestingly, miR-29 family miRNAs have distinct subcellular locations. miR-29a is predominantly localized in the cytoplasm, whereas miR-29b and miR-29c are significantly enriched in the nucleus (Hwang, Wentzel, and Mendell 2007; Liao et al. 2010). The difference in cytosolic and nuclear location suggests that the biological effects of miR-29 family miRNAs are likely associated with targeting protein localization. Although the role of miR-29 family miRNAs in placental trophoblast cells remains largely unknown, increased expression of all three miR-29 family miRNAs (miR-29a, miR-29b, and miR-29c) is found in term placentas compared with first-trimester placentas (Table 26.1).

miR-29 family miRNAs have been identified to be potent immune modulators. The roles of miR-29 family miRNAs in adaptive immunity have been demonstrated through several mechanisms (Liston et al. 2012). For example, in thymic epithelial cells, miR-29 family miRNAs could control T-cell production by tuning type I interferon (IFN) signaling. These miRNAs could also balance Th1–Th2 cell fate decision and create a neutral threshold for T-cell polarization. Regulation of B-cell oncogenic transformation has also been demonstrated by the miR-29 family miRNAs. Beyond the adaptive immune system, miR-29 family miRNAs also play roles in cancer biology as tumor suppressor (Cui et al. 2011; Nguyen et al. 2011) through regulation of p53 signaling and induction of apoptosis by targeting Mcl-1 (Mott et al. 2007), a member of the B-cell lymphoma (Bcl)-2 family.

The expression of miR-29b was found to be significantly increased in placental tissues in pregnancy complicated with preeclampsia (Li et al. 2013), a hypertensive disorder in human pregnancy. Increased miR-29b expression is associated with reduced expression of matrix protein (MCL 1) and MMP-2, as well as angiogenic factors vascular endothelial growth factor (VEGF) A and integrin beta 1 (ITGB1), in preeclamptic placental tissues. All of them are targets of miR-29b. The role of miR-29b in trophoblast cell lines HTR-8/SVneo, BeWo, and JAR cells was also studied (Li et al. 2013). miR-29b not only induces cell apoptosis in trophoblast cells but also reduces the invasiveness and decreases the formation of capillary tube and network in HTR-8/SVneo cells (Li et al. 2013). Their data, combined with the up-regulation of miR-29a/b/c expression in the term placenta (Gu et al. 2013), indicate that miR-29 family miRNAs participate a diverse role in normal placenta development and in pathophysiological process such as suppression of angiogenic function of placental trophoblasts at term.

26.2.6 MiR-34 Family

The miR-34 family consists of three members: miR-34a, miR-34b, and miR-34c; miR-34a is located on chromosome 1p36.22, whereas miR-34b and miR-34c are located on chromosome 11q23.1. The molecular effects of miR-34 family miRNAs have been intensively studied in cancer research. It is well known that miR-34 miRNAs are tumor suppressors by directly or indirectly targeting p53 signaling pathway molecules and antagonize many different oncogenic processes. For example, regulator gene (c-MYC), group of genes (E2F), cyclin-dependent kinase 4 (CDK4), and cyclin-dependent kinase 6 (CDK6) are molecules participating in G1/S transition. Bcl-2 and sirtuin 1 (SIRT1) are involved in antiapoptosis. c-MET regulates invasion processes (Misso et al. 2014). All of them are targets of miR-34 family miRNAs. Thus, miR-34 family miRNAs play critical roles in inducing cell cycle arrest and apoptosis and inhibiting cell growth.

Only a few studies have been done with miR-34 family miRNAs to the placental function. Gu et al. found that the expression of all three miR-34 family miRNAs (miR-34a, miR-34b, and miR-34c) is increased in term placentas compared with first-trimester placentas (Gu et al. 2013). Doridot et al. (2014) compared miR-34a expression in placentas from normal pregnancies and from women with preeclampsia, and they found that miR-34a expression was decreased in preeclamptic placentas. They also found that ectopic overexpression of miR-34a in JEG-3 cells down-regulates serpin peptidase inhibitor, clade A, member 3 (SERPINA3) expression (Doridot et al. 2014). SERPINA3 is a serine protease inhibitor, and altered placental SERPINA3 expression has been considered a potential marker of preeclampsia (Chelbi et al. 2007). Therefore, reduced miR-34a expression could be an important mechanism contributing to SERPINA3 deregulation in IUGR and preeclampsia (Chelbi et al. 2007). The expression of miR-34a was also found to be down-regulated in placenta accrete (Umemura et al. 2013). It is speculated that deregulation of miR-34 family miRNA expression is associated with abnormal placental development in pregnancy disorders.

26.2.7 MiR-188 CLUSTER

The miR-188 cluster contains five miRNAs (miR-188, miR-501, miR-362, miR-532, and miR-660) and is located on chromosome Xp11.23. The expression of several miR-188 cluster miRNAs is increased in the term placenta (Table 26.1). miR-188 is considered a potent tumor suppressor. The role of miR-188 cluster miRNAs has been reported in tumor cells and neurons, but not in placental cells. In human nasopharyngeal carcinoma CNE cells, G1/S transition can be suppressed by miR-188 through targeting multiple cyclin/CDK complex (Wu et al. 2014). miR-188 inhibits both mRNA and protein expression of CCND1, CCND3, CCNE1, CCNA2, CDK4, and CDK2. All of them are cell cycle control regulators. miR-188 could also suppress Rb phosphorylation and down-regulate E2F target genes (Wu et al. 2014). In colorectal cancer HCT116 cells, miRNA-362-3p can induce cell cycle arrest by targeting of E2F1, upstream transcription factor 2 (USF2), and protein tyrosine phosphatase, non-receptor type 1 (PTPN1) (Christensen et al. 2013). E2F1 and USF2 are transcriptional factors and play a crucial role in controlling the cell cycle and act on tumor suppressor proteins. PTPN1 is known as protein-tyrosine phosphatase 1B (PTP1B) and is a negative regulator of the insulin-signaling pathway. PTP1B is present in the placenta (Tonks, Diltz, and Fischer 1988). An animal study found that miR-188 serves to fine-tune synaptic plasticity by targeting neuropilin-2 (Nrp-2) expression in the nervous system (Lee et al. 2012). Nrp-2 is a receptor for Sema-3F and interacts with VEGF. Nrp-2 plays a role in cardiovascular development and axon guidance and is a negative regulator of spine development and synaptic structure. miR-188 is able to reverse the Nrp-2-induced reduction in dendritic spine density and rescue the Nrp-2-induced reduction in basal synaptic transmission (Lee et al. 2012). Whether placenta miR-188 expression is associated with fetal CNS development is not known.

26.2.8 LET-7 FAMILY MiRNAs

The *let-7* family has eight members (Roush and Slack 2008). They are *let-7a, let-7b, let-7c, let-7d, let-7e, let-7f, let-7g,* and *let-7i*. All of them were found to be up-regulated in term placentas compared with first-trimester placentas (Gu et al. 2013). The *let-7* family miRNAs have been intensively studied in cancer cells and tumor tissues. They are characterized as key miRNA regulators in developmental and cancer biology (Jérôme et al. 2007). The two major functions of *let-7* family miRNAs are promotion of cell differentiation and tumor suppression. A study has shown that in *Caenorhabditis elegans* (*C. elegans*), up-regulation of *let-7* mediates terminal differentiation "larval-to-adult switch" (Ambros 2011). *Let-7* expression is up-regulated during mouse brain development (Wulczyn et al. 2007). In HeLa cells, overexpression of *let-7* inhibits cell proliferation and promotes G1 to S transition via regulation of key cell cycle proto-oncogenes, including RAS, cell division cycle 25 homolog A (CDC25a), CDK6, and cyclin D (Johnson et al. 2007). In prostate cancer cells, overexpression of *let-7* induces G2-M phase cell-cycle arrest (Liu et al. 2012). In contrast, down-regulation or lack of expression of *let-7* family miRNAs has been demonstrated in several types of cancers, including prostate cancer (Nadiminty et al. 2012), breast cancer (Zhao et al. 2011), lung cancer (Osada and Takahashi 2011), ovarian cancer (Helland et al. 2011), etc. *Let-7* associated with trophoblast differentiation was demonstrated in mouse trophoblast stem cells (Seabrook et al. 2013), in which increased *let-7* expression was seen when mouse trophoblast stem cells were induced to differentiate into mouse trophoblast giant cells (Seabrook et al. 2013). This observation is consistent with the finding of up-regulation of *let-7* family miRNA expression in term placental tissue (Gu et al. 2013). Chan et al. (2013) also examined lin28 and *let-7* miRNA expression in term placentas delivered by caesarean section with or without labor and they found that the expression of lin28 protein and *let-7* miRNA did not vary significantly with labor onset and delivery in term placenta, although *let-7* miRNA and lin28 displayed tissue-specific expression in the placenta, choriodecidua, and amnion. The findings that transient overexpression of *let-7a* in first-trimester placental explants significantly attenuated the proportion of Ki67-positive cytotrophoblasts and reduced basal cytotrophoblast proliferation (Farrokhnia et al. 2014) provide further evidence that the homeostasis of *let-7* family miRNAs likely play a vital role in regulating placental cell differentiation/maturation.

26.3 TROPHOBLAST EXOSOMES—miRNA TRANSPORTER

The first study of trophoblast secretion of miRNAs was reported by Luo et al. (2009). In that study, miRNAs were analyzed in both placental tissues and maternal plasma samples from first-trimester and full-term pregnant women. By small RNA library sequencing, these investigators found that most placenta-specific miRNAs were linked to a miRNA cluster on chromosome 19 (C19MC). They also found that 10 miRNAs (including miR-23a, miR-25, miR-29a, miR-143, miR-484, miR-503, miR-517a, miR-518b, miR-526b, and let-7a) detected in the maternal plasma might be pregnancy-dominant miRNAs because these miRNAs were at a much lower frequency in plasma samples from healthy nonpregnant women (Luo et al. 2009). Their results suggest that placental trophoblasts secrete miRNAs. Trophoblast secretion of placental-specific miRNAs was further demonstrated by examination of exosomes isolated from BeWo cells with or without transfection of miR-519a, a member of C19MC miRNAs (Luo et al. 2009). Placental exosomes carrying C19MC miRNAs were subsequently confirmed by Donker et al. (2012) in primary isolated placental trophoblast cells and in cultured human placental choriocarcinoma JEG-3 and BeWo cells. A reduction in maternal levels of C19MC miRNAs after delivery provides additional evidence that placental syncytiotrophoblasts could be the major source of C19MC miRNAs shed into the maternal circulation. In fact, extracellular miRNAs can be shed or secreted in different forms: enclosed with apoptotic bodies or microvesicles, bonded with protein or lipid complexes, and packed in exosomes (Turchinovich, Weiz, and Burwinkel 2012; Xu, Yang, and Ai 2013; Ouyang et al. 2014). Figure 26.1 shows a schematic of extracellular miRNAs derived from placental trophoblasts.

Exosomes are bioactive vesicles derived from endosomal membranes and are involved in the intercellular communication by their specific cargos of proteins, mRNAs, and miRNAs. Proteomic analysis of placental exosomes has identified numerous proteins in exosomes (Mincheva-Nilsson and Baranov 2010), including ribosomal proteins 60S and 40S, signal transduction proteins 14-3-3 and RhoA, integrins α5 and β1, cytoskeleton proteins myosin and tubulin, membrane fusion protein annexins, enzymes dipeptidyl peptidases, immunoregulators CD9 and CD63, etc. (Mincheva-Nilsson and Baranov 2010). Exosomes also carry human leukocyte antigen G (HLA-G) and B7

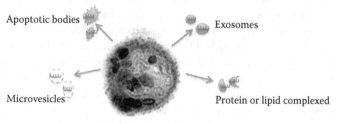

FIGURE 26.1 A schematic of extracellular miRNAs derived from placental villous trophoblasts. miRNAs can be shed or released from syncytiotrophoblasts in different forms: enclosed with apoptotic bodies or microvesicles, bonded with protein or lipid complexes, and packed in exosomes.

family immunomodulators. These immunomodulators play an important role in modulating the functions of leukocyte cytokine activities (Petroff et al. 2002; Hunt et al. 2005). Exosomes exert their effects probably through different mechanisms, such as mediating receptor–ligand interactions, fusion with a target cell and donation of intravesicular and membrane-associated contents, and/or being engulfed by phagocytes. In fact, exosomes derived from syncytiotrophoblasts are considered "The Good Guys" (Mincheva-Nilsson and Baranov 2014). They are immunosuppressive and pluripotent and able to down-regulate cytotoxicity, modulate T-cell signaling, induce apoptosis, and mediate TGF-β effects on recipient cells (Mincheva-Nilsson and Baranov 2014).

In the immune system, exosomes have two major functional directions: either with immunoactivating or with tolerance/immune-suppressive properties. Trophoblasts exosome-C19MC miRNAs are considered immune-suppressive. These small noncoding RNAs could regulate placental–maternal communication and play significant roles in directing maternal adaptation to pregnancy (Bullerdiek and Flor 2012). Trophoblast exosome miRNAs can specifically target immune cells in their local environment, such as decidua, as well as those in the systemic circulation, thereby transferring their signals when interacting with or endocytosed by the membrane of recipient cells and subsequently reprogram recipient cells in the maternal system (Mincheva-Nilsson and Baranov 2014; Ouyang et al. 2014). This raises the intriguing possibility that exosome C19MC miRNAs may serve as messengers for paternally inherited placental antigens that are ultimately cross-presented to maternal T cells by antigen-presenting cells and mediate adaptation of maternal system to pregnancy.

26.4 ROLES OF miRNAs IN EMT IN PLACENTAL DEVELOPMENT

The EMT was first recognized as a feature of embryogenesis. EMT and its reverse process, mesenchymal–epithelial transition (MET), are crucial for the development of many tissues and organs in the developing embryo as well as in the placenta. EMT is a process by which epithelial cells undergo remarkable morphological changes (Thiery 2003). Cells undergoing EMT acquire a mesenchymal phenotype, which is characterized by an epithelial-to-mesenchymal switch in marker expression, such as the loss of epithelial markers (e.g., E-cadherin, claudin, and occludin) and the gain of mesenchymal markers (e.g., vimentin and N-cadherin) (Guo et al. 2014). Loss of epithelial marker expression is a key hallmark of EMT. The process of EMT involves a disassembly of cell–cell junctions, reorganization of cell actin cytoskeleton, and an increase in cell motility and invasion and production of ECM components (Kong et al. 2011). In this process, EMT is regulated by a variety of signaling pathways, including TGF-β, hepatocyte growth factor, platelet-derived growth factor, epithelial growth factor, and integrin engagement, all of which converge at the level of key transcription factors ZEB, Snail, and Twist (Kalluri and Weinberg 2009).

EMT is considered an important physiological remodeling process in placental development, especially during the early pregnancy. In this process, extravillous trophoblasts invade into maternal decidua of the uterine wall. These cytotrophoblasts originate as epithelial cells and are subsequently triggered to change from an epithelial- to a mesenchymal-like migratory phenotype. They become loosely attached, lose their tight epithelial assembly and phenotype, and subsequently invade the maternal decidua as interstitial cytotrophoblasts (Kokkinos et al. 2010). Recent evidence indicates that miRNAs are powerful regulators of EMT. Numerous miRNAs have been identified to regulate EMT by repressing E-cadherin expression through targeting transcriptional factors, including ZEB, Snail, and Twist. As shown in Figure 26.2, ZEB1/2 is targeted by miR-130, miR-150, miR-192, miR-200, and miR-205; Snail1/2 is targeted by miR-29b, miR-30, miR-34, miR-203, and miR-182; and Twist1/2 is targeted by let-7, miR-29b, miR-214, miR-675, etc. (Guo et al. 2014). All of these miRNAs are found strongly expressed in both first-trimester and term placental tissues (Gene Expression Omnibus [GEO] Series accession number GSE42915, http://www.ncbi.nlm.nih.gov/geo/query/acc.cgi?acc=GSE42915). Interestingly, among the eight miRNA-gene networks (miR-25, miR-200a, miR-141, miR101, miR-29c, miR-506, miR-128, and miR-182) that are identified and involved in EMT in serous ovarian cancer cells (Yang et al. 2013; Guo et al. 2014), miR-25 and miR-182 expressions

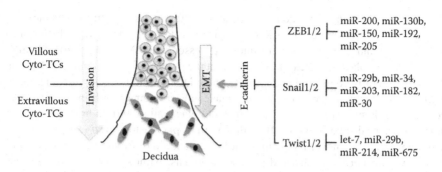

FIGURE 26.2 In the processes of implantation and placental remodeling of the uterine vasculature during early pregnancy, specialized epithelial cells (cytotrophoblasts, Cyto-TCs) that arise from the placenta invade and migrate into the maternal decidua. The process is considered an epithelial–mesenchymal transition (EMT), which involves a functional transition of polarized epithelial cells into mobile and ECM component associated with loss of epithelial cell adhesion molecule E-cadherin expression. E-cadherin expression can be repressed by several transcriptional factors including ZEB1/2, Snail1/2, and Twist1/2. The function of these transcriptional factors is regulated by numerous miRNAs.

are up-regulated in first-trimester placentas, whereas miR-29c expression is up-regulated in term placentas (Gu et al. 2013). The expressions of miR-200a, miR-141, and miR-128 are strongly expressed in both first-trimester and term placental tissues. In contrast, miR-506 and miR-101 are weakly expressed in both first-trimester and term placentas (GEO Series accession number GSE42915, http://www.ncbi.nlm.nih.gov/geo/query/acc.cgi?acc=GSE42915). It seems that miR-506 has an opposite effect on EMT, since miR-506 can augment E-cadherin expression, inhibit cell migration and invasion, and prevent TGF-β-induced EMT by targeting Snail2, a transcriptional repressor of E-cadherin (Yang et al. 2013). E-cadherin plays an important role in EMT and placental development (Kokkinos et al. 2010). Altered E-cadherin expression has been found in placentas from preeclamptic pregnancies (Zhou, Damsky, and Fisher 1997), suggesting that deregulation of EMT process during placental development might contribute to placenta deficiency in pregnancy disorders such as in preeclampsia.

Very little information is available as to MET in the placenta. However, several miRNAs that were reported to inhibit EMT process in cancer cells were increased in their expression in term placentas compared with first-trimester placentas, such as miR-150 and miR-34 cluster miRNAs (Gu et al. 2013). It was reported that miR-150 could inhibit EMT in esophageal squamous cell carcinoma, through targeting ZEB1, an EMT inducer (Yokobori et al. 2013). The inhibition of EMT by p53 has also been described as a new model of tumor suppression. miR-34 family miRNAs (miR-34a/b/c) could activate p53 and subsequently down-regulate the EMT-inducing transcription factor Snail. Prevention of TGF-β-induced EMT by miR-34a was also observed in the colorectal cancer cell line HCT116 (Siemens et al. 2011). Besides the direct down-regulation of Snail by miR-34, indirect inhibition of Snail through down-regulation of histone deacetylase-1 (HDAC1) was also reported (Kaller et al. 2011). HDAC1 functions as a co-repressor of Snail (Peinado et al. 2004). Moreover, attenuation of EMT associated with the expression of connective tissue growth factor, α-SMA, collagen type 1, collagen type 3, and fibronectin by miR-34c was also reported in mice (Morizane et al. 2014). Interestingly, the expression of all three members of the miR-34 family miRNAs is increased in term placentas. It is possible that miRNAs dynamically regulate the balance between EMT and the reverse process MET during placental development. miRNA-mediated cell differentiation and tumor suppression could probably be parts of mechanisms of MET that takes place in term placenta.

26.5 CONCLUSION AND PERSPECTIVES

miRNAs are emerging as major players in gene regulation and contribute to diverse biological processes. The discovery of placental-specific miRNAs heralds a new and exciting era in trophoblast biology, immunology, and maternal-fetal communication during pregnancy. Activation of oncomiR and stem cell marker miRNAs such as miR-17-92 and miR-371 clusters in first-trimester placentas and up-regulation of tumor suppressor miRNAs such as miR-29, miR-34, and *let-7* families in term placentas clearly point out that the pattern of placental miRNA production is spatially and temporally controlled and directly related to placental developmental programming, i.e., dominant angiogenic activity to promote placental vascular growth in the first and second trimesters and the dominant angiostatic state to limit placental growth in pregnancy toward term. The finding of paternal-inherited C19MC miRNAs in trophoblast-derived exosomes in the maternal circulation provides a novel mechanism of how adaptation of maternal system to pregnancy is regulated by the paternally inherited placental antigens. Although the precise mechanisms of miRNAs that regulate placental and innate/adaptive immune function during pregnancy remain unknown, it is believed that the endogenous autoregulatory circuit that controls miRNA production is dynamic and regulated on multiple levels during placental development. As "micro-managers" of gene expression, there is no doubt that placental miRNAs could serve as valuable biomarkers of placental function and molecular regulators acting on the maternal systemic vasculature and immune system.

REFERENCES

Aguado-Fraile, Elia, Edurne Ramos, David Sáenz-Morales, Elisa Conde, Ignacio Blanco-Sánchez, Konstantinos Stamatakis, Luis del Peso, Edwin Cuppen, Bernhard Brüne, and María Laura García Bermejo. 2012. "miR-127 protects proximal tubule cells against ischemia/reperfusion: Identification of kinesin family member 3B as miR-127 target." *PLoS One* 7:e44305.

Altuvia, Yael, Pablo Landgraf, Gila Lithwick, Naama Elefant, Sébastien Pfeffer, Alexei Aravin, Michael J. Brownstein, Thomas Tuschl, and Hanah Margalit. 2005. "Clustering and conservation patterns of human microRNAs." *Nucleic Acids Res* 33 (8):2697–2706.

Ambros, Victor. 2011. "MicroRNAs and developmental timing." *Curr Opin Genet Dev* 21 (4):511–517.

Bartel, David P. 2004. "MicroRNAs: Genomics, biogenesis, mechanism, and function." *Cell* 116 (2): 281–297.

Belair, Cédric, Jessica Baud, Sandrine Chabas, Cynthia M. Sharma, Jörg Vogel, Cathy Staedel, and Fabien Darfeuille. 2011. "Helicobacter pylori interferes with an embryonic stem cell micro RNA cluster to block cell cycle progression." *Silence* 2 (1):7.

Bernstein, Emily, Sang Yong Kim, Michelle A. Carmell, Elizabeth P. Murchison, Heather Alcorn, Mamie Z. Li, Alea A. Mills, Stephen J. Elledge, Kathryn V. Anderson, and Gregory J. Hannon. 2003. "Dicer is essential for mouse development." *Nat Genet* 35 (3):215–217.

Boettger, Thomas and Thomas Braun. 2012. "A new level of complexity: The role of microRNAs in cardiovascular development." *Circ Res* 110 (7):1000–1013.

Bortolin-Cavaillé, Marie-Line, Marie Dance, Michel Weber, and Jérôme Cavaillé. 2009. "C19MC microRNAs are processed from introns of large Pol-II, non-protein-coding transcripts." *Nucleic Acids Res* 37 (10):3464–3473.

Bouillet, Philippe, Jared F. Purton, Dale I. Godfrey, Li-Chen Zhang, Leigh Coultas, Hamsa Puthalakath, Marc Pellegrini, Suzanne Cory, Jerry M. Adams, and Andreas Strasser. 2002. "BH3-only Bcl-2 family member Bim is required for apoptosis of autoreactive thymocytes." *Nature* 415 (6874):922–926.

Bullerdiek, Jörn and Inga Flor. 2012. "Exosome-delivered microRNAs of 'chromosome 19 microRNA cluster' as immunomodulators in pregnancy and tumorigenesis." *Mol Cytogenet* 5 (1):27.

Chan, Hsiu-Wen, Martha Lappas, Sarah W. Yee, Kanchan Vaswani, Murray D. Mitchell, and Gregory E. Rice. 2013. "The expression of the let-7 miRNAs and Lin28 signalling pathway in human term gestational tissues." *Placenta* 34 (5):443–448.

Chelbi, Sonia T., Françoise Mondon, Hélène Jammes, Christophe Buffat, Thérèse-Marie Mignot, Jorg Tost, Florence Busato et al. 2007. "Expressional and epigenetic alterations of placental serine protease inhibitors: SERPINA3 is a potential marker of preeclampsia." *Hypertension* 49 (1):76–83.

Chen, Chang-Zheng, Ling Li, Harvey F. Lodish, and David P. Bartel. 2004. "MicroRNAs modulate hematopoietic lineage differentiation." *Science* 303 (5654):83–86.

Choong, Meng Ling, Henry He Yang, and Ian McNiece. 2007. "MicroRNA expression profiling during human cord blood-derived CD34 cell erythropoiesis." *Exp Hematol* 35 (4):551–564.

Christensen, Heidi Tobiasen, Anja Holm, Troels Schepeler, Marie S. Ostenfeld, Kasper Thorsen, Mads H. Rasmussen, Karin Birkenkamp-Demtroeder et al. 2013. "MiRNA-362-3p induces cell cycle arrest through targeting of E2F1, USF2 and PTPN1 and is associated with recurrence of colorectal cancer." *Int J Cancer* 133 (1):67–78.

Cochella, Luisa and Oliver Hobert. 2012. "Diverse functions of microRNAs in nervous system development." *Curr Top Dev Biol* 99:115–143.

Cui, Yun, Wen-Yu Su, Jing Xing, Ying-Chao Wang, Ping Wang, Xiao-Yu Chen, Zhi-Yong Shen, Hui Cao, You-Yong Lu, and Jing-Yuan Fang. 2011. "MiR-29a inhibits cell proliferation and induces cell cycle arrest through the downregulation of p42.3 in human gastric cancer." *PLoS One* 6 (10):e25872.

Cullen, Bryan R. 2004. "Transcription and processing of human microRNA precursors." *Molecular Cell* 16 (6):861–865.

Das, Radhika, Yew Kok Lee, Ruslan Strogantsev, Shengnan Jin, Yen Ching Lim, Poh Yong Ng, Xueqin Michelle Lin et al. 2013. "DNMT1 and AIM1 imprinting in human placenta revealed through a genome-wide screen for allele-specific DNA methylation." *BMC Genomics* 14:685.

Delorme-Axford, Elizabeth, Rogier B. Donker, Jean-Francois Mouillet, Tianjiao Chu, Avraham Bayer, Yingshi Ouyang, Tianyi Wang et al. 2013. "Human placental trophoblasts confer viral resistance to recipient cells." *Proc Natl Acad Sci U S A* 110 (29):12048–12053.

Dews, Michael, Jamie L. Fox, Stacy Hultine, Prema Sundaram, Wenge Wang, Yingqiu Y. Liu, Emma Furth et al. 2010. "The myc-miR-17~92 axis blunts TGF{beta} signaling and production of multiple TGF{beta}-dependent antiangiogenic factors." *Cancer Res* 70 (20):8233–8246.

Donker, Rogier B., Jean-Francois Mouillet, Tianjiao Chu, Carl A. Hubel, Donna B. Stolz, Adrian E. Morelli, and Yoel Sadovsky. 2012. "The expression profile of C19MC microRNAs in primary human trophoblast cells and exosomes." *Mol Hum Reprod* 18 (8):417–424.

Doridot, Ludivine, Dorothée Houry, Harald Gaillard, Sonia T. Chelbi, Sandrine Barbaux, and Daniel Vaiman. 2014. "miR-34a expression, epigenetic regulation, and function in human placental diseases." *Epigenetics* 9 (1):142–151.

Duester, Gregg. 2008. "Retinoic acid synthesis and signaling during early organogenesis." *Cell* 134 (6):921–931.

Farrokhnia, Farkhondeh, John D. Aplin, Melissa Westwood, and Karen Forbes. 2014. "MicroRNA regulation of mitogenic signaling networks in the human placenta." *J Biol Chem* 289 (44):30404–30416.

Flavin, Richard J., Paul C. Smyth, Alexandros Laios, Sharon A. O'Toole, Ciara Barrett, Stephen P. Finn, Susan Russell et al. 2009. "Potentially important microRNA cluster on chromosome 17p13.1 in primary peritoneal carcinoma." *Mod Pathol* 22:197–205.

Flor, Inga, Armin Neumann, Catharina Freter, Burkhard Maria Helmke, Marc Langenbuch, Volkhard Rippe, and Jörn Bullerdiek. 2012. "Abundant expression and hemimethylation of C19MC in cell cultures from placenta-derived stromal cells." *Biochem Biophys Res Commun* 422 (3):411–416.

Gilad, Shlomit, Eti Meiri, Yariv Yogev, Sima Benjamin, Danit Lebanony, Noga Yerushalmi, Hila Benjamin et al. 2008. "Serum microRNAs are promising novel biomarkers." *PLoS One* 3 (9):e3148.

Graham, Charles H., Jeffrey J. Lysiak, Keith R. McCrae, and Peeyush K. Lala. 1992. "Localization of transforming growth factor-beta at the human fetal-maternal interface: Role in trophoblast growth and differentiation." *Biol Reprod* 46 (4):561–572.

Gu, Yang, Jingxia Sun, Lynn J. Groome, and Yuping Wang. 2013. "Differential miRNA expression profiles between the first and third trimester human placentas." *Am J Physiol Endocrinol Metab* 304 (8):E836–E843.

Guo, Fei, Brittany C. Parker Kerrigan, Da Yang, Limei Hu, Ilya Shmulevich, Anil K. Sood, Fengxia Xue, and Wei Zhang. 2014. "Post-transcriptional regulatory network of epithelial-to-mesenchymal and mesenchymal-to-epithelial transitions." *J Hematol Oncol* 7:19.

He, Xiaoping, Yang Cao, Lihua Wang, Yingli Han, Xiuying Zhong, Guixiang Zhou, Yongping Cai, Huafeng Zhang, and Ping Gao. 2014. "Human fibroblast reprogramming to pluripotent stem cells regulated by the miR19a/b-PTEN axis." *PLoS One* 9 (4):e95213.

Helland, Åslaug, Michael S. Anglesio, Joshy George, Prue A. Cowin, Cameron N. Johnstone, Colin M. House, Karen E. Sheppard et al. 2011. "Deregulation of MYCN, LIN28B and LET7 in a molecular subtype of aggressive high-grade serous ovarian." *PLoS One* 6 (4):e18064.

Hermeking, Heiko. 2010. "The miR-34 family in cancer and apoptosis." *Cell Death Differ* 17:193–199.

Hernandez, Arturo, Steven Fiering, Elena Martinez, Valerie Anne Galton, and Donald St. Germain. 2002. "The gene locus encoding iodothyronine deiodinase type 3 (Dio3) is imprinted in the fetus and expresses antisense transcripts." *Endocrinology* 143 (11):4483–4486.

Houbaviy, Hristo B., Michael F. Murray, and Phillip A. Sharp. 2003. "Embryonic stem cell-specific MicroRNAs." *Dev Cell* 5 (2):351–358.

Hromadnikova, Ilona, Katerina Kotlabova, Jindrich Doucha, Klara Dlouha, and Ladislav Krofta. 2012. "Absolute and relative quantification of placenta-specific microRNAs in maternal circulation with placental insufficiency-related complications." *J Mol Diagn* 14 (2):160–167.

Hunt, Joan S., Margaret G. Petroff, Ramsey H. McIntire, and Carole Ober. 2005. "HLA-G and immune tolerance in pregnancy." *FASEB J* 19 (7):681–693.

Hwang, Hun-Way, Erik A. Wentzel, and Joshua T. Mendell. 2007. "A hexanucleotide element directs microRNA nuclear import." *Science* 315 (5808):97–100.

Inukai, Sachi, Alexandre de Lencastre, Michael Turner, and Frank Slack. 2012. "Novel microRNAs differentially expressed during aging in the mouse brain." *PLoS One* 7 (7):e40028.

Jérôme, Torrisani, Parmentier Laurie, Buscail Louis, and Cordelier Pierre. 2007. "Enjoy the silence: The story of let-7 microRNA and cancer." *Curr Genomics* 8 (4):229–233.

Johnson, Charles D., Aurora Esquela-Kerscher, Giovanni Stefani, Mike Byrom, Kevin Kelnar, Dmitriy Ovcharenko, Mike Wilson et al. 2007. "The let-7 microRNA represses cell proliferation pathways in human cells." *Cancer Res* 67 (16):7713–77122.

Jones, Rebecca L., Chelsea Stoikos, Jock K. Findlay, and Lois A. Salamonsen. 2006. "TGF-beta superfamily expression and actions in the endometrium and placenta." *Reproduction* 132 (2):217–232.

Kagami, Masayo, Kentaro Matsuoka, Toshiro Nagai, Michiko Yamanaka, Kenji Kurosawa, Nobuhiro Suzumori, Yoichi Sekita et al. 2012. "Paternal uniparental disomy 14 and related disorders: Placental gene expression analyses and histological examinations." *Epigenetics* 7 (10):1142–1150.

Kaller, Markus, Sven-Thorsten Liffers, Silke Oeljeklaus, Katja Kuhlmann, Simone Röh, Reinhard Hoffmann, Bettina Warscheid, and Heiko Hermeking. 2011. "Genome-wide characterization of miR-34a induced changes in protein and mRNA expression by a combined pulsed SILAC and microarray analysis." *Mol Cell Proteomics* 10 (8):M111.

Kalluri, Raghu and Robert A. Weinberg. 2009. "The basics of epithelial–mesenchymal transition." *J Clin Invest* 119 (6):1420–1428.

Keklikoglou, Ioanna, Cindy Koerner, Christian Schmidt, Jitao David Zhang, Doreen Heckmann, Anna Shavinskaya, Heike Allgayer et al. 2012. "MicroRNA-520/373 family functions as a tumor suppressor in estrogen receptor negative breast cancer by targeting NF-κB and TGF-β signaling pathways." *Oncogene* 31 (37):4150–4163.

Khuu, Cuong, Anne-Marthe Jevnaker, Magne Bryne, and Harald Osmundsen. 2014. "An investigation into anti-proliferative effects of microRNAs encoded by the miR-106a-363 cluster on human carcinoma cells and keratinocytes using microarray profiling of miRNA transcriptomes." *Front Genet* 5:246.

Kim, Hyesoo, Gabsang Lee, Yosif Ganat, Eirini P. Papapetrou, Inna Lipchina, Nicholas D. Socci, Michel Sadelain, and Lorenz Studer. 2011. "miR-371-3 expression predicts neural differentiation propensity in human pluripotent stem cells." *Cell Stem Cell* 8 (6):695–706.

Kokkinos Maria I., Padma Murthi, Razan Wafai, Erik W. Thompson, and Donald F. Newgreen. 2010. "Cadherins in the human placenta–epithelial–mesenchymal transition (EMT) and placental development." *Placenta* 31 (9):747–755.

Kong, Dejuan, Yiwei Li, Zhiwei Wang, and Fazlul H. Sarkar. 2011. "Cancer stem cells and epithelial-to-mesenchymal transition (EMT)-phenotypic cells: Are they cousins or twins?" *Cancers (Basel)* 3 (1):716–729.

Kumar, Premlata, Yanmin Luo, Carmen Tudela, James M. Alexander, and Carole R. Mendelson. 2013. "The c-Myc-regulated microRNA-17~92 (miR-17~92) and miR-106a~363 clusters target hCYP19A1 and hGCM1 to inhibit human trophoblast differentiation." *Mol Cell Biol* 33 (9):1782–1796.

Labialle, Stéphane, Virginie Marty, Marie-Line Bortolin-Cavaillé, Magali Hoareau-Osman, Jean-Philippe Pradère, Philippe Valet, Pascal G. P. Martin, and Jérôme Cavaillé. 2014. "The miR-379/miR-410 cluster at the imprinted Dlk1-Dio3 domain controls neonatal metabolic adaptation." *EMBO J* 33: 2216–2230.

Lagos-Quintana, Mariana, Reinhard Rauhut, Abdullah Yalcin, Jutta Meyer, Winfried Lendeckel, and Thomas Tuschl. 2002. "Identification of tissue-specific microRNAs from mouse." *Curr Biol* 12 (9):735–739.

Laurent, Louise C., Jing Chen, Igor Ulitsky, Franz-Josef Mueller, Christina Lu, Ron Shamir, Jian-Bing Fan, and Jeanne F. Loring. 2008. "Comprehensive microRNA profiling reveals a unique human embryonic stem cell signature dominated by a single seed sequence." *Stem Cells* 26 (6):1506–1516.

Lee, Rosalind C., Rhonda L. Feinbaum, and Victor Ambros. 1993. "The C. elegans heterochronic gene lin-4 encodes small RNAs with antisense complementarity to lin-14." *Cell* 75 (5):843–854.

Lee, Kihwan, Joung-Hun Kim, Oh-Bin Kwon, Kyongman An, Junghwa Ryu, Kwangwook Cho, Yoo-Hun Suh, and Hye-Sun Kim. 2012. "An activity-regulated microRNA, miR-188, controls dendritic plasticity and synaptic transmission by downregulating neuropilin-2." *J Neurosci* 32 (16):5678–5687.

Li, Steven Shoei-Lung, Sung-Liang Yu, Li-Pin Kao, Zong Yun Tsai, Sher Singh, Bo Zhi Chen, Bing-Ching Ho, Yung-Hsien Liu, and Pan-Chyr Yang. 2009a. "Target identification of microRNAs expressed highly in human embryonic stem cells." *J Cell Biochem* 106 (6):1020–1030.

Li, Zhaoyong, Mohammad Q. Hassan, Mohammed Jafferji, Rami I. Aqeilan, Ramiro Garzon, Carlo M. Croce, Andre J. van Wijnen, Janet L. Stein, Gary S. Stein, and Jane B. Lian. 2009b. "Biological functions of miR-29b contribute to positive regulation of osteoblast differentiation." *J Biol Chem* 284 (23): 15676–15684.

Li, Pengfei, Wei Guo, Leilei Du, Junli Zhao, Yaping Wang, Liu Liu, Yali Hu, and Yayi Hou. 2013. "microRNA-29b contributes to pre-eclampsia through its effects on apoptosis, invasion and angiogenesis of trophoblast cells." *Clin Sci (Lond)* 124 (1):27–40.

Liang, Zhongxing, Yuhua Li, Ke Huang, Nicholas Wagar, and Hyunsuk Shim. 2011. "Regulation of miR-19 to breast cancer chemoresistance through targeting PTEN." *Pharm Res* 28 (12):3091–3100.

Liao, Jian-You, Li-Ming Ma, Yan-Hua Guo, Yu-Chan Zhang, Hui Zhou, Peng Shao, Yue-Qin Chen, and Liang-Hu Qu. 2010. "Deep sequencing of human nuclear and cytoplasmic small RNAs reveals an unexpectedly complex subcellular distribution of miRNAs and tRNA 3′ trailers." *PLoS One* 5 (5):e10563.

Lindsay, Mark A. 2008. "microRNAs and the immune response." *Trends Immunol* 29 (7):343–351.

Liston, Adrian, Aikaterini S. Papadopoulou, Dina Danso-Abeam, and James Dooley. 2012. "MicroRNA-29 in the adaptive immune system: Setting the threshold." *Cell Mol Life Sci* 69 (21):3533–3541.

Liu, Yong, Norman E. Taylor, Limin Lu, Kristie Usa, Allen W. Cowley Jr., Nicholas R. Ferreri, Nan Cher Yeo, and Mingyu Liang. 2010. "Renal medullary microRNAs in Dahl salt-sensitive rats: miR-29b regulates several collagens and related genes." *Hypertension* 55 (4):974–982.

Liu, Can, Kevin Kelnar, Alexander V. Vlassov, David Brown, Junchen Wang, and Dean G. Tang. 2012. "Distinct microRNA expression profiles in prostate cancer stem/progenitor cells and tumor-suppressive functions of let-7." *Cancer Res* 72 (13):3393–3404.

Luo, Shan-Shun, Osamu Ishibashi, Gen Ishikawa, Tomoko Ishikawa, Akira Katayama, Takuya Mishima, Takami Takizawa et al. 2009. "Human villous trophoblasts express and secrete placenta-specific microRNAs into maternal circulation via exosomes." *Biol Reprod* 81 (4):717–729.

Mayor-Lynn Kathleen, Tannaz Toloubeydokhti, Amelia C. Cruz, and Nasser Chegini. 2011. "Expression profile of microRNAs and mRNAs in human placentas from pregnancies complicated by preeclampsia and preterm labor." *Reprod Sci* 18 (1):46–56.

Mazan-Mamczarz, Krystyna, X. Frank Zhao, Bojie Dai, James J. Steinhardt, Raymond J. Peroutka, Kimberly L. Berk, Ari L. Landon et al. 2014. "Down-regulation of eIF4GII by miR-520c-3p represses diffuse large B cell lymphoma development." *PLoS Genet* 10 (1):e1004105.

Miao, Hui-Lai, Chang-Jiang Lei, Zhi-Dong Qiu, Zhong-Kao Liu, Ran Li, Shi-Ting Bao, and Ming-Yi Li. 2014. "MicroRNA-520c-3p inhibits hepatocellular carcinoma cell proliferation and invasion through induction of cell apoptosis by targeting glypican-3." *Hepatol Res* 44 (3):338–348.

Mincheva-Nilsson, Lucia and Vladimir Baranov. 2010. "The role of placental exosomes in reproduction." *Am J Reprod Immunol* 63 (6):520–533.

Mincheva-Nilsson, Lucia and Vladimir Baranov. 2014. "Placenta-derived exosomes and syncytiotrophoblast microparticles and their role in human reproduction: Immune modulation for pregnancy success." *Am J Reprod Immunol* 72 (5):440–457.

Misso, Gabriella, Maria Teresa Di Martino, Giuseppe De Rosa, Ammad Ahmad Farooqi, Angela Lombardi, Virginia Campani, Mayra Rachele Zarone et al. 2014. "Mir-34: A new weapon against cancer?" *Mol Ther Nucleic Acids* 3:e194.

Miura, Kiyonori, Shoko Miura, Kentaro Yamasaki, Ai Higashijima, Akira Kinoshita, Koh-Ichiro Yoshiura, and Hideaki Masuzaki. 2010. "Identification of pregnancy-associated microRNAs in maternal plasma." *Clin Chem* 56 (11):1767–1771.

Morizane, Ryuji, Shizuka Fujii, Toshiaki Monkawa, Ken Hiratsuka, Shintaro Yamaguchi, Koichiro Homma, and Hiroshi Itoh. 2014. "miR-34c attenuates epithelial–mesenchymal transition and kidney fibrosis with ureteral obstruction." *Sci Rep* 4:4578.

Mott, Justin L., Shogo Kobayashi, Steven F. Bronk, and Gregory J. Gores. 2007. "mir-29 regulates Mcl-1 protein expression and apoptosis." *Oncogene* 26 (42):6133–6140.

Murphy, Susan K., Zhiqing Huang, and Cathrine Hoyo. 2012. "Differentially methylated regions of imprinted genes in prenatal, perinatal and postnatal human tissues." *PLoS One* 7 (7):e40924.

Nadiminty, Nagalakshmi, Ramakumar Tummala, Wei Lou, Yezi Zhu, Xu-Bao Shi, June X. Zou, Hongwu Chen et al. 2012. "MicroRNA let-7c is downregulated in prostate cancer and suppresses prostate cancer growth." *PLoS One* 7 (3):e32832.

Nguyen, Tung, Christine Kuo, Michael B. Nicholl, Myung-Shin Sim, Roderick R. Turner, Donald L. Morton, and Dave S. Hoon. 2011. "Downregulation of microRNA-29c is associated with hypermethylation of tumor-related genes and disease outcome in cutaneous melanoma." *Epigenetics* 6 (3):388–394.

Noguer-Dance, Marie, Sayeda Abu-Amero, Mohamed Al-Khtib, and Annick Lefèvre. 2010. "The primate-specific microRNA gene cluster (C19MC) is imprinted in the placenta." *Hum Mol Genet* 19 (18):3566–3582.

O'Connor, Liam, Andreas Strasser, Lorraine A. O'Reilly, George Hausmann, Jerry M. Adams, Suzanne Cory, and David C. Huang. 1998. "Bim: A novel member of the Bcl-2 family that promotes apoptosis." *EMBO J* 17 (2):384–395.

Ogata, Tsutomu, and Masayo Kagami. 2008. "Molecular mechanisms leading to the phenotypic development in paternal and maternal uniparental disomy for chromosome 14." *Clin Pediatr Endocrinol* 17 (4):103–111.

Osada, Hirotaka and Takashi Takahashi. 2011. "let-7 and miR-17-92: Small-sized major players in lung cancer." *Cancer Sci* 102 (1):9–17.

Ouyang, Yingshi, Jean-Francois Mouillet, Carolyn B. Coyne, and Yoel Sadovsky. 2014. "Review: Placenta-specific microRNAs in exosomes—Good things come in nano-packages." *Placenta* 35 Suppl:S69–S73.

Peinado, Hector, Esteban Ballestar, Manel Esteller, and Amparo Cano. 2004. "Snail mediates E-cadherin repression by the recruitment of the Sin3A/histone deacetylase 1 (HDAC1)/HDAC2 complex." *Mol Cell Biol* 24 (1):306–319.

Petrocca, Fabio, Andrea Vecchione, and Carlo M. Croce. 2008. Emerging role of miR-106b-25/miR-17-92 clusters in the control of transforming growth factor beta signaling. *Cancer Res* 68 (20):8191–8194.

Petroff, Margaret G., Lieping Chen, Teresa A. Phillips, and Joan S. Hunt. 2002. "B7 family molecules: Novel immunomodulators at the maternal–fetal interface." *Placenta* 23 Suppl A:S95–S101.

Pickering, Mary T., Bradford M. Stadler, and Timothy F. Kowalik. 2009. "miR-17 and miR-20a temper an E2F1-induced G1 checkpoint to regulate cell cycle progression." *Oncogene* 28 (1):140–145.

Pineles, Beth L., Roberto Romero, Daniel Montenegro, Adi L. Tarca, Yu Mi Han, Yeon Mee Kim, Sorin Draghici et al. 2007. "Distinct subsets of microRNAs are expressed differentially in the human placentas of patients with preeclampsia." *Am J Obstet Gynecol* 196 (3):261.e1–261.e6.

Qi, Junlin, Jenn-Yah Yu, Halyna R. Shcherbata, Julie Mathieu, Amy Jia Wang, Sudeshna Seal, Wenyu Zhou et al. 2009. "microRNAs regulate human embryonic stem cell division." *Cell Cycle* 8 (22):3729–3741.

Río, Paula, Xabier Agirre, Leire Garate, Rocío Baños, Lara Álvarez, Edurne San José-Enériz, Isabel Badell et al. 2012. "Down-regulated expression of hsa-miR-181c in Fanconi anemia patients: Implications in TNFα regulation and proliferation of hematopoietic progenitor cells." *Blood* 119:3042–3049.

Rosenbluth, Evan M., Dawne N. Shelton, Amy E. Sparks, Eric Devor, Lane Christenson, and Bradley J. Van Voorhis. 2013. "MicroRNA expression in the human blastocyst." *Fertil Steril* 99 (3):855–861.

Roush, Sarah and Frank J. Slack. 2008. "The let-7 family of microRNAs." *Trends Cell Biol* 18 (10):505–506.

Schilling, Birte and John Yeh. 2000. "Transforming growth factor-beta(1), -beta(2), -beta(3) and their type I and II receptors in human term placenta." *Gynecol Obstet Invest* 50 (1):19–23.

Schonrock, Nicole, David T. Humphreys, Thomas Preiss, and Jürgen Götz. 2012. "Target gene repression mediated by miRNAs miR-181c and miR-9 both of which are down-regulated by amyloid-β." *J Mol Neurosci* 46:324–335.

Seabrook, Jill L., Jeremy D. Cantlon, Austin J. Cooney, Erin E. McWhorter, Brittany A. Fromme, Gerrit J. Bouma, Russell V. Anthony, and Quinton A. Winger. 2013. "Role of LIN28A in mouse and human trophoblast cell differentiation." *Biol Reprod* 89 (4):95.

Seitz, Hervé, Hélène Royo, Marie-Line Bortolin, Shau-Ping Lin, Anne C. Ferguson-Smith, and Jérôme Cavaillé. 2004. "A large imprinted microRNA gene cluster at the mouse Dlk1-Gtl2 domain." *Genome Res* 14 (9):1741–1748.

Sekita, Yoichi, Hirotaka Wagatsuma, Kenji Nakamura, Ryuichi Ono, Masayo Kagami, Noriko Wakisaka, Toshiaki Hino et al. 2008. "Role of retrotransposon-derived imprinted gene, Rtl1, in the feto–maternal interface of mouse placenta." *Nat Genet* 40 (2):243–248.

Siemens, Helge, Rene Jackstadt, Sabine Hünten, Markus Kaller, Antje Menssen, Ursula Götz, and Heiko Hermeking. 2011. "miR-34 and SNAIL form a double-negative feedback loop to regulate epithelial–mesenchymal transitions." *Cell Cycle* 10 (24):4256–4271.

Sylvestre, Yannick, Vincent De Guire, Emmanuelle Querido, Utpal K. Mukhopadhyay, Véronique Bourdeau, François Major, Gerardo Ferbeyre, and Pascal Chartrand. 2007. "An E2F/miR-20a autoregulatory feedback loop." *J Biol Chem* 282 (4):2135–2143.

Tay, Yvonne M., Wai-Leong Tam, Yen-Sin Ang, Philip M. Gaughwin, Henry Yang, Weijia Wang, Rubing Liu et al. 2008. "MicroRNA-134 modulates the differentiation of mouse embryonic stem cells, where it causes post-transcriptional attenuation of Nanog and LRH1." *Stem Cells* 26 (1):17–29.

Thiery, Jean P. 2003. "Epithelial–mesenchymal transitions in development and pathologies." *Curr Opin Cell Biol* 15 (6):740–746.

Toffanin, Sara, Yujin Hoshida, Anja Lachenmayer, Augusto Villanueva, Laia Cabellos, Beatriz Minguez, Radoslav Savic et al. 2011. "MicroRNA-based classification of hepatocellular carcinoma and oncogenic role of miR-517a." *Gastroenterology* 140 (5):1618–1628.

Tonks, Nicholas K., Curtis D. Diltz, and Edmond H. Fischer. 1988. "Purification of the major protein-tyrosine-phosphatases of human placenta." *J Biol Chem* 263 (14):6722–6730.

Tsai, Kuo-Wang, Hsiao-Wei Kao, Hua-Chien Chen, Su-Jen Chen, and Wen-Chang Lin. 2009. "Epigenetic control of the expression of a primate-specific microRNA cluster in human cancer cells." *Epigenetics* 4 (8):587–592.

Turchinovich, Andrey, Ludmila Weiz, and Barbara Burwinkel. 2012. "Extracellular miRNAs: The mystery of their origin and function." *Trends Biochem Sci* 37 (11):460–465.

Umemura, Kota, Shin-Ichi Ishioka, Toshiaki Endo, Yoshiaki Ezaka, Madoka Takahashi, and Tsuyoshi Saito. 2013. "Roles of microRNA-34a in the pathogenesis of placenta accreta." *J Obstet Gynaecol Res* 39 (1):67–74.

Ventura, Andrea, Amanda G. Young, Monte M. Winslow, Laura Lintault, Alex Meissner, Stefan J. Erkeland, Jamie Newman. 2008. "Targeted deletion reveals essential and overlapping functions of the miR-17 through 92 family of miRNA clusters." *Cell* 132 (5):875–886.

Ventura, Walter, Keiko Koide, Kyoko Hori, Junko Yotsumoto, Akihiko Sekizawa, Hiroshi Saito, and Takashi Okai. 2013. "Placental expression of microRNA-17 and -19b is down-regulated in early pregnancy loss." *Eur J Obstet Gynecol Reprod Biol* 169 (1):28–32.

Voorhoeve, P. Mathijs, Carlos le Sage, Mariette Schrier, Ad J. Gillis, Hans Stoop, Remco Nagel, Ying-Poi Liu et al. 2007. "A genetic screen implicates miRNA-372 and miRNA-373 as oncogenes in testicular germ cell tumors." *Adv Exp Med Biol* 124 (6):1169–1181.

Woods, Keith, J. Michael Thomson, and Scott M. Hammond. 2007. "Direct regulation of an oncogenic micro-RNA cluster by E2F transcription factors." *J Biol Chem* 282 (4):2130–2134.

Wu, Jiangbin, Qing Lv, Jie He, Haoxiang Zhang, Xueshuang Mei, Kai Cui, Nunu Huang, Weidong Xie, Naihan Xu, and Yaou Zhang. 2014. "MicroRNA-188 suppresses G 1 /S transition by targeting multiple cyclin/CDK complexes." *Cell Commun Signal* 12 (1):66.

Wulczyn, F. Gregory, Lena Smirnova, Agnieszka Rybak, Christine Brandt, Erik Kwidzinski, Olaf Ninnemann, Michael Strehle, Andrea Seiler, Stefan Schumacher, and Robert Nitsch. 2007. "Post-transcriptional regulation of the let-7 microRNA during neural cell specification." *FASEB J* 21 (2):415–426.

Xiao, Changchun, Lakshmi Srinivasan, Dinis Pedro Calado, Heide Christine Patterson, Baochun Zhang, Jing Wang, Joel M. Henderson, Jeffrey L. Kutok, and Klaus Rajewsky. 2008. "Lymphoproliferative disease and autoimmunity in mice with increased miR-17-92 expression in lymphocytes." *Nat Immunol* 9 (4):405–414.

Xie, Lan, Jean-Francois Mouillet, Tianjiao Chu, W. Tony Parks, Elena Sadovsky, Martin Knöfler, and Yoel Sadovsky. 2014. "C19MC microRNAs regulate the migration of human trophoblasts." *Endocrinology* 155 (12):4975–4985.

Xu, Shunbin, P. Dane Witmer, Stephen Lumayag, Beatrix Kovacs, and David Valle. 2007. "MicroRNA (miRNA) transcriptome of mouse retina and identification of a sensory organ-specific miRNA cluster." *J Biol Chem* 282 (34):25053–25066.

Xu, Ling, Bao-Feng Yang, and Jing Ai. 2013. "MicroRNA transport: A new way in cell communication." *J Cell Physiol* 228 (8):1713–1719.

Yang, Wei J., Derek D. Yang, Songqing Na, George E. Sandusky, Qing Zhang, and Genshi Zhao. 2005. "Dicer is required for embryonic angiogenesis during mouse development." *J Biol Chem* 280 (10):9330–9335.

Yang, Da, Yan Sun, Limei Hu, Hong Zheng, Ping Ji, Chad V. Pecot, Yanrui Zhao et al. 2013. "Integrated analyses identify a master microRNA regulatory network for the mesenchymal subtype in serous ovarian cancer." *Cancer Cell* 23 (2):186–199.

Yokobori, Takehiko, Shigemasa Suzuki, Naritaka Tanaka, Takanori Inose, Makoto Sohda, Akihiko Sano, Makoto Sakai et al. 2013. "MiR-150 is associated with poor prognosis in esophageal squamous cell carcinoma via targeting the EMT inducer ZEB1." *Cancer Sci* 104 (1):48–54.

Zhang, Xiaoying, Hui Wang, Sheng Zhang, Jie Song, Yupei Zhang, Xiujuan Wei, and Zhichun Feng. 2012. "MiR-134 functions as a regulator of cell proliferation, apoptosis, and migration involving lung septation." *In Vitro Cell Dev Biol Anim* 48:131–136.

Zhao, Yingchun, Caishu Deng, Jiarui Wang, Jing Xiao, Zoran Gatalica, Robert R. Recker, and Gary G. Xiao. 2011. "Let-7 family miRNAs regulate estrogen receptor alpha signaling in estrogen receptor positive breast cancer." *Breast Cancer Res Treat* 127 (1):69–80.

Zhou, Yan, Caroline H. Damsky, and Susan J. Fisher. 1997. "Preeclampsia is associated with failure of human cytotrophoblasts to mimic a vascular adhesion phenotype. One cause of defective endovascular invasion in this syndrome?" *J Clin Invest* 99:2152–2164.

Index

Page numbers followed by f and t indicate figures and tables, respectively.